W. A. Newman (William Alexander Newman) Dorland

American Pocket Medical Dictionary

W. A. Newman (William Alexander Newman) Dorland

American Pocket Medical Dictionary

ISBN/EAN: 9783742831347

Manufactured in Europe, USA, Canada, Australia, Japa

Cover: Foto ©Lupo / pixelio.de

Manufactured and distributed by brebook publishing software (www.brebook.com)

W. A. Newman (William Alexander Newman) Dorland

American Pocket Medical Dictionary

American Pocket Medical Dictionary

EDITED BY

W. A. NEWMAN DORLAND, A.M., M.D.
ASSISTANT OBSTETRICIAN TO THE HOSPITAL OF THE UNIVERSITY OF PENNSYLVANIA; FELLOW OF THE AMERICAN ACADEMY OF MEDICINE, ETC.

CONTAINING THE PRONUNCIATION AND DEFINITION OF OVER 26,000 OF THE TERMS USED IN MEDICINE AND THE KINDRED SCIENCES, ALONG WITH OVER 60 EXTENSIVE TABLES

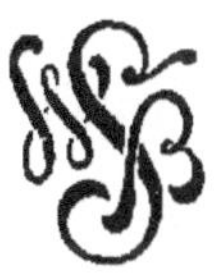

PHILADELPHIA
W. B. SAUNDERS
925 WALNUT STREET
1898

PREFACE.

THIS small volume is the outcome of a need for a pocket dictionary which, though handy in size, should be so full and complete as to supply the wants of the practising physician no less than those of the student of medicine. It is not the editor's intention to attempt to take the place of the larger dictionaries indispensable to a thorough understanding of the language of medicine, but he has striven to develop the possibilities of the pocket lexicon to a degree not heretofore attained.

The chief aim has been to make the selection of words as complete as possible. To this end the larger dictionaries have been freely used, and a systematic gleaning has been made through the latest medical literature, so that the vocabulary may be said to be strictly up to date. Of necessity the definitions of terms are brief, but the endeavor has been to make them clear, adequate, and to the point.

The order of arrangement of matter is strictly alphabetical. In cases of a phrase, consisting of a noun and qualifying adjective, the definition will usually be found under the noun, under which all the phrases containing that noun have been grouped.

Besides the ordinary dictionary words it has seemed desirable to insert a considerable amount of matter in tabular form. This matter, it is believed, will prove of value to students for memorizing in preparing for examinations, besides serving to group correlated facts in a convenient form for quick consultation.

SEPTEMBER, 1898.

INDEX TO THE TABLES

THE

AMERICAN POCKET MEDICAL DICTIONARY.

A.

A. 1. Abbreviation for *anterior* and *anode*. 2. Symbol for *argon*.

A-. A prefix signifying "without" or "not."

ĀĀ, āā. An abbreviation used in prescriptions and meaning "of each."

Ab. A Latin preposition meaning "from."

Ab'aca (ab'ak-a). Manila hemp.

Abac'tus ven'ter. Induced abortion.

Abadie's sign (ah-bah-deez'). Spasm of the levator palpebræ superioris, indicative of exophthalmic goiter.

Abaissement (ah-bās-maw'). 1. Depression. 2. Couching.

Aba'lienated (ab-a'lyen-a-ted). Mentally deranged.

Abaliena'tion (ab-a-lyen-a'shun). Decay of the mental faculties.

Ab'anet (ab'an-et). A girdle-like bandage.

Abaptis'ton. A trephine so shaped as not to penetrate the brain.

Abarthro'sis. Same as *Abarticulation*.

Abartic'ular. Not affecting a joint; at a distance from a joint.

Abarticula'tion. 1. Same as *Diarthrosis*. 2. A dislocation.

Aba'sia (ah-ba'ze-ah). Inability to walk from loss of co-ordination.

Aba'sic. Pertaining to or affected with abasia.

Abate'ment. Decrease in severity of a pain or symptom.

Abattoir (ah-bat-wah'). A slaughter-house.

Abax'ial. Not situated in the axis of the body.

Abbé's catgut rings. Oval rings of catgut for intestinal anastomosis. **A.'s condenser** or **illuminator,** a number of non-achromatic lenses attached to a microscope for strong illumination. **A.'s operation,** lateral anastomosis of the intestine with catgut rings.

A. B. C. method. Deodorization of sewage with alumina, blood, and charcoal.

Abdo'men (ab-do'men). The portion of the body lying between the thorax and the pelvis. **Pendulous a.,** a relaxed condition of abdominal walls. **Scaphoid a.,** abdomen whose anterior wall is hollowed.

Abdom'inal (ab-dom'in-al). Pertaining to the abdomen.

Abdom'ino-ante'rior. With the abdomen forward: said of fetus in utero.

Abdominocys'tic. Pertaining to abdomen and bladder.

Abdominogen'ital nerves. The ilio-inguinal and ilio-hypogastric nerves.

Abdominohysterec'tomy, Abdominohysterot'omy. Hysterectomy or hysterotomy through an abdominal incision.

Abdominoposte'rior. With the belly backward: said of fetus in utero.

Abdominos'copy. Examination or inspection of the abdomen.

Abdominoscro'tal muscle. The cremaster muscle.

Abdominothora'cic arch. The lower boundary of the front of the thorax.

Abdomino-uterot'omy. Same as *Abdominohysterotomy.*

Abdominoves'ical pouch. Fold of peritoneum which includes the urachal folds.

Abdu'cens (ab-du'senz). 1. External rectus muscle of the eye. 2. Sixth cranial nerve. **A. labio'rum.** Same as *A. oris.* **A. oc'uli,** external rectus of eye. **A. o'ris,** levator anguli oris muscle.

Abdu'cent (ab-du'sent). Abducting.

Abduct'. To draw away from the median line.

Abduc'tion. The act of abducting; the state of being abducted.

Abduc'tor. A muscle which performs abduction. See *Muscle Table.*

Ab'ernethy's fascia. A layer of areolar tissue around external iliac artery.

Aber'rant. Wandering from the normal or usual course.

Aberra'tio. Metastasis, as of the humors, milk, or menses.

Aberra'tion (ab-er-a'shun). 1. Deviation from the usual course. 2. Imperfect refraction or focalization of a lens. **Chromatic a.,** unequal refraction of different colored rays producing a blurred image. **Distantial a.,** blurring of vision due to distance. **Mental a.,** mental unsoundness not sufficient to constitute insanity. **Spherical a.,** imperfect focalization of a convex lens.

Abevacua'tion (ab-e-vak-u-a'shun). Incomplete evacuation.

Abey'ance (ab-a'ans). A condition of suspended activity.

A'bies (a'be-ēz). Genus of trees, including firs, spruces, etc.

Abi'etene (ab-i'et-ēn). Liquid hydrocarbon, C_7H_{16}, from a species of *Abies.*

Abiet'ic or **Abietin'ic acid.** Crystalline substance, $C_{20}H_{30}O_2$, from rosin.

Ab'ietin (ab'i-et-in). A resin, $C_{53}H_{70}O_8$, from Canada balsam.

Ab'ietite. A sugar, $C_4H_8O_3$, from *Abies pectinata.*

Abiogen'esis. Production of life from matter not alive.

Abiolog'ical (ab-i-o-loj'ik-al). Having no relation to biology.

Abio'sis (ab-bi-o'sis). Absence or deficiency of life.

Abir'ritant (ab-ir'it-ant). Diminishing irritation; soothing.

Abirrita'tion. Diminished irritability; atony.

Ablacta'tion (ab-lak-ta'shun). Weaning.

Ablastem'ic. Not concerned with germination.

Ablate'. To remove, especially by cutting.

Abla'tio ret'inæ. Detachment of the retina.

Abla'tion (ab-la'shun). Removal, especially by cutting.

Ablepha'ria. Total or partial absence of the eyelids.

Ableph'arous (ab-lef'ar-us). Having no eyelids.

Ablep'sia (ab-lep'se-ah). Lack of sight; blindness.

Ab'luent. Detergent; cleansing.

Ablu'tion (ab-lu'shun). A washing.

Abnor'mal. Not normal; contrary to the usual structure or condition.

Abnormal'ity. 1. The state of being abnormal. 2. A malformation.

Abnor'mity. Same as *Abnormality.*

Aboiment (ah-bwah-maw'). The utterance of barking sounds.

Aboli'tion. Destruction of a part or suppression of a function.

Aboma'sum, Aboma'sus. The fourth stomach of ruminants.

Abo'rad (ab-o'rad). In an aboral direction.

Abo'ral (ab-o'ral). Opposite to, or remote from, the mouth.

Abort' (ab-ort'). 1. To miscarry. 2. To arrest the development of disease. 3. An aborted fetus.

Abort'icide. The killing of a fetus within the uterus.

Abor'tient (ab-or'shent). Causing abortion; abortifacient.

Abortifa'cient. Causing abortion; also, a drug so acting.

Abor'tion. 1. Expulsion of a fetus before it is viable. 2. Premature arrest of a morbid or a natural process. Abortion is termed **accidental** or **spontaneous**, when due to accident; **artificial** or **induced**, when brought on purposely; **criminal**, when not necessary for therapeutic reasons; **embryonic**, when it occurs before the fourth month; **fetal**, when after the fourth month; **habitual**, when repeated in successive pregnancies; **incomplete**, when the placenta is retained; **inevitable**, when the embryo is dead or there is rupture of the ovum; **missed**, when the fetus is dead, but is not expelled within two weeks; **ovular**, when occurring within the first three weeks.

Abor'tionist. One who makes a business of producing abortions.

Abor'tive. 1. Incompletely developed. 2. Abortifacient.

Abor'tus. An aborted fetus; abortion.

Abouchement (ah-boosh-maw'). The termination of a vessel in a larger one.

Abou'lia, Abouloma'nia. See *Abulia*, *Abulomania*.

Abra'chia (ah-ra'ke-ah). The condition of having no arms.

Abrachiocepha'lia. Absence of the head and arms.

Abra'chius. A monster fetus without arms.

Abra'sio cor'neæ. The scraping off of corneal excrescences.

Abra'sion (ab-ra'zhun). 1. A rubbing off or scraping off. 2. A spot rubbed bare of skin or mucous membrane.

A'brin (a'brin). The poisonous principle of jequirity.

Abrot'anum. Southernwood, a plant which is tonic vermifuge.

A'brus (a'brus). A genus of plants, including jequirity, *q. v.*

Ab'scess (ab'ses). A localized collection of pus in a cavity formed by the disintegration of tissue. **Alveolar a.**, abscess of the gum. **Chronic** or **Cold a.**, one of slow, non-inflammatory development. **Embolic a.**, one formed in the clot of an embolus. **Ischiorectal a.**, abscess in ischiorectal fossa. **Mammary a.**, abscess of the breast. **Metastatic a.** Same as *Embolic a.* **Primary a.**, one formed at the seat of infection. **Psoas a.**, one in which pus descends in sheath of psoas muscle. **Residual a.**, one developed from the residues of former inflammations. **Scrofulous a.**, a collection of pus from tuberculous degeneration of bone or lymph-glands. **Secondary a.** Same as *Embolic a.* **Stitch a.**, an abscess developed about a stitch or suture. **Thecal a.**, an abscess in the sheath of a tendon.

Absci'ssæ. The transverse lines cutting vertical ones at right angles to show in a diagram the relations of two series of parts.

Abscis'sion. Removal of a part or growth by cutting.

Ab'sinthe. A French liqueur containing oil of wormwood.

Absin'thin. Bitter crystalline principle, $C_{20}H_{28}O_4$, from wormwood.

Absin'thism. A condition similar to alcoholism, from excessive use of absinthe.

Absin'thium. Wormwood, the leaves and tops of *Artemis'ia absin'thium:* stomachic tonic and heart-stimulant.

Absin'thol. Oily principle, $C_{10}H_6O$, from oil of wormwood.

Ab'solute alcohol. Alcohol free from water and impurities. **A. agraphia.** See *Agraphia*. **A. near-point.** See *Near-point*. **A. temperature**, temperature measured from the A. zero. **A. zero**, the lowest possible temperature, 273.7° below zero Cent.

Absor'bent. 1. Sucking up; taking up by suction. 2. A lacteal or lymphatic. 3. A medicine producing absorption of diseased tissue.

Absorptiom'eter. Device for measuring the layer of liquid absorbed between two glass plates; used as a hematoscope.

Absorp'tion (ab-sorp'shun). The act of taking up by suction. **A. lines.** Same as *Fraunhofer's lines.* **A. spectrum,** a spectrum obtained by passing light through a gas, which gas absorbs the same rays that its own spectrum consists of.

Absorp'tive. Having the power of absorption.

Abster'gent. Cleansing or detergent; also a cleansing agent.

Abster'sion (ab-ster'shun). The act or process of cleansing.

Abster'sive. Same as *Abstergent.*

Ab'stract, Abstrac'tum. A powder made from a drug mixed with milk-sugar, and having twice the strength of the original drug.

Abstrac'tion (ab-strak'shun). 1. Concentration of mind. 2. Venesection.

Abter'minal. Passing from tendinous to muscular tissue: said of electric currents.

Abu'lia (ab-u'le-ah). Lack or defect of will-power.

Abu'lic (ab-u'lik). Affected with abulia.

Abulioma'nia. Mental disease with loss of will-power.

Aca'cia (ak-a'she-ah). 1. A genus of trees furnishing gum arabic and catechu. 2. Gum arabic, a white transparent gum from bark of *Aca'cia Sen'egal:* demulcent and used as a vehicle.

Acal'ypha (ak-al'if-ah). Genus of plants. **A. frutico'sa** of India and **A. his'pida** are tonic in diarrhea and dyspepsia. **A. in'dica** is expectorant and emetic. **A. virgin'ica** is diuretic and expectorant.

Acamp'sia. Rigidity of part of a limb.

Acan'tha. A spinous process of a vertebra.

Acanthesthe'sia. A feeling as if a sharp point were pricking the body.

Acan'thia lectula'ria. The common bed-bug.

Acan'thion. A point at the base of the anterior nasal spine.

Acanthoceph'ala. An order of worms, including Echinorrhynchus.

Acanthol'ysis. Atrophy of the prickle layer of the skin.

Acantho'ma. A tumor in the prickle layer of the skin.

Acantho'sis. Any disease of the prickle layer of the skin. **A. nig'ricans,** general pigmentation of the skin with papillary growths.

Acar'dia. Congenital absence of the heart.

Acardi'acus. A fetus without a heart.

Acari'asis (ak-ar-i'as-is). Same as *Mange.*

Acar'icide (ak-ar'is-id). A medicine that destroys acari.

Ac'arid, Acar'idan. A tick or mite; an acarus.

Acarino'sis. Any disease caused by acari.

Acarodermati'tis. Dermatitis caused by acari.

Ac'aroid resin. A yellow aromatic resin from Australia: used as digestive tonic and stimulant.

Acaropho'bia. Insane dread of the itch.

Ac'arus. A genus of insects including mites, ticks, etc.

Acatamathe'sia. Lack of power to understand speech.

Acatapha'sia. Inability to speak in an orderly manner; agrammatism.

Acathec'tic jaundice. Jaundice from pathogenic changes in the liver-cells, which become unable to retain their secretion.

Acau'dal, Acau'date. Having no tail.

A. C. C. An abbreviation for *anodal closure contraction.*

Accel'erans nerve. See *Nerves, Table of.*

Accelera'tion. Quickening, as of the pulse or the respiration.

Accelera'tor. That which hastens. **A. uri'næ.** See *Muscle Table.*

Accentua'tion. Increased loudness or distinctness.

Accesso'rius. 1. The spinal accessory nerve (**A. Willis'ii**). 2. A muscle which assists another.

Acces'sory. Additional; supplementary: said of muscles, ducts, nerves, arteries, etc.

Accip'iter. A facial bandage with tails like the claws of a hawk.

Acclimata'tion, Acclima'tion, Acclimatiza'tion. Process of becoming accustomed to new climate, soil, and water.

Accommoda'tion. Adjustment; especially, adjustment of the eye for various distances of vision. **Absolute a.**, the accommodation of either eye separately. **Histologic a.**, changes in the morphology and function of cells following changed conditions. **Negative a.**, adjustment of the eye for long distances by relaxation. **A. phosphenes**, streaks of light seen in the dark after accommodation. **Positive a.**, adjustment of eye for short distances by contraction. **Range of a.**, distance between the nearest point of distinct vision and the farthest point. **A. reflex**, Argyll-Robertson pupil.

Accom'modative iridoplegia. See *Iridoplegia.*

Accouchement (ah-koosh-maw'). Act of being delivered. **A. forcé**, forcible delivery with the hand.

Accoucheur (ah-koo-sher'). One skilled in midwifery.

Accoucheuse (ah-koo-shuz'). A midwife.

Accrementi'tion. Growth by addition of similar tissue.

Accre'tion (ak-re'shun). Accumulation of matter to a part.

Accu'mulator. Apparatus for accumulating and storing electricity.

A. C. E. mixture. An anesthetic mixture consisting of 1 part alcohol, 2 parts chloroform, and 1 part ether.

Acen'tric. Not originating in a nerve-center; peripheric.

Acepha'lia, Aceph'alism. Absence of the head.

Acephalobra'chia. Absence of the head and arms.

Acephalocar'dia. Absence of the head and heart.

Acephalocar'dius. Monster without head or heart.

Acephalochi'ria. Absence of the head and hands.

Aceph'alocyst, Acephalocys'tis. A sterile echinococcus cyst. **A. racemo'sa**, a hydatid mole of the uterus.

Acephalogas'ter. A monster without head or stomach.

Acephalogas'tria. Absence of the head and stomach or belly.

Acephalopo'dia. Absence of the head and feet.

Acephalopo'dius. Monster with neither head nor feet.

Acephalora'chia. Absence of head and spinal column.

Acephalosto'mia. Absence of head with presence of mouth-aperture on the upper aspect.

Acephalothora'cia. Absence of head and thorax.

Aceph'alous (ah-sef'al-us). Headless.

Aceph'alus (ah-sef'al-us). A monster fetus without a head.

Acerato'sis. Deficiency in formation of horny tissue.

Acervulo'ma (as-er-vu-lo'mah). Same as *Psammoma.*

Acer'vulus, Acer'vulus cer'ebri. Sandy matter about the pineal gland and other parts of the brain; brain-sand.

Aces'cence (as-es'ans). The state of being sour; sourness.

Acesto'ma. A mass of granulations.

Acetab'ular. Pertaining to the acetabulum.

Acetab'ulum. Cup-shaped cavity in the innominate bone receiving the head of the femur.

Ac'etal (as'et-al). Diethylacetal; a colorless liquid, $C_6H_{14}O_2$: used as a hypnotic.

Acetal'dehyd. Normal aldehyd; ethaldehyd.

Acetam'id. White crystalline solid, C_2H_5NO.

Acetan'ilid. Colorless crystalline antipyretic powder, C_8H_4NO; called also *antifebrin.*

Ac'etate (as'et-āt). Any salt of acetic acid.

Acet'ic acid. The acid of vinegar, $C_2H_4O_2$.

Ac'etin (as'et-in). A glyceryl acetate, $C_3H_5(C_2H_3O_2)_3$.

Aceto-acet'ic acid. Same as *Diacetic acid.*

Acetom'eter. Instrument for measuring acetic acid.

Ac'etone (as'et-ōn). Colorless inflammable liquid, C_3H_6O, or dimethyl ketone; anesthetic and anthelmintic.

Acetonemia (as-et-o-ne'me-ah). Presence of acetone in the blood.

Acetoni'tril. Methyl cyanid, CH_3CN, a colorless acid.

Acetonu'ria (as-et-o-nu're-ah). Presence of acetone in the urine.

Acetophenet'idin. Same as *Phenacetin.*

Acetophe'none. Hypnone, C_8H_8O, a pungent fluid: used as a hypnotic and antiseptic.

Ac'etous (as'et-us). Resembling or pertaining to vinegar.

Acetphenet'idin. Same as *Phenacetin.*

Acet-to'luid. An antipyretic, $C_9H_{11}NO$, resembling acetanilid.

Ace'tum (as-e'tum). 1. Vinegar. 2. A medicine prepared with vinegar. **A. aromat'icum.** See *Aromatic vinegar.*

Acet'yl peroxid. A thick liquid, $(C_2H_3O)_2O_2$; powerful oxidizing agent.

Acet'ylene (as-et'il-ēn). A colorless, combustible gas, C_2H_2, with unpleasant odor.

Acetylphenylhydra'zin. Same as *Pyrodin.*

Acetyltan'nin. Same as *Tannigen.*

Achalybe'mia. Deficiency of iron in the blood.

Achei'lia. Congenital absence of one or both lips.

Achei'lous. Having no lips.

Achei'ria. Congenital absence of one or both hands.

Achil'lea. Genus of plants, of which *A. millefo'lium* or yarrow is used as a bitter tonic.

Achil'lein. Active principle of *Achillea.*

Achil'les tendon. The cord at the back of the heel, the tendon of the gastrocnemius and soleus muscles. **A. t. reaction,** contraction of muscles of the calf on tapping the Achilles tendon.

Achillobursi'tis. Inflammation of the bursæ about the Achilles tendon.

Achillodyn'ia (ak-il-o-din'e-ah). Pain in the Achilles tendon.

Achillotenot'omy, Achillot'omy. Section of the Achilles tendon.

Achlorhyd'ria. Absence of hydrochloric acid from gastric juice.

Achlorop'sia. Blindness to green colors.

Acho'lia (ak-o'le-ah). Absence of bile-secretion.

Achondropla'sia, Achon'droplasty. Condition in rickets marked by defective development of cartilage at the epiphyses of the long bones.

Acho'rion. Genus of fungi. *A. keratoph'agus* produces onychomycosis, *A. Leber'tii* produces tinea tonsurans, *A. Schönlei'nii* produces favus.

Achroacyto'sis. Excessive development of lymph-cells (colorless cells).

Achroiocythe'mia. Lack of hemoglobin in red corpuscles.

Achro'ma (ak-ro'mah). Absence of color.

Achromat'ic lens. Lens for neutralizing chromatic aberration. **A. spindle,** spindle-shaped figure in karyokinesis.

Achro'matin. The faintly staining ground-work of a cell-nucleus.

Achro'matism. Absence of chromatic aberration.

Achromatop'sia. Color-blindness.

Achromato'sis. Any disease marked by deficiency of pigmentation.

Achromatu'ria. Colorless state of the urine.

Achro'mia (ak-ro'me-ah). Achroma.

Achromoder'mia. Colorless state of the skin.

Achromotrich'ia. Colorless condition of the hair.

Achroodex'trin. A kind of dextrin not colored by iodin.

Achy'lia, Achylo'sis. Absence of chyle. **A. gas'trica,** absence of ferments of the gastric juice.

Achy'lous (ak-i'lus). Deficient in chyle.

Achymo'sis. Deficient formation of chyme.

Acic'ular (as-ik'u-lar). Needle-shaped.

Acid (as'id). 1. Sour. 2. A compound of an electronegative element with one or more hydrogen atoms which are replaceable by electropositive atoms. **Abietic a., Abietinic a.,** crystalline substance, $C_{20}H_{30}O_2$, from rosin. **Abric a.,** crystalline acid, $C_{12}H_{24}N_3O$, from jequirity. **Acetic a.,** crystalline acid, $C_2H_4O_2$, the acid of vinegar. **Aconitic a.,** crystalline acid, $C_6H_6O_6$, from *Aconitum Napellus* and other plants. **Adipic a.,** crystalline acid, $C_6H_{10}O_4$, formed by oxidizing fats with nitric acid. **Agaric a., Agaricic a.,** acid, $C_{16}H_{30}O_5+H_2O$, from *Polyporus officinalis:* used in night sweats. **Amido-acetic a.,** glycocoll. **Amidobenzoic a.,** acid, $C_7H_7NO_2$, sometimes found in urine. **Amidosuccinic a.,** asparagin. **Angelic a.,** crystalline acid, $C_5H_8O_2$, from roots of *Angelica archangelica.* **Anisic a.,** acid, $C_8H_8O_3$, from anise seed. **Anticyclic a.,** white powder with antiseptic properties. **Arabic a.,** acid, $C_{12}H_{22}O_{11}$, from gum arabic. **Aromatic a's.,** certain organic acids from resins, balsams, etc. **Arsenic a., Arsenous a.** See *Arsenic.* **Asparaginic a., Aspartic a.,** crystalline acid, $C_4H_7NO_4$, from beet-root, and found in the body. **Auric a.,** gold trihydroxid, $Au(OH)_3$. **Benzoic a.,** white, crystalline acid, $C_7H_6O_2$, from certain resins. **Boracic a., Boric a.,** white antiseptic powder, H_3BO_3, from borax. **Butyric a.,** rancid, viscid acid, $C_4H_8O_2$, from butter, urine, feces, and perspiration. **Caffeic a.,** crystalline acid, $C_9H_8O_4$, from coffee. **Cahincic a.** Same as *Cahincin.* **Camphoric a.,** crystalline acid, $C_{10}H_{16}O_4$, from camphor: used in night sweats. **Capric a.,** crystalline acid, $C_{10}H_{20}O_2$, from butter. **Caprylic a.,** fatty acid, $C_8H_{16}O_2$, from butter and cocoanut oil. **Carbamic a.,** monobasic acid, $CO.NH_2.OH$. **Carbazotic a.** Same as *Picric a.* **Carbolic a.,** crystalline acid, C_6H_6O, from coal-tar: disinfectant and antiseptic. **Carbonic a.,** carbon dioxid, CO_2, colorless, odorless gas. **Carminic a.,** coloring matter, $C_{17}H_{18}O_{10}$, from buds of certain plants and cochineal insect. **Cathartic a., Cathartinic a.,** active principle from *Cassia.* **Cerotic a.,** fatty acid, $C_{27}H_{54}O_2$, from beeswax and Chinese wax. **Chloracetic a.,** caustic combination of chlorin and acetic acid. **Chloric a.,** an acid, $HClO_3$, known only in its compounds. **Cholalic a., Cholic a.,** crystalline acid, $C_{24}H_{42}O_5$, from bile. **Chromic a.** 1. The compound, H_2CrO_4. 2. Chromium trioxid, CrO_3: escharotic. **Chrysophanic a.,** yellow, crystalline acid, $C_{15}H_{10}O_4$, from lichen, senna, and rhubarb. **Cinnamic a.,** compound, $C_9H_8O_2$, from balsams and resins: used in tuberculosis. **Citric a.,** crystalline acid, $C_6H_8O_7$, from lemons, currants, and other fruits. **Cresolsulphuric a.,** acid, $C_7H_7O.SO_2.O_4$, found in small quantities in urine. **Cresylic a.** Same as *Cresol.* **Cyanic a.,** acid, $CNHO$, stable only at low temperatures. **Diacetic a.,** acid, $C_4H_6O_3$, found in urine in diabetes and other diseased conditions. **Fatty a.,** monobasic acid produced by oxidation of a primary alcohol, and having the general formula, CnH_2nO_2. **Formic a.,** colorless, pungent liquid, CH_2O_2, from secretion of ants, nettles, etc. **Gallic a.,** crystalline acid, $C_7H_6O_5$, found in nut-galls, fruit, and tea: astringent and disinfectant. **Glycocholic a.,** crystalline acid, $C_{26}H_{43}NO_{61}$, found in bile. **Glycuronic a.,** an acid, $C_6H_{10}O_7$, which has been found in the urine. **Hippuric a.,** crystalline acid, $C_9H_9NO_3$, from urine of herbivorous animals. **Hydriodic a.,** gaseous acid, HI: used in aqueous solution and in syrup as an alterative. **Hydrobromic a.,** irritating gaseous acid, HBr: used diluted in nervous conditions. **Hydrochloric a.,** colorless gas, HCl, used in aqueous solution as an aid to digestion. **Hydrocyanic a.,** a volatile poisonous liquid, HCN, from bitter almonds, peach leaves, cherry leaves, etc.; used diluted as a sedative. **Hydrofluoric a.,** colorless caustic liquid, HF. **Hydrosulphuric a.,** stinking gas, H_2S, formed during the putrefaction of albuminoid substances. **Hypochlorous a.,** unstable compound, $HClO$: used as disinfectant and bleaching agent. **Hypophosphorous a.,** an acid, $PH(OH)_2$, forming salts called hypophosphites. **Indoxyl-sulphuric a.,** acid which combined with potassium, occurs in the urine as indican. **Iodic a.,** monobasic acid, HIO_3: used in dilute solution as an alterative. **Lactic a.,** syrupy liquid, $HC_3H_5O_3$, produced in the fermentation of milk. **Linoleic a.,** acid, $C_{16}H_{28}O_2$, found as a glycerid in drying oils. **Malic a.,** crystalline acid, $C_4H_6O_5$, from juices of many fruits and plants. **Maloric a.,** acid, $C_3H_4O_4$, from beet. **Meconic a.,** white crystalline acid, $C_7H_4O_7$, from opium. **Metaphosphoric a.,** solid compound, HPO_3, used as a test for albumin in urine. **Muriatic a.** Same as *Hydrochloric a.* **Myronic a.,** acid, $C_{10}H_{19}NSO_{10}$, found in combination in black mustard. **Nitric a.,** colorless, fuming liquid, HNO_3, used as a cauterizing agent. **Nitrohydrochloric a., Nitromuriatic a.,** yellow, fuming mixture of nitric acid and hydrochloric acid. **Oleic a.,** colorless, crystallizable oil, $C_{18}H_{34}O_2$, found in many fats and oils. **Organic a.,** an acid containing the group, CO.OH, or carboxyl. **Orthophosphoric a.,** ordinary phosphoric acid, H_3PO_4. **Osmic a.,** osmium oxid, OsO_4, in yellow crystals: used in cancer, strumous glands, etc., and as a stain and fixing agent in histology. **Oxalic a.,** colorless, crystalline, poisonous acid, $C_2H_2O_4$, from wood-sorrel, sugar, and other substances. **Palmitic a.,** acid, $C_{16}H_{32}O_2$, found in palm oil and solid fats. **Phosphoric a.,** an acid, H_3PO_4, crystalline when pure, but ordinarily a syrupy liquid. **Phosphorous a.,** acid, H_3PO_3. **Picric a.,** yellow, crystalline acid, $C_6H_3N_3O_7$, used as a dye and as a fixing agent: also said to be antiperiodic and anthelmintic. **Prussic a.** Same as *Hydrocyanic a.* **Pyroboric a.,** acid, $H_2B_4O_7$, obtained by heating boric acid. **Pyrogallic a.,** white, crystalline, poisonous compound, $C_6H_6O_3$, used in skin diseases. **Pyroligneous a.,** clear liquid from the destructive distillation of wood, etc. **Pyrophosphoric a.,** crystalline acid, $2H_2O.P_2O_5$, one of the forms of phosphoric acid. **Quinic a.,** crystalline acid, $C_7H_{12}O_6$, from cinchona. **Rosolic a.,** compound, $C_{20}H_{16}O_3$: used as a dye and as a test for acids. **Salicylic a.,** crystalline acid, $C_7H_6O_3$, found in various plants and made from carbolic acid: antipyretic, antirheumatic, and antiseptic. **Salicylsulphonic a.,** crystalline substance: used as a test for proteids. **Sarcolactic a.,** acid, $C_3H_6O_3$, found in muscles and blood and in urine in phosphorus poisoning. **Sclerotinic a.,** one of the active principles of ergot. **Stearic a.,** wax-like acid, $C_{18}H_{36}O_2$, from fats. **Succinic a.,** acid, $C_4H_6O_4$, distilled from amber. **Sulphanilic a.,** crystalline acid, $C_6H_4(NH_2)SO_3H$, used as a reagent. **Sulphocarbolic a.,** compound, $C_6H_6SO_4$: antiseptic and antipyretic. **Sulphuric a.,** colorless, caustic liquid, H_2SO_4. **Sulphurous a.,** colorless liquid, $H2SO_3$: used as oxidizing and bleaching agent, and as a lotion in diphtheria, stomatitis, etc. **Tannic a.,** an astringent powder, $C_{14}H_{10}O_9$, from nut-galls: astringent and hemostatic. **Tartaric a.,** white powder, $C_4H_6O_6$, from juice of grape and other plants. **Taurocholic a.,** crystalline acid, $C_{24}H_{45}NOS_7$, from the bile. **Trichloracetic a.,** crystalline, caustic compound, $HC_2Cl_3O_2$. **Uric a.,** crystalline acid, $C_5H_4N_4O_3$, found in urine and in some organs of the body.

Valerianic a., Valeric a., colorless, oily, pungent liquid, $C_5H_{10}O_2$: used in nervous diseases.

Acid'ifiable. Capable of being made acid.

Acidifica'tion. The act of making acid ; conversion into an acid.

Acidim'eter. Instrument for performing acidimetry.

Acidim'etry. The determination of the amount of free acid in a liquid.

Acid'ity (as-id'it-e). 1. The state of being acid. 2. The combining power of a base.

Acid'ophil, Acidoph'ilic (as-id'o-fil, as-id-o-fil'ik). Easily stained with acid dyes.

Acidos'teophyte (as-id-os'te-o-fit). A sharp osteophyte.

Acid'ulated (as-id'u-la-ted). Somewhat sour or acid.

Acid'ulous (as-id'u-lus). Moderately sour.

Ac'idum (as'id-um). Latin for acid.

Acine'sia (as-in-e'ze-ah). See *Akinesia.*

Acinet'ic (as-in-et'ik). 1. Affected with acinesia. 2. Diminishing muscular power.

Acin'iform (as-in'if-orm). Grape-like.

A'cinous, A'cinose (as'in-us, -ōs). Made up of acini.

A'cinus (as'in-us), pl. *a'cini.* One of the smallest lobules of a compound gland.

Acleitocar'dia. Open state of the foramen ovale.

Ac'me (ak'me). The critical stage or crisis of a disease.

Ac'ne (ak'ne). Any inflammatory disease of the sebaceous glands. **A. al'bida,** milium. **A. artificia'lis,** acne due to external irritation. **A. atroph'ica.** Same as *A. varioliformis.* **A. cilia'ris,** acne of the edges of the eyelids. **A. dissemina'ta.** Same as *A. vulgaris.* **A. genera'lis,** acne over the whole surface of the body. **A. hypertroph'ica.** a. rosacea with thickening of the tips and sides of the nose. **A. indura'ta.** variety of a. vulgaris with chronic livid indurations. **Iodin a.,** eruption from continued use of iodids. **A. kerato'sa,** variety in which a horny plug takes the place of the comedo. **A. mentag'ra,** sycosis. **A. papulo'sa,** acne with the formation of papules. **A. picia'lis,** tar-acne, a variety due to the irritation of tar or its vapor. **A. rosa'cea,** a chronic inflammatory state of the nose and contiguous parts of the face in drunkards. **A. scorbu'tica,** a papular eruption in scurvy. **A. sim'plex.** Same as *A. vulgaris.* **A. tar'si,** acne of the sebaceous glands of the eyelids. **A. variolifor'mis,** variety in which pustules appear in groups about the forehead and scalp. **A. vulga'ris,** common acne.

Acne'mia (ak-ne'me-ah). Atrophy of the calves.

Aco'mia (ak-o'me-ah). Baldness.

Ac'onin. An alkaloid, $C_{26}H_{41}NO_{11}$, from aconitin.

Ac'onite (ak'o-nit). Poisonous drug from the root and leaves of *Aconi'tum Napel'lus:* cardiac, sedative, antipyretic, diaphoretic, and diuretic.

Aconit'ic acid. Crystalline acid, $C_6H_6O_6$, from aconite and sugar-cane.

Acon'itin. Deadly white alkaloid, $C_{33}H_{45}NO_{12}$, from aconite.

Aconi'tum (ak-o-ni'tum). See *Aconite.*

Aconure'sis (ak-on-u-re'sis). Involuntary urination.

Aco'rea (ak-o're-ah). Absence of the pupil.

Aco'ria (ak-o're-ah). Insatiable appetite.

Acor'mus. A monster fetus with scarcely any trunk.

Ac'orus (ak'o-rus). See *Calamus.*

Acou'meter, Acouom'eter. Instrument for measuring the hearing power.

Acouopho'nia. Auscultatory percussion.

Acous'ma. The hearing of imaginary sounds.

Acous'tic (ak-oos'tik or ak-kow'stik). Relating to sound or the sense of hearing.
Acous'ticon. A variety of ear-trumpet.
Acous'tics (ak-oos'tiks or ak-kow'stiks). The science of sound and hearing.
Acqui'red. Obtained after birth; not congenital.
Acracon'itin. Same as *Pseudaconitin.*
Acral'dehyd (ak-ral'de-hid). Same as *Acrolein.*
Acra'nia. Partial or complete absence of the cranium.
Acra'nial. Having no cranium.
Acratnre'sis. Inability to urinate from atony of the bladder.
Ac'rid (ak'rid). Irritating; pungent.
Ac'ridin. Crystalline alkaloid, $C_{12}H_9N$, from anthracene.
Acrit'ical (ak-rit'ik-al). Having no crisis.
Acritochro'macy. Color-blindness.
Acroæsthe'sia. See *Acroesthesia.*
Acroanesthe'sia. Anesthesia of the extremities.
Acroasphyx'ia. Asphyxia of the extremities; Raynaud's phenomenon.
Acrobysti'tis (ak-ro-bis-ti'tis). Inflammation of prepuce.
Ac'roblast (ak'ro-blast). The external layer of the mesoblast.
Acrocepha'lia. Pointed condition of the top of the head.
Acrocephal'ic. Marked by acrocephalia.
Acrocine'sis. Excessive motility; abnormal freedom of movement.
Acrocinet'ic (ak-ro-sin-et'ik). Marked by acrocinesis.
Acrodyn'ia (ak-ro-din'e-ah). A disease marked by pricking pains in the palms and soles, hyperesthesia, and eruption on hands and feet.
Acroesthe'sia. 1. Exaggerated sensitiveness. 2. Pain in the extremities.
Acro'lein. A volatile, oily liquid, C_3H_4O, from decomposition of glycerol.
Acroma'nia. Incurable or extreme mania.
Acromasti'tis. Inflammation of the nipple.
Acromega'lia, Acromeg'aly. A disease marked by enlargement of the tissues of the face, hands, and feet.
Acro'mial (ak-ro'me-al). Pertaining to the acromion.
Acromic'ria. Abnormal smallness of the extremities.
Acromioclavic'ular. Pertaining to acromion and clavicle.
Acromiohu'meral. Pertaining to the acromion and the humerus. **A. muscle,** the deltoid muscle.
Acro'mion. The outward extension of the spine of the scapula, forming the point of the shoulder.
Acromiothora'cic. Pertaining to the acromion and the thorax.
Acrom'phalus. 1. Bulging of the navel as the first stage of umbilical hernia. 2. The center of the navel.
Acronarcot'ic. Both acrid and narcotic.
Acroneuro'sis. Any neurosis of the extremities.
Acroparal'ysis. Paralysis of the extremities.
Acroparesthe'sia. 1. Paresthesia of the extremities. 2. Extreme paresthesia.
Acropathol'ogy. Pathology of the extremities.
Acrop'athy (ak-rop'ath-e). Any disease of the extremities.
Acropho'bia. Morbid fear of being at a great height.
Acroposthi'tis. Inflammation of the prepuce.
Acrot'ic. Pertaining to acrotism.
Ac'rotism. Defect or failure of the pulse.
Acrytal'dehyd (ak-rit-al'de-hid). Same as *Acrolein.*
Actæ'a. Genus of plants furnishing cohosh and cimicifuga.
Actin'ic (ak-tin'ik). Producing chemical action: said of rays of light beyond the violet of the spectrum.

Ac'tinism. The chemical property of light-rays.
Actin'ograph. A skiagraph.
Actinomy'ces (ak-tin-o-mi'sēz). A genus of fungi, of which *A. bo'vis* is the cause of actinomycosis.
Actinomyco'sis. An infectious disease of cattle and man, characterized by formation of tumors in the jaws and tongue.
Actinomycot'ic. Pertaining to or caused by actinomycosis.
Ac'tion of arrest. Inhibition. **Reflex a.,** involuntary action produced by a stimulus which is conveyed to the nervous system and reflected to the periphery.
Ac'tive treatment. See *Treatment.*
Ac'tol. Silver lactate, used as an antiseptic.
Ac'tual cautery (ak'tshu-al). Cautery by red heat.
Acu'ity. Sharpness or clearness, especially of vision.
Acu'meter. An instrument for measuring hearing.
Acu'minate. Sharp-pointed.
Acupres'sion, Ac'upressure. Compression of a blood-vessel by inserted needles.
Ac'upuncture. Therapeutic insertion of needles.
A'cus (a'kus). A needle, or needle-like process.
Acus'ticus. The auditory nerve.
Acute'. 1. Sharp. 2. Having severe symptoms and a short course. **A. decubitus.** See *Decubitus.*
Acutenac'ulum. Same as *Needle-holder.*
Acutor'sion. Acupressure with twisting of a bleeding vessel.
Acyanop'sia, Acyanoblep'sia. Same as *Blue-blindness.*
Acye'sis. 1. Sterility in woman. 2. Absence of pregnancy.
Acys'tia (as-is'te-ah). Congenital absence of bladder.
Acystoner'via, Acystoneu'ria. Paralysis of bladder.
A. D. For L. *au'ris dex'tra*, right ear.
Adac'rya (ad-ak're-ah). Deficiency in lacrimal secretion.
Adactyl'ia. Congenital lack of fingers or toes.
Adac'tylous (ad-ak'til-us). Lacking fingers or toes.
Ad'am's apple. Same as *Pomum Adami.*
Adanso'nin. A febrifugal alkaloid from *Adanso'nia digita'ta*, the baobab of Africa.
Adapta'tion. Adjustment of pupil to light.
Addepha'gia (ad-ef-a'je-ah). Same as *Bulimia.*
Ad'dison's disease. Tuberculous disease of suprarenal capsules, with discoloration of skin and anemia. **A.'s keloid.** Same as *Morphea.*
Addu'cens oc'uli. See *Rectus internus*, in *Muscles, Table of.*
Adduct'. To draw entad, or toward a center.
Adduc'tion. Act of drawing together, or toward a median line.
Adduc'tor. Any adducting muscle. See *Muscles, Table of.*
Adelomor'phous. Of indefinite form.
Adel'photaxy. The assumption by cells of a definite arrangement.
Adenal'gia, Adenal'gy. Pain in a gland.
Aden'dric. Without dendrons: used of cells.
Adenec'tomy (ad-en-ek'to-me). Surgical removal of a gland.
Adenecto'pia. Displacement of a gland.
Adenemphrax'is. Obstruction of the duct of a gland.
Ade'nia (ad-e'ne-ah). Same as *Lymphoma.*
Aden'iform. Gland-shaped.
Ad'enin. A leucomain, $C_5H_5N_5$, mainly found in various glands.
Adeni'tis. Inflammation of a gland.
Adeniza'tion. Assumption of an abnormal gland-like appearance.
Ad'enoblast. 1. A gland-cell, secretory or excretory. 2. Embryonic cell whence gland-tissue is derived.
Adenocarcino'ma. A cancerous or malignant adenoma.

Ad'enocele (ad'en-o-sēl). A cystic, adenomatous tumor.
Adenochondro'ma. Adenoma mixed with chondroma.
Ad'enocyst. A cyst developed from rudimentary structures.
Adenocysto'ma (ad-en-o-sis-to'mah). Adenoma blended with cystoma.
Adenodyn'ia (ad-en-o-din'e-ah). Pain in a gland.
Adenofibro'ma. Adenoma blended with fibroma.
Adenog'raphy. Anatomy, physiology, histology, and pathology of glands.
Ad'enoid (ad'en-oid). 1. Resembling a gland. 2. Adenoma.
Adenologadi'tis. Ophthalmia neonatorum.
Adenol'ogy. Sum of knowledge regarding glands.
Adenolympho'ma (ad-en-o-lim-fo'mah). Adenoma of a lymph-gland.
Adeno'ma. Tumor composed of glandular tissue. **A. des'truens,** a destructive variety of adenoma. **A. seba'ceum,** a yellowish tumor on the face, containing a mass of yellowish glands. **A. sim'plex,** glandular hyperplasia.
Adenomala'cia. Undue softness of a gland.
Adenomyo'ma. Adenoma combined with myoma.
Adenomyxo'ma. Adenoma blended with myxoma.
Adenomyxosarco'ma. Myxosarcoma of a gland.
Adenop'athy. Any disease of glands.
Adenopharyngi'tis. Inflammation of tonsils and pharynx.
Adenophleg'mon. Phlegmonous inflammation of glands.
Adenophthal'mia. Inflammation of the Meibomian glands.
Adenosarco'ma. Adenoma complicated with sarcoma.
Adenosclero'sis. Hardening of a gland.
Adeno'sis (ad-en-o'sis). Any disease of a gland.
Adenot'omy. 1. Anatomy of the glands. 2. Incision of a gland.
Ad'eps (ad'eps). Lard; axungia. **A. anseri'nus,** goose-grease. **A. benzoina'tus,** benzoinated lard. **A. la'næ,** lanolin, wool-fat. **A. la'næ hydro'sus,** hydrous lanolin. **A. ovil'lus,** sheep's suet or tallow.
Ader'mia. Defect or absence of the skin.
Adermogen'esis. Imperfect development of skin.
Adermotro'phia. Deficient nutrition of the skin.
Adhe'sion. 1. Abnormal joining of parts to each other. 2. Band or patch by which parts abnormally cohere. **Primary a.,** healing by first intention. **Secondary a.,** healing by second intention.
Adhe'sive. Sticking closely.
Adhe'sol. A form of surgical dressing similar to collodion.
Adian'tum. Maiden-hair fern; a pectoral demulcent.
Adiaphore'sis. Deficiency of the perspiration.
Adiapneus'tia. Defect or absence of perspiration.
Adip'ic acid. A crystalline acid, $C_6H_{10}O_4$, from fats.
Ad'ipocere (ad'ip-o-sēr). A waxy substance from bodies long dead; grave-wax.
Adipofibro'ma. A fibrous tumor with fatty elements.
Adipog'enous (ad-ip-oj'en-us). Producing fat.
Adipo'ma (ad-ip-o'mah). Same as *Lipoma.*
Ad'ipose. Of a fatty nature; fatty.
Adipo'sis doloro'sa. A disease marked by painful localized fatty degenerations and various nerve-lesions. **A. hepat'ica,** fatty degeneration of liver.
Adiposu'ria. The occurrence of fat in the urine.
Adip'sia (ad-ip'se-ah). Abnormal avoidance of drinking.
Adip'sous (ad-ip'sus). Quenching the thirst.
Ad'itus. An entrance or opening. **A. ad an'trum,** the recess which lodges the head of the malleus. **A. laryn'gis,** the entrance to the larynx.

Adjust'ment. The mechanism for raising and lowering the tube of a microscope.

Ad'juvant. An auxiliary remedy.

Ad lib. Abbreviation for L. *ad lib' itum*, at pleasure.

Adna'ta (ad-na'tah). Same as *Tunica adnata*.

Adneu'ral. Occurring or situated at a nerve.

Adnex'a. Appendages; adjunct parts. **A. oc'uli,** the lacrimal glands. **A. u'teri,** the oviducts and ovaries.

Adoles'cence (ad-o-les'ens). Youth.

Adon'idin. A poisonous glucosid from *Adonis vernalis*.

Ado'nis verna'lis. A poisonous herb; cardiant and acrid stimulant.

Ado'ral. Situated or occurring at or near the mouth.

Adoscula'tion. Impregnation without penetration.

Adre'nal. 1. Near the kidney. 2. A suprarenal capsule.

Ad'rae (ad'ra-e). See *Cyperus*.

Adus'tion. 1. Cauterization. 2. A dry, fevered state.

Advance'ment (ad-vans'ment). Detachment of an eye-muscle, and reattachment at an advanced point: an operation for strabismus. **Capsular a.,** attachment of capsule of Tenon in front of its normal position.

Adventi'tia (ad-ven-tish'ah). Outer coat of an artery.

Adventit'ious (ad-ven-tish'us). Acquired; not normal to a part.

Adyna'mia (ad-i-na'me-ah). Lack of vital powers.

Adynam'ic. Characterized by adynamia; asthenic.

Aeby's plane (e'bēz). Plane through basion and nasion, and perpendicular to median plane.

Ægophony and other words in **Æ.,** see *Egophony*, etc.

A'erated blood (a'er-a-ted). The arterial blood.

Aera'tion. The purification of blood in the lungs.

Aereadocar'dia. Gas or air in the heart.

Aerhemocto'nia. Death caused by air in a blood-vessel.

Ae'rial (a-e're-al). Pertaining to the air.

Aerif'erous (a-er-if'er-us). Conveying air.

Aer'iform (a-er'if-orm). Resembling air; gaseous.

Aero'bia (a-er-o'be-ah). Microphytes which require air or oxygen.

Aero'bic. Unable to live without oxygen.

Aero'bion. An aerobic organism. **Facultative a.,** an organism which is able to live without oxygen under some conditions, but which normally uses it. **Obligate a.,** one which always requires oxygen to live.

Aerobio'sis. Life that requires free oxygen.

Aerobiot'ic. Growing only in the presence of air.

Aerocystos'copy. Examination of the bladder by means of the aero-urethroscope.

Aerodermecta'sia. Subcutaneous or surgical emphysema.

Aerodynam'ics. Science of motion of gases.

Aerohydrop'athy. Therapeutic use of air and water.

Aerol'ogy (a-er-ol'o-ge). The science of air and its qualities.

Aerom'eter (a-er-om'et-er). Instrument for estimating gaseous density.

Aerom'icrobe. Any aerobic microphyte.

Aeroperito'nia. Air or gas in the peritoneal cavity.

Aeroph'agy (a-er-of'aj-e). Habitual swallowing of air.

Aeropho'bia. Morbid dread of drafts of air.

A'erophore (a'er-o-fōr). Device for inflating the lungs of still-born infants.

A'erophyte. Microbe, or other plant, that lives upon air.

Aeroplethys'mograph. Apparatus for graphically recording the expired air.

A'eroscope. Instrument for testing the purity of air.

Aerostat'ics. Science of air, or gases, at rest.

Aerotherapeu'tics, Aerother'apy. Treatment of disease by air.

Aerotho'rax (a-er-o-tho'raks). Same as *Pneumothorax.*

Aerotonom'eter. A device used in measuring the tension of the blood-gases.

Aerotym'panal. Performed by the agency of the air and the tympanum.

Aero-ureth'roscope. An instrument for use in aero-urethroscopy.

Aero-urethros'copy. Examination of the urethra by means of the aero-urethroscope.

Aerteriver'sion (a-er-ter-iv-er'shun). Surgical eversion of the coats of a bleeding artery.

Aerteriver'ter (a-er-ter-iv-er'ter). An instrument used in performing aerteriversion.

Æs-, Æt-. For words thus beginning, see *Es-, Et-.*

Afeb'rile (af-eb'ril). Without fever.

Affec'tion. Morbid condition or diseased state.

Af'ferent (af'er-ent). Centripetal or esodic.

Affin'ity. 1. Inherent likeness. 2. Chemical attraction. **Chemic a.,** the force that unites atoms of different substances. **Elective a.,** that force by which a substance chooses to unite with one substance rather than another.

Af'flux, Afflux'ion. Rush of blood to a part.

Affu'sion. The pouring of water on the body for cooling or cleansing.

Af'rican lethargy. Nelavan or sleeping sickness: said to be a form of filariasis.

Af'ter-birth. Placenta with umbilical cord. **A.-brain,** the metencephalon. **A.-cataract,** recurrent or secondary cataract. **A.-hearing,** hearing of sounds after the stimulus has ceased. **A.-image,** the retention of a retinal impression after the real object has ceased to be visible. **A.-pains,** pains which follow the expulsion of the placenta. **A.-perception,** perception of after-sensations. **A.-sensation,** sensation which persists after cessation of the stimulus.

Agalac'tia (ag-al-ak'she-ah). Failure or absence of milk secretion.

Agamogen'esis. Reproduction by an asexual process.

Ag'ar, Ag'ar-Ag'ar. Gelatin of various seaweeds: used in making culture-media.

Ag'aric. A fungus or mushroom of the genus *Agaricus,* of which several species are medicinal.

Agar'ic acid. Agari'cic acid. An acid from *Polyporus officinalis,* a fungus; used in night-sweats.

Agar'icin. A poisonous principle from *Agaricus albus;* used in night-sweats.

Agastroneu'ria. Lack of nervous tonicity in the stomach.

Ag'athin. An analgesic medicine not unlike salicylic acid.

Aga've (ag-a've). A genus of American plants: diuretic and antisyphilitic.

Agene'sia. Lack of sexual development; impotence.

Agenoso'mia. Imperfect development of sexual organs.

Ageu'sia, Ageus'tia. Loss or lack of the sense of taste.

Agglom'erated. Crowded into a mass.

Agglu'tinant, Agglu'tinative. 1. Acting like glue. 2. A substance which promotes union of parts.

Agglutina'tion. A joining together. **Immediate a.,** healing by first intention. **Mediate a.,** healing by formation of plastic material.

Ag'gregate, Ag'gregated. Huddled together. **A. glands.** Same as *Peyer's patches.*

Aglobu'lia. Decrease in the proportion of blood-corpuscles.
Aglos'sia. Congenital absence of the tongue.
Agluti'tion (ag-lu-tish'un). Inability to swallow.
Agmatol'ogy. The sum of what is known regarding fractures.
Ag'minate glands (ag'min-āt). Same as *Peyer's patches.*
Ag'nail. Same as *Hangnail.*
Agna'thia (ag-na'the-ah). Absence of a jaw-bone.
Ag'nin. A proprietary wool-fat preparation.
Agomphi'asis. Loose state of the teeth.
Ag'ony (ag'o-ne). 1. Death-struggle. 2. Extreme suffering.
Agorapho'bia. 1. Morbid dread of open spaces. 2. Dread of crowds of people.
Agre'mia, Agræ'mia. Gouty diathesis.
Agram'matism. Loss of power of uttering words.
Agraph'ia (ag-raf'e-ah). Inability to express thoughts by writing, owing to a central lesion. **Absolute a.,** inability to form letters. **Verbal a.,** ability to form letters, but not to write words.
Agraph'ic. Affected with, or pertaining to, agraphia.
Ag'ria. An obstinate pustular eruption.
Ag'rimony. The plant *Agrimonia eupatoria;* astringent and tonic.
Agrippi'nus par'tus. Footling presentation.
Agroma'nia (ag-ro-ma'ne-ah). Insane desire for solitude.
Agryp'nia (ag-rip'ne-ah). Abnormal wakefulness; insomnia.
Agrypnot'ic. A drug that promotes wakefulness.
A'gue (a'gu). Malarial fever. **Brass-founders' a.,** disease of brass-founders, with symptoms resembling intermittent fever. **Brow a.,** intermittent neuralgia of brow. **A. cake,** enlargement of spleen from chronic malaria. **Catenating a.,** ague associated with other diseases. **A. drop,** Fowler's solution. **Dumb a., Masked a.,** ague without well-marked chill and with only slight periodicity. **A. spleen.** Same as *A. cake.*
Ah. Symbol for *Hypermetropic astigmatism.*
Ahyp'nia. Sleeplessness; insomnia.
Aichmopho'bia. Insane dread of pointed instruments.
Ailan'thus glandulo'sa. A tree with tonic and anthelmintic bark and leaves.
Ainhum (in-yoon'). Tropical disease in which a little toe drops off.
Ai'odin (ah-i'o-din). An extract of thyroid gland, not containing iodin.
Air. The gaseous mixture which makes up the atmosphere. **Complemental a.,** the air in excess of the tidal air which may be drawn into the lungs by forced respiration. **Residual a.,** air that stays in the lungs after the strongest possible expiration. **Supplemental a.,** air which may be expelled from the lungs in excess of that normally breathed out. **Tidal a.,** air that is carried to and fro in normal respiration. **A.-cell.** Same as *A.-vesicle.* **A.-douche,** injection of air into a cavity. **A.-hunger,** dyspnea which affects both inspiration and expiration. **A.-passage,** any passage through which air passes in breathing. **A.-pump,** instrument used in producing a vacuum. **A.-sac.** Same as *A.-vesicle.* **A.-vesicle,** any normal saccule in lung-tissue into which air is drawn in breathing.
Air'ol. A green antiseptic powder; used externally.
Akanthesthe'sia, and other words in Ak., see under *Ac.*
Akine'sia. Loss of power of motion. **A. al'gera,** paralysis caused by the intense pain of muscular movement.
A'la (a'lah), pl. *a'læ.* Any wing-like process. **A. mag'na,** the great wing of the sphenoid bone. **A. na'si,** the cartilaginous flap on the outer side of either nostril. **A. par'va,** the lesser wing of the sphenoid. **A. vespertilio'nis** ("bat's wing"), the broad ligament of the uterus.
Ala'lia. Lack of power of speech not due to central lesion.

Alant-camphor. A camphor, $C_{10}H_{16}O$, found in elecampane.

Alan'tol. Oily antiseptic principle, $C_{15}H_{20}O_2$, from elecampane.

A'lar (a'lar). 1. Pertaining to or like a wing. 2. Pertaining to the axilla.

Albar'as. A skin disease with formation of white anesthetic patches on which the hair turns white.

Albe'do (al-be'do). Whiteness. **A. ret'inæ,** edema of retina.

Al'bert's disease. Achillodynia or achillobursitis.

Al'bicans. Either one of the corpora albicantia.

Albidu'ria. Discharge of white or colorless urine.

Al'binism. White condition of hair, skin, eyes, etc.

Albi'no (al-bi'no). A person affected with albinism.

Al'bolin. Oily emollient liquid used in spraying nose and throat.

Albugin'ea (al-bu-jin'e-ah). The tunica albuginea. **A. oc'uli.** Same as *Sclera.* **A. ova'rii,** the outer layer of the ovarian stroma. **A. pe'nis,** the outer envelop of the corpora cavernosa.

Albugini'tis. Inflammation of the albuginea of the penis.

Albu'go. White opacity of the cornea of the eye.

Albu'kalin. A principle derivable from leukemic blood.

Albu'men. The white of eggs.

Albumim'eter. Same as *Albuminimeter.*

Albu'min. A proteid found in nearly every animal tissue and fluid. **Acid a.,** albumin altered by action of acid. **Blood-a.** Same as *Serum-a.* **Circulating a.,** that found in the bodily fluids. **Derived a.,** albumin altered by action of chemicals. **Egg-a.,** albumin of the animal body. **Floating a.** Same as *Circulating a.* **Native a.,** any normal albumin of the organism. **Serum-a.,** a. of the body, especially of the blood. **Vegetable a.,** that of vegetable tissues.

Albu'minate. A compound of albumin with a base.

Albuminatu'ria. Excess of albuminates in the urine.

Albuminif'erous. Yielding albumin.

Albuminim'eter. Instrument for discovering the proportion of albumin present.

Albuminip'arous (al-bu-min-ip'ar-us). Producing albumin.

Albu'minoid. 1. Resembling albumin. 2. Any one of a large class of proteids.

Albu'minone. A principle from albuminoids, soluble in alcohol.

Albuminorrhe'a. Excessive excretion of albumins.

Albu'minose. Same as *Albumose.*

Albumino'sis. Abnormal excess of albuminous elements.

Albu'minous. Charged with or resembling albumin.

Albuminuret'ic. 1. Producing albuminuria. 2. Drug which so acts.

Albuminu'ria. Presence of albumin in the urine. **A. of adolescence.** See *Cyclic a.* **Cardiac a.,** that caused by valvular disease. **Cyclic a.,** occurrence of small quantity of albumin in the urine, especially of the young, at regular times each day. **False a.,** mixture of albumin with the urine during its course through the urinary passages. **Functional a.** Same as *Cyclic a.* **Mixed a.,** combined true and false a. **Paroxysmal a.** Same as *Cyclic a.* **Physiologic a.,** albumin in normal urine without disease of the system. **Simple a.** Same as *Cyclic a.* **True a.,** that due to excretion of some of the albuminous elements of the blood with the urine.

Al'bumose. Any primary product of the digestion of a proteid; further digestion converts the albumoses into peptones.

Albumosu'ria. Presence of an albumose in the urine.

Al'cock's canal. The sheath of obturator fascia which envelops the internal pudic nerve.

Al'cohol. 1. Ethyl hydrate, C_2H_5OH, a liquid distilled from products of vinous ferments. 2. Any compound of a hydrocarbon with hydroxyl: a term further extended to various substitution products. **Absolute a.**, a. with not over 1 per cent. of water. **Amyl a.**, fusel oil. **Ethyl a.**, ordinary alcohol. **Methyl a.**, wood spirit, CH_4O. **Primary, Secondary, Tertiary a.**, one formed by replacement, 1, 2, or 3 hydrogen atoms in carbinol with alkyls.

Al'coholate. A compound or a preparation containing alcohol.

Alcohol'ature (al-ko-hol'at-ur). An alcoholic tincture.

Alcohol'ic. Containing or pertaining to alcohol.

Al'coholism. Morbid effects of excess in using alcoholic drinks.

Al'coholize. 1. To treat with alcohol. 2. To transform into alcohol.

Alcoholom'eter. Instrument for finding percentage of alcohol present.

Alcoholophil'ia (al-ko-hol-o-fil'e-ah). Morbid appetite for alcoholic drink.

Al'dehyd. Any one of a class of partly dehydrogenated alcohols. **Acetic a.**, C_2H_4O, an anesthetic and antiseptic liquid.

Al'der (all'der). See *Alnus*.

Ale'cithal (al-es'ith-al). Having no distinct yolk: used of the ovum of mammals.

Alem'bic. Utensil used in distilling.

Alem'broth. A compound of mercuric and ammonium chlorids: antiseptic.

Alep'po boil, button, or **sore.** Same as *Oriental sore*.

Al'etrin. A precipitate from *Aletris farinosa*: diuretic.

Al'etris farinosa. Star-grass; a tonic and diuretic herb.

Aleucocyto'sis. See *Aleukocytosis*.

Aleuke'mia. Paucity of white corpuscles in the blood.

Aleukocyto'sis. Diminished production of white corpuscles in the blood.

Aleu'ronat. A vegetable albumin used for bread in diabetes.

Alexan'der's operation. Shortening the round ligaments for cure of uterine displacements.

Alex'ia. Inability to read, due to a central lesion. **Musical a.**, inability to read music.

Alex'in. A defensive proteid in the leukocytes of the body.

Alexiphar'mac. Warding off the ill effects of a poison.

Alexipyret'ic. Febrifuge; preventive of fevers.

Al'gæ (al'je). A group of plants living in the water.

Algefa'cient (al-je-fa'shent). Cooling or refrigerant.

Alge'sia (al-je'se-ah). Sensitiveness to pain; hyperesthesia.

Algesichronom'eter. Instrument for ascertaining the time required to produce a painful impression.

Algesim'eter (al-je-sim'et-er). An instrument used in measuring the degree of sensitiveness. **Boas's a.**, instrument for determining the sensitiveness over the epigastrium.

Algesthe'sis (al-jes-the'sis). A painful sensation.

Al'gid (al'jid). Chilly; cold. **A. stage,** period of a disease in which the temperature is low.

Algogen'ic (al-go-jen'ik). 1. Causing pain. 2. Lowering the temperature.

Algom'eter. Device used in testing the sensitiveness of a part.

Algopho'bia (al-go-fo'be-ah). Morbid dread of pain.

Al'gor. Chill or rigor.

Al'ible. Nutritive; good for food.

Al'ices (al'is-ēs). Spots which precede the small-pox eruption.

Aliena'tion (a-lyen-a'shun). Mental derangement; insanity.

A'lienism (a'lyen-izm). The study or treatment of insanity.

A'lienist (a'lyen-ist). One skilled in treating medical disorders.

Al'iform (al'if-orm). Shaped like a wing.

Al'iment (al'im-ent). Food; nutritive material.

Alimen'tary. Serving as food; nutritious.

Alimenta'tion. Act of giving or receiving nourishment. **Rectal a.,** feeding by injection of nutriment into rectum.

Alina'sal. Pertaining to either wing of the nose.

Alisphe'noid. Pertaining to the great wing of the sphenoid.

Aliz'arin. A red coloring principle, $C_{14}H_8O_4$, obtained from coal-tar or from madder.

Alkales'cent. Having a tendency to alkalinity.

Al'kali (al'kal-i). Any one of a class of compounds which form salts with acids and soaps with fats. **A. albumin,** albumin which has been treated with alkalies. **Caustic a.,** hydroxid of sodium or potassium in solid form. **A. metals,** potassium, sodium, lithium, rubidium, cesium, etc.

Alkalim'eter. Instrument used in measuring the alkali contained in a mixture.

Alkalim'etry. Measurement of alkalies present.

Al'kaline (al'kal-in). Having the reactions of an alkali.

Alkalin'ity. The quality of being alkaline.

Alkalinu'ria. An alkaline condition of the urine.

Alkaliza'tion. Act of making alkaline.

Al'kaloid. Any alkaline principle of organic origin. **Animal a.,** alkaloid substance formed in decomposition of animal tissues. **Cadaveric** or **Putrefactive a.,** a ptomain.

Al'kanet. The root of *Anchusa tinctoria*, affording a red color.

Al'kanin. Red coloring matter from alkanet.

Alkap'ton. A nitrogenous principle sometimes occurring in urine.

Alkaptonu'ria. Presence of alkapton in urine.

Allantia'sis. Sausage-poisoning; botulism.

Allanto'ic. Pertaining to allantois.

Allan'toin. Crystalline substance, $C_4H_6N_4O_3$, from allantoic fluid and fetal urine.

Allan'tois. One of the membranes enclosing the fetus, the lower part developing into the bladder, and the upper into the urachus.

Allantotox'icon. The poison of decaying sausages.

Allesthe'sia. Same as *Allocheiria*.

Allia'ceous (al-e-a'shus). Resembling garlic.

Al'lium. The garlic: also the genus to which garlic and onion belong.

Allochei'ria. State in which, if stimulus is applied to one side, the patient refers the consequent sensation to the other side.

Allochesthe'sia. Same as *Allocheiria*.

Allola'lia. Any defect of speech of central origin.

Al'lopath, Allop'athist. Incorrect title for a regular practitioner.

Allop'athy. Erroneous name for the regular system of practice.

Allorrhyth'mia. Irregular rhythm of the pulse.

Allotox'in. A substance arising within the body which serves as a defence against toxins.

Allotriodon'tia. 1. Transplanting of teeth from one person to another. 2. Presence of teeth in abnormal places.

Allotriogeus'tia (al-ot-re-o-joos'te-ah). Perverted sense of taste.

Allotrioph'agy. Craving for unnatural food; pica.

Allotriu'ria. Passage of any unusual or strange substance in urine.

Allot'ropism, Allot'ropy. Existence of an element in two or more distinct forms.

Allox'an. A substance, $C_4H_2N_2O_4$, derivable from uric acid.

Alloxan'tin. A derivative from alloxan.

Allox'in. Any one of a class of bases derived from the nuclein of cell-nuclei, and on oxidation producing uric acid.

Alloy' (al-oy'). A mixture obtained by fusing metals together.

All'spice. Same as *Pimenta*.

Allylam'in. A liquid derivative, $NH_2(C_3H_5)$, from oil of mustard.

Almén's tests (ahl-mênz'). Three tests of urine, for blood, albumin, and sugar.

Al'mond (ah'mund). Fruit of *Prunus amygdala.* See also *Amygdala.*

Al'nuin. Resinoid from species of *Alnus:* tonic and resolvent.

Al'nus (al'nus). Genus of trees and shrubs; alders; tonic and astringent.

Alo'chia (al-o'ke-ah). Absence or suppression of the lochia.

A'loe (al'o-e). Genus of plants which afford aloes.

Al'oes (al'ōz). Dried juice of various species of *Aloe:* cathartic.

Aloet'ic (al-o-et'ik). A preparation containing aloes.

Aloe'tin. Medicinal preparation of aloes.

Alo'gia (al-o'je-ah). Inability to speak, due to lesion of nerve-substance.

Al'oin. Purgative glucosid from aloes of various kinds.

Alope'cia (al-o-pe'se-ah). Baldness from disease. **A. adna'ta,** congenital a. **A. area'ta, A. circumscrip'ta,** condition in which bald patches appear on hairy regions of body. **Congenital a.,** baldness from absence of hair-bulbs. **A. furfura'cea,** baldness with hyperemia, itching, and exfoliation of scales. **A. loca'lis, A. neurit'ica,** that occurring at site of injury or in the course of a nerve. **A. pityro'ides universa'lis,** rapid, general loss of hair in debilitated conditions. **A. sim'plex,** premature baldness. **A. universa'lis,** general falling out of hairs of the body.

Aloxan'thin. Yellow substance, $C_{15}H_{10}O_6$, from Barbadoes aloes.

Al'pha-leukocyte. Leukocyte which disintegrates during the coagulation of blood.

Al'pha-naph'tol. A non-official variety of naphtol.

Al'phol. A principle, $C_{17}H_{12}O_3$; anodyne and antiseptic.

Al'phos. A variety of psoriasis or lepra.

Alpin'ia. See *Galangal.*

Alsto'nia schola'ris. Oriental tree which yields dita bark; a tonic febrifuge.

Al'stonin. Alkaloid, $C_{21}H_{20}N_2O_4$, from alstonia.

Al'terant, Al'terative. Re-establishing healthy functions of the system.

Al'ternate hemiplegia. See under *Hemiplegia.*

Al'ternating current. See *Current.*

Alterna'tion of generation. Reproduction in which one generation is sexually developed, and the next asexually.

Althæ'a officina'lis. The plant marshmallow; demulcent.

Al'um. An aluminium and potassium (or ammonium) sulphate; astringent. **A.-hematoxylon,** purple tissue-stain. **A.-whey,** whey from milk boiled with alum.

Alu'men (al-u'men). L. for *alum.* **A. exsicca'tum,** dried or burnt alum.

Alu'mina (al-u'min-ah). Aluminum oxid Al_2O_3.

Alu'minated (al-u'min-a-ted). Containing alum.

Alumin'ium. Same as *Aluminum.*

Alumino'sis. A lung disease of alum-workers.

Alu'minoid. A white astringent antiseptic powder.

Alu'minol. A white powder; astringent and antiseptic.

Alu'minum. A very light whitish metal; symbol Al.

Alum'nol. Same as *Aluminol.*

Alvegniat's pump (ahl-ven-yahz'). Pump for abstracting gases from the blood.

Alve'olar. Pertaining to an alveolus.

Alve'oli (al-ve'o-li). Plural of *Alveolus.*

Alveoli'tis. Inflammation of an alveolus, as of a tooth.

Alveoloden'tal. Pertaining to the teeth and their sockets.

Alve'olus (al-ve'o-lus), pl. *alve'oli.* A little hollow; socket of a tooth. **A. of a gland,** any follicle of a racemose gland. **A. of lung-tissue.** Same as *Air-vesicle.* **A. of the stomach,** any one of the honeycomb cells of the gastric mucous membrane.

Al'vine (al'vin). Pertaining to the belly. **A. concretion,** calculus in intestine. **A. flux.** Same as *Diarrhea.*

Alym'phia (ah-lim'fe-ah). Absence or lack of lymph.

Am. Symbol for *Myopic astigmatism.*

Am'acrine-cells, Am'acrines. Branched retinal structures.

Am'adou (am'ad-oo). A fungus used in surgery.

Amal'gam. A compound of mercury with another metal.

Aman'itin. A poisonous alkaloid from fly-agaric.

Ama'ra (am-a'rah). Bitter medicines.

Am'arin. Alkaloid, $C_{21}H_{18}N_2$, from bitter almonds.

Amase'sis. Lack of power to chew the food.

Amas'tia. Absence of mammary glands.

Amauro'sis. Blindness from disease of the optic nerve or of the retina. It may be **albuminuric** or due to renal disease; **cerebral** or due to brain-disease; **congenital,** when existing from birth; **diabetic,** when associated with diabetes; **reflex,** caused by reflex action of remote irritation; **saburral,** when occurring in an attack of acute gastritis; **uremic,** when due to uremia.

Amaurot'ic. Of the nature of amaurosis. **A. cat's-eye,** retinal glioma.

Amaxopho'bia. Morbid dread of carriages and wagons.

Ama'zia. Congenital absence of the breasts.

Am'ber. A fossil resin; its volatile oil is antispasmodic and stimulant.

Am'bergris. A gray substance from the sperm whale's intestines: somewhat useful as a nerve-stimulant.

Ambidex'trous. Working effectively with either hand.

Ambio'pia. Same as *Diplopia.*

Amblo'sis (am-blo'sis). Abortion.

Amblot'ic. 1. Producing abortion. 2. An abortifacient.

Amblya'phia (am-ble-a'fe-ah). Dulness or bluntness of the sense of touch.

Amblyo'pia. Dimness of vision that cannot be relieved. **A. exanop'sia,** weakness of sight from long disuse. **Crossed a.,** amblyopia of one eye with hemianesthesia of the same side. **Postmarital a.,** that due to sexual excess.

Ambro'sia. A genus of plants, bitter, stimulant, and styptic.

Am'bulance. Wagon for the sick and wounded.

Am'bulant, Am'bulatory. Walking.

Ambus'tial (am-bus'tshal). Pertaining to a burn.

Ambus'tion (am-bus'tshun). A burn or scald; act of burning.

Ame'ba (am-e'bah). A minute one-celled protozoan animal; also, genus (*Amœba*) of such organisms; also, a phase of protozoan development. **A. co'li,** the ameba of dysentery.

Ame'bic. Of the nature of an ameba.

Ame'bicide (am-e'bis-id). Destructive to amebæ.

Ame'boid. Resembling, or having the movements of an ameba. **A. movements,** changes of shape peculiar to amebæ.

Amebu'ria, Amœbu'ria. Discharge of amebæ with the urine.

Ame'lia. Congenital absence of a limb or limbs.

Amel'oblast. A cell of the group whence dental enamel is formed.

Am'elus (am'el-us). Fetus born with no limbs.

Ame'nia (am-e'ne-ah). Absence of the menses; amenorrhea.

Amenoma'nia, Amenoma'nia. Insanity with agreeable hallucinations.

Amenorrhe'a. Absence, or abnormal stoppage of, the menses.

A'ment. An idiot; a person with no mind.

Amen'tia (am-en'she-ah). Absence of intellect; idiocy.

Amet'ria. Congenital absence of the womb.
Ametrohe'mia. Lack of uterine blood-supply.
Ametrom'eter. Instrument for measuring degree of ametiopia.
Ametro'pia. Imperfection in the refractive powers of the eye.
Ametrop'ic. Affected with, or pertaining to, ametropia.
Amianth'inopsy. Inability to see violet tints.
Amicro'bic. Not produced by microbes.
Am'id (am'id). Any compound derived from ammonia by substituting an acid radical for hydrogen.
Am'idin. One of the constituents of starch-granules.
Amido-ace'tic acid. Same as *Glycocoll*.
Amidoben'zene. Same as *Anilin*.
Amid'ogen (am-id'o-jen). The hypothetic radical, NH_2, of amids.
Amidomy'elin. A derivative from brain-substance, $C_{44}H_{92}K_2PO_{10}$; also, any compound of the class to which it belongs.
Amid'ulin. A soluble starch; granulose separated from its envelop of amylocellulose.
Amim'ia. Loss of the power of expression by the use of signs.
Am'in. Any compound formed from ammonia by replacing hydrogen with an alcohol radical.
Am'inol. An antiseptic and deodorant preparation.
Amito'sis. Direct nuclear or cell division.
Amitot'ic. Not occurring by karyokinesis; of the nature of amitosis.
Ammone'mia. See *Ammoniemia*.
Ammo'nia. 1. A colorless alkaline gas, NH_3. 2. Also water charged with the same, called also *ammonia water;* stimulant.
Ammo'niac. A fetid gum-resin: stimulant and expectorant.
Ammonie'mia. The presence of ammonia in the blood.
Ammo'niated. Combined with ammonia.
Ammo'nium. The radical, NH_4, of ammonia.
Ammoniu'ria. Excess of ammonia in the urine.
Am'monol. A combination of ammonia with acetanilid.
Ammother'apy. Treatment by sand-bath; psammotherapy.
Amne'sia (am-ne'ze-ah). Lack or loss of memory. **Auditory a.**, word-deafness. **Visual a.**, word-blindness.
Amne'sic. Characterized by loss of memory. **A. aphasia.** Same as *Amnesia*.
Amniocho'rial. Pertaining to amnion and chorion.
Am'nion. Innermost fetal membrane, with the bag of waters.
Amniorrhe'a. Escape of amniotic waters.
Am'niote (am'ne-ōt). Any animal with amnion.
Amniot'ic. Relating to the amnion.
Amnioti'tis. Same as *Amnitis*.
Am'niotome (am'ne-o-tōm). Instrument for cutting fetal envelops.
Amni'tis (am-ni'tis). Inflammation of the amnion.
Amœba and words in **Amœ-**. See *Ameba*, etc.
Amo'mum. Genus of plants affording cardamoms.
Amor'phism (am-or'fizm). State of being amorphous.
Amor'phous. Having no definite form; shapeless.
Amor'phus. A shapeless acardiac monster.
Ampelop'sin. Tonic resinoid from *Ampelopsis quinquefolia*.
Ampelother'apy. Therapeutic use of grapes and grape-products; grape-cure.
Am'perage. The number of amperes in use.
Ampere (ahm-pār'). Unit of electric current strength; current yielded by one volt of electromotive force against one ohm of resistance.
Ampere'meter. Instrument for measuring amperage.
Amphiar'kyochrome. A nerve-cell with peculiar staining qualities.

Amphiarthro'sis. A joint in which the surfaces are connected by disks of fibrocartilage, as between vertebræ.

Am'phiaster (am'fe-as-ter). Same as *Diaster*.

Amphib'ia. A class of animals living both on land and in water, as frog, newt, etc.

Amphiblas'tula. A blastula with unequal segments.

Amphibo'lia. The uncertain period of a fever or disease.

Amphib'olous. Changeable; uncertain.

Amphicœ'lous. Concave on either side or end.

Amphicra'nia. Headache affecting both sides of head.

Amphicre'atin. A leucomain from muscle.

Amphicreat'inin. A poisonous leucomain from muscle.

Amphicyt'ula. The ovum in its cytula stage.

Amphidiarthro'sis. A joint having the nature of both ginglymus and arthrodia, as that of the lower jaw.

Amphigas'trula. Gastrula of the human ovum at an advanced stage.

Amphikrea'tin. See *Amphicreatin.*

Amphikreat'inin. See *Amphicreatinin.*

Amphimicro'bian. Both aerobic and anaerobic.

Amphimix'is. Union of germ nuclei in reproduction.

Amphipep'tone. Antipeptone mixed with hemipeptone.

Amphis'toma hom'inis. A rare trematode worm from human intestine.

Amphodiplo'pia. Double vision in each eye.

Amphopep'tone. See *Amphipeptone.*

Am'phophil, Amphoph'ilous (am'fo-fil, am-fof'il-us). Staining with either acid or basic dyes.

Amphor'ic. Pertaining to a bottle. **A. breathing, A. respiration,** a breathing, auscultatory sound like that made by blowing across the mouth of a bottle. **A. bubble,** a sound like the noise of a liquid poured from a bottle; a sign of hydropneumothorax.

Amphoroph'ony. Amphoric sound of voice.

Amphoter'ic, Amphot'erous. Affecting both red and blue litmus.

Amphoterodiplo'pia. Same as *Amphodiplopia.*

Amplifica'tion. Enlargement of visual area of a microscope.

Am'plifier. Apparatus for increasing magnification of a microscope.

Am'plitude. Largeness, fulness: widest range or extent.

Ampul'la. Any flask-like dilatation; the dilated end of the semicircular canal of the ear. **Lieberkuhn's a.,** the fluid termination of lacteals in the villi of the intestines. **A. of rectum,** part above the perineal flexure. **A. of Vater,** dilatation at entrance of common bile duct and pancreatic duct into duodenum.

Amputa'tion. Surgical cutting off of a limb or other part. **Accidental a.,** separation of a limb by some accident. **Bloodless a.,** one in which there is little loss of blood, the circulation being controlled by mechanical means. **Circular a.,** one performed by making a single flap, by circular incision, in a direction vertical to the long axis of the limb. **Coat-sleeve a.,** circular a., in which the skin-flap is made very long, the end being closed by a tape. **Congenital a.,** amputation of parts of fetus by constricting bands. **A. in contiguity,** amputation at a joint. **A. in continuity,** amputation of a limb elsewhere than at a joint. **Consecutive a.,** an amputation during or after the period of suppuration. **Diclastic a.,** a. in which bone is broken by osteoclast and the soft tissues divided by an écraseur. **Double-flap a.,** one in which two flaps are formed. **Dry a.** See *Bloodless a.* **Elliptical a.,** one in which the cut has an elliptical outline, on account of the oblique direction of the incision. **Flap a.,** one in which flaps are made from the soft tissues, the division being oblique. **Flapless a.**, one in which flaps cannot be formed. **Galvano-caustic a.**, one in which the soft parts are divided with the galvano-cautery. **Immediate a.**, one performed within twelve hours after the injury. **Intermediary**, or **Intermediate a.**, one done during the period of reaction, and before suppuration. **Intrapyretic a.** Same as *Intermediary a.* **Intra-uterine a.** See *Congenital a.* **Mediate a.** See *Intermediary a.* **Mixed a.**, one done by a combination of the circular and flap methods. **Multiple a.**, amputation of two or more parts at the same time. **Oval a.**, one in which the incision consists of two reversed spirals. **Primary a.**, one performed after the period of shock and before the development of inflammation. **Racket a.**, one in which there is a single longitudinal incision continuous below with a spiral incision on either side of the limb. **Secondary a.**, one performed during suppuration. **Spontaneous a.** See *Congenital a.* **Subperiosteal a.**, one in which the cut end of the bone is covered by periosteal flaps. **Synchronous a.** See *Multiple a.*

Amu'sia (ah-mu'se-ah). Inability to produce (**motor a.**) or to comprehend (**sensory a.**) musical sounds.

Am'ussat's operation. Left lumbar colotomy.

Amyelenceph'alus (am-i-e-len-sef'a-lus). Same as *Amyencephalus*.

Amye'lia. Absence of the spinal cord.

Amyelin'ic. 1. Without myelin. 2. Having no spinal cord.

Amyelot'rophy (am-i-el-ot'ro-fe). Atrophy of spinal cord.

Amy'elus (am-i'el-us). Fetus with no spinal cord.

Amyenceph'alus. Fetus with neither brain nor myelon.

Amyg'dala (am-ig'dal-ah). 1. Fruit of *Amygdalus communis*, almond. **A. ama'ra**, bitter almond; **a. dul'cis**, sweet almond. 2. A tonsil. 3. A lobule of the cerebellum.

Amyg'dalin (am-ig'dal-in). A principle from bitter almonds.

Amyg'daline (am-ig'dal-in). Pertaining to tonsils.

Amygdali'tis (am-ig-dal-i'tis). Same as *Tonsillitis*.

Amyg'daloid fossa. A depression lodging the tonsil. **A. tubercle**, mass of gray matter at end of descending cornu of lateral ventricle.

Amygdal'olith (am-ig-dal'o-lith). Calculus in a tonsil.

Amygdalop'athy. Any disease of a tonsil.

Amyg'dalotome. Instrument for cutting a tonsil.

Amygdalot'omy. Same as *Tonsillotomy*.

Am'ykos (am'e-kos). A Russian antiseptic fluid.

Am'yl (am'il). The radical C_5H_{11}. **A. nitrite**, an antiseptic liquid; used as a vasodilator.

Amyla'ceous. Composed of or resembling starch.

Amylam'in. Poisonous base, $C_5H_{13}N$, from cod-liver oil.

Am'ylene (am'il-ēn). Poisonous hydrocarbon, C_5H_{10}; dangerous anesthetic. **A. hydrate**, **A. alcohol**, hypnotic liquid, $C_5H_{12}O$.

Amyleniza'tion. Anesthesia produced by amylene.

Amyl'ic alcohol. Same as *Fusel oil*.

Am'yline (am'il-in). The same as *Amidin*.

Amy'loform (am-i'lo-form). White antiseptic and deodorizing powder, a compound of starch with formaldehyd.

Amylogen'ic. Producing starch.

Am'yloid (am'il-oid). Starch-like; amylaceous.

Amylol'ysis. Digestive change of starch into sugar.

Amylolyt'ic. Effecting the digestion of starch.

Amy'loplast. A starch-forming vegetable leucoplastid.

Amylop'sin. One of the pancreatic ferments.

Am'ylose (am'il-ōs). Any carbohydrate other than a glucose or saccharose.

Amy'lum (am-i'lum). L. for *starch.*
Amyocar'dia. Weakness of the heart-muscle.
A'myon (ah'me-on). Absence of muscular tissue.
Amyosta'sia. Nervous tremor of the muscles.
Amyosthe'nia. Failure of muscular strength.
Amyosthen'ic. 1. Characterized by amyosthenia. 2. A medicine which diminishes muscular power.
Amyotro'phia. Atrophy of a muscle or muscles.
Amyotroph'ic. Pertaining to amyotrophia.
Amy'ous (am-i'us). Deficient in muscular tissue.
Ana. Symbol meaning "of each."
Anab'asis (an-ab'as-is). The stage of increase in a disease.
Anabat'ic. Increasing, as a stage of fever.
Anabio'sis (an-ab-i-o'sis). Restoration to consciousness.
Anabol'ergy (an-ab-ol'er-je). The work done in anabolism.
Anabol'ic. Pertaining to constructive metabolism. **A. nerves,** nerves which control constructive processes.
Anab'olin. Any product of a constructive process.
Anab'olism. Any constructive process, or anabolic change; assimilation.
Anacamptom'eter. An instrument for measuring the reflexes.
Anacar'dium. Genus of tropical trees furnishing cashew gum and oil.
Anacid'ity (an-as-id'it-e). Abnormal lack or deficiency of acid.
Anacrot'ic. Characterized by anacrotism. **A. limb,** up-stroke of sphygmographic record.
Anac'rotism. The existence of two or more expansions of an artery in one beat.
Anacu'sis. Same as *Anakusis.*
Anade'nia (an-ad-e'ne-ah). Defect of glandular action.
Anadicrot'ic. Characterized by double indentation of the ascending wave of the sphygmographic record.
Anadip'sia (an-ad-ip'se-ah). Intense thirst.
Anæ'mia. See *Anemia.*
Ana'erobe. Anaero'bion (an-a'er-ōb, an-a-er-o'be-on). Any microbe which thrives with no access to the air.
Anaerob'ic, Anaerobiot'ic. Thriving best without air.
Ana'eroplasty. Exclusion of air from wounds by applying water.
Anæsthe'sia, etc. See *Anesthesia.*
Anaku'sis. Deafness due to a nervous or central lesion.
A'nal (a'nal). Relating to the anus.
Analep'tic. 1. Restorative; cordial. 2. A restorative medicine.
Anal'gen (an-al'jen). A crystalline, antipyretic, and analgesic preparation, $C_{18}H_{16}N_2O_2$.
Analge'sia (an-al-je'ze-ah). Absence of sensibility to pain.
Analge'sic (an-al-je'sik). 1. Relieving pain. 2. Of the nature of analgesia.
Analge'sin (an-al-je'sin). Same as *Antipyrin.*
Anal'gia (an-al'je-ah). Painlessness.
Anal'gic (an-al'jik). Same as *Analgesic.*
Anal'gin (an-al'jin). Same as *Creolin.*
An'alogue (an'al-og). A part resembling another in function, but not in structure.
Anal'ysis (an-al'is-is). Separation into component parts. **Gasometric a.,** analysis of gaseous compounds. **Gravimetric a.,** determination by weight of the quantity of the elements of a compound. **Organic a.,** analysis of animal and vegetable tissues. **Proximate a.,** determination of the simpler constituents of a substance. **Qualitative a.,** determination of the nature of the constituents of a compound. **Quantitative a.,** determination of the proportionate quantities of the constituents

of a compound. **Ultimate a.,** determination of the ultimate elements of a compound. **Volumetric a.,** quantitative analysis by volume.

An'alyzer. The Nicol prism in a polarimeter.

An'am ulcer. Phagedena common in hot countries.

Anamne'sis. The past history of any particular case of disease.

Anamniot'ic. Having no amnion.

Anapeirat'ic. Due to excessive use or over-exercise.

An'aphase (an'af-āz). That phase of karyokinesis just before the formation of the daughter-stars.

Ana'phia (an-a'fe-ah). Lack or loss of the sense of touch.

Anaphrodis'ia. Absence or loss of sexual desire.

Anaphrodis'iac. 1. Repressing sexual appetite. 2. A drug that allays sexual desires.

Anaplas'tic. Restoring a lost or absent part.

An'aplasty. Plastic or restorative surgery.

Anap'nograph. Device which registers the speed and pressure of the respired air-current.

Anapno'ic (an-ap-no'ik). Relieving dyspnea.

Anapnom'eter. Same as *Spirometer.*

Anapoph'ysis. An accessory vertebral process.

Anar'cotin. Alkaloid of opium, said to be a valuable antiperiodic.

Anarith'mia. Inability to count, due to a central lesion.

Anar'thria. Inability to pronounce distinctly. **A. litera'lis,** stuttering.

Anasar'ca. General dropsy of the cellular tissues.

Anaspa'dias. Condition in which the urethra opens upon the dorsum of the penis.

Anastal'tic. Styptic; highly astringent.

An'astate (an'as-tāt). Any substance, or condition, characteristic of an anabolic process.

Anas'tole (an-as'to-le). Retraction, as of the lips of a wound.

Anastomo'sis. 1. Communication between vessels. 2. Surgical or pathologic formation of a passage between any two normally distinct spaces. **Crucial a.,** an arterial anastomosis in the upper part of the thigh. **Intestinal a.,** establishment of a communication between two portions of the intestine.

Anastomot'ic. Pertaining to, or of the nature of, anastomosis.

Anastomot'ica mag'na. A branch of the femoral artery.

Anatherapeu'sis. Treatment by increasing doses.

Anatom'ic, Anatom'ical. Pertaining to anatomy. **A. tubercle.** Same as *Dissection tubercle.*

Anat'omist. One who is skilled in anatomy.

Anat'omy (an-at'o-me). The science of the structure of organized bodies. **Applied a.,** anatomy as applied to diagnosis and treatment. **Comparative a.,** comparison of structure of different animals and plants one with another. **Descriptive a.,** study of the individual parts of the body. **Gross a.,** that dealing with structures that can be distinguished with the naked eye. **Microscopic** or **Minute a.,** that studied with the microscope. **Morbid** or **Pathologic a.,** anatomy of diseased tissues. **Regional a.,** study of limited portions or regions of the body. **Topographical a.,** study of parts in relation to surrounding parts.

Anatricrot'ic. Causing three indentations on the ascending curve of the sphygmogram.

Anatrip'tic. A medicine applied by rubbing.

Anazotu'ria. Too little urea in the urine.

An'azyme. A proprietary preparation used like iodoform.

An'chorage (ang'ko-rāj). Surgical fixation of a displaced viscus.

Anchylo-. See under *Ankylo-.*

Ancip'ital (an-sip'it-al). Two-edged.

An'conad (ang-ko-nad). Toward the elbow or olecranon.
Anconag'ra (ang-ko-nag'rah). Gouty seizure of the elbow.
An'conal (ang'ko-nal). Pertaining to the elbow.
Ancone'us (ang-ko-ne'us). See *Muscles, Table of.*
Ancylo-. See *Ankylo-.*
An'cyroid (an'sir-oid). Anchor-shaped.
An'da Gome'sii. Tree of Brazil, which yields a purgative oil.
An'dersch's ganglion. Inferior ganglion of glossopharyngeal nerve.
An'derson's pill. Compound pill of gamboge.
Androgalactoze'mia. Secretion of milk from male breast.
Andro'gynous (an-droj'in-us). Hermaphrodite; of double or doubtful sex.
Androl'ogy. The science of man, or human nature.
Androma'nia. Same as *Nymphomania.*
Andromedotox'in. Poisonous hypnotic principle from ericaceous plants.
Andropho'bia. Insane dread of the male sex.
Anec'tasin. A substance produced by bacteria not antagonistic to the true bacterial action.
Anelec'trode. Positive pole of a battery.
Anelectrot'onus. Lessened irritability of a nerve at the anode during the passage of electric current.
Anel's operation (ah-nelz'). Ligation of an artery on the proximal side of aneurysmal sac. **A.'s probe,** a fine probe for the lacrimal passages.
Ane'mia (an-e'me-ah). Deficient quantity or quality of the blood. **Essential a., Idiopathic a.,** that due to disease of the blood or the blood-producing organs. **A. lymphat'ica,** Hodgkin's disease. **Miners' a.,** ankylostomiasis. **Primary a.** Same as *Idiopathic a.* **Secondary** or **Symptomatic a.,** that due to, or symptomatic of, some distinct cause, as cancer, hemorrhage, etc. **A. splen'ica,** anemia with enlarged spleen. **Tunnel a.,** ankylostomiasis.
Anem'ic (an-em'ik). Affected with anemia.
Anemom'eter. Instrument for measuring velocity of wind.
Anem'one (an-em'o-ne). Genus of plants. See *Pulsatilla.*
Anem'onin. A poisonous principle from pulsatilla.
Anemop'athy. Treatment of disease by inhalation.
Anemot'rophy. Insufficient nourishment of the blood.
Anencepha'lia. Absence of the brain.
Anencephalohe'mia. Insufficient supply of blood to the brain.
Anenceph'alous (an-en-sef'al-us). Having no brain.
Aner'gic (an-er'jik). Characterized by inactivity. **A. stupor,** acute dementia.
An'eroid barometer. See *Barometer.*
Anerythrop'sia. Inability to distinguish red colors.
Anesthe'sia (an-es-the'ze-ah). Loss of feeling or sensation. **Bulbar** or **Central a.,** that due to lesion of the nerve centers. **Crossed a.,** that occurring on one side of the body from central lesion of other side. **A. doloro'sa,** severe pain after the occurrence of complete paralysis. **Infiltration a.,** local anesthesia produced by injecting solutions beneath the skin. **Local a.,** that confined to a part of the body. **Muscular a.,** lack of muscular sense. **Primary a.,** temporary a. occurring in the beginning of anesthesia.
Anesthesim'eter. 1. Instrument for testing degree of insensitiveness. 2. Device for regulating the amount of anesthetic given.
Anesthet'ic. 1. Without the sense of touch. 2. A drug that produces anesthesia.
Anestheiza'tion. Production of insensibility to pain.
Anes'thetizer. One who administers an anesthetic.

Ane'thol. A principle, $C_{10}H_{12}O$, from oil of fennel.

Ane'thum. A genus of plants, including fennel and dill.

Aneu'ria (an-u're-ah). Deficiency of nervous energy.

An'eurysm (an'u-rizm). A sac formed by the dilatation of part of an artery, and filled with blood. **Abdominal a.**, a. of abdominal aorta. **A. by anastomosis**, dilatation of a number of vessels forming a pulsating tumor beneath the skin. **Arteriovenous a.**, simultaneous rupture of an artery and vein, the blood being retained in the surrounding tissue. **Bérard's a.**, varicose a. in tissues around the vein. **Cirsoid a.**, dilatation and tortuous lengthening of part of an artery. **Compound a.**, one in which some of the coats are ruptured and others merely dilated. **Dissecting a.**, one in which blood is forced between the coats of an artery. **False** or **Spurious a.**, one in which all the coats are ruptured and the blood is retained in surrounding tissues. **Fusiform a.**, a spindle-shaped a. **Innominate a.**, a. of innominate artery. **Mixed a.**, a compound a. **Park's a.**, arteriovenous a. in which the arterial dilatation communicates with two veins. **Pott's a.**, an aneurysmal varix. **Racemose a.** Same as *A. by anastomosis*. **Rodrigues's a.**, varicose a. in which the sac is contiguous to the artery. **Sacculated a.**, a sac-like a. **Spurious a.** Same as *False a.* **Varicose a.**, one formed by rupture of an aneurysm into a vein. **Verminous a.**, one containing hematozoa.

Aneurys'mal. Pertaining to an aneurysm.

Anfractuos'ity. A cerebral sulcus.

Anfract'uous (an-frakt'u-us). Convoluted; sinuous.

Angei'tis (an-ge-i'tis). Same as *Angiitis*.

Angel'ica. Genus of aromatic plants; root tonic and stimulant.

An'gel's wing. Deformity in which both scapulæ are prominent.

Angiec'tasis. Dilatation of a vessel, whether from aneurysm, varix, or angioparalysis.

Angii'tis (an-ge-i'tis). Inflammation of a vessel.

Angileuci'tis. See *Angioleucitis*.

An'gina (an'jin-ah). Any disease marked by spasmodic suffocative attacks. **A. acu'ta, A. sim'plex**, sore throat. **A. laryn'gea**, laryngitis. **A. Ludovi'ci, A. Ludwig'ii**, purulent inflammation seated around the submaxillary gland. **A. parotid'ea**, mumps. **A. pec'toris**, paroxysmal thoracic pain, with suffocation and syncope, due to vasomotor spasm. **Streptococcus a.**, a. due to streptococci. **A. tonsilla'ris**, quinsy. **A. trachea'lis**, croup.

An'ginoid (an'jin-oid). Resembling angina.

Anginopho'bia. Morbid dread of angina pectoris.

An'ginose (an'jin-ōs). Characterized by angina.

Angioatax'ia. Irregular tension of the blood-vessels.

An'gioblast (an'je-o-blast). Embryonic cell-form whence the vessels are derived.

Angiocardi'tis. Inflammation of heart and great blood-vessels.

Angiocav'ernous. Pertaining to or like angioma cavernosum.

Angiocholi'tis. Inflammation of biliary ducts.

Angiodystro'phia ova'rii. Disease of ovaries with disease of and increase in number of blood-vessels.

Angioelephanti'asis. Extensive angiomatous condition of subcutaneous tissues.

Angiogen'esis (an-je-o-jen'es-is). Development of the vessels.

Angioglio'ma. A form of vascular glioma.

An'giograph (an'je-o-graf). A variety of sphygmograph.

Angiog'raphy (an-je-og'raf-e). A treatise on the vessels.

Angiokerato'ma. Angioma blended with keratoma of the skin.

Angioleuci'tis (an-je-o-lu-si'tis). Inflammation of a lymph-vessel; lymphangitis.

Angiolith'ic neoplasm. One marked by mineral deposits and hyaline degeneration of the coats of the vessels.

Angiol'ogy (an-je-ol'o-je). Scientific account of the vessels.

Angiolymphi'tis. Same as *Angioleucitis*.

Angiolympho'ma. Tumor made up of lymph-vessels.

Angio'ma. Tumor composed of blood-vessels. **A. caverno'-sum.** Same as *Erectile tumor*. **A. serpigino'sum,** skin disease marked by minute vascular points arranged in rings on the skin. **Telangiectatic a.,** one made up of dilated blood-vessels.

Angiomala'cia (an'je-o-mal-a'se-ah). Softening of walls of the vessels.

Angiom'atous. Of the nature of angioma.

Angiom'eter (an-je-om'et-er). Instrument for measuring diameter and tension of blood-vessels.

Angiomyo'ma. Angioma blended with myoma.

Angioneuro'sis. Angioparalysis, angiospasm, or other neurosis primarily affecting blood-vessels.

Angioneurot'ic edema. Circumscribed edematous patches arising from an angioneurosis.

Angiono'ma. Ulceration of blood-vessels.

Angioparal'ysis. Paralysis of blood-vessels from vasomotor defect.

Angiopar'esis. Vasomotor paresis.

Angiop'athy (an-je-op'ath-e). Any disease of the vessels.

Angiorrhex'is. Rupture of a blood-vessel.

Angiosarco'ma. Sarcoma containing many vessels.

Angioscloro'sis. Hardening of the walls of blood-vessels.

Angiosiali'tis. Inflammation of a salivary duct.

Angio'sis. Same as *Angiopathy*.

An'giospasm. Spasmodic contraction of blood-vessels.

Angiospas'tic. Of the nature of angiospasm.

Angiosteno'sis. Narrowing of caliber of blood-vessels.

Angiotelec'tasis. Dilatation of blood-vessels.

Angioti'tis. Inflammation of the vessels of the ear.

Angiot'omy. Dissection or anatomy of the vessels.

An'gle (ang'gl). Sharp bend formed by the meeting of two borders or surfaces. **Acromial a.,** that between head of humerus and clavicle. **A. alpha,** that formed by intersection of visual line with optic axis. **A. of aperture,** angle between two lines from the focus of a lens to the ends of its diameter. **Basiopic a.,** angle between nasobasilar line and Meissner's horizontal. **Biorbital a.,** that formed by the intersection of the axes of the orbits. **Costal a.,** angle between the meeting ribs at the ensiform cartilage. **A. of deviation,** that between a refracted ray and the incident ray prolonged. **A. of elevation,** that between the visual plane when moved upward or downward and its normal position. **Facial a.,** an angle indicating the slope of the forehead. **A. of incidence,** the angle at which a light-ray strikes a denser medium. **A. of jaw,** the junction of the lower edge with the posterior edge of the lower jaw. **Louis's** or **Ludwig's a.,** that between manubrium and gladiolus. **Optic a.** Same as *Visual a.* **A. of pubes,** that between the pubic bones at the symphysis. **A. of reflection,** that which a reflected ray makes with a line perpendicular to the reflecting surface. **A. of refraction,** that between a refracted ray and a line perpendicular to the refracting surface. **Sternoclavicular a.,** that between the sternum and the clavicle. **Visual a.,** the angle between two lines from the point of vision on the retina to the extremities of the object seen.

An'glesey leg. A kind of jointed artificial leg.

An'glicus su'dor. English sweating fever; a deadly pestilential fever which several times ravaged England.

Angophra'sia. A drawling and broken form of speech.

Anguil'lula stercora'lis. A nematode intestinal parasite of hot climates.

An'gular. Having corners or angles; bent sharply.

Angula'tion (ang-gu-la'shun). Formation of sharp obstructive bend in the intestine.

Angustu'ra. Bark of *Galipea casparia* of tropical America; it is stimulant and bitter tonic.

Angustu'rin. Medicinal alkaloid, $C_{10}H_{40}NO_{14}$, from angustura.

Anha'phia (an-ha'fe-ah). Same as *Anaphia*.

Anhela'tion. Shortness of breath; panting, or dyspnea.

Anhemato'sis. Defective blood-formation.

Anhidro'sis. Abnormal deficiency of sweat.

Anhidrot'ic (an-hid-rot'ik). Checking the flow of sweat.

Anhis'tic, Anhis'tous. Of uniform formation; structureless.

Anhydre'mia. Lack of water in the blood.

Anhy'drid (an-hi'drid). Compound derived from an acid by abstraction of a molecule of water.

Anhy'drous (an-hi'drus). Containing no water.

Anian'thinopsy. Inability to distinguish violet tints.

Anid'eus (an-id'e-us). A parasitic monster fetus consisting of a shapeless mass of flesh.

Anidro'sis. Same as *Anhidrosis*.

An'ilid (an'il-id). Any compound formed from anilin by substituting a radical for the hydrogen of NH_2.

An'ilin. An amin, $C_6H_5NH_2$, from coal-tar and indigo; poisonous and nervine. **A.-rash,** a skin inflammation due to anilin poison. **A. stains,** anilin pigments used in staining microscopic preparations.

Anilin'ophil, Anilinoph'ilous. Staining readily with anilin dyes.

An'ilism (an'il-izm). Anilin poisoning.

An'imal. A living organism having sensation and power of voluntary movement.

Animal'cule (an-im-al'kūl). A minute animal organism.

An'ime (an'im-e). A resin of various origin; little used in medicine.

An'imin. Substance derivable from bone-oil.

An'ion. The element which in electrolysis passes to the positive pole.

Anirid'ia. Congenital absence of the iris.

An'isated (an'is-a-ted). Flavored with anise.

Anischu'ria (an-is-ku're-ah). Enuresis.

An'ise (an'is). Fruits of *Pimpinella anisum;* expectorant and carminative.

Anis'ic acid. Antirheumatic and antiseptic substance, $C_8H_8O_3$, from anethol.

An'isin. Alkaloid, $C_{22}H_{24}N_2O_3$, from anise.

Anisoco'ria. Inequality of the two pupils.

An'isol. Phenyl-methyl ether, $C_7H_8O_3$.

Anisome'lia. Inequality between paired limbs.

Anisometro'pia. Inequality in refractive power of the two eyes.

Anisometrop'ic. Having eyes which are unlike in refraction.

Aniso'pia. Inequality of visual power in the two eyes.

Anisosthen'ic. Not having equal power: said of muscles.

Anisot'ropal, Anisotrop'ic. Doubly refracting or polarizing.

Ani'sum (an-i'sum). L. for *anise*.

An'kle (ang'kl). Part of leg just above the foot. **A. bone,** the astragalus. **A. clonus, A. jerk,** succession of rhythmical foot-contractions on pushing the foot.

Ankylobleph'aron. Adhesion of eyelids.

Ankylochi'lia. Adhesion of the lips.

Ankyloglos'sia. Same as *Tongue-tie.*

Ankyloproc'tia (ang-kil-lo-prok'she-ah). Stricture of the anus.

An'kylosed (ang'kil-ōzd). Affected with ankylosis.

Ankylo'sis (ang-kil-o'sis). Abnormal immobility and consolidation of a joint. **Extracapsular a.,** that caused by rigidity of parts outside the joint. **False** or **Spurious a.,** that caused by rigidity of surrounding parts. **Intracapsular a.,** that from rigidity of structures within the joint. **True a.,** that in which the connecting material is bone.

Ankylos'toma duodena'lis. A dangerous intestinal nematode.

Ankylostomi'asis. Disease not unlike idiopathic anemia, due to presence of *Ankylostoma.*

Ankylo'tia (ang-kil-o'she-ah). Closure of external meatus of ear.

Ankyl'otome (ang-kil'o-tōm). Knife for operating on tongue-tie.

Ankylure'thria. Stricture of the urethra.

An'kyrism. Hook-like articulation or suture.

An'kyroid cavity (ang'kir-oid). The descending cornu of lateral ventricle.

An'lage (ahn'lah-ge). The embryonic area in which traces of any part first appear.

Annat'to (an-at'o). See *Annotto.*

Annec'tant gyri. Gyri between parietal and occipital lobes.

Annid'alin. A substance not unlike aristol.

Annot'to. A red color or stain from *Bixa Orellana.*

An'nuens (an'u-enz). Rectus capitis anticus minor muscle.

An'nular. Ring-shaped.

An'nulus. A ring-shaped organ or area. **A. abdomina'lis,** either of the openings of the inguinal canal. **A. cilia'ris,** boundary between iris and choroid. **A. mi'grans,** eruption of circles spreading over the tongue. **A. ova'lis,** margin of the septum of the foramen ovale of fetal heart. **A. tympan'icus.** Same as *Tympanic bone.* **A. umbil'icus,** the umbilical ring.

Anococcy'geal (a-no-kok-sij'e-al). Pertaining to anus and coccyx.

An'odal closure contraction. Contraction of muscles at anode on closure of electric circuit.

An'ode (an'ōd). A positive electrode.

Anod'mia. Lack or loss of sense of smell.

Anodon'tia (an-o-don'she-ah). Absence of teeth.

An'odyne (an'o-dīn). 1. Relieving pain. 2. A medicine that eases pain.

Anodyn'ia (an-o-din'e-ah). Freedom from pain.

Anoi'a (an-oi'ah). Idiocy.

Anom'alous (an-om'al-us). Contrary to natural or normal order.

Anom'aly. Deviation from normal standard.

Anonych'ia (an-o-nik'e-ah). Absence of the nails.

Anon'ymous (an-on'im-us). Innominate; unnamed.

Anoop'sia (an-o-op'se-ah). An upward strabismus.

Anophthal'mia. Absence of the eyes. **A. cyclo'pia,** rudimentary condition of eye-socket and orbit.

Anop'sia. 1. Anoopsia. 2. Defect of vision.

Anor'chism. Congenital absence of testicles.

Anor'chus. A person with no testes or with undescended testes.

Anorec'tal. Pertaining to anus and rectum.

Anorex'ia. Lack or loss of appetite for food. **A. nervo'sa,** hysteric aversion to food.

Anortho'pia. Unsymmetrical or distorted vision.

Anos'mia, Anosphra'sia. Absence of the sense of smell.

Anospi'nal center. Center in the cord which controls defecation.

Anosto'sis. Defective formation of bone.
Ano'tus (an-o'tus). Fetus with no ears.
Anou'rous (an-u'rus). Without a tail.
Anoves'ical. Pertaining to the anus and bladder.
Anoxe'mia. Lack of sufficient oxygen in the blood.
An'sa (an'sah). A loop; a handle. **A. hypoglos'si,** loop in the neck formed by descendens noni nerve and 2d and 3d cervical nerves. **A. lenticula'ris,** tract between the crusta and lenticular nucleus.
An'serine (an'ser-in). Pertaining to a goose.
Anta'cid (ant-as'id). Good against acidity.
Anta'cidin (ant-as'id-in). Saccharate of lime.
Antac'rid (ant-ak'rid). Good against acridity.
Antag'onism. Opposition or contrariety, as between muscles or medicines.
Antag'onist. A medicine or a muscle which counteracts the effects of another medicine or muscle.
Antal'gic (ant-al'jik). Anodyne or analgesic.
Antal'kaline (ant-al'kal-in). Neutralizing alkalinity.
Antaphrodis'iac. Abrogating the sexual impulse.
Antapoplec'tic. Relieving apoplexy.
Antarthrit'ic (ant-ar-thrit'ik). Good against gout.
Antasthen'ic (ant-as-then'ik). Restoring strength.
Antasthmat'ic. Affording relief for asthma.
Antatroph'ic (ant-at-rof'ik). Correcting atrophy.
Antebra'chium (an-te-bra'ke-um). The forearm.
Antecur'vature (an-te-ker'va-tūr). A slight anteflexion.
Anteflex'ion. Abnormal forward curvation.
Anteloca'tion. Displacement of an organ forward.
Antemet'ic (an-tem-et'ik). Tending to arrest vomiting.
An'te mor'tem. L. for *before death.*
An'te par'tum. L. for *before delivery,* or *childbirth.*
Antephial'tic (ant-ef-e-al'tik). Preventing nightmare.
Antepyret'ic. Done before the stage of traumatic fever.
An'terograde (an'ter-o-grād). Extending or moving backward.
Antero-infe'rior. Situated in front and below.
Anterolat'eral. Situated before and to one side.
Anterome'dian. Situated in front and on the middle line.
Anteropari'etal. Corresponding to the forward part of the parietal bone.
Anteroposte'rior. Extending from before backward.
Anterosupe'rior. Situated in front and above.
Antever'sion. Forward tipping or tilting of an organ.
An'thelix (an'the-lix). Same as *Antihelix.*
Anthelmin'tic (an-thel-min'tik). Destructive to worms.
An'themis (an'them-is). See *Chamomile.*
Anthemorrha'gic. Good against hemorrhage.
An'ther. The male sexual organ in plants.
Anthi'arin (an-thi'ar-in). Same as *Antiarin.*
Anthoris'ma (an-tho-riz'mah). A diffuse swelling.
Anthrace'mia (an-thras-e'me-ah). 1. Asphyxia, as from carbon monoxid poisoning. 2. Presence of *Bacillus anthracis* in the blood.
An'thracene (an'thras-ēn). Crystalline hydrocarbon, $C_{14}H_{10}$, from coal-tar.
Anthra'cia (an-thra'se-ah). Diseases marked by formation of carbuncles.
An'thracin. A poisonous ptomain from cultures of anthrax.
An'thracoid (an'thrak-oid). Resembling anthrax.
Anthracom'eter. Instrument for measuring carbon dioxid in the air.
Anthraconecro'sis. Degeneration of tissue into a black mass.

Anthraco'sis. Lung-disease from inhaling coal-dust.

Anthraqui'none. Yellow substance, $C_{14}H_8O_2$, from anthracene.

Anthraro'bin. Yellow-white powder, $C_{14}H_{10}O_3$, from alizarin: used in skin-disease.

An'thrax. Infectious disease of cattle, caused by *Bacillus anthracis*. It may occur in man. **Malignant a.** Same as *Anthrax*. **Symptomatic a.,** disease of cattle in summer, marked by emphysematous, subcutaneous pustules.

Anthropo'geny (an-thro-poj'en-e). Development or evolution of man.

An'thropoid (an'thro-poid). Resembling a man.

Anthropol'ogy. The science of man.

Anthropom'etry. Comparative measurement of man.

Anthropoph'agy. Cannibalism.

Anthropopho'bia. Morbid dread of society.

Anthroposomatol'ogy. Sum of knowledge regarding the human body.

Anthropotox'in. Poison excreted by human lungs.

Anthydrop'ic (ant-hi-drop'ik). Relieving dropsy.

Anthypnot'ic (ant-hip-not'ik). Hindering or preventing sleep.

Anthyster'ic (ant-his-ter'ik). Relieving hysteria.

Antial'bumate, Antial'bumid. A product of incomplete digestion of albumin.

Antialbu'min. A constituent of albumin: gastric digestion changes it into antialbumose.

Antial'bumose. A digestion-product convertible into antipeptone.

Antiapoplec'tic. Affording relief to, or preventing, apoplexy.

Anti'arin. Poisonous principle, $C_{14}H_{20}O_5+2H_2O$, from bohun upas; heart-depressant.

Antiarthrit'ic (an-te-ar-thrit'ik). Same as *Antarthritic*.

Antibacte'rial. Checking the growth of bacteria.

Antibech'ic (an-te-bek'ik). Relieving cough; bechic.

Antibil'ious (an-te-bil'yus). Good against bilious conditions.

Antibiot'ic (an-te-bi-ot'ik). Destructive of life.

Antiblennorrha'gic. Preventing or relieving gonorrhea.

An'tibody. A protective body in the blood of immune animals.

Antibra'chium (an-te-bra'ke-um). The forearm.

Antibro'mic. Deodorant; overcoming ill smells.

Antical'culous. Curative of calculus.

Antican'crin. Same as *Cancroin*.

Antical'dium. Pit of stomach; scrobiculus cordis.

Antica'rious (an-te-ka're-us). Preventive of caries.

Anticheirot'onus. Spasmodic inflexion of thumb.

Antichol'erin (an-te-kol'er-in). Substance from cholera-bacillus cultures: used against cholera.

Antic'ipating intermittent. Intermittent with paroxysms recurring at an earlier hour each day.

Anticli'nal vertebra. Tenth or eleventh thoracic vertebra.

Anticonvul'sive. Good against convulsions.

Anti'cus (an-ti'kus). Anterior.

Anticyc'lic acid (an-te-sik'lik). An antipyretic medicine.

Antidiabet'icum. Glycosolvol, a remedy for diabetes.

Antidiabe'tin. A sugar for diabetics, composed of saccharin and mannite.

Antidin'ic (an-te-din'ik). Relieving giddiness or vertigo.

Antidiph'therin (an-te-dif'ther-in). A derivative from cultures of diphtheria bacillus; used against diphtheria.

Antido'tal. Serving as an antidote.

An'tidote (an'te-dōt). A remedy for poisoning. Antidotes are distinguished as **chemical,** or those that change the chemical nature of the poison; **mechanical,** or those that prevent ab-

sorption of the poison; and **physiologic**, or those that counteract the effects of the poison by producing other effects.
Antidyscrat'ic (an-te-dis-krat'ik). Good against a dyscrasia.
Antidysenter'ic. Relieving, curing, or preventing dysentery.
Antiemet'ic. Preventing or arresting vomiting.
Antien'zyme (an-te-en'zim). Neutralizing an enzyme.
Antiephial'tic. Same as *Antephialtic*.
An'tifat. An agent that removes excess of fat.
Antifeb'rile (an-te-feb'ril). Allaying or diminishing fever.
Antifeb'rin (an-te-feb'rin). Same as *Acetanilid*.
Antifer'ment. Agent preventing fermentation.
Antifermen'tative. Same as *Antizymotic*.
Antigalac'tic (an-te-gal-ak'tik). Diminishing secretion of milk.
Antihe'lix. Curved ridge opposite the helix of the ear.
Antihemicra'nin. Same as *Antimigraine*.
Antihidrot'ic. Same as *Anhidrotic*.
Antihydrop'ic. Relieving dropsical conditions.
Antihy'dropin. Diuretic substance obtained from cockroaches.
Anti-icter'ic. Relieving icterus, or jaundice.
Antikam'nia. Proprietary antipyretic and anodyne remedy.
An'tikol. Proprietary antipyretic medicine.
Antile'mic (an-te-le'mik). Curative of the plague.
Antilep'sis. Revulsive or derivative treatment.
Antilethar'gic (an-te-leth-ar'jik). Hindering sleep.
Antilith'ic. Preventing the formation of calculus or stone.
Antilo'bium. The tragus of the ear.
Antiluet'ic (an-te-lu-et'ik). Serviceable against syphilis.
Antilys'sic. Affording relief to hydrophobia.
An'timere (an'te-mēr). One of the segments of the body bounded by planes at right angles to the body.
Antimetro'pia. Hypermetropia of one eye, with myopia in the other.
Antimiasmat'ic. Serviceable against miasmatic disorders.
Antimicro'bic. Checking the growth of microbes.
Antimi'graine. Mixture of caffein, antipyrin, and sugar: used in migraine.
Antimo'nial. Pertaining to, or containing, antimony.
An'timony. A crystalline metallic element with various medicinal and poisonous salts.
Antimycot'ic (an-te-mi-kot'ik). Same as *Antibacterial*.
Antinarcot'ic. Relieving narcotism.
Antinau'sea. Proprietary remedy for sea-sickness.
Antinephrit'ic (an-te-nef-rit'ik). Serviceable in kidney diseases.
Antiner'vin. Proprietary remedy for neuralgia.
Antineural'gic (an-te-nu-ral'jik). Curative of neuralgia.
Antin'ion. Frontal pole of the head.
Antinon'nin. A remedy destructive to external parasites.
Antino'sin. A substance whose solution is an external antiseptic.
Antiparalyt'ic. Relieving paralytic symptoms.
Antiparasit'ic. Destructive to parasites.
Antiparastati'tis. Inflammation of Cowper's glands.
Antipath'ic (an-te-path'ik). Opposite in nature.
Antip'athy (an-tip'ath-e). Dislike or aversion.
Antipep'tone (an-te-pep'tōn). Peptone derived from antialbumose by digestion.
Antiperiod'ic. Serviceable against malarial or periodic recurrences. **A. tincture**, Warburg's tincture.
Antiperistal'sis. Peristaltic action from below upward.
Antiperistal'tic. Pertaining to antiperistalsis.
Antiphlogis'tic. Diminishing inflammation.
Antiphthis'ic (an-te-tiz'ik). Checking or alleviating phthisis.
Antiphthi'sin. A form of modified tuberculin.

Antip'ilus. A proprietary depilatory.
Antiplas'tic (an-te-plas'tik). Unfavorable to healing.
Antipneumotox'in. An antitoxin antagonistic to pneumotoxin.
Antip'odal cells. A group of four cells in early embryo.
Antipros'tate (an-te-pros'tāt). Cowper's gland.
Antiprostati'tis. Inflammation of Cowper's glands.
Antiprurit'ic (an-te-pru-rit'ik). Relieving or preventing itching.
Antipso'ric (an-te-so'rik). Curative of the itch.
Antiputrefac'tive. Good against putrefaction.
Antipy'ic (an-te-pi'ik). Preventing suppuration.
Antipy'onin. Sodium polyborate used in ophthalmology.
Antipyre'sis. The employment of antifebrile remedies.
Antipyret'ic. Relieving fever; cooling; febrifuge.
Antipy'rin (an-ti-pi'rin). An antipyretic coal-tar derivative, $C_{11}H_{12}N_2O$. **A. salicylate.** Same as *Salipyrin.*
Antipyrot'ic. Curative of, or relieving, burns.
Antirab'ic. Preventive of, or curing, rabies; antilyssic.
Antirheumat'ic. Relieving or preventing rheumatism.
Antirheu'matin. A combination of sodium salicylate and methylene-blue.
Antiscorbu'tic. Correcting or curing scurvy.
Antisep'sin. Monobromacetanilid, C_8H_8BrNO; an antipyretic, antiseptic, and analgesic.
Antisep'sis. 1. Use of antiseptic measures. 2. Absence of septic tendency.
Antisep'tic. 1. Preventing decay or putrefaction. 2. A substance destructive of poisonous germs. **A. dressing,** dressing charged with antiseptic substances.
Antisep'ticism. Systematic employment of antisepsis.
Antisep'tin. A white antiseptic compound.
Antisep'tol. Cinchonin iodosulphate: used externally.
Antisial'agogue, Antisial'ic. Checking the flow of saliva.
Antispas'min. A proprietary analgesic and hypnotic.
Antispasmod'ic, Antispas'tic. Relieving spasm.
Antispas'tic. 1. Counter-irritant. 2. Antispasmodic.
Antistreptococ'cic, Antistreptococ'cous. Opposed to streptococcus.
Antistreptococ'cin. The antitoxin of diphtheria streptococcus.
Antisu'doral. Preventing or relieving sweating.
Antisu'dorin. A remedy to correct sweating.
Antisyphilit'ic. Curative of, or useful against, syphilis.
Antith'enar. Placed opposite to the palm or sole.
Antither'mic. Antipyretic; antifebrile.
Antither'min. An antipyretic coal-tar derivative, $C_{11}H_{14}N_2O_2$.
Antitox'ic (an-te-tok'sik). Good against a poison.
Antitox'in. Any defensive principle developed in the body as a result of the implantation of a poison.
Antitrag'icus (an-te-traj'ik-us). A muscle passing from the antitragus to the caudate process.
Antit'ragus. Prominence on the ear fronting the tragus.
Antitris'mus. Spasm which prevents the closure of the mouth.
An'titrope (an'te-trōp). An organ which forms a symmetrical pair with another.
Antituberculot'ic. Checking the advance of tuberculosis.
Antiven'ene. Blood-serum from an animal immunized against snake-bite.
Antivene'real. Antisyphilitic.
Antizymot'ic. Opposing action of ferments or ferment-like germs.
Antodontal'gic (ant-o-don-tal'jik). Relieving toothache.

Au'tozone. The disinfectant, hydrogen peroxid.
An'tracele (an'tras-ēl). Accumulation of fluid in the maxillary antrum.
An'tral (an'tral). Of, or pertaining to, an antrum.
Antrec'tomy. Removal of the walls of the mastoid antrum.
Antri'tis (an-tri'tis). Inflammation of an antrum, especially of that of Highmore.
An'trophore (an'tro-fōr). A soluble medicated bougie.
An'troscope. Instrument for inspecting antrum of Highmore.
Antros'copy. The use of the antroscope.
An'trotome. Instrument for performing antrotomy.
Antrot'omy. Cutting open of an antrum.
Antrotympani'tis. Chronic purulent middle-ear disease.
An'trum. A chamber or cavity in a bone. **A. of Highmore, A. maxilla're,** a cavity in upper maxilla, communicating with nose. **A. mastoi'deum.** recess in the mastoid process, communicating with the tympanum.
Anuret'ic. Affected with anuria.
Anu'ria (an-u're-ah). Too scanty urine.
A'nus (a'nus). Distal end and outlet of rectum. **Artificial a.,** an opening from the bowel formed by operation. **Imperforate a.,** closure of the natural opening of the anus. **A. of Rusconi.** Same as *Blastopore*. **Vulvovaginal a.,** a combined vulvar and anal opening.
An'vil (an'vil). See *Incus*.
Anydre'mia (an-id-re'me-ah). Deficiency of water in the blood.
Anyp'nia (an-ip'ne-ah). Sleeplessness.
A. O. C. Abbreviation of *anodal opening contraction*.
Aor'ta. Great artery springing from left ventricle. **Abdominal a.,** part of aorta below the diaphragm. **Arch of a.,** the proximal portion of aorta, consisting of an *ascending*, a *transverse*, and a *descending* part. **Thoracic a.,** part of aorta below the arch and above the diaphragm.
Aor'tal, Aor'tic. Of, or pertaining to, the aorta. **A. arches,** five fetal aortic bows; visceral arches. **A. murmur,** auscultatory sign of aortic valvular disease. **A. opening.** 1. The entrance of the aorta from left ventricle. 2. Passage for aorta through diaphragm. **A. plexus,** nerve-plexus on front and sides of aorta. **A. valves,** three semilunar valves at the aortic orifice in the left ventricle.
Aorti'tis (a-or-ti'tis). Inflammation of aorta.
Aortomala'cia (a-or-to-mal-a'se-ah). Softening of the aorta.
Aortosteno'sis. Narrowing of the aorta.
Apacon'itin. Poisonous base derived from aconitin.
Ap'athy (ap'ath-e). Lack of feeling or emotion; indifference.
Apat'ropin. A derivative, $C_{17}H_{21}NO_2$, from atropin.
Ape-fissures. Those fissures in the human brain which are found also in apes. **A.-hand, a** hand with the thumb permanently extended.
Apel'lous (ah-pel'us). Skinless.
Apep'sia. Cessation or failure of digestive function. **A. nervo'-sa.** Same as *Anorexia nervosa*.
Ape'rient. 1. Mildly cathartic. 2. A gentle purgative.
Aperistal'sis. Absence of peristaltic action.
Ap'erture (ap'er-tūr). An opening or orifice.
A'pex. Top or pointed end of a conical part. **A. beat,** heart-beat felt in 5th left intercostal space. **A. murmur,** a murmur over the apex of the heart.
Apha'cia, Apha'kia (af-a'se-ah, af-a'ke-ah). Absence of the lens of the eye.
Apha'cic, Apha'kic (af-a'sik, af-a'kik). Destitute of the crystalline lens.

Apha'gia (af-a'je-ah). Loss of the power of swallowing.

Apha'kia. See *Aphacia.*

Apha'sia (af-a'zhah). Defect or loss of the power of expression by speech, writing, or signs. **Amnesic a.**, inability to remember words. **Ataxic a.**, aphasia in which the patient knows what he wishes to say, but cannot utter the words. **Conduction a.**, aphasia due to lesion of path between sensory and motor speech-centers. **Gibberish a.**, aphasia with utterance of meaningless phrases. **Mixed or Total a.**, union of motor and sensory aphasia. **Motor a.** Same as *Ataxic a.* **Sensory a.**, inability to understand or to remember words.

Apha'sic (af-a'zik). Pertaining to, or affected with, aphasia.

Aphe'mia. Loss of power of speech due to a central lesion.

Aphepho'bia. Morbid dread of being touched.

Aph'eter (af'et-er). Supposed material which gives to inogen the stimulus that decomposes it and thus causes muscular contraction.

Apho'nia. Loss of voice not due to a central lesion. **A. clerico'rum**, clergyman's sore throat.

Aphon'ic. 1. Of, or pertaining to, aphonia. 2. Without audible sound.

A'phose (ah'fōs). Any subjective visual sensation due to absence or interruption of light sensation.

Aphra'sia. Dumbness of whatever kind (except aphonia). **A. parano'ica**, stubborn and wilful silence.

Aphrodis'iac. 1. Exciting sexual impulses. 2. Drug that arouses the sexual instinct.

Aph'thæ (af'the). Thrush, or the whitish spots that characterize it. **Bednar's a.**, two ulcers on hard palates of cachectic infants. **Cachectic a.**, aphthæ beneath the tongue, with severe constitutional symptoms.

Aphthen'xia. Impairment of power to express articulate sounds.

Aphthon'gia (af-thon'je-ah). Aphasia due to spasm of the speech-muscles.

Aph'thous (af-thus). Pertaining to, or characterized by, aphthæ.

Ap'ical (ap'ik-al). Of, or pertaining to, an apex.

A'piol (a'pe-ol). An oil, $C_{12}H_{14}O_4$, from parsley seed: useful in disorders of menstruation.

A'piolin (a'pe-o-lin). An emmenagogue, active principle of parsley.

A'pium. A genus of umbelliferous plants. See *Celery* and *Parsley.*

Aplacen'tal (ah-pla-sen'tal). Having no placenta.

Aplanat'ic. Correcting, or not affected by, spherical aberration.

Apla'sia. Defective formation or development.

Aplas'tic. Having no tendency to develop into new tissue.

Apne'a, Apnœ'a (ap-ne'ah). 1. The cessation of respiration which follows forced respiration. 2. Asphyxia.

Apneumato'sis. Collapse of the air-cells.

Apneu'mia. Congenital absence of the lungs.

Apoacon'itin. Same as *Apaconitin.*

Apochromat'ic. Same as *Achromatic.*

Apoco'dein. Alkaloid, $C_{18}H_{19}NO_2$, derived from codein.

Apo'cynin (ap-os'in-in). Alkaloid, also a precipitate, from apocynum; both actively medicinal.

Apo'cynum cannabi'num. Canadian hemp (not to be confounded with *cannabis*); anthydropic tonic and cathartic.

Apo'dia. Absence of feet.

Apo'lar. Having neither poles nor processes; without polarity.

Apollina'ris water. An effervescent table water.

Apol'ysin (ap-ol'is-in). A phenatidin citrate; used like phenacetin.

Apomor'phin. A powerfully emetic alkaloid, $C_{17}H_{17}NO_2$, from morphin.

Apomy'elin. A principle from brain-substance.

Ap'one (ap'ōn). Anodyne preparation of various composition with capsicum as a basis.

Aponeurol'ogy. The study of aponeuroses.

Aponeuro'sis. A firm gristly membrane serving mainly as an investment for muscles and other organs.

Aponeurosi'tis. Inflammation of an aponeurosis.

Aponeurot'ic. Pertaining to, or of the nature of, an aponeurosis.

Aponeu'rotome (ap-o-nu'ro-tōm). Knife for cutting an aponeurosis.

Aponeurot'omy. Surgical division of an aponeurosis.

Apophys'eal. Of, or pertaining to, an apophysis.

Apoph'ysis (ap-of'is-is). A process of a bone which has never been entirely distinct from the body of the bone. **A. of Ingrassias**, the lesser wing of the sphenoid bone. **A. ravia'na**, the gracile process of the malleus. **A. of Rau**, the long process of the malleus.

Apoplec'tic. Pertaining to, or affected with, apoplexy.

Apoplec'tiform, Apoplec'toid. Resembling apoplexy.

Apoplectig'enous. Producing apoplexy.

Ap'oplexy (ap'o-plek-se). 1. Sudden paralysis and coma from cerebral effusion or extravasation of blood. 2. Copious extravasation into any organ. **Capillary a.**, that due to rupture of capillaries. **Ingravescent a.**, apoplexy with progressive loss of consciousness from gradual escape of blood. **Pulmonary a.**, escape of blood into parenchyma of lungs. **Spinal a.**, rupture of a blood-vessel of the spinal cord. **Splenic a.**, malignant anthrax.

Apore'tin. Purgative resin from rhubarb.

Apo'sia (ah-po'ze-ah). Absence of thirst.

Aposit'ia (ap-o-sit'e-ah). Disgust or loathing of food.

Apos'tasis. 1. An abscess. 2. An exfoliation.

Aposte'ma (ap-os-te'mah). An abscess.

Apos'thia (ah-pos'the-ah). Absence of the prepuce.

Apos'toli's method. Electrotherapy of diseases of women.

Apoth'ecaries' weight. See *Weights, Table of.*

Apoth'ecary. A druggist or pharmacist. In England, some apothecaries are also authorized physicians.

Ap'othem, Ap'otheme. The dark deposit which appears in decoctions or infusions exposed to the air.

Apoth'eter (ap-oth'et-er). A navel string repositor.

Ap'ozeme (ap'o-zēm). A medicinal or medicated decoction.

Appara'tus. 1. Mechanical appliances used in operations and experiments. 2. The complex of parts which unite in any function. 3. Cystotomy or lithotomy. **A. ma'jor**, median lithotomy. **A. mi'nor**, lateral lithotomy. **Clover's a.**, apparatus for administering ether or chloroform.

Appendec'tomy, Appendicec'tomy. Removal of the vermiform appendix.

Appen'dices epiplo'icæ. Peritoneal pouches containing fat and joined to the large intestine.

Appendi'cial, Appendic'ular. Pertaining to the appendix vermiformis. **A. colic**, acute local pain in early stage of appendicitis.

Appendici'tis. Inflammation of appendix vermiformis. **A. oblit'erans**, appendicitis marked by obliteration of the cavity of the appendix.

Appen'dix. An appendage. **Auricular a.**, forward prolongation of the auricle of the heart. **Ensiform a.**, the lowermost piece of the sternum. **A vermifor'mis**, **Vermiform a.**, worm-shaped process of the cecum. **Xiphoid a.** Same as *Ensiform a.*

Appercep'tion. Conscious perception of a sensory impression.

Ap'petite. Desire; chiefly desire for food.

Applana'tio cor'neæ. Undue flatness of the cornea.

Ap'ple-head. The broad, thick skull of a dwarf.

Ap'plicator. Instrument for making local applications.

Apposi'tion (ap-o-zish'un). Contact of adjacent parts.

Aprax'ia. Insane performance of preposterous acts.

Aproc'tia (ah-prok'she-ah). Absence or imperforation of the anus.

A'pron, Hottentot. Artificial elongation of the nymphæ.

Aprosex'ia. Inability to fix the mind upon any subject.

Aproso'pia. Congenital absence of the face.

Apselaphe'sia. Lack or loss of the sense of touch.

Apsithy'ria. Inability to whisper: it is usually hysteric.

Apsych'ia (ap-sik'e-ah). Lack or loss of consciousness.

Aptya'lia, Apty'alism. Deficiency or absence of saliva.

A'pus (a'pus). Fetus which has no feet.

Apy'onin (ap-i'o-nin). A yellow antiseptic powder.

Apyret'ic (ap-i-ret'ik). Without fever.

Apyrex'ia. Absence or intermission of fever.

A'qua (a'kwah). *L.* for *Water.* **A. ammo'niæ,** water charged with ammonia; antacid and stimulant. **A. chlo'ri,** water charged with chlorin; antiseptic and cleansing. **A. destil-la'ta,** distilled water. **A. for'tis,** nitric acid. **A. labyrin'-thi,** the clear fluid in the labyrinth of the ear. **A. oc'uli,** aqueous humor of eye. **A. re'gia,** nitrohydrochloric acid.

Aquacapsuli'tis. Same as *Aquocapsulitis.*

Aquapunc'ture. Subcutaneous injection of water.

Aq'ueduct (ak'we-dukt). Any canal or passage. **A. of coch-lea,** foramen in temporal bone for a vein from the cochlea. **A. of Fallopius,** canal for facial nerve in petrous portion of temporal bone. **A. of Sylvius,** a canal which connects 3d and 4th ventricles of brain.

A'queous (a'kwe-us). Watery; prepared with water.

Aquocapsuli'tis. Serous inflammation of the iris.

Ar'abic acid, Ar'abin. A carbohydrate, $C_{12}H_{22}O_{11}$, from gum arabic.

Ar'abinose. Gum-sugar; a carbohydrate, $C_5H_{10}O_5$, from arabin.

Arachni'tis. Inflammation of arachnoid membrane.

Arach'noid. 1. Like a spider's web. 2. The arachnoid membrane.

Arachnoidi'tis. Same as *Arachnitis.*

Arachnopi'a. Pia and arachnoid together; the pia-arachnoid.

Aræom'eter. See *Areometer.*

Aran-Duchenne's disease (ah-ran-des-shenz). Same as *Progressive muscular atrophy.*

Aran'tius's body, A.'s nodule. A tubercle on each of the six semilunar valves. **A.'s ventricle,** small sac in the medulla oblongata, being the lower end of fourth ventricle.

Araro'ba. Tree or wood that produces Goa powder.

Ar'bor vi'tæ. 1. Tree-like outlines seen on median section of cerebellum. 2. Series of ridges within cervix uteri. 3. See *Thuja.*

Arbores'cent (ar-bo-res'ent). Branching like a tree.

Arboriza'tion. Branching terminus of a nerve-cell process.

Arbu'tin. Diuretic glucosid, $C_{24}H_{32}O_{14} + H_2O$, from uva ursi.

Arcade', Flint's. An arteriovenous arch at the base of the renal pyramids.

Arca'num. A secret remedy or nostrum.

Ar'cate (ar'kāt). Curved; bow-shaped.

Arec'in (ar-se'in). Arecolin hydrobromate, an energetic myotic.

Arch (artsh). A structure of bow-like or curved outline. **A. of aorta.** See *Aorta.* **Aortic a's., Branchial a's.,** a series of four cartilaginous arches of the fetus in the region of the neck.

A's. of Corti, series of arches made up of rods of Corti. **Crural a., Femoral a.,** Poupart's ligament. **Dental a.,** the arch of the alveolar process of the jaw. **Hemal a.,** arch formed by bodies of vertebræ, ribs, and sternum. **Hyoid a.,** the second branchial arch. **Neural a.,** arch of a vertebra enclosing the cord. **Palmar a.,** the arch of the radial and ulnar arteries in the palm of the hand. **Pharyngeal a's.** Same as *Branchial a's.* **Plantar a.,** arch formed by external plantar artery. **A. of pubes,** portion of pelvis formed by the rami of the ischia and the pubes on each side. **Supra-orbital a.,** curved margin of frontal bone forming upper boundary of orbit. **Tarsal a's.,** arches of palpebral arteries around the tarsal cartilages. **A. of vertebra,** the portion of a vertebra enclosing the spinal foramen. **Visceral a's.** Same as *Branchial a's.* **Zygomatic a.,** arch formed by malar and temporal bones.

Ar'chæocyte (ar'ke-o-sīt). See *Archeocyte.*

Archam'phiaster. Amphiaster forming polar globules.

Archebio'sis, Archegen'esis (ar-ke-bi-o'sis, ar-ke-jen'es-is). Spontaneous origin of life.

Archen'teron (ark-en'ter-on). Entodermal sac of the gastrula.

Ar'cheocyte. A wandering cell; a form of ameboid cell.

Archepy'on (ar-ke-pi'on). Very thick pus.

Archespo'rium. The cells which give rise to spore mother-cells.

Ar'chetype (ar'ke-tip). An original or ideal type.

Ar'chiblast (ar'ke-blast). Same as *Discus proligerus.*

Archiblas'tic. Derived from, or pertaining to, the archiblast.

Archiblasto'ma. Tumor from the epiblast.

Archigas'ter. The primitive alimentary canal of embryo.

Ar'chil (ar'kil). The lichen *Rocella tinctoria;* also, the violet-red stain obtained from it.

Archineph'ron (ar-ke-nef'ron). Same as *Wolffian body.*

Archineu'ron. The neuron at which efferent impulse starts.

Ar'chistome (ar'kis-tōm). The blastopore.

Archi'tis (ar-ki'tis). Inflammation of lower rectum; proctitis.

Ar'chocele (ar'ko-sēl). Hernia of the rectum.

Archopto'sis. Prolapse of lower rectum; proctoptosis.

Archorrha'gia, Archorrhe'a. Free hemorrhage from rectum.

Archosteno'sis, Archostegno'sis. Stricture of the rectum.

Ar'ciform (ar'sif-orm). Shaped like an arch or bow.

Arcta'tion (ark-ta'shun). Contraction of any opening canal.

Arc'tium (ark'she-um). The burdock. See *Lappa.*

Ar'cuate (ar'ku-āt). Bent like a bow; arciform.

Arcua'tion (ar-ku-a'shun). Curvature.

Ar'culus. A bed-cradle to protect a part.

Ar'cus. L. for *arch* or *bow.* **A. denta'lis,** the dental arch. **A. seni'lis,** circular corneal opacity in aged persons.

Ar'dent (ar'dent). Hot; feverish.

Ar'dor uri'næ. Sensation of scalding in passing urine.

A'rea (a're-ah). A limited space or plane surface. **Auditory a.,** the auditory center. **Broca's a.,** area of gray matter between middle olfactory root and peduncle of corpus callosum. **A. Cel'si.** See *Alopecia areata.* **Cohnheim's a's.,** dark areas outlined by bright matter, seen on cross-section of a muscle-fiber. **Embryonal a.** Same as *A. germinativa.* **A. germina-ti'va,** part of ovum where the embryo is formed. **Motor a.,** ascending frontal and ascending parietal convolutions. **Occipital a.,** area of brain below occipital bone. **A. opa'ca,** outer opaque part of a. germinativa. **A. pellu'cida,** central clear part of a. germinativa. **Rolandic a.,** the excitomotor region of the brain. **A. vasculo'sa,** part of a. opaca, where the blood-vessels are first seen. **A. vitelli'na,** yolk-area beyond the vasculous area in mesoblastic eggs.

Ar'eca. Genus of Asiatic palms. *A. cat'echu* affords betel-nut and an inferior catechu.

Ar'ecain. A poisonous and medicinal alkaloid from betel-nut.

Are'calin. Vermifugal alkaloid, $C_8H_{13}NO_2$, from betel-nut.

Arece'tin (ar-es-e'tin). Same as *Arecalin.*

Ar'ecin. An alkaloid, $C_{23}H_{26}N_2O$, from cinchona bark.

Arena'tion (ar-en-a'shun). Treatment by hot sand-bath; ammotherapy.

Are'ola (ar-e'o-lah). Darkened ring around a part. **A. of breast,** pigmented ring about the nipple.

Are'olar. Containing minute spaces. **A. tissue,** connective tissue which occupies the interspaces of the body.

Areom'eter. Instrument for measuring specific gravity of fluids.

Argamblyo'pia. Amblyopia from disease of the eye.

Argentam'id. An astringent and antiseptic silver preparation.

Argentam'in (ar-jen-tam'in). Antiseptic solution of silver phosphate in ethylendiamin.

Argenta'tion (ar-jen-ta'shun). Staining with silver.

Argen'tic, Ar'gentine (ar-jen'tik, ar'jen-tin). Containing silver.

Argen'tum (ar-jen'tum). L. for *Silver.*

Argil'la. L. for *Clay.*

Ar'ginin (ar'jin-in). A base, $C_6H_{14}N_4O_2$, from lupine.

Ar'gol, Ar'gols. Crude cream of tartar.

Ar'gon. A gaseous chemical element from the air.

Ar'gonin. A disinfectant and antiseptic silver preparation.

Argyll-Robertson pupil. A pupil which does not respond to light, but contracts in accommodation: seen in locomotor ataxia.

Argyria, Argyro'sis (ar-jir'e-ah, ar-jir-o'sis). Discoloration of skin or tissues from free use of silver preparations.

Arhinencepha'lia. Same as *Cyclopia.*

Arhin'ia (ah-rin'e-ah). Absence of nose.

Arhyth'mia (ah-rith'me-ah). Lack of rhythm in the beating of the heart.

Arhyth'mic (ah-rith'mik). Irregular.

Ar'ica bark. A variety of cinchona bark.

Ar'icin (ar'is-in). A cinchona alkaloid, $C_{23}H_{26}N_2O_4$.

Ar'istol. A reddish powder, dithymol iodid: used like iodoform.

Aristolo'chia (ar-is-to-lo'ke-ah). Same as *Serpentaria.*

Aristolo'chin. A bitter derivative from serpentaria.

Arithmoma'nia. Insane habit of counting, with worriment about numbers.

Arlt's ointment. Ointment of mercury with belladonna.

Arm. Upper extremity from shoulder to hand. **A. center,** cortical center at middle third of fissure of Rolando, controlling arm movements.

Armamenta'rium, Arma'rium. Outfit of a practitioner or institution, such as medicines, instruments, books, etc.

Ar'mature (ar'mat-ūr). Iron bar across end of a horse-shoe magnet.

Armil'la. The annular enlargement of the wrist.

Arm-to-arm vaccination. Transfer of vaccine virus from one patient to another.

Ar'my itch. Chronic itch prevalent in United States during Civil War.

Ar'nica monta'na. Plant with vulnerary and stimulant leaves and flowers.

Ar'nicin (ar'nis-in). A glucosid, $C_{26}H_{30}O_4$, from arnica.

Ar'nold's canal. Passage in petrous bone for A.'s nerve. **A.'s ganglion,** near foramen ovale. **A.'s nerve,** the auricular branch of pneumogastric nerve.

Aromat'ic. 1. Having a spicy fragrance. 2. A stimulant, spicy medicine.

Aro'min. A fragrant principle from urine.
Arrecto'res pilo'rum. Minute involuntary muscles of the skin.
Arrhin'ia. See *Arhinia.*
Arrhyth'mia (ar-ith'me-ah). Absence of rhythm.
Ar'row-root. Nutrient starch from rhizome of *Maranta arundinacea*, etc.
Ar'senate. Any salt of arsenic acid.
Arsenau'ro. An antiluetic solution of gold and arsenic bromids.
Arseni'asis. Arsenical poisoning; arsenicism.
Ar'senic, Arsen'icum. 1. A metal whose salts are poisonous and medicinal. 2. Popular name for arsenous acid. **White a.,** arsenous acid.
Arsen'ical. Of, or pertaining to, arsenic.
Arsen'icism (ar-sen'is-izm). Arsenical poisoning.
Arsenicoph'agy (ar-sen-ik-of'aj-e). Habit of eating arsenic.
Arsen'oblast. Male element of sexual cell; a masculonucleus.
Ar'senous acid. White arsenic, $HAsO_2$: exceedingly poisonous.
Ar'tarin. Alkaloid from artar, the root of *Xanthoxylum senegalense*: a heart stimulant.
Ar'tefact. A structure or change which is not natural, but due to manipulation.
Artemis'ia. Genus of plants. *A. abrot'anum* of southernwood is stimulant, tonic, and vermifuge.
Arte'ria. L. for *Artery.*
Arteriag'ra. Neuralgia of an artery.
Arte'rial. Pertaining to an artery. **A. varix,** a varicose artery.
Arterializa'tion. The change of venous into arterial blood.
Ar'terin. The pigment of arterial blood.
Arteriocap'illary fibrosis. The narrowing of capillaries and minute arteries by internal fibrosis.
Arteriofibro'sis. Same as *Arteriocapillary fibrosis.*
Arte'riogram. Same as *Sphygmogram.*
Arteriog'raphy. A description of the arteries.
Arteri'olæ rec'tæ. Branches of the arteries of kidney going to the medullary pyramids.
Arte'riole (ar-te're-ōl). Any minute arterial branch.
Arteriol'ogy. Sum of knowledge regarding the arteries.
Arteriomala'cia (ar-te-re-o-mal-a'se-ah). Softening of the arterial coats.
Arteriop'athy. Any disease of an artery.
Arterioscl ero'sis. Hardening of arterial walls.
Arteriosteno'sis. Narrowing of the caliber of an artery.
Arte'ritome. Instrument for arteriotomy.
Arteriot'omy. Surgical division of an artery.
Arteriove'nous. Both arterial and venous.
Arteriover'sion. See *Aerteriversion.*
Arteriover'ter. Instrument for performing arterioversion.
Arteri'tis. Inflammation of an artery. **A. defor'mans,** chronic endarteritis. **A. oblit'erans.** See *Endarteritis obliterans.*
Ar'tery. An efferent blood-vessel. [See *Table of the Arteries*, pp. 46-50.] **A.-constrictor,** instrument for compressing arteries. **A.-forceps,** forceps for seizing and compressing arteries.
Arthral'gia (ar-thral'je-ah). Pain or gout of a joint.
Arthrec'tomy. Excision of a joint.
Ar'thric (ar'thrik). Pertaining to a joint.
Arthrit'ic. Pertaining to gout or arthritis.
Arthri'tis. Gout, or any joint-inflammation. **A. defor'mans,** rheumatoid arthritis with consequent deformity. **A. fungo'sa,** tuberculous disease of the joints. **Gonorrheal a.,** a form of gonorrheal infection. **Rheumatoid a.,** chronic joint-disease with overgrowth of articular cartilages and synovial membranes.

A TABLE OF THE ARTERIES.

ARTERY.	ORIGIN.	DISTRIBUTION.	BRANCHES.
Acromiothorac'ic.	Axillary.	Shoulder, arm, upper front part of chest.	Acromial, humeral, pectoral, clavicular.
A'lar thorac'ic.	Second part of the axillary.	Lymphatic glands of axilla.	
Anastomot'ica mag'na.	Brachial.	Elbow.	Posterior and anterior.
Anastomot'ica mag'na.	Superficial femoral.	Knee.	Superficial and deep.
An'gular.	Termination of the facial.	Lacrimal sac and inferior orbicularis palpebrarum.	Phrenic, celiac axis, suprarenal, superior mesenteric, lumbar, renal, spermatic, inferior mesenteric, common iliac, middle sacral.
Aor'ta (abdominal).	Thoracic aorta.	Two common iliacs.	Phrenic, celiac axis, mesenteric, suprarenal, renal, spermatic, lumbar, sacral, right and left common iliac.
Aor'ta (arch).	Left ventricle.	Thoracic aorta.	Coronary, innominate, l. common carotid, l. subclavian.
Aor'ta (thoracic).	Arch of the aorta.	Abdominal aorta.	Pericardiac, bronchial, esophageal, mediastinal, intercostals.
Auric'ular, posterior.	External carotid.	Back of ear, scalp, and neck.	Stylomastoid, auricular.
Ax'illary.	Subclavian.	Upper extremity, pectoral muscles, axilla.	Superior thoracic, acromiothoracic, long thoracic, alar thoracic, subscapular.
Bas'ilar.	Right and left vertebral.	Brain.	Transverse, right and left posterior cerebral.
Bra'chial.	Axillary.	Arm and forearm.	Superior and inferior profunda, nutrient, anastomotica magna, muscular, radial, ulnar.
Carot'id, common.	Innominate (on rt. side), arch of aorta (on lt. side).	External and internal carotid.	External and internal carotid.

Carot′id, external.	Common carotid.	Front of neck, face, side of head, meninges, middle ear, thyroid gland, tongue, tonsils.	Superior thyroid, lingual, facial, occipital, posterior auricular, ascending pharyngeal, temporal, internal maxillary.
Carot′id, internal.	Common carotid.	Large part of brain, eye, internal ear, forehead, nose.	Tympanic, arteriæ receptaculi, anterior meningeal, ophthalmic, posterior communicating, anterior choroid, anterior cerebral, middle cerebral.
Ce′liac axis.	Abdominal aorta.	Esophagus, stomach, duodenum, spleen, pancreas, liver, gallbladder.	Gastric, hepatic, splenic.
Cor′onary (of heart).	Anterior sinus of Valsalva.	Heart.	Auricular, interventricular, preventricular, marginal, transverse, terminal.
Dorsa′lis pe′dis.	Anterior tibial.	Foot.	Tarsal, metatarsal, dorsalis hallucis, communicating.
Epigas′tric.	External iliac.	Abdominal wall, femoral ring, and cremaster.	Cremasteric, pubic, muscular, and terminal branches.
Fa′cial.	External carotid.	Pharynx and face.	Inferior palatine, tonsillar, submaxillary, submental, muscular, inferior labial, coronary of lips, latera′lis na′si, angular.
Fem′oral.	External iliac.	Lower part of abdominal wall, upper thigh, genitals.	Superficial epigastric, superficial external iliac, external pudic, profun′da fem′oris, muscular, anastomot′ica mag′na, popliteal.
Gas′tric.	Celiac axis.	Stomach, liver, esophagus.	Esophageal, cardiac, gastric, hepatic.
Gastroduode′nal.	Hepatic.	Pylorus, pancreas, stomach, duodenum.	Pyloric, gastroepiploic, pancreaticoduodenal.
Glu′teal.	Internal iliac.	Gluteal muscles.	Superficial, deep.
Hepat′ic.	Celiac axis.	Liver, pancreas, duodenum, stomach.	Pyloric, gastroduodenal, cystic, right and left hepatic.
Il′iac, common.	Abdominal aorta.		External and internal iliac, unnamed branches.
Il′iac, external.	Common iliac.	Integument and muscles of abdomen, generative organs, lower extremity.	Epigastric, circumflex, unnamed, femoral.
Il′iac, internal.	Common iliac.	Pelvis, generative organs, gluteal region.	Anterior and posterior trunk.

A TABLE OF THE ARTERIES (*continued*).

ARTERY.	ORIGIN.	DISTRIBUTION.	BRANCHES.
Il′iac, internal (anterior trunk).	Internal iliac.	Pelvis, genitals, thigh.	Vesical, middle hemorrhoidal, uterine, vaginal, obturator, internal pudic, sciatic.
Il′iac, internal (posterior trunk).	Internal iliac.	Muscles of the hip and sacrum.	Iliolumbar, lateral sacral, gluteal.
Innom′inate.	Arch of aorta.		Right carotid, right subclavian.
Intercos′tal, superior.	Subclavian.	Neck, upper part of the thorax.	Profun′da cervi′cis, first and second intercostal, arte′ria aber′rans.
Interos′seous.	Ulnar.	Deep structures of the forearm.	Anterior and posterior interosseous.
Lin′gual.	External carotid.	Muscles of the hyoid, sublingual gland, mouth, tongue.	Hyoid, dorsa′lis lin′guæ, sublingual, ranine.
Mam′mary, internal.	Subclavian.	Structures of the thorax.	Co′mes ner′vi phren′ici, mediastinal, pericardiac, sternal, anterior intercostal, perforating, musculophrenic, superior epigastric.
Max′illary, internal.	External carotid.	Structures indicated by the names of the branches.	Tympanic, middle meningeal, small meningeal, inferior dental, deep temporal, pterygoid, masseteric, buccal, posterior palatine, Vidian, pterygopalatine, sphenopalatine, alveolar, infraorbital.
Mesenter′ic, inferior.	Abdominal aorta.	Descending colon, sigmoid flexure, rectum.	Col′ica sinis′tra, sigmoid, superior hemorrhoidal.
Mesenter′ic, superior.	Abdominal aorta.	Small intestine, colon, cecum, ileum.	Inferior pancreaticoduodenal, colica dextra and media, ileocolic, vasa intestini tenuis.
Na′sal.	Ophthalmic.	Lacrimal sac and integument of the nose.	Lacrimal and transverse nasal.
Obtura′tor.	Internal iliac.	Pelvis and thigh.	Iliac, vesical, pubic, external and internal pelvic.
Occip′ital.	External carotid.	Muscles of the neck and scalp, auricle, meninges.	Muscular, auricular, meningeal, prin′ceps cervi′cis, cranial branches.

Ophthal'mic.	Internal carotid.	Eye, adjacent structures, portion of face.	Lacrimal, supraorbital, anterior and posterior ethmoid, superior and inferior palpebral, muscular, anterior, long and short ciliary, central artery of retina, frontal, nasal.
Pal'mar arch (deep).	Radial.	Palm and fingers.	Perforating, palmar interosseous, recurrent.
Pal'mar arch (superficial).	Ulnar.	Palm and fingers.	Communicating, digital, branch to radialis indicis.
Pharyn'geal, ascending.	External carotid.	Neck, pharynx, meninges.	External, pharyngeal, meningeal.
Plan'tar arch.	External plantar.	Anterior part of foot and toes.	Unnamed, posterior perforating, digital.
Plan'tar, external.	Posterior tibial.	Sole and toes.	Muscular, calcaneal, cutaneous, anastomotic, posterior perforating, plantar arch.
Poplit'eal.	Femoral.	Thigh, knee, and leg.	Superior and inferior muscular, cutaneous, superior external and superior internal articular, azygos articular, inferior external and inferior internal articular, anterior and posterior tibial.
Profun'da fem'oris.	Femoral.	Thigh.	External and internal circumflex, first, second, third, and fourth perforating.
Pu'dic, internal.	Internal iliac (anterior trunk).	Genital organs.	Inferior hemorrhoidal, superficial and transverse perineal, artery of the bulb, artery of the corpus cavernosum, dorsalis penis.
Pul'monary.	Right ventricle.	Lungs.	Right and left pulmonary.
Ra'dial.	Brachial.	Forearm, wrist, and hand.	Radial recurrent, muscular, superficial volar, anterior and posterior carpal, metacarpal, dorsa'lis pol'licis, dorsa'lis in'dicis, prin'ceps pol'licis, radia'lis in'dicis.
Re'nal.	Abdominal aorta.	Kidney.	Inferior suprarenal, capsular, ureteral.
Sciat'ic.	Internal iliac.	Muscles and viscera of pelvis.	Muscular, vesical, coccygeal, hemorrhoidal, inferior gluteal, co'mes ner'vi ischiad'ici, articular.
Splen'ic.	Celiac axis.	Pancreas, great curvature of stomach, spleen.	Small and large pancreatic, gastric, left gastroepiploic, splenic branches.

A TABLE OF THE ARTERIES (*continued*).

ARTERY.	ORIGIN.	DISTRIBUTION.	BRANCHES.
Subcla′vian.	Innominate (right side), arch of aorta (left side).	Neck, thorax, arms, brain, meninges.	Vertebral, thyroid axis, internal mammary, superior intercostal, axillary.
Suprascap′ular.	Thyroid axis.	Muscles of the shoulder.	Inferior sternomastoid, nutrient, suprasternal, acromial, articular, etc.
Tem′poral.	External carotid.	Forehead, parotid gland, masseter muscle, ear, etc.	Transverse facial, anterior auricular, middle temporal, anterior and posterior temporal.
Thy′roid axis.	Subclavian.	Shoulder, neck, thorax, spine.	Inferior thyroid, suprascapular, transversa′lis col′li.
Thy′roid, inferior.	Thyroid axis.	Larynx, esophagus, neck, thyroid gland.	Laryngeal, tracheal, esophageal, ascending cervical.
Thy′roid, superior.	External carotid.	Omohyoid, sternohyoid, sternothyroid, thyroid gland.	Hyoid, sternomastoid, superior laryngeal, cricothyroid.
Tib′ial, anterior.	Popliteal.	Knee, leg, and ankle.	Recurrent tibial, muscular, internal and external malleolar, dorsalis pedis.
Tib′ial, posterior.	Popliteal.	Leg, ankle, foot.	Peroneal, muscular, nutrient, communicating, internal calcaneal, external and internal plantar.
Transversa′lis col′li.	Thyroid axis.	Muscles of neck and back.	Superficial cervical, posterior scapular.
Ul′nar.	Brachial.	Forearm, wrist, and hand.	Anterior and posterior ulnar recurrent, interosseous, muscular, anterior and posterior carpal, superficial palmar arch.
U′terine.	Uterus.	Branch of the internal iliac.	Cervical, vaginal, azygos.
Ver′tebral.	Subclavian.	Neck, cord, cerebrum, cerebellum.	Lateral spinal, muscular, posterior meningeal, anterior and posterior spinal, inferior cerebellar, basilar.
Vid′ian.	Internal maxillary.	Roof of the pharynx, Eustachian tube, tympanum.	Pharyngeal, Eustachian, tympanic.

Urethral a., gonorrheal rheumatism. **A. urit'ica,** arthritis from gout.

Ar'thritism. Gouty or rheumatic diathesis.

Arthrobacte'rium. A bacterium which is reproduced by separation of joints.

Arthroc'ace (ar-throk'as-e). Ulceration of a joint or joints.

Ar'throcele (ar'thro-sēl). A joint-swelling.

Arthrochondri'tis. Inflammation of cartilages of a joint.

Arthrocla'sia. Breaking up of an ankylosis.

Arthrode'sis. Surgical fixation of a joint.

Arthro'dia. Diarthrosis which allows a gliding motion.

Arthrodyn'ia. Same as *Arthralgia.*

Arthrog'raphy. A treatise on the joints.

Arthrogrypo'sis. 1. Persistent flexure of a joint. 2. Tetanoid spasm. **Tetanilla a.,** tetany.

Arthrol'ogy. Sum of what is known regarding the joints.

Arthromeningi'tis. Same as *Synovitis.*

Arthroneural'gia. Neuralgia of a joint.

Ar'thropathy. 1. Any joint-disease. 2. Effusion of fluid into joints in tabes dorsalis: called also *Charcot's arthropathy.*

Arthrophy'ma. A joint-swelling.

Ar'throphyte. Abnormal growth of a joint-cavity.

Ar'throplasty. Plastic surgery of a joint.

Arthropyo'sis. Formation of pus in a joint-cavity.

Arthrorheu'matism. Articular rhematism.

Arthro'sis. Articulation.

Ar'throspore. A bacterial spore formed by fission.

Ar'throtome. A stout knife for operating on joints.

Arthrot'omy. Incision of a joint.

Arthroty'phoid. Typhoid beginning with symptoms of acute rheumatism.

Arthroxe'sis (ar-throx-e'sis). Scraping of joints.

Ar'tiad. An element of an even-numbered valency.

Artic'ular. Of, or pertaining to, a joint.

Artic'ulate. 1. To unite by joints; to join. 2. United by joints; jointed. **A. speech.** utterance of words and sentences.

Articula'tion. 1. A joint or arthrosis. 2. Enunciation of words and sentences. **Confluent a.**, speech in which syllables are run together.

Artic'ulatory. Relating to utterance.

Artic'ulo mor'tis. At the point or moment of death.

Artifi'cial (ar-tif-ish'al). Formed by art; not natural.

Aryepiglot'tic or **Aryepiglottid'ean folds.** Folds of mucous membrane extending between arytenoid cartilage and epiglottis.

Arytæno-epiglottid'eus. See *Muscles, Table of.*

Arytænoi'deus. See *Muscles, Table of.*

Aryte'noid (ar-it-e'noid). Shaped like a jug or pitcher.

Arytenoidi'tis. Inflammation of arytenoid muscles or cartilage.

As. 1. Abbreviation for *Astigmatism.* 2. Symbol for *Arsenic.*

A. S. L. *Aura sinistra.*

Asafet'ida, Asafœt'ida, Fetid gum-resin from *Ferula fœtida:* antispasmodic and expectorant.

Asa'phia. Indistinctness of utterance.

As'aprol. An antipyretic and antiseptic powder, $Ca(C_{10}H_6OHSO_3)_2$.

As'arol. A principle, $C_{10}H_{18}O$, from asarum.

As'arum. Genus of plants with emetic and cathartic properties.

Asbes'tos. Fibrous magnesium and calcium silicate.

Ascar'icide (as-kar'is-id). A drug destructive to ascarides.

Ascaridi'asis. Infestation with ascarides.

As'caris, pl. *ascar'ides.* A genus of intestinal worms.

Ascen'ding (as-en'ding). Having an upward course.
As'cherson's vesicles. Globules formed by shaking oil with albumin.
As'cia (as'e-ah). A spiral bandage without reverses.
Asci'tes (as-i'têz). Dropsy of the abdominal cavity. **A. chylo'-sus,** ascites in which the fluid contains chyle.
Ascit'ic (as-sit'ik). Affected with, or pertaining to, ascites.
Asclepi'adin. Poisonous glucosid of *Asclepias.*
Ascle'pias. Genus of herbs; *A. tubero'sa* is expectorant, diaphoretic, or cathartic.
Asclep'idin. A poisonous principle from asclepiadin; also, a deobstruent precipitate from *Asclepias tuberosa.*
Ascococ'cus. A genus of schizomycetes; *A. cit'reus* occurs in the skin in seborrhea.
Ascomyce'tes (as-ko-mi-se'têz). A genus of fungi.
As'cospore (as'ko-spōr). A spore contained or produced in an ascus.
As'cus. The spore case of certain fungi.
Asel'lin. Basic principle, $C_{25}H_{32}N_5$, from cod-liver oil.
Asema'sia. Loss of power of expression by signs or by words.
Ase'mia. Inability to understand or make use of signs or speech.
Asep'sin (as-ep'sin). Same as *Antisepsin.*
Asep'sis. Absence of septic matter, or freedom from infection.
Asep'tic. Not septic; free from septic material.
Aseptic-antiseptic. Aseptic as well as antiseptic.
Asep'ticize. To render aseptic; to free from pathogenic materials.
Asep'tol. A brown, oily antiseptic, $C_6H_6SO_3$; sulphocarbolic acid.
Asep'tolin. A preparation of phenol and pilocarpin; used for phthisis and intermittent fevers.
Asex'ual. Having no sex; not sexual.
Asia'lia (ah-si-a'le-ah). Absence or deficiency of saliva.
Asiat'ic cholera. See *Cholera.*
Asit'ia (ah-sit'e-ah). Loathing of food.
Aso'mata. Monster without a trunk.
Aspar'agin. Diuretic amid, $C_4H_8N_2O_3$, from asparagus and other plants.
Asparagin'ic acid, Aspar'tic acid. See *Acid.*
Aspar'agus. Genus of plants whose roots are mild diuretic.
As'pect. 1. That part of a surface which looks in any particular direction. 2. The look or appearance.
Aspergil'lin. Black pigment from *Aspergillus* spores.
Aspergil'lus. A genus of fungi (moulds) of which several species are endoparasitic and probably pathogenic. **A. mycosis,** disease of ear caused by aspergillus.
Asper'matism, Asper'mia. Deficient secretion of semen.
Asper'sion (as-per'shun). The act of sprinkling.
Asphyx'ia (as-fik'se-ah). Suspended animation as from suffocation, or carbon monoxid in inhalation. **A. carbon'ica,** suffocation from the inhalation of coal-gas or water-gas. **Local a.,** the congestive stage of Raynaud's disease. **A. neonato'rum,** imperfect breathing in new-born infants.
Asphyx'ial (as-fik'se-al). Characterized by asphyxia.
Asphyx'iate. To put into a state of more or less complete asphyxia.
Aspid'ium. A genus of ferns; several species are vermifugal.
Aspidosa'min. Emetic principle from quebracho bark.
Aspidosper'ma. See *Quebracho.*
Aspidosper'min. An alkaloid, $C_{22}H_{30}N_2O_2$, from quebracho.
Aspira'tion. Withdrawal of liquids by the aspirator.
As'pirator. Instrument for evacuating pus or serum.
Asple'nium. Genus of ferns; some species have limited medicinal uses.
Asporogen'ic. Not producing spores.

Assafet'ida, Assafœt'ida. See *Asafetida.*

Assana'tion. Sanitation; improvement of sanitary conditions.

Assim'ilable. Capable of being assimilated.

Assimila'tion. Transformation of food into tissues.

Asso'ciated movements. Involuntary coincident movements of associated muscles. **A. paralysis,** paralysis of associated muscles. **A. spasm,** coincident spasm of associated muscles.

Associa'tion center. The nerve-center which controls associated movements.

As'surin. Complex substance from brain-tissue.

Asta'sia. Motor incoordination with inability to stand. **A. aba'sia,** inability to stand or walk.

Asteato'sis. Deficiency or absence of sebaceous secretion. **A. cu'tis,** a variety resulting in dry, fissured condition of skin.

As'ter. Star-shaped structure around the centrosome; also, a star-shaped group of chromosomes.

Aste'rion (as-te're-on). The junction of occipital, parietal, and temporal bones.

Aster'nal. Not joined to the sternum.

Aster'nia. Absence of the sternum.

As'teroid (as'ter-oid). Star-shaped.

Asthe'nia. Debility; lack or loss of strength.

Asthen'ic (as-then'ik). Characterized by debility.

Asthenom'eter. Device used in measuring muscular asthenia.

Astheno'pia. Weakness and speedy tiring of visual organs. **Accommodative a.,** due to strain of ciliary muscle. **Muscular a.,** due to weakness of external ocular muscles.

Asthenop'ic. Characterized by asthenopia.

Asth'ma (az'mah). Intermittent dyspnea, with wheezing, cough, and sense of constriction. **Cardiac a.,** dyspnea from heart-disease. **A. convulsi'vum,** bronchial asthma. **A. crystals,** acicular crystals in sputum of asthma patients. **A. dyspep'ticum,** asthma due to nervous reflexes. **Heberden's a.,** angina pectoris. **Kopp's a.,** spasm of the glottis. **Renal a.,** dyspnea occurring in Bright's disease.

Asthmat'ic. Pertaining to, or affected with, asthma.

Astigmat'ic. Pertaining to, or affected with, astigmatism.

Astig'matism (as-tig'mat-izm). Defect in which light-rays are not brought to a proper focus by the unaided eye. **Compound a.,** a. complicated with hypermetropia or with myopia. **Corneal a.,** that due to unequal curvature of the cornea. **Irregular a.,** that in which different portions of a meridian have different refracting powers. **Lenticular a.,** that due to imperfections of the lens. It may complicate hypermetropia (**hyperopic** or **hypermetropic a.**) or myopia (**myopic a.**). **Mixed a.,** that in which one principal meridian is myopic and the other hyperopic. **Regular a.** is that in which the two principal meridians are at right angles to each other.

Astigmatom'eter, Astigmom'eter. Apparatus used in measuring astigmatism.

Asto'matous, Asto'mous. Without an oral aperture.

Astragalec'tomy. Surgical removal of the astragalus.

Astrag'alus. Bone of the foot which articulates with the tibia.

Astrapho'bia, Astrapopho'bia. Morbid fear of lightning.

Astric'tion. 1. The action of an astringent. 2. Constipation.

Astrin'gent (as-trin'jent). 1. Causing contraction and arresting discharges. 2. An agent that arrests discharges.

As'trocyte (as'tro-sit). A bone corpuscle; so-called from its star-shape.

Astrokinet'ic motions. Movements of the centrosome.

Astu'rian rose. See *Pellagra.*

Asy'lum ear. Hematoma auris.

Asymbo'lia. Same as *Asemia.*
Asym'metry (as-im'et-re). Lack or absence of symmetry.
Asyn'clitism. Oblique presentation of the head in parturition
Asyn'ergy (as-in'er-je). Lack of coordination.
Asyne'sia (as-in-e'ze-ah). Dulness of intellect; stupidity.
Asyno'via. Absence or insufficiency of synovia.
Asystemat'ic. Not confined to one system; diffuse.
Asys'tole (as-is'to-le). Imperfect or incomplete systole.
Asysto'lia (as-is-to'le-ah). Same as *Asystole.*
Atac'tic (at-ak'tik). Same as *Ataxic.*
At'avism. Inheritance of characters from remote ancestors.
Ataxapha'sia. Ability to utter words, but not sentences.
Atax'ia. Failure of muscular coordination. **Briquet's a.,** hysteric condition with anesthesia of skin and leg-muscles. **Family a., Hereditary a.** See *Friederich's disease.* **Hysterical a.,** ataxia of leg-muscles in hysteria. **Locomotor a.,** degeneration of posterior columns of spinal cord, marked by flashes of pain, incoordination, disturbances of sensation, loss of reflexes, etc. **Motor a.,** inability to coordinate the muscles properly. **Thermal a.,** irregular changes in the body temperature.
Atax'iagram. Tracing drawn by an ataxic patient.
Atax'iagraph. Apparatus used in diagnosis of extent of ataxia.
Ataxiamne'sia. Characterized by ataxia and amnesia.
Atax'ic, Atax'ial. Pertaining to, or affected with, ataxia.
Ataxophe'mia. Lack of coordination of speech-muscles.
Ataxopho'bia. Morbid dread of disorder.
Atax'y (at-ak'se). Same as *Ataxia.*
Atelec'tasis. Imperfect expansion of lungs at birth; also, partial collapse of lung.
Ate'lia (ah-te'le-ah). Incomplete development.
Atelocar'dia. Incomplete development of the heart.
Atelocepn'alous. Having an incomplete skull.
Atelochei'lia. Congenital defect of the lip.
Ateloglos'sia. Abnormality or defect of the tongue.
Atelomye'lia. Imperfect formation of the spinal cord.
Atelorrachid'ia. Imperfect development of spinal column.
Athero'ma. 1. Degeneration of coats of blood-vessels. 2. Distention of sebaceous follicles.
Atheroma'sia. Atheromatous degeneration.
Athero'matous. Pertaining to, or affected with, atheroma.
Ath'etoid. 1. Not unlike athetosis. 2. Affected with athetosis.
Atheto'sis. Affection marked by continuous movements of fingers and toes.
Ath'lete's heart. Aortic incompetence due to strain in athletic exercise.
Athrep'sia. Insufficient nutrition of infants.
Athy'ria (ath-i're-ah). Myxedema.
Atlan'tad. Toward the atlas.
Atlan'tal. Of, or pertaining to, the atlas.
At'las. First cervical vertebra.
Atlo-ax'oid. Pertaining to atlas and axis.
Atlod'ymus. Monster with two heads and one body.
Atmiat'rics, Atmi'atry. Treatment by medicated vapors.
At'mograph. Instrument for recording respiratory movements.
Atmol'ysis (at-mol'is-is). Separation of mixed gases.
Atmom'eter. Instrument for measuring exhaled vapors.
At'mosphere. 1. Air encircling the earth. 2. Pressure of air at sea-level, being 15 pounds to the square inch.
Atmospher'ic. Of, or pertaining to, the atmosphere.
Ato'cia (at-o'se-ah). Sterility in the female.
At'om. Any one of the ultimate particles of a molecule or of matter.

Atom'ic (at-om'ik). Pertaining to an atom.
Atomi'city. Chemical valency or quantivalence.
At'omizer. Instrument for throwing a jet or spray.
Aton'ic. Characterized by lack of normal tone.
At'ony (at'o-ne). Absence or lack of normal tone.
Atopomenorrhe'a. Vicarious menstruation.
Atrabil'iary. Pertaining to dark bile. **A. capsules,** supra-renal capsules.
Atre'mia. 1. Absence of tremor. 2. Hysterical inability to walk.
Atre'sia. Imperforation; absence of a normal opening.
Atre'sic (at-re'sik). Characterized by atresia.
Atrich'ia. Atricho'sis. Absence of hair.
Atrioventric'ular. Pertaining to the auricle and ventricle.
A'trium (a'tre-um). 1. The auricle of the heart. 2. Main part of the tympanic chamber.
At'ropa belladon'na. See *Belladonna*.
Atro'phia (at-ro'fe-ah). L. for *Atrophy*.
Atroph'ic (at-rof'ik). Pertaining to, or characterized by, atrophy.
Atrophoder'ma. Atrophy of the skin or of a part of it.
At'rophy (at'ro-fe). A wasting or diminution of size. **Acute yellow a.,** atrophy and yellow discoloration of liver, with jaundice. **Brown a.,** atrophy in which the organ takes on a brownish hue. **Compression a.,** atrophy of part from constant compression. **Correlated a.,** atrophy of a part following destruction of another part. **Cruveilhier's a.,** progressive muscular atrophy. **A. of disuse,** wasting from lack of normal exercise. **Gray a.,** degeneration of optic disk, in which it becomes gray. **Idiopathic muscular a.,** progressive wasting affecting groups of muscles and due to changes in the muscles themselves. **Landouzy-Déjerine a.,** atrophy of muscles of face and scapulohumeral region. **Muscular a.,** wasting of muscles. **Progressive muscular a.,** disease with progressive wasting of muscles and paralysis, due to degeneration of anterior gray horns of spinal cord. **Red a.,** atrophy from chronic congestion. **Senile a.,** atrophy of old age. **Trophoneurotic a.,** atrophy due to disease of the nerves or center supplying a part. **Unilateral facial a.,** progressive wasting of the tissues of one side of the face. **White a.,** atrophy of nerve, leaving only white connective tissue.
At'ropin. Poisonous alkaloid, $C_{17}H_{23}NO_3$, of belladonna: mydriatic and narcotic.
Atropi'na. Same as *Atropin*.
At'ropinism, At'ropism. Condition produced by use of atropin.
Atropiniza'tion. 1. Subjection to influence of atropin. 2. Atropism.
At'ropinize. To put under the influence of atropin.
At'tar of roses. Volatile oil from rose-petals.
Atten'uant. A medicine that thins the blood.
Atten'uated virus. Virus rendered less pathogenic by repeated inoculation.
Attenua'tion. 1. Act or process of thinning. 2. Medicine or virus that has been attenuated.
At'tic. Part of tympanum above the atrium. **A. disease,** chronic suppurative inflammation of attic.
Attol'lens. Raising; lifting up. **A. au'rem.** See *Muscles, Table of*.
Attrac'tion, capillary. The force by which liquids rise in fine tubes.
At'trahens. Drawing toward or forward. **A. au'rem.** See *Muscles, Table of*.
Attrit'ion (at-rish'un). Friction; abrasion; also, friction-sound.
Atyp'ic (at-ip'ik). Not conforming to the type.

Au. Symbol for gold (*aurum*).

Audiom'eter. Device to test hearing power.

Audiom'etry. Testing of the sense of hearing.

Au'diphone. A device for aiding deafness.

Audi'tion (aw-dish'un). Perception of sound; hearing. **Chromatic a., A. colorée.** Same as *Chromesthesia.*

Au'ditory. Pertaining to the sense of hearing. **A. area,** the auditory center. **A. capsule,** cartilaginous embryonic structure which forms the external ear. **A. center,** center for hearing in superior temporal convolution. **A. dysesthesia.** Same as *Dysacusis.* **A. field,** space within which sounds are audible. **A. hairs,** epithelial hairs of internal ear. **A. meatus.** See *Meatus auditorius.* **A. nerve,** eighth cranial nerve. **A. nuclei,** nuclei in oblongata whence auditory nerves arise. **A. ossicles,** the incus, malleus, stapes, and orbiculare. **A. pit,** depression on each side of after-brain of embryo, forming labyrinth of ear. **A. teeth,** tooth-like points in the cochlea. **A. vesicle,** epiblastic expansion which becomes the membranous labyrinth.

Au'erbach's plexus. Complex of nerves between the longitudinal and circular fibers of intestine.

Augna'thus. A fetus with double lower jaw.

Au'la (aw'lah). Forward part of third ventricle.

Aulate'la. The covering membrane of the aula.

Auliplex'us. Part of choroid plexus in the aula.

Au'lix (aw'liks). The sulcus of Monro.

Au'ra (aw'rah). Cool sensation which foreruns an epileptic attack. **A. elec'trica,** breezy sensation on reception of static electricity. **Epigastric a.,** painful sensations in epigastrium preceding an epileptic attack.

Au'ral (aw'ral). Pertaining to the ear. **A. vertigo.** Same as *Ménière's disease.*

Auram'in. Same as *Yellow pyoktanin.*

Auran'tium. L. for *Orange.*

Au'ric (aw'rik). Pertaining to gold.

Au'ricle (aw'rik-l). 1. The flap of the ear. 2. The upper chamber on either side of the heart.

Auric'ular. Pertaining to an auricle. **A. appendix,** anterior prolongation of auricle of heart. **A. artery.** See *Arteries, Table of.* **A. point,** center of entrance of the external meatus of the ear.

Auricula'ris mag'nus. See *Nerves, Table of.*

Auriculotem'poral nerve. See *Nerves, Table of.*

Auriculoventric'ular. Pertaining to an auricle and ventricle.

Au'ripuncture (aw'rip-ungk-tūr). Puncture of membrana tympani.

Au'ris (aw'ris). The ear.

Au'riscope (aw'ris-kōp). Instrument for examining the ear.

Au'rist (aw'rist). Specialist in ear-diseases.

Au'rum (aw'rum). L. for *Gold.*

Aus'cult, Aus'cultate. To examine by listening.

Ausculta'tion (aws-kul-ta'shun). Listening for sounds within the body. **Immediate a.,** auscultation without the stethoscope. **Mediate a.,** auscultation performed by the aid of instruments. **A. tube,** a kind of stethoscope.

Auscul'tatory. Of, or pertaining to, auscultation. **A. percussion,** auscultation combined with percussion.

Autech'oscope. Instrument for auscultating one's own body.

Aute'cic. See *Autœcic.*

Au'toblast. A separate, independent bioblast, as a bacterium.

Autocath'eterism. Passage of the catheter by the patient.

Autoch'thonous. Found in the place of formation; not removed to a new site.

Au'toclave (aw'to-klāv). A variety of steam sterilizer.

Autodiges'tion. Same as *Autopepsia.*

Autœ'cic (aw-te'sik). Always living upon the same organism.

Autogen'esis (aw-to-jen'es-is). 1. Spontaneous generation. 2. Origination within the organism.

Autogenet'ic. Auto'genous. Originated within the body.

Autog'raphism. Hysterical state in which marks or words written upon the skin leave more or less persistent traces.

Autohyp'notism. Hypnotic state voluntarily self-induced.

Auto-infec'tion. Infection by a virus generated in the organism.

Auto-inocula'tion. Inoculation with a virus from one's own body.

Auto-intoxica'tion. Poisoning by some uneliminated matter (toxins) formed within the body.

Autolaryngos'copy. Observation of one's own larynx.

Automat'ic. Spontaneous; done by no act of the will.

Autom'atism. Performance of acts without conscious volition.

Automysopho'bia. Insane dread of personal uncleanness.

Auton'omous. Having independent functions.

Auton'omy. Functional independence of other parts.

Auto-ophthal'moscope. Ophthalmoscope for examining one's own eyes.

Auto-ophthal'moscopy. The use of the auto-ophthalmoscope.

Autopathog'raphy. Description of the phenomena of one's own disease.

Autopep'sia. Digestion of stomach-wall by its own secretion.

Autoph'agy (aw-tof'aj-e). The eating of one's own tissues in insanity.

Autopho'bia. Insane dread of solitude or of one's self.

Autoph'ony. 1. Observation of one's own voice as transmitted through a patient's chest. 2. State in which the patient's voice seems to himself abnormal or too loud.

Autophthal'moscope. See *Auto-ophthalmoscope.*

Au'toplasty. Repair of diseased or injured parts by pieces taken from another part.

Au'topsy. Post-mortem examination of a dead body.

Au'toscope. Instrument for examination of one's own organs.

Autos'copy. Examination of one's own organs.

Au'tosite (aw'to-sīt). 1. A monster or teratism capable of independent life. 2. A teratism upon or within which a parasitic twin lives.

Autosteth'oscope. Stethoscope for use on one's own chest.

Autosugges'tion. Peculiar mental state with loss of will, in which suggestions become easy. It often follows shock or accident.

Autotem'nous. Capable of spontaneous fission.

Autother'apy. Spontaneous cure of disease.

Autotoxe'min. Autotoxico'sis. Poisoning by ferment or virus generated within the body.

Autotox'in. Any pathogenic principle developed within the body.

Autotransfu'sion. The forcing of blood into vital parts by bandaging or elevating the limbs.

Autovaccina'tion. Vaccination of a patient with his own virus.

Au'tumn catarrh. A variety of hay fever.

Auxocar'dia. 1. Diastole. 2. Enlargement of the heart.

A'va. A'va-ka'va. Same as *Kava.*

Av'alanche theory. Doctrine that nervous impulses accumulate force in passing along an efferent nerve.

Avas'cular (ah-vas'ku-lar). Not vascular; bloodless.

Avasculariza'tion. Expulsion of blood, as by bandaging.

Ave′na sati′va. The plant which bears oats. See *Oat.*

Ave′nin. Stimulant and tonic preparation from oats.

Avogad′ro's law. Equal volumes of gases, with same pressure and temperature, contain the same number of molecules.

Avoirdupois (ah-vwah-doo-polz′). See *Weights.*

Avul′sion. The tearing away of a structure or part.

Ax′ial, Ax′ile. Of, or pertaining to, an axis. **A. current,** the colored central part of the blood-stream. **A. neuritis.** See *Neuritis.*

A′xil, Axil′la. The armpit.

Axilem′ma. Sheath of the axis-cylinder.

Ax′illary (ak′sil-ar-e). Of, or pertaining to, the armpit.

Ax′in (ak′sin). Varnish-like substance from an insect, *Coccus axinus:* vulnerary and resolvent.

Ax′is (ak′sis). 1. Straight line through a center. 2. Second cervical vertebra. **Basicranial a.,** line from basion to gonion. **Basifacial a.,** line from gonion to subnasal point. **Binauricular a.,** line joining the two auricular points. **Celiac a.,** a thick branch from the abdominal aorta. **Cerebrospinal a.,** the central nervous system. **A.-cylinder,** the core or central part of a nerve-fiber. **A.-cylinder process,** nerve-cell process continuous with the axis-cylinder. **Frontal a.,** imaginary line running from right to left through center of eyeball. **Neural a.** Same as *Cerebrospinal a.* **Sagittal a.,** imaginary line extending through the eye from before backward. **A.-traction forceps, A.-tractor,** instrument for making traction on the fetus in the course of the pelvic axis. **Visual a.,** line from point of vision of retina to the object of vision.

Axolem′ma. Same as *Axilemma.*

Ax′on. Same as *Axis-cylinder process.*

Axonom′eter. Apparatus for rapid determination of the cylindrical axis of a lens.

Ax′oplasm. Material by which fibrils of the axis-cylinder are surrounded.

Axun′gia (ak-sun′je-ah). Lard.

Azalein. Same as *Fuchsin.*

Azed′arach. Medicinal root-bark of *Melia azedarach*, an Asiatic tree.

Az′erin. Ferment from various insectivorous plants.

Azoben′zene. A derivative, $C_{12}H_{10}N_2$, from nitrobenzene.

Azo′ic (ah-zo′ik). Destitute of living organisms.

Azolit′min. A red coloring principle from litmus.

Azoösper′mia. Lack or absence of spermatozoa in semen.

A′zote (a′zōt). Old name of nitrogen.

Azote′mia (a-zo-te′me-ah). Same as *Uremia.*

Azotene′sis. A disease due to excess of nitrogen in system, as scurvy, gangrene, etc.

A′zotized. Containing or charged with nitrogen.

Azotu′ria (a-zo-tu′re-ah). Excess of urea in the urine.

Azoxyben′zene. A product, $C_{12}H_{10}N_2O$, of the reduction of nitrobenzene.

Az′ulene. Blue coloring matter, $C_{16}H_{26}O$, from certain volatile oils.

Az′ulin. A blue anilin color or dye.

Az′ygos (az′ig-us). Any unpaired part.

Az′ygous (az′ig-us). Having no fellow; unpaired. **A. ganglion.** Same as *Ganglion impar.* **A. muscle,** the uvularis muscle. See *Muscles, Table of.* **A. veins,** three veins in front and near sides of vertebral column.

Az′ymia (az-im′e-ah). Absence of ferment.

Azym′ic (az-im′ik). Not giving rise to fermentation.

B.

B. Symbol of *boron.*

Ba. Symbol of *barium.*

Bab'bit metal. An alloy somewhat used in dentistry.

Ba'by-farm. A place where infants are reared.

Bac'ca (bak'ah). A berry; a berry-like fruit.

Baccel'li's sign (bat-shel'ēz). Aphonic pectoriloquy: a sign of pleural effusion.

Bac'charin. Poisonous alkaloid from *Baccharis cordifolia.*

Bac'chia (bak'e-ah). Acne rosacea.

Bacillæ'mia. See *Bacillemia.*

Bac'illar, Bac'illary (bas'il-ar, bas'il-ar-e). Pertaining to bacilli, or to rod-like forms. **B. layer,** the rod-and-cone layer of the retina.

Bacille'mia. Condition in which the blood contains bacilli.

Bacil'licidal, Bacillicid'ic. Destructive to bacilli.

Bacil'licide (bas-il'is-īd). A drug that destroys bacilli.

Bacil'liculture. The propagation of bacilli.

Bacil'liform. Shaped like a bacillus.

Bacillip'arous (bas-il-ip'ar-us). Producing bacilli.

Bacillopho'bia. Insane dread of microbes.

Bacillu'ria. State in which the urine contains bacilli.

Bacil'lus (bas-il'us), pl. *bacil'li.* A genus of schizomycetic organisms, consisting of non-motile, rod-like forms. **B. ace'ti, B. acet'icus,** b. found in air and vinegar and causing acetic fermentation. **B. ac'idi lac'tici,** found in air and sour milk, and causing lactic-acid fermentation. **B. acidofor'mans,** pathogenic b. from liver of yellow-fever cadaver. **B. actinobac'ter.** Same as *B. butyricus.* **B. aero'genes,** one of three forms—I, II, III—from the alimentary canals of healthy persons. **B. aero'genes capsula'tus,** non-pathogenic b. from blood-vessels in a case of thoracic aneurysm. **B. aeroph'ilus,** non-pathogenic b. from air. **B. al'bicans paterifor'mis,** species from the skin in seborrhea. **B. albu'minis,** non-pathogenic b. from feces. **B. al'bus,** white, non-pathogenic b. from water. **B. al'bus cadav'eris,** pathogenic b. from blood of a cadaver. **B. al'bus pu'tridus,** non-pathogenic species from water. **B. allanto'-ides,** non-pathogenic b. from air. **B. al'lii,** non-pathogenic b. found in decaying onions. **B. al'vei,** pathogenic b. from diseased bees. **B. amylobac'ter.** Same as *B. butyricus.* **B. anaero'bicus liquifa'ciens,** species from intestine of yellow-fever corpse. **B. an'thracis,** the b. of anthrax. **B. aquat'ilis** non-pathogenic species from well water. **B. arbores'cens,** non-pathogenic b. from hydrant water, forming orange color. **B. argentophosphores'cens,** either of three species—I, II, III—from sea water, phosphorescent fish, and cuttle-fish. **B. auranti'acus,** b. from well water, forming yellow pigment. **B. au'reus,** b. from water and the skin in seborrhea. **B. beriber'icus,** species found in persons with beri-beri. **B. Bienstock'ii,** pathogenic b. from human feces. **B. bras'sicæ,** non-pathogenic b. from infusions of cabbage-leaves. **B. bronchit'idis pu'tridæ,** the b. of putrid bronchitis. **B. brun'neus,** non-pathogenic species from water. **B. bucca'lis,** non-pathogenic b. from buccal secretions of healthy persons. **B. butyl'icus, B. butyri'cus,** non-pathogenic b. from milk, old cheese, water, soil, dust, etc., producing butyric-acid fermentation. **B. cadav'eris,** pathogenic b. from yellow-fever cadavers. **B. cana'lis capsula'tus,** pathogenic b. from sewer water. **B. cana'lis par'vus,** pathogenic species from sewer water. **B. can'dicans,** non-pathogenic b. from soil. **B. capsula'tus,** pathogenic b. from blood of guinea-pig. **B. capsula'tus mu-**

co'sus, pathogenic b. from nasal secretions of influenza patient. **B. carabifor'mis,** non-pathogenic b. from stomach of meat-fed dog. **B. carota'rum,** non-pathogenic b. from cooked carrots and beets. **B. caten'ula,** non-pathogenic b. from cheese. **B. Caucas'icus,** non-pathogenic b. from Kefir grains. **B. ca'viæ fortu'itus,** non-pathogenic b. from guinea-pigs inoculated with yellow fever. **B. cavici'dus,** pathogenic b. from human feces. **B. Chauvæ'i,** b. causing symptomatic anthrax in cattle. **B. chlori'nus,** non-pathogenic b. from decaying vegetable matter. **B. chol'eræ Asiat'icæ,** the spirillum of Asiatic cholera. **B. chol'eræ gallina'rum.** Same as *B. septicæmiæ*. **B. cho'væi,** the b. of symptomatic anthrax. **B. chromo-aromat'icus,** pathogenic b. from carcass of a diseased dog. **B. clavifor'mis,** pathogenic b. from fermenting casein. **B. cloa'cæ,** non-pathogenic b. from sewage. **B. cœru'leus,** saprophytic b. from water. **B. co'li commu'nis,** pathogenic b. from intestines of man and animals. **B. constric'tus,** a b. from hydrant water, producing yellow pigment. **B. copro'genes fœ'tidus,** b. from intestines of pigs with hog-cholera. **B. copro'genes par'vus,** pathogenic b. from human feces. **B. cras'sus,** the broadest b. known. **B. cras'sus sputig'enus,** pathogenic b. from sputum of man. **B. cunea'tus,** pathogenic species from blood and viscera of animals dead of sepsis. **B. cuniculici'dus.** Same as *B. septicæmiæ hæmorrhagicæ*. **B. cyano'genus,** the b. of blue milk. **B. cystifor'mis,** non-pathogenic b. from urine of cystitis patient. **B. denitrif'icans,** b. from sewage and soil; decomposes nitrates. **B. denta'lis vir'idans,** pathogenic b. from carious teeth. **B. devo'rans,** non-pathogenic b. from well water. **B. diffu'sus,** non-pathogenic b. from soil. **B. diphthe'riæ,** pathogenic b. from diphtheritic membranes. **B. diphthe'riæ columba'rum,** the b. of pigeon-diphtheria. **B. diphthe'ria spu'rius,** b. similar to b. diphtheriæ from healthy pharynx. **B. diphthe'riæ vitulo'rum,** pathogenic b. from mouths of calves with diphtheria. **B. distor'tus,** species from milk and cheese. **B. dysente'riæ,** b. from viscera of person dead of dysentery. **B. dyso'des,** b. causing souring of bread. **B. endocardi'tidis capsula'tus,** pathogenic b. from viscera of endocarditis corpses. **B. endocardi'tidis gris'eus,** pathogenic b. from heart in case of ulcerative endocarditis. **B. enteri'tidis,** pathogenic b. from cow dead of enteritis. **B. epider'midis,** b. from epidermis of spaces between the toes. **B. erysipel'atos lep'oris,** b. of erysipelas in the rabbit. **B. erysipel'atos su'is,** pathogenic b. of hog-erysipelas. **B. erythros'poros,** non-pathogenic species from albuminous fluids. **B. ex pneumo-enterit'ide su'is,** the b. of hog-cholera. **B. figu'rans,** saprophytic b. from air and water. **B. filifor'mis,** non-pathogenic b. from cheese and milk. **B. of Flocca,** pathogenic b. from saliva of dogs and cats. **B. fitzia'nus,** saprophytic b. from infusions of hay. **B. fla'vus,** b. from water producing yellow pigment. **B. fluores'cens liquifa'ciens,** saprophytic b. from air and water. **B. fluores'cens pu'tidus,** non-pathogenic b. from air and water, producing repulsive odor. **B. fœ'tidus,** pathogenic b. from sweating feet and cow-dung. **B. fœ'tidus oze'næ,** pathogenic species from secretions of ozena patients. **B. ful'vus,** b. from hydrant water, producing yellow pigment. **B. fus'cus,** b. from water, forming brown pigment. **B. fus'cus limba'tus,** non-pathogenic b. from rotten eggs. **B. gallina'rum,** pathogenic b. from blood of chickens dead of a disease resembling chicken-cholera. **B. genicula'tus,** non-pathogenic b. from the stomach. **B. gingi'væ pyo'genes,** pathogenic species from foul mouth and decaying dental pulp. **B. gra'cilis,** non-pathogenic species from water. **B. grave'olens,** non-pathogenic b. from between the toes. **B. Hansen'ii,** b. from water, producing yellow pigment. **B. hemineerobioph'ilus,** pathogenic b. from cheesy lymph-glands. **B. hydroph'ilus fus'cus,** b. from lymph-disease of frogs. **B. ian'thinus,** b. from hydrant water and sewage, producing violet pigment. **B. in'dicus,** pathogenic b. from stomach of monkey. **B. indigo'genus,** pathogenic b. from leaves of indigo-plant. **B. influen'zæ,** the specific b. of influenza. **B. lac'ticus.** Same as *B. acidi lactici.* **B. lac'tis aero'genes,** pathogenic b. from intestine of animals fed on milk. **B. lac'tis erythro'genes,** the b. of red milk. **B. lac'tis visco'sus,** non-pathogenic b. from ropy milk. **B. lep'ræ,** pathogenic b. from leprous tubercles. **B. lioder'mos,** b. from milk, peptonizing casein. **B. liquefa'ciens,** non-pathogenic b. from water. **B. liquefa'ciens bo'vis,** pathogenic b. from lungs of diseased ox. **B. liquefa'ciens mag'nus,** non-pathogenic b. from mice inoculated with garden soil. **B. liquefa'ciens par'vus,** non-pathogenic b. from same source as last. **B. lu'teus.** Same as *Bacterium luteum.* **B. mala'riæ,** probably pathogenic b. from blood of malarial patients. **B. mal'lei,** pathogenic b. from the nodules of glanders. **B. megate'rium,** non-pathogenic b. from boiled cabbage. **B. melanos'poros,** b. from air, producing black pigment. **B. mesenter'icus fus'cus,** saprophytic b. from air, water, and potato-peelings. **B. mesenter'icus ru'ber,** b. causing pink color on potatoes. **B. mesenter'icus vulga'tus,** b. from potatoes, milk, and human feces. **B. mirab'ilis,** b. causing putrefaction of animal matter. **B. multipedic'ulus,** non-pathogenic b. from air and water. **B. murisep'ticus.** Same as *B. erysipelatos suis.* **B. murisep'ticus pleomor'phus,** pathogenic b. from uterine discharges of pyemia. **B. musco'ides,** non-pathogenic b. from soil, old cheese, and cow-dung. **B. myco'ides,** non-pathogenic b. from soil and water. **B. neapolita'nus.** Same as *B. coli communis.* **B. œdem'atis malig'ni,** pathogenic b. from dust, foul water, and putrefying matter. **B. oxyto'cus pernicio'sus,** pathogenic b. from stale milk. **B. par'vus ova'tus,** pathogenic b. from pig dying with swine-plague. **B. Pasteuria'nus,** b. from beer, causing acetic fermentation. **B. phosphores'cens gel'idus,** non-pathogenic b. from phosphorescent fish. **B. pneumo'niæ,** pathogenic b. sometimes found in exudates of pneumonia. **B. pneumon'icus a'gilis,** pathogenic b. from vagus-pneumonia of rabbit. **B. polymyx'a,** b. from fermenting infusions of potatoes, etc. **B. polypifor'mis,** non-pathogenic b. from cow-dung, and exudates of mice inoculated with garden soil. **B. prodigio'sus,** non-pathogenic b. found on various foods. **B. pseudopneumon'icus,** pathogenic b. from pus. **B. pyocya'neus,** pathogenic b. from blue pus. **B. pyo'genes fœ'tidus,** pathogenic b. from pus of an abscess. **B. radia'tus,** non-pathogenic b. from exudates of mice and guinea-pigs inoculated with garden soil. **B. ramo'sus liquefa'ciens,** non-pathogenic b. from the air. **B. rhinosclerom'atis,** pathogenic b. from tubercles of rhinoscleroma. **B. ru'ber,** saprophytic b. from the air. **B. saliva'rius sep'ticus,** the diplococcus of pneumonia. **B. sapro'genes,** a b. in three forms, from fetid sweat of feet, putrefying pus, gangrenous tissue. **B. sca'ber,** non-pathogenic species from cheese. **B. Schäf'feri,** non-pathogenic b. from cheese and fermenting potato. **B. of Scheurlein,** non-pathogenic b. from cancer and from healthy breast. **B. of septicæ'mia,** saprophytic b. from the blood. **B. septicæ'miæ hæmorrha'gicæ,** the b. of chicken-cholera. **B. sep'ticus acumina'tus,** pathogenic b. from blood and organs of child dead from septicemia. **B. sep'ticus sputi'genus,** the diplococcus of pneumonia. **B. sim'ilis**, non-pathogenic b. from human feces. **B. sol'idus**, non-pathogenic b. from mice inoculated with garden soil. **B. stolona'tus**, non-pathogenic b. from water. **B. subti'lis**, non-pathogenic b. from air, water, soil, and decaying matter. **B. subti'lis sim'ulans.** Same as *B. similis*. **B. synog'onus**, non-pathogenic b. from blue milk. **B. synxan'thus**, non-pathogenic b. from yellow milk. **B. syphil'idis**, b. from syphilitic tissue; not yet proved pathogenic. **B. ten'uis**, non-pathogenic b. from cheese, causing albuminoid decomposition. **B. ter'mo.** Same as *Bacterium termo*. **B. tet'ani**, pathogenic b. from soil and pus of tetanus. **B. thermoph'ilus**, non-pathogenic b. from intestine of man and animals and from soil. **B. trem'ulus**, saprophytic b. from decaying infusions of plants. **B. tuberculo'sis**, pathogenic b. of tuberculosis. **B. tumes'cens**, non-pathogenic b. from beets and turnips. **B. tur'gidus**, saprophytic b. from air. **B. tus'sis convulsi'væ**, pathogenic b. from sputum of whooping-cough. **B. typho'sus**, **B. ty'phi abdomina'lis**, pathogenic b. of typhoid fever. **B. ul'na**, non-pathogenic b. from healthy sputum. **B. ure'æ.** See *Bacterium ureæ*. **B. uroceph'alus**, b. from putrefying animal matter, causing albuminoid fermentation. **B. Utpadel**, pathogenic b. from small intestine of man. **B. varico'sus conjuncti'va**, pathogenic b. from healthy conjunctiva. **B. viola'ceus**, b. from river water, producing violet pigment. **B. vi'rens**, found in stagnant water, forming green pigment. **B. vires'cens**, non-pathogenic b. from green sputum. **B. vir'gula**, b. causing albuminoid fermentation of casein. **B. vir'idis**, found in a polyporus-fungus in water. **B. visco'sus**, b. from river water and soil, producing green pigment. **B. vitulo'rum**, pathogenic b. from diphtheria of calves. **B. vulga'ris**, b. causing putrefaction of animal matter. **B. X**, pathogenic species from yellow-fever cadavers. **B. xantho'genus.** Same as *B. synxanthus*. **B. xero'sis**, non-pathogenic b. from xerosis. **B. Zenk'eri**, b. causing putrefaction. **B. Zop'fii**, b. from intestine of chickens and blood of ducks. **B. zurnia'num**, non-pathogenic b. from water.

Back-cut of Salmon. Incision or slitting of an anal fistula.

Back'ward progression. Tendency to walk backward in some cases of central nervous lesion.

Ba'cony degeneration or **infiltration.** Amyloid degeneration. **B. spleen**, a spleen affected with amyloid degeneration.

Bactere'mia. Same as *Bacteriemia*.

Bacte'ria. Schizomycetes or vegetable micro-organisms.

Bacte'rial. Pertaining to, or produced by, bacteria.

Bacterici'dal. Destructive to bacteria.

Bacter'icide. Anything which destroys bacteria.

Bacterie'mia. The presence of schizomycetes in the blood.

Bacte'rioid. Resembling a bacterium.

Bacteriolog'ic, Bacteriolog'ical. Pertaining to bacteria.

Bacteriol'ogist. An expert in the study of bacteria.

Bacteriol'ogy. The science of bacteria.

Bacteriopro'tein. A toxalbumin formed by bacteria.

Bacteriopur'purin. Peach-colored pigment in *Beggiatoa*.

Bacterioscop'ic. Pertaining to the microscopy of bacteria.

Bacterios'copy. The microscopic study of bacteria.

Bacteriotherapeu'tic. Pertaining to bacteriotherapy.

Bacteriother'apy. The cure of disease by introducing bacteria into the system.

Bacteritox'in. A substance destructive to bacteria.

Bacte'rium, pl. *bacte'ria*. A genus of schizomycetes of short, rod-like form. **B. ace'ti.** Same as *Bacillus aceti*. **B. a'cidi lac'tici.** Same as *Bacillus acidi lactici*. **B. aero'genes**, the bacillus aerogenes. **B. al'lii.** Same as *Bacillus allii.* **B. auranti'-acum**, a chromogenic bacterium. **B. brun'neum**, a species from putrid infusion of Indian corn. **B. buty'ri colloi'deum**, a species from butter. **B. capita'tum**, a species from infusions of albuminous matter. **B. caten'ula**, species from putrid wine and decaying blood. **B. co'li commu'ne.** Same as *Bacillus coli communis.* **B. decal'vans**, a species said to cause alopecia areata. **B. farina'ceum**, a species from sour dough. **B. glis-chro'genum**, a species from viscid urine. **B. gum'mis**, a species causing the gummy disease of fig, orange, and almond trees. **B. Hes'sii**, a species causing ropy state of milk. **B. hyacin'thi**, pathogenic b. from diseased hyacinth-bulbs. **B. line'ola**, non-pathogenic species from water, soil, and vegetables. **B. lu'teum**, species from water, producing orange-pigment. **B. merismopedio'ides**, a b. from the mud of sewage. **B. o'leæ**, a species causing disease of olives. **B. periplane'-tæ**, a species causing disease of cockroaches. **B. radicic'ola**, species found in soil and roots of leguminous plants: said to cause their growth. **B. rosa'ceum metallo'ides**, species producing gas in urine. **B. sulphu'reum**, a species found in urine and producing hydrogen sulphid. **B. ter'mo**, non-pathogenic species from healthy saliva. **B. tholoid'eum**, species from intestinal contents of healthy persons. **B. ul'na.** Same as *Bacillus ulna.* **B. ure'æ**, a non-pathogenic species from ammoniacal urine. **B. viola'ceum**, species from putrefying solutions of egg-albumen. **B. xyli'num**, species from solutions of carbohydrates, producing acetic acid.

Bacteriu'ria. The existence of bacteria in the urine.

Bac'teroid (bak'ter-oid). Resembling a bacterium.

Bael (bel). The dried fruit of *Æ'gle mar'melos*, or Bengal quince; used in diarrhea and dysentery.

Baer's vesicle (bārz). A Graafian follicle containing an ovum.

Bag. A sack or pouch. **Barnes's b.**, a lyre-shaped rubber bag for dilating uterine cervix. **Politzer's b.**, a soft bag of rubber for inflating the middle ear. **B. of waters**, the membranes enclosing the liquor amnii of the fetus.

Ba'ker-leg. Knock-knee.

Ba'kers' itch. Eczema of the hands from irritation of yeast. **B.'s salt**, ammonium carbonate. **B.'s stigmata**, callosities on the hands from kneading dough.

Bal'ance. 1. An instrument for weighing. 2. Harmonious adjustment of parts.

Balan'ic. Pertaining to the glans penis or glans clitoridis.

Bal'anism. Treatment with pessaries or suppositories.

Balani'tis (bal-an-i'tis). Inflammation of the glans penis.

Balanoblennorrhe'a. Gonorrheal balanitis.

Bal'anoplasty. Plastic surgery of the glans penis.

Balanoposthi'tis. Inflammation of the glans and prepuce.

Balanoprepu'tial. Pertaining to the glans and foreskin.

Balantid'ium co'li. A protozoan parasite in intestine of pigs and man, causing diarrhea.

Balbu'ties (bal-bu'she-ēz). Stammering.

Bald'ness. Lack of hair. See *Alopecia.*

Ball-and-socket joint. Same as *Enarthrosis.*

Ball thrombus. See *Thrombus.*

Balloon'ing. The distention of a cavity by air or otherwise.

Ballottement (bal-ŏt-maw'). Diagnosis of pregnancy by pushing the uterus with the finger inserted into the vagina, causing the embryo to rise and fall.

Balm. 1. A balsam. 2. A soothing or healing medicine. **B. of Gilead.** 1. Mecca balsam. 2. Canada balsam. 3. Resin of poplar buds.

Balneog'raphy. Treatise on baths.

Balneol'ogy. Science of baths.

Balneother'apy. Treatment of disease with baths.

Bal'neum, pl. *bal'nea.* A bath. **B. are'næ,** a sand-bath. **B. lu'teum,** a mud-bath.

Bal'sam (bawl'sam). A semifluid, fragrant, resinous, vegetable juice. **B.-apple,** plant *Momor' dica balsami' na,* with a purgative and vulnerary fruit. **B. of Mecca,** balsam from *Balsamoden'dron opobal' samum.* **B. of Peru,** balsam from *Toluif' era Perei'ræ:* expectorant, soothing, stimulant, and antiseptic. **B. of tolu,** a resinous, expectorant balsam from *Toluifera balsamum.*

Balsam'ic. Of the nature of balsam. **B. tincture,** compound tincture of benzoin.

Bal'ser's fatty necrosis. Fatty degeneration of pancreas, omentum, and mesentery.

Bam'berger's fluid. A mercurial compound for syphilis.

Ban'dage. A piece or strip of gauze or other fabric for wrapping any part or member. **Desault's b.,** a bandage for fractured clavicle. **Figure-of-8 b.,** a bandage in which the turns cross each other like a figure 8. **Hueter's b.,** a spica bandage for the perineum. **Langier's b.,** a many-tailed paper bandage. **Larrey's b.,** a many-tailed bandage with the edges glued together. **Maisonneuve's b.,** a plaster-of-Paris bandage made of folded cloth held in place by other bandages. **Martin's b's.,** India-rubber bandages for varicose veins. **Recurrent b.,** a bandage over the end of a stump. **Richet's b.,** plaster-of-Paris bandage to which gelatin has been added. **B. of Scultetus,** a bandage applied in strips overlapping each other in shingle fashion. **Suspensory b.,** a bandage for supporting the scrotum. **T.-bandage,** a bandage shaped like a letter **T.** **Theden's b.,** a roller bandage applied from below upward over a graduated compress to control hemorrhage. **Velpeau's b.,** a bandage to support the arm in fracture of the clavicle.

Ban'dl's ring. A thickening of the uterus above the internal os during labor.

Ban'dy-leg. Same as *Bow-leg.*

Bang. Same as *Cannabis indica.*

Ban'ting cure, Ban'tingism. Treatment of corpulence by diet.

Bap'tin. Aperient glucosid from *Baptisia tinctoria.*

Baptis'ia tincto'ria. Wild indigo, a plant of N. America: febrifugal, laxative, antiseptic.

Bap'tisin. Cathartic extractive of *Baptisia tinctoria.*

Baptitox'in. A poisonous alkaloid from *Baptisia tinctoria.*

Barba'does leg. Elephantiasis.

Barbalo'in. Aloin from Barbadoes aloes.

Bar'bary gum. Gum arabic from the Barbary provinces.

Bar berry. The *Berberis vulgaris* and its fruit. See *Berberis.*

Bar'bers' itch. Tinea sycosis.

Bar'botine. Barbary worm-seed.

Bar'egin. See *Glairin.*

Baresthesiom'eter. Instrument for estimating sense of weight or pressure.

Ba'ric. Pertaining to barium.

Baril'la. Impure sodium carbonate; pulverin.

Bar'ium. A metallic element, salts of which are medicinal.

Bark, Jesuits'. Popular name for cinchona.

Bar'kow's ligaments. The anterior and posterior ligaments of the elbow.

Bar'low's disease. Infantile scurvy.

Bar'nes's curve. The segment of a circle whose center is the sacral promontory, its concavity being backward. **B.'s dilators,**

caoutchouc bags used in inducing premature labor by dilating the cervix uteri.

Bar'ograph. A self-registering barometer.

Barom'eter. Instrument indicating the atmospheric pressure. **Aneroid b.**, one containing no mercury or other fluid.

Bar'oscope. A delicate or highly sensitive form of barometer.

Baros'ma. See *Buchu.*

Baros'min. Diuretic precipitate from buchu.

Bar'rel chest. A somewhat cylindrical form of thorax.

Bar'ren. Sterile; incapable of having offspring.

Bartholini'tis. Inflammation of Bartholin's glands.

Bar'tholin's duct. A duct of the sublingual gland. **B.'s glands**, the vulvovaginal glands.

Bar'ton's bandage. Double figure-of-8 bandage for lower jaw. **B.'s fracture**, fracture of lower end of radius.

Baru'ria. High specific gravity of urine.

Baryecoi'a. Dulness of hearing.

Baryglos'sia. Thickness of vocal utterance.

Baryla'lia. Same as *Baryglossia.*

Barypho'nia. Difficulty of utterance.

Bary'ta, Bary'tes. Poisonous oxid of barium.

Barythym'ia. Melancholy.

Ba'sad (ba'sad). Toward a basal aspect.

Ba'sal (ba'sal). Pertaining to a base. **B. ganglion**, the corpora striata and optic thalami.

Bascula'tion. Replacement of a retroverted uterus by swinging it into place.

Bas'cule movement. Systolic recoil of the heart.

Base. 1. The lower part of anything. 2. Main ingredient of a compound. 3. Non-acid part of a salt.

Bas'edow's disease. Same as *Exophthalmic goiter.*

Base'ment membrane. A delicate subepidermic or subepithelial layer.

Bas-fond (bah-fong') [Fr.]. A fundus, especially of the urinary bladder.

Bash'am's mixture. Same as *Liquor ferri et ammonii acetatis.*

Ba'sial. Pertaining to the basion.

Basiarachni'tis. Inflammation of the basal part of the arachnoid.

Basibregmat'ic axis. Vertical line from the basion to the bregma.

Ba'sic (ba'sik). Pertaining to, or having qualities of, a base. **B. salt**, a salt with excess of a basic element.

Basic'ity (ba-sis'it-e). The quality of being basic; power of combining with a base.

Basicra'nial axis. Straight line from the basion to the gonion.

Basid'ia. The reproductive organs of certain fungi.

Basifa'cial axis. Straight line from the gonion to the subnasal point.

Basihy'al, Basihy'oid. The body of the hyoid.

Bas'ilad. Toward the basilar aspect.

Bas'ilar. Pertaining to the base. **B. artery.** See *Arteries, Tables of.* **B. membrane**, the lower boundary of the scala media of the ear. **B. process**, a forward projection of the occipital bone. **B. suture**, suture between the basilar process of the occipital bone and the sphenoid.

Basilat'eral. Both basilar and lateral.

Basilem'ma. 1. Basement membrane. 2. Neuroglia.

Basil'ic vein. Large vein on inner aspect of arm.

Basil'icon ointment. Ceratum resinæ, or resin cerate.

Basil'ysis. The fracture of the base of the fetal skull in craniotomy.

Bas'ilyst. An instrument for performing a basilysis.
Basioccip'ital bone. Pertaining to the basilar process.
Basioglos'sus. Portion of hyoglossus attached to the base of the hyoid bone.
Ba'sion. The mid-point of anterior border of foramen magnum.
Basiot'ic bone. Small fetal bone between basisphenoid and basioccipital bones.
Ba'siotribe. An instrument for effecting basiotripsy.
Ba'siotripsy. Crushing of the head of the fetus.
Basirrhin'al fissure. A cerebral fissure at base of the olfactory lobe.
Ba'sis (ba'sis). Same as *Base*.
Basisphe'noid. An embryonic bone which becomes the back part of the body of the sphenoid.
Basisyl'vian fissure. Transverse basilar portion of Sylvian fissure.
Ba'sophil, Ba'sophilic, Basoph'ilous. Staining with alkaline dyes.
Basopho'bia. Morbid dread of walking.
Bass-deaf'ness. Deafness to low musical tones.
Bas'sora gum. A substance like gum arabic, from Persia.
Bas'sorin. A principle, $C_{12}H_{20}O_{10}$, found in tragacanth.
Bast. Inner bark of exogenous plants; used in surgery.
Ba'syl (ba'sil). An electropositive chemical element.
Bate'man's drops. Tinctura pectoralis; preparation of catechu, camphor, and opium.
Bath. Water or other medium in which the body is immersed for therapeusis or for cleansing. **Acid-b.**, bath containing nitric and hydrochloric acids. **Air-b.**, bath in which little water is used, the body being exposed to the air. **Alkaline b.**, bath containing potassium or sodium carbonate; used in skin-diseases. **Bog-b.**, a bath containing bog-earth. **Bran-b.**, bath containing boiled bran. **Brand b.**, the cold bath for treating typhoid fever. **Graduated b.**, one in which the temperature is gradually lowered. **Hip-b.** See *Sitz b.* **Mercurial b.**, bath in vapor of mercury for syphilis. **Mud-b.**, bath containing mud for rheumatism. **Russian b.**, a vapor bath. **Sand-b.**, immersion in warm, dry sand. **Sitz b.**, one in which the buttock and hips alone are immersed. **Sun-b.**, exposure to the sun's rays. **Turkish b.**, bath in which the person is placed successively in rooms of higher temperature, then rubbed and stimulated by a cold plunge.
Bath'mism. The force which controls growth and nutrition.
Batopho'bia. 1. Morbid dread of high objects. 2. Acrophobia.
Bat'rachoplasty. Plastic surgical operation for ranula.
Bat'rasin. Poison obtainable from the skin of toads.
Bat'tarism (bat'ar-izm). Stuttering or stammering.
Bat'tery. Series of cells affording galvanic currents.
Bat'tey's operation. Removal of healthy ovaries.
Bat'tledore placenta. Placenta with cord attached near edge.
Bat'tley's sedative. A mild opiate liquid preparation.
Baudelocque's diameter (bo-dloks'). External conjugate diameter of pelvis.
Bauhin's valve (bo-anz'). The ileocecal valve.
Baun'scheidtism (bown'shid'tism). Form of acupuncture by several short needles dipped in irritant liquid.
Bava'rian splint. An immovable dressing consisting of plaster of Paris between two flannel cloths.
Baycu'ru. The root of *Stat'ice brazilien'sis*: astringent.
Bay'onet-leg. Ankylosis of knee following backward displacement of tibia and fibula.
Bay'-rum. Same as *Spiritus myrciæ*.

Ba′zin (ba′zin). Molluscum contagiosum.
Bazin's disease (bah-zanz′). Psoriasis of the inside of the cheek.
Bdellepithe′cium. A tube used in leeching.
Bdel′lium. A myrrh-like gum-resin of various origin.
Bea′ker (be′ker). A form of glass cup used by chemists and apothecaries. **B.-cells.** Same as *Goblet-cells.*
Beal's fiber. A form of spiral nerve-fiber.
Bear′berry. Same as *Uva ursi.*
Bear′ing down. The expulsive effort of a parturient woman.
Beat (bēt). A throb, as of the heart or pulse. **Apex-b.,** the beat of the apex of the left ventricle of the heart against the chest-wall.
Bebeer′in. The alkaloid, $C_{18}H_{21}NO_3$, from bebeeru bark: tonic.
Bebee′ru. The greenheart tree, *Nectandra rodiæi,* of tropical America.
Bech′ic. 1. Relieving a cough. 2. A medicine for a cough.
Bech′terew's nucleus. The accessory auditory nucleus.
Béclard's hernia (ba-klahrz′). Femoral hernia at the saphenous opening.
Becquerel's gout pills (bek-relz′). Pills of colchicum, quinin, and digitalis.
Bed′bug. Same as *Cimex lectularius.*
Bed-case. Case of hysteria with voluntary and persistent lying in bed. **B.-pan,** a vessel for excreta, to be used in bed. **B.-sore,** gangrenous sore caused by long lying in bed.
Bed′nar's aphthæ. Aphthous ulceration of the hard palate of young children.
Beef-tea. An infusion of lean beef: nutrient and analeptic.
Beer. Fermented infusion of malted barley and hops.
Beer's knife. Knife with triangular blade for corneal incision.
Bees′wax. Wax from honey-comb. See *Cera.*
Beggiato′a (bej-e-at-o′ah). A species of water fungus.
Be′hen, oil of. Same as *Ben, oil of.*
Beh′ring's serum. Serum containing antitoxin of diphtheria.
Bei′gel's disease (bi′gelz). Hysterical chorea.
Be′læ fruc′tus. The fruit of *Ægle marmelos.* See *Bael.*
Belch′ing. Eructation of wind.
Belladon′na. The leaves and root of *Atropa belladonna:* poisonous, but much valued as a narcotic remedy. It affords atropin.
Belladon′nin. Alkaloid, $C_{17}H_{23}NO_3$, from belladonna.
Belli′ni's ducts. The ducti recti, or excretory ducts of the kidney.
Bell′-metal resonance. A metallic sound heard in pneumothorax.
Bellocq's cannula (bel-loks′). An instrument for plugging the posterior nares.
Bel′lows murmur. Bruit de soufflet.
Bell sound. Bell-metal resonance.
Bell's disease. Acute periencephalitis. **B.'s law,** the fact that anterior roots of spinal nerves are motor and posterior ones sensory. **B.'s nerves,** internal and external respiratory nerves. **B.'s paralysis,** facial paralysis of peripheral causation. **B.'s spasm.** Same as *Convulsive tic.*
Belly of muscle. The thick and non-tendinous part of a muscle.
Belonepho′bia. Insane dread of pins and needles.
Ben, oil of. Colorless oil from the seed of *Moringa pterygosperma.*
Ben′edikt's syndrome. Paralysis on one side of parts supplied by the third cranial nerve, with tremors of upper extremity on other side.
Beng. Same as *Cannabis indica.*
Benign (be-nin′). Not malignant; not recurrent.
Ben′ne oil (ben′e). Oil of sesamum.
Benza′cetin. Acetamidomethylsalicylate, used for neuralgia.

Benzal'dehyd. Bitter almond oil, colorless liquid, C_7H_6O.

Benzanal'gen. An antineuralgic and antiseptic, $C_{18}H_{16}N_2O_2$, from chinolin.

Benzan'ilid. A crystalline antipyretic, $C_6H_5NH(C_7H_5O)$.

Ben'zene. A liquid hydrocarbon, C_6H_6, from coal-tar.

Ben'zin, Benzi'num. A liquid obtained from petroleum: a solvent for rubber, fats, oils, etc.

Ben'zoate. Any salt of benzoic acid.

Ben'zoated. Charged with benzoic acid or benzoin.

Benzo'ic acid. See *Acid.*

Benzo'in. A resin from *Styrax benzoin:* expectorant, stimulant, and soothing.

Benzo'inated lard. Lard charged with benzoin.

Benzo'inol. Excipient and emollient oily liquid.

Ben'zol, Ben'zole. Same as *Benzene.*

Benzonaph'tol, Benzoyl naph'tol. An intestinal antiseptic, $C_{17}H_{12}O_2$, from beta-naphtol. **B. bismuth,** a combination of the above with bismuth.

Benzopheno'neid. A non-irritant germicide.

Benzosal'icin. A benzoyl derivative of salicin; populin.

Benzo'sol. A colorless powder, $C_{14}H_{12}O_3$: antipyretic and a creosote substitute.

Benzoyl-pseudotro'pein. A locally anesthetic alkaloid from coca. **B.-quin'in,** a benzoyl compound with local anesthetic properties. **B.-tropein,** a local anesthetic.

Bérard's aneurysm (ba-rahrz'). A varicose aneurysm whose sac is developed in the tissues surrounding the vein. **B.'s ligament,** the suspensory ligament of the pericardium. **B.'s valve,** a fold at the beginning of the nasolacrimal duct.

Ber'berin. An alkaloid, $C_{20}H_{17}NO_4$, from the bark of barberry; a useful tonic.

Ber'beris. A genus of shrubs. See *Barberry.*

Ber'gamot. The orange-like fruit of *Citrus bergamia;* its oil is used in perfumery.

Ber'gamot camphor, Bergap'tin. The stearaptene of bergamot oil, $C_{12}H_8O_4$.

Ber'genin (ber'je-nin). A crystalline nerve-tonic from saxifrage.

Ber'geron's disease. A hysterical form of chorea.

Ber'iberi. An endemic and infective form of polyneuritis, chiefly seen in Japan and India.

Berlin blue. Ferric ferrocyanid, $Fe_43Fe(C_6N_6)_2$.

Bernard's granular layer (ber-nards'). Stratum of cells lining the acini of the pancreas.

Bertillonage (ber-te-yo-nahzh'). The systematic measurement and recorded description of criminals.

Ber'tin's bones. Sphenoturbinal bones. **B.'s columns,** cortical substance between the pyramids of the kidney. **B.'s ligament,** the iliofemoral ligament.

Besoin de respirer (ba-zwan du res-pe-ra'). The sensation which prompts the act of breathing.

Bes'tiality. Sexual connection with an animal.

Bes'tucheff's tincture. Same as *Tincture ferri chloridi ætherea.*

Be'ta (be'tah). The genus of plants to which the beet belongs. **B.-naphtol.** See *Naphtol.*

Be'tacism. Excessive use of *b* sound in speaking.

Beta'in (be-ta'in). An emmenagogue alkaloid, $C_5H_{11}NO_2$, from beets.

Be'tel. A masticatory prepared from the nut of *Areca catechu,* lime, and betel-leaf. **B.-leaf,** the leaf of *Piper betel;* pan, or pawn.

Be'tin. A precipitate from beet-root: recommended as a substitute for ergot.

Be'tol. A compound, $C_{10}H_7O.C_7H_5O_2$, useful in rheumatism and cystitis.

Bet'ula. The genus which contains the birch trees.

Bet'ulin. A resin, $C_{36}H_{60}O_3$, from white-birch bark.

Bezo'ar. A concretion of various character from the stomachs of different animals: formerly highly valued as a medicine.

Bhang (bang). Same as *Cannabis indica.*

Bi. Symbol of bismuth.

Biaster'ic. Pertaining to the two asteria.

Biba'sic (bi-ba'sik). Doubly basic.

Bib'ulous paper. Paper having the property of absorbing moisture.

Bicar'bonate. A salt containing two equivalents of carbonic acid and one of a basic substance.

Bicau'dal, Bicau'date. Having two tails.

Bicel'lular (bi-sel'u-lar). Made up of two cells.

Biceph'alus (bi-sef'al-us). A two-headed monster.

Bi'ceps (bi'seps). Having two heads: said of a muscle of the arm and thigh. See *Muscles, Table of.*

Bichat's canal (be-shahz'). The small subarachnoid passage which transmits the veins of Galen. **B.'s fat-ball**, fatty mass behind the buccinator muscle. **B.'s fissure**, the cleft which separates the cerebrum from the cerebellum. **B.'s foramen**, foramen between subarachnoid space and third ventricle. **B.'s tunic**, the intima of blood-vessels.

Bichlo'rid. A chlorid containing two equivalents of chlorin.

Bicip'ital (bi-sip'it-al). Having two heads; pertaining to a biceps muscle. **B. tuberosity**, tuberosity beneath the neck of the radius.

Bicon'cave. Having two concave surfaces.

Bicon'vex. Having two convex surfaces.

Bicor'nute. Having two horns.

Bicoro'nial. Pertaining to the two coronia.

Bicus'pid, Bicus'pidate. Having two cusps or teeth.

Bidet (be-da') [Fr.]. A form of sitz bath-tub.

Bier'mer's sign (bēr'merz). See *Gerhardt's sign.*

Bifa'cial paralysis. See *Paralysis.*

Bi'fid (bi'fid). Cleft into two parts. **B. spine.** See *Spina bifida.* **B. tongue**, a tongue cleft lengthwise.

Bifo'cal spectacles. Spectacles having a reading lens cemented below the distance lens.

Bifo'rate. Having two holes or foramens.

Bifur'cate (bi-fer'kāt). Forked; divided into two like a fork.

Bifurca'tion. Division into two branches.

Big'elow's ligament. The iliofemoral ligament. **B.'s septum**, the calcar femorale.

Bigem'ina, Bigem'inal bodies. Embryonal structures which develop into the corpora quadrigemina. **B. pulse.** See *Pulse.*

Bigem'inum (bi-jem'in-um). A bigeminal body.

Bi'labe. An instrument for taking small calculi from the bladder through the urethra.

Bilat'eral. Having two sides; pertaining to both sides. **B. symmetry**, reversed symmetry like that which characterizes paired organs.

Bilat'eralism. Bilateral symmetry.

Bile (bil). The substance secreted by the liver; gall. **B. duct.** See *Duct.*

Bilhar'zia hæmato'bia. A fluke or trematode sometimes found in human blood-vessels.

Bilharzi'asis, Bilharzio'sis. Disease due to the presence of bilharzia.

Bil'iary (bil-e-a're). Pertaining to the bile. **B. acids**, taurocholic and glycocholic acids. **B. colic,** colic caused by gall-stones. **B. diabetes.** See *Hanot's disease.* **B. ducts.** See *Duct.*

Bilicy'anin. A blue pigment derivable from bilirubin.

Bilifica'tion. The formation or secretion of bile.

Bilifla'vin. A yellow pigment from biliverdin.

Biliful'vin. Same as *Bilirubin.*

Bilifus'cin. A dark principle from gall-stones.

Bilihu'min. A brown principle from gall-stones.

Bi'lin. A gummy substance, essentially mixture of sodium salts of the bile acids: it is the principal constituent of bile.

Bilineu'rin. Same as *Cholin.*

Bil'ious (bil'yus). Characterized by bile. **B. fever,** remittent fever with vomiting of bile. **B. remittent,** a form of remittent fever.

Bil'iousness. Malaise accompanied with seeming excess of bile.

Biliphe'in. A bile coloring-matter said to be the same as bilirubin.

Bilipra'sin. Green pigment from gall-stones.

Bilipur'pin, Bilipur'purin. A purple color from biliverdin.

Bilirn'bin. A red bile-pigment sometimes found in the urine.

Biliver'din. A green pigment, $C_{12}H_{20}N_2O_5$, from bilirubin.

Bill'roth's mixture (bil'rōt). Anesthetic mixture of 3 parts chloroform and 1 part each of ether and alcohol.

Bilo'bate, Bi'lobed. Having two lobes.

Bilob'ular. Having two lobules.

Biloc'ular. Having two compartments.

Biman'ual. With both hands.

Bimas'toid. Pertaining to both mastoid processes.

Bin'ary (bin'ar-e). Made up of two elements.

Binau'ral. Pertaining to both ears. **B. arc,** the arc across the top of the head from one aural point to another.

Binauric'ular. Pertaining to both auricles.

Bin'der (bin'der). Abdominal girdle for women in childbed.

Bind'web. Same as *Neuroglia.*

Binoc'ular. Pertaining to both eyes. **B. vision,** normal use of both eyes.

Binot'ic. Same as *Binaural.*

Binu'clear Binu'cleate. Having two nuclei.

Binu'cleolate. Having two nucleoli.

Bi'oblast. A corpuscle that has not yet become a cell.

Biochem'istry. Chemistry of living organisms.

Biodynam'ics. The doctrine or science of living force.

Bi'ogen (bi'o-jen). Same as *Bioplasm.*

Biogen'esis. The origination of living beings from things already living.

Biolog'ic, Biolog'ical. Pertaining to biology.

Biol'ogist. A professional student of biology.

Biol'ogy (bi-ol'o-je). The science of living organisms or of plant and animal life.

Biolyt'ic (bi-o-lit'ik). Destructive to life.

Biom'etry. Computation of probable duration of life.

Bi'on (bi'on). An individual living organism.

Bion'di's fluid. A histological stain of orange-G., methyl-green, and acid fuchsin.

Bion'omy. The science of the laws of life.

Bioph'agism, Bioph'agy. The eating or absorbing of living matter.

Bi'ophore (bi'o-fōr). One of the smallest particles exhibiting vital forces.

Biophysiol'ogy. Portion of biology including organogeny, morphology, and physiology.

Bi'oplasm. The more vital or essential part of protoplasm.

Bioplas'mic. Pertaining to bioplasm.

Bi'oplast (bi'o-plast). A living cell or bioplasmic particle.

Bior'bital angle. The angle between the lines of sight.

Bios'copy. Examination with respect to viability or to the extinction of life.

Biostat'ics. Static biology; the anatomy and physics of living bodies.

Biotax'is, Bi'otaxy. 1. The selecting and arranging powers of living cells. 2. Systematic classification of organisms.

Biot'ics. The science of the qualities of living organisms.

Biot'omy. Vivisection.

Bipalat'inoid. A gelatin capsule with two compartments.

Biparasit'ic. Living parasitically upon a parasite.

Bipari'etal diameter. Straight line between the two parietal eminences.

Bip'arous. Producing two at a birth.

Bipen'niform. Doubly feather-shaped.

Biper'forate (bi-per'fo-rāt). Twice perforated.

Bipo'lar. Having two poles; pertaining to both poles. **B. nerve-cells,** nerve-cells with two axis-cylinder processes.

Bipubiot'omy. Same as *Ischiopubiotomy.*

Birch. Any tree of the genus *Betula.* The tarry oil of *B. alba* (white birch) and the volatile oil of *B. lenta* are used in medicine.

Bird's-nest bodies. A set of peculiar cellular structures seen in epithelioma.

Birefrac'tive, Birefrin'gent. Doubly refractive.

Birth. Act or process of being born. **B.-mark,** congenital nevus; mother's mark. **B.-palsy,** palsy from injury occurring at birth.

Bisacro'mial. Pertaining to the two acromial processes.

Bis'cara button. Same as *Oriental sore.*

Bis'cuit, diabetic. A form of bran-cake for the use of diabetic patients.

Bisec'tion (bi-sek'shun). A cutting into two parts.

Bisex'ual. Pertaining to both sexes; hermaphrodite.

Bisfe'rious. Dicrotic; having two beats.

Bisil'iac. Pertaining to the two ilia.

Bis in d., Bis in die. Twice a day.

Bisischiat'ic. Pertaining to the two ischia.

Bis'kra button. Aleppo boil, or furunculus orientalis.

Bis'mark brown. A brown anilin dye used in microscopy.

Bis'muth. A silvery-white metallic element; symbol Bi: its salts are much used in medicine.

Bis'muthol. An antiseptic and astringent compound containing bismuth and salicylic acid.

Bismutho'sis. The absorption of bismuth and its deposits in the tissues.

Bistephan'ic. Pertaining to the two stephania.

Bis'tort. The plant *Polygonum bistorta;* root astringent.

Bis'toury. A long narrow surgical knife.

Bisul'phate. An acid sulphate; one with twice the proportion of acid found in a normal sulphate.

Bisvi'gum (bis-ve'gum). A concentrated food used in the French army.

Bitem'poral. Pertaining to both temples or temporal bones.

Bitrochanter'ic. Pertaining to both trochanters.

Bit'noben. An East Indian panacea containing salt, iron, and an astringent.

Bit'ter almond. See *Amygdala amara.* **B. elixir,** an aromatized wormwood preparation. **B. tincture,** an aromatic tincture of gentian and centaury; stomach drops. **B. wine of iron,** a solution of white wine, citrate of iron, quinin, and syrup.

Bit'ters. Medicines for increasing the tone of the gastro-intestinal mucous membrane. **Aromatic b.,** medicines having the properties of aromatics and simple bitters. **Simple b.,** medicines which simply stimulate the digestive tract. **Styptic b.,** medicine having styptic and astringent properties as well as those of bitters.

Bit'tersweet. Same as *Dulcamara.*

Bitu'men. Any one of various natural and artificial solid or dry petroleum products.

Biu'ret. A crystalline urea derivative, $C_2O_2N_3H_5$; used in testing for urea and proteids.

Biv'alent (biv'al-ent). Having a valency of two.

Bi'valve speculum. Speculum of two valves.

Biven'ter. A two-bellied muscle. See *Muscles, Table of.*

Biven'tral. Having two bellies; digastric.

Bix'in. An orange dye, $C_{16}H_{20}O_2$, from annatto.

Bizygomat'ic. Pertaining to the two zygomata.

Bizzoze'ro's corpuscles (bit-so-tsa'roz). Lymphoid cells of spleen and bone-marrow.

Black. Reflecting no light or true color; of the darkest hue. **B. alder.** Same as *Prinos.* **B. cancer,** melanotic cancer; melanosis. **B. death,** bubonic plague. **B. draught,** compound infusion of senna; infusum sennæ compositum. **B. drop,** vinegar of opium. **B.-head.** Same as *Comedo.* **B. measles,** measles, of severe type, with dark-hued eruption. **B. lead,** graphite or plumbago. **B. tongue,** glossophytia. **B. vomit,** the characteristic symptom of yellow fever. **B. wash,** lotion of calomel and lime-water for syphilis.

Black'berry. Fruit of various species of *Rubus.* See *Rubus.*

Black'water fever. A fatal infectious disease of tropical countries, with chills, irregular fever, dyspnea, vomiting, and jaundice.

Blad'der. The membranous sac which contains the urine. **Atony of b.,** inability to pass urine from deficient muscular power. **Catarrh of b.,** cystitis. **Extrophy of b.** See *Extropy.* **Irritable b.,** state of bladder marked by constant desire to urinate. **Neck of b.,** the narrowed portion continuous with the urethra. **Nervous b.,** condition with constant desire to urinate, but without power to do so completely. **Sacculated b.,** bladder with pouches between the hypertrophied muscular fibers. **Stammering b.,** a bladder which acts spasmodically, causing irregular urination. **B.-worm.** See *Cysticercus* and *Hydatid.* **B.-wrack.** Same as *Fucus vesiculosus.*

Blain'ville's ear. Congenital deformity in which the two ears are of different shape or size.

Blan'card's pills. Pills of iodid of iron.

Blandin's glands (blan-danz'). Same as *Nuhn's glands.*

Blaste'ma. Rudimentary substance from which cells, tissues, and organs are formed.

Blas'tid, Blas'tide. The first indication of a nucleus in a fertilized ovum.

Blas'tocele (blas'to-sēl), **Blastoce'le.** The cavity within a blastosphere.

Blastoce'lic. Pertaining to a blastocele.

Blas'tochyle (blas'to-kīl). Fluid within the blastosphere, or the blastodermic vesicle.

Blas'tocyst, Blastocys'tinx. The germinal vesicle.

Blas'toderm. The delicate membrane which lines the zona pellucida of the impregnated ovum.

Blastoder'mic membrane. The blastoderm. **B. rim,** the thickened edge of the germinal disk. **B. vesicle,** the sphere into which the impregnated ovum first expands.

Blasto'ma. A morbid growth due to a micro-organism.

Blas'tomere. Any cell or cell-mass of the blastoderm.

Blas'tophore (blas'to-fōr). That part of a sperm-cell that is not converted into spermatozoa.

Blastophyl'lum. A primitive germ-layer.

Blas'topore (blas'to-pōr). The small opening into the notochordal canal.

Blas'tosphere. The ovum after it has passed the morula-stage.

Blas'tula (blas'tu-lah). The blastosphere.

Blas'tular. Pertaining to a blastula.

Blastula'tion (blas-tu-la'shun). The formation of the blastula.

Blat'tic acid. A diuretic principle from cockroaches.

Bland's pills (blōz). Pills of ferrous carbonate.

Bleach'ing powder (blētsh'ing). Chlorinated lime: disinfectant.

Blear-eye. Marginal blepharitis; lippitudo.

Bleb. A bulla or skin-vesicle filled with fluid.

Blee'der (ble'der). 1. One who bleeds easily. 2. One who lets blood.

Blee'der's disease. Hemophilia; hemorrhagic diathesis.

Blennorrha'gia, Blennorrhe'a. 1. Free discharge of mucus. 2. Gonorrhea.

Blennorrhe'al. Same as *Gonorrheal.*

Blennotho'rax. Mucus in the chest.

Blennu'ria (blen-u're-ah). Mucus in the urine.

Blepharadeni'tis. Inflammation of the Meibomian glands.

Bleph'aral. Pertaining to the eyelids.

Bleph'arism (blef'ar-izm). Spasm of the eyelid.

Blephari'tis (blef-ar-i'tis). Inflammation of the eyelids. **B. cilia'ris**, inflammation of the hair-follicles of the eyelids. **B. margina'lis**, inflammation of the margins of the eyelids. **B. ulcero'sa**, an ulcerous form of marginal blepharitis.

Blepharo-adeno'ma. Adenoma of the margins of the eyelids.

Blepharo-athero'ma. Encysted tumor of an eyelid.

Blepharochromidro'sis. Discoloration of the eyelid in patches.

Blepharophimo'sis. Narrowing of the slit between the eyelids.

Bleph'aroplasty (blef'ar-o-plas-te). Plastic surgery of an eyelid.

Blepharople'gia (blef-ar-o-ple'je-ah). Paralysis of an eyelid.

Blepharopto'sis. Drooping of the upper eyelid from paralysis.

Blepharor'rhaphy. Surgical closure of the slit between the eyelids.

Bleph'arospasm. Spasm of the orbicular muscle of the eyelids.

Bleph'arostat. An instrument for holding the eyelids apart.

Blepharosteno'sis. Narrowing of the palpebral slit.

Blepharosyne'chia. Growing together of the eyelids.

Blepharot'omy. Surgical cutting of an eyelid.

Bles'sed thistle. Same as *Carduus benedictus.*

Blind. Not having the sense of sight. **B.-spot**, the spot on the retina where the optic nerve enters.

Blind'ness. Lack or loss of sight. **Blue-b.**, color-blindness for blue. **Color-b.**, inability to appreciate differences of color. It may be *complete* or *partial*. **Cortical b.**, blindness due to lesion of cortical visual center. **Day-b.**, vision which is better by night than by day. **Mind-b.** Same as *Psychic b.* **Night-b.**, defect of vision in the dark or at night. **Object-b.**, apraxia. **Psychic b.**, blindness from brain-lesion. **Red-b.**, blindness to red tints. **Snow-b.**, dimness of vision due to glare of the sun upon snow. **Soul-b.** Same as *Psychic b.* **Word-b.**, inability to recognize written words as symbols of ideas.

Blink'ing. The act of winking.

Blis'ter. 1. Collection of serous, bloody, or watery fluid under the skin. 2. An epispastic agent. **Fly-b.,** blister of cantharides. **Flying b.,** a blister applied long enough to produce redness, but not vesication.

Blis'tering cerate. Cantharidal cerate. **B. collodion,** cantharidal collodion. **B. liquid,** liniment of cantharides. **B. paper,** paper saturated with cantharides.

Blood. The fluid which circulates through the heart, arteries, and veins. **B.-casts,** microscopic threads of blood in urine. **B.-cell,** a blood-corpuscle. **B.-clot,** a coagulum of blood. **B.-corpuscles, red,** the biconcave floating disks found in blood. **B.-corpuscles, white,** the leukocytes or ameboid protoplasmic blood-cells. **B.-crasis,** the mixture of the constituents of the blood. **B.-crystals,** crystals of hematoidin in the blood. **B.-cyst.** See *Hematocyst.* **B.-disk,** a blood-platelet. **B.-islands,** groups of corpuscles in the mesoblast in early fetal life. **B.-plaques.** Same as *B.-platelets.* **B.-plasma,** the colorless fluid of the blood; liquor sanguinis. **B.-platelets,** disks found in the blood, less than half the size of the red blood-corpuscles. **B.-poisoning,** toxemia. **B.-pressure,** tension on the walls of blood-vessels, derived from the blood-currents. **B.-tumor,** a hematoma; also an aneurysm. **B.-vessel,** an artery, vein, or sinus.

Blood'less operation. Surgical operation in which the blood is expelled and kept out of the part to be operated upon.

Blood'letting. Therapeutic withdrawal of blood. **General b.,** venesection. **Local b.,** cupping, leeching, or scarification.

Blood'root. See *Sanguinaria.*

Blood'shot. Congested with blood.

Blood'y flux. Dysentery. **B. sweat,** hematidrosis.

Blow'ing respiration. Same as *Bruit de soufflet.*

Blue baby. An infant affected with cyanosis. **B.-blindness,** inability to distinguish the color blue. **B. disease,** cyanosis. **B. edema.** See *Edema.* **B. flag,** the plant *Iris versicolor.* **B.-gum,** the *Eucalyptus globulus,* an Australian tree. **B.-mass,** mass of mercury. **B.-ointment,** mercurial ointment. **B.-pill,** blue-mass in the form of pills. **B.-stone, B.-vitriol,** sulphate of copper.

Blunt'-hook. A hook used in embryotomy.

Bo'as's reagent. Resorcin, 5; sugar, 3; dilute alcohol, 100 parts; for testing for hydrochloric acid in gastric juice.

Boat'-belly. Same as *Scaphoid abdomen.*

Boch'dalek's ganglion. A node at junction of the anterior and middle dental nerves.

Bo'do. A genus of protozoans: endoparasitic and probably pathogenic.

Bod'y (bod'e). 1. Any mass of matter. 2. The trunk. **Amylaceous b's.** See *Corpora amylacea.* **B.-cavity.** See *Celom.* **Cavernous b's.,** the corpora cavernosa. **Ciliary b.,** that part of the vascular coat of the eye including the ciliary muscle and processes. **Dentate b.** See *Corpus dentatum.* **Foreign b.,** a body which is not normal to the place where it is found. **Geniculate b.** See *Corpus geniculatum.* **Highmore's b.,** the mediastinum testis. **Hyaloid b.** Same as *Vitreous b.* **Laveran's b's.,** plasmodia of malaria. **B.-louse.** See *Pediculus corporis.* **Malpighian b's.,** small bodies in the kidney at the commencement of the uriniferous tubules. **Olivary b's.,** oval prominences on the sides of the anterior pyramids of the medulla oblongata. **Pacchionian b's.,** small eminences of arachnoid tissue under the dura mater of the brain. **Pituitary b.,** a reddish body in a depression of the sphenoid bone. **Polar**

b., two small bodies protruded from the ovum at time of impregnation. **Restiform b.**, lateral column of medulla oblongata extending to cerebellum. **Rosenmüller's b.**, the parovarium. **Suprarenal b.**, a flat, triangular organ on the upper side of the kidney. **Vitreous b.**, the transparent substance contained in a hyaloid membrane between the lens and the retina. **Wolffian b's.**, the primitive kidney or excretory organ of the embryo.

Bog'gy swelling. One that is soft and puffy.

Bo'hun upas. The *Antiaris toxicaria*, poison-tree of Java; also its deadly gum-resin.

Boil. See *Furuncle*, *Aleppo boil*.

Boiler-makers' deafness. See *Deafness*.

Bol'din. Anesthetic and hypnotic alkaloid of boldo.

Bol'do. Leaves of *Boldoa fragrans*, a tree of Chili: tonic and sedative. **B., oil of**, volatile oil, useful in catarrhal states.

Boldoglu'cin. Narcotic glucosid from boldo.

Bol'dus. Same as *Boldo*.

Bole (bōl). A name for various earths, formerly valued as medicines.

Bole'tus. A genus of agarics, some of them poisonous: several were once esteemed as remedies.

Bo'lus. A large pill. **Alimentary b.**, the mass of food made ready by mastication for swallowing.

Bon'duc. Seeds of two species of *Guilandina*: antiperiodic and stimulant.

Bone. The material of the skeleton of most vertebrate animals. (For varieties of bones, see the adjectives.) **B.-cartilage.** Same as *Ossein*. **B.-conduction**, the perception of sound through the bones of the head. **B.-cyst**, a cystic tumor of a bone.

Bone'let. An ossicle or small bone.

Bone'set. See *Eupatorium perfoliatum*.

Bone'setter. A non-authorized person who professes skill in reducing fractures and luxations.

Bon'net's capsule. Same as *Tenon's capsule*.

Borac'ic acid (bo-ras'ik). See *Acid*.

Bo'ral. Aluminum borotartrate; astringent and antiseptic.

Bo'rate. Any salt of boric acid.

Bo'rated. Containing borax or boric acid.

Bo'rax. A refrigerant, soothing, and diuretic salt; sodium pyroborate. **B.-carmin**, a solution of borax and carmin in water: used as a stain.

Borboryg'mus. The noise made by flatus in the bowels.

Bo'ric acid. See *Acid*.

Bo'rism. Poisoning by a boron compound.

Bor'neene. Valerene, readily convertible into borneol.

Bor'neo camphor. A peculiar camphor from Borneo.

Bor'neol. $C_{10}H_{18}O$; artificial Borneo camphor.

Borobo'rax. An antiseptic preparation of borax and boric acid.

Boroglyc'erid (bo-ro-glis'er-id). Antiseptic paste of boric acid and glycerin.

Boroglyc'erol (bo-ro-glis'er-ol). Liquid formed of boroglycerid and glycerin.

Bo'ron. Non-metallic element, the base of borax and boric acid.

Borophe'nol. Borax and carbolic acid combination; disinfectant.

Borosalicyl'ic acid. An antiseptic preparation of borax and salicylic acid.

Boss. A roundish eminence.

Bos'selated. Covered with bosses or knobs.

Bossela'tion. One of a set of small elevations or bosses.

Bot. The larva of a gad-fly, often found in the stomach of a horse.

Bot'alism (bot'a-lizm). Sausage-poisoning.

Botal'lo's duct. The ductus arteriosus. **B.'s foramen,** the foramen ovale. **B.'s ligament,** a persistent relic of the ductus arteriosus.

Bothrioceph'alus la'tus. The most common tapeworm of man found in European countries.

Botriotherapeu'tics, Botryother'apy. Grape-cure.

Bot'ryoid (bot're-oid). Shaped like a bunch of grapes.

Bött'cher's annuli (bet'kerz). Ring-shaped meshes in the lamina over the organ of Corti. **B.'s crystals,** little crystals produced by treating prostatic fluid with ammonium phosphate.

Bot'tle-nose. Acne rosacea, with hypertrophy of the nose.

Botulin'ic acid. A principle found in putrid sausage.

Bot'ulism (bot'u-lizm). Sausage-poisoning.

Bouchard's nodules (boo-sharz'). Nodules seen on the fingers and toes of patients with gastrectasis.

Bouchut's tubes (boo-shuz'). Tubes for intubation.

Bougard's paste (boo-garz'). Caustic paste for cancer.

Bou'gie (boo'zhe). An instrument for introduction into the urethra or other natural orifice to dilate it. **B. à boule,** a bulbous b. **Armed b.,** a b. with a piece of caustic attached to its end. **Bulbous b.,** a b. with a bulb-shaped top. **Filiform b.,** a b. of very small diameter. **Soluble b.,** b. composed of matter that will dissolve at the temperature of the body.

Bouillon (boo-yon'). Soup or broth prepared from meat. **B.-culture,** a bacteriological culture of which bouillon is the basis.

Boul'ton's solution (bōl'tnz). Liquor iodi carbolatus: an iodin and carbolic-acid preparation.

Bouquet (boo-ka'). The characteristic flavor and aroma of a wine.

Bourdin's paste (boor-danz'). An escharotic mixture of nitric acid and flowers of sulphur.

Bourdonnement (boor-dŏn-maw'). A buzzing or humming sound.

Boutonnière operation (boo-tŏn-yăr'). Incision through perineum behind the place of an impervious stricture.

Bo'vine heart. Same as *Cor bovinum*. **B. lymph,** vaccine virus from a heifer.

Bo'vinine. A proprietary medicated meat-juice preparation.

Bovis'ta. A fungus used as a styptic and in nervous diseases.

Bow'el. The gut or intestine.

Bow-leg. Outward curve at or below the knee.

Bow'man's capsule. Same as *Malpighian's capsule*. **B.'s disks,** discoid plates in striated muscular fiber. **B.'s glands,** tubular glands of the olfactory mucous membrane. **B.'s lamina. B.'s membrane,** the basement membrane which underlies the corneal epithelium. **B.'s muscle,** the ciliary muscle. **B.'s probe,** a probe for dilating the lacrimal duct.

Boy'er's bursa. Subhyoid bursa. **B.'s cyst,** cyst of Boyer's bursa.

Boyle's law. Volume of a gas varies inversely with the pressure.

Boze'man's catheter. Double-current uterine catheter.

Br. Symbol of *Bromin*.

Bra'chial (bra'ke-al). Pertaining to the arm. **B. artery,** extension of the axillary artery on the inner side of the arm. **B. glands,** lymphatic glands of the arm. **B. plexus,** nerve plexus supplying the upper extremity. **B. veins,** veins of the arm accompanying the brachial artery.

Brachial'gia (bra-ke-al'je-ah). Pain in the arm.

Brach'inin. A principle from a beetle, *Brachinus crepitans*: used in rheumatism.

Brachiocephal'ic. Pertaining to the arm and head.

Brachiocru'ral. Pertaining to arm and leg.

Brachiofa'cial. Pertaining to arm and face.

Brachioradia'lis. Supinator longus muscle.

Brachiot'omy. The surgical cutting or removal of an arm.

Bra'chiplex. The brachial plexus.

Bra'chium (bra'ke-um), pl. *bra'chia.* 1. The arm. 2. Any one of certain white tracts of the brain.

Brach-Romberg symptom. See *Romberg's symptom.*

Brachycar'dia. Same as *Bradycardia.*

Brachycephal'ic, Brachyceph'alous. Having a head with a short anteroposterior diameter.

Brachyceph'alism, Brachyceph'aly. The quality or fact of being brachycephalic.

Brachygna'thia. Abnormal shortness of the under jaw.

Brachymetro'pia. Myopia; near-sightedness.

Brachymetrop'ic. Myopic; near-sighted.

Bradyar'thria. Abnormal slowness in vocal articulation.

Bradycar'dia. Abnormal slowness of the pulse.

Bradydiasto'lia. Abnormal prolongation of the diastole.

Bradyecoi'a. Partial deafness.

Bradyesthe'sia (bra-de-es-the'ze-ah). Dulness of perception.

Bradyla'lia. Slow utterance due to a central lesion.

Bradypep'sia. Abnormally slow digestion.

Bradypha'sia. Slow utterance from central lesion.

Bradyphra'sia. Slowness of speech due to mental defect.

Bradysper'matism. Abnormally slow ejaculation of semen.

Bradyu'ria. Slow discharge of urine.

Braid'ism (bra'dizm). Hypnotism.

Brain. The nervous mass within the skull. **B.-fag,** exhaustion from overwork of the brain. **B.-fever,** cerebritis or cerebral meningitis. **B.-sand.** See *Acervulus cerebri.* **B.-storm,** sudden and severe cerebral disturbance. **B.-tire,** brain exhaustion from excessive functional activity.

Bran bath. See *Bath.*

Bran'chial (brang'ke-al). Pertaining to, or resembling, gills. **B. arches.** See *Arch.* **B. clefts** or **openings,** a series of clefts which lie between the branchial arches.

Branchiog'enous (brang-ke-oj'en-us). Derived from a branchial cleft.

Branchiom'erism. Metameric division of the entoderm.

Brand bath. See *Bath.*

Bran'dy. Alcoholic stimulant from wine; spiritus vini.

Bras'dor's operation. Distal ligation of an artery near the aneurysm.

Brash. Burning sensation in the stomach; pyrosis.

Brass-founders' disease. Chronic poisoning to which workers in brass-foundries are liable.

Braw'ny induration. An inflammatory hardening and thickening of tissues.

Braye'ra. The flowers and tops of *Brayera anthelmintica.* See *Kousso.*

Bra'yerin. An anthelmintic resin from brayera.

Bread-crumb. Bread used as a vehicle in making pills. **B.-paste,** a culture-medium prepared from bread.

Breadth-feeling. That element in vision by which breadth is perceived.

Break. Interruption of an electric current. See *Make.*

Break-bone fever. Dengue.

Breast. 1. The thorax, and chiefly its anterior aspect. 2. The mamma. **B.-bone,** the sternum. **Broken b.,** abscess of mammary gland. **Chicken b.,** a deformity consisting of prominence of the sternum. **Gathered b.,** mammary abscess. **B.-pang.** Same as *Angina pectoris.* **B.-pump,** apparatus for drawing milk from the mammary gland.

Breath. Air taken in and expelled from the lungs. **B.-sounds,** breathing-sounds heard on auscultation.

Breath'ing. See *Respiration.* **Abdominal b.,** breathing performed by the abdominal muscles and diaphragm. **B. capacity,** the air that can be expelled from the lungs after a full inspiration. **Interrupted b.,** an interrupted breathing from nervousness or irregular contraction of muscles. **Puerile b.,** breathing with exaggerated respiratory murmur, as in the normal breathing of children. **Suppressed b.,** entire absence of breath-sounds. **Thoracic b.,** respiration in which the thoracic walls are actively moved.

Breech. The buttock. **B.-presentation,** presentation of the breech or sacrum in labor.

Breeze, static. See *Static breeze.*

Breg'enin. A principle, $C_{40}H_{87}NO_6$, derivable from the brain.

Breg'ma. Junction of coronal and sagittal sutures.

Bregmat'ic. Pertaining to the bregma.

Breis'ky's disease. Kraurosis vulvæ.

Breschet's veins (bra-shāz'). Four veins of the diploe.

Brew'ers' yeast (bru'erz). Ferment obtained in brewing beer; used as a stimulant and in poultices.

Brick-dust deposit. Reddish sediment of urates in urine.

Brick-layers' itch. Prurigo on the hands of brick-layers.

Brick-makers' disease. Ankylostomiasis.

Bri'dle. A fold or band across a canal or ulcer. **B. stricture,** stricture formed by a band across the urethra.

Bright'ic (brit'ik). 1. Affected with Bright's disease. 2. One who is ill of Bright's disease.

Bright's disease (brits). Any kidney-disease with albuminuria.

Brim. The edge of the superior strait of the pelvis.

Brim'stone. Sulphur.

Briquet's ataxia (bre-kāz'). Hysterical ataxia.

Brisement forcé (brēz-maw for-sa'). The forcible breaking up of an ankylosis.

Brise-pierre (brēz-pe-ār'). An instrument for breaking stones in the bladder.

Bris'tle cells. Ciliary cells in the distribution of the auditory nerve.

Brit'ish gum. Same as *Dextrin.*

Broad ligament. 1. Double layer of peritoneum which supports the uterus. 2. The suspensory ligament of the liver.

Bro'ca's area. Patch of gray matter between the middle olfactory root and the peduncle of the callosum. **B.'s center,** the speech-center. **B.'s convolution,** third left frontal convolution. **B.'s point,** the auricular point.

Bro'die's abscess (bro'dēz). Circumscribed abscess of the head of a bone. **B.'s disease, B.'s joint, B.'s knee,** a form of chronic synovitis.

Bro'kaw ring. A ring for intestinal anastomosis, made of portion of rubber tube threaded with catgut.

Bro'ken breast. Mammary abscess.

Bro'mal. Poisonous hypnotic liquid, $CBr_3.CHO$. **B. hydrate,** an oily liquid, $CBr_3CHO + H_2O$, resembling chloral hydrate.

Bro'malin. A formal and bromin compound, serviceable in epilepsy.

Bromalo'in. A derivative containing bromin and barbaloin.

Broman'id. An antipyretic and analgesic.

Bro'mate. Any salt of bromic acid.

Bro'mated. Charged with bromin.

Bro'melin. Ferment from pine-apples.

Brometh'yl. Same as *Ethyl-bromid.*

Bromethyl-for'malin. Same as *Bromalin.*

Bro'mic acid. The compound $HBrO_3$.

Bro'mid. Any binary compound of bromin. Several bromids are useful in epilepsy.

Bromid'ia. Proprietary anodyne and hypnotic.

Bromidrosipho'bia. Morbid delusions as to bodily odors.

Bromidro'sis (bro-mid-ro'sis). Fetid sweating.

Bro'min (bro'min). A reddish-brown liquid element, giving off a suffocating vapor. Its salts are used as sedatives.

Bro'minism. Bro'mism. Poisoning by bromin or a bromid.

Bromocaf'fein. Proprietary bromin and caffein preparation.

Bro'moform. A formyl bromid, $CHBr_3$, anesthetic and antispasmodic.

Bromo-i'odism. Poisoning by bromids and iodids.

Bro'mol (bro'mol). Tribromphenol; caustic and antiseptic.

Bromoma'nia. Insanity from misuse of bromids.

Bromophe'nol. A liquid used to make an ointment for erysipelas.

Bro'mum (bro'mum). Same as *Bromin.*

Bron'chi (brong'ki), pl. of *bronchus.*

Bron'chia (brong'ke-ah). The bronchial tubes smaller than the bronchi.

Bron'chial (brong'ke-al). Pertaining to the bronchia. **B. fluke,** distoma Ringeri. **B. gland,** lymphatic glands along the bronchi. **B. crises.** See *Crisis.* **B. respiration.** See *Respiration.*

Bronchiarc'tia. Stenosis of the bronchial tubes.

Bronchiec'tasis. Dilatation of bronchia.

Bron'chiole (brong'ke-ōl). A minute bronchial tube.

Bronchioli'tis. Inflammation of the bronchioles. **B. exudati'va,** a form with exudation.

Bronchiosteno'sis. Same as *Brachiactia.*

Bronchit'ic. Pertaining to bronchitis.

Bronchi'tis (brong-ki'tis). Inflammation of the bronchial tubes. **Capillary b.,** inflammation of the minuter bronchial tubes. **Catarrhal b.,** a form with profuse mucopurulent discharge. **Fibrinous** or **Plastic b.,** bronchitis with expectorated casts of fibrin. **Mechanic b.,** variety caused by inhalation of particles, dust, etc. **Putrid b.,** chronic b. with offensive sputum.

Bronchocav'ernous. Both bronchial and cavernous.

Bron'chocele (brong'ko-sēl). Same as *Goiter.*

Bronchoegoph'ony. Same as *Egobronchophony.*

Bron'cholith (bron'ko-lith). Bronchial calculus.

Bronchomyco'sis. Bronchial disease due to microbes.

Bronchop'athy (brong-kop'ath-e). Disease of the air-passages.

Bronchoph'ony (brong-kof'o-ne). The sound of the voice as heard through the stethoscope applied over a healthy bronchus. **Whispered b.,** bronchophony with the patient whispering.

Bron'choplasty (brong'ko-plas-te). Plastic surgery of the trachea.

Bronchopneumo'nia (brong-ko-nu-mo'ne-ah). Inflammation of the lungs and bronchia; lobar pneumonia.

Bronchopul'monary. Pertaining to the bronchi and lungs.

Bronchorrha'gia. Hemorrhage from the bronchi.

Bronchorrhe'a. Bronchitis with profuse expectoration.

Bron'chotome (brong'ko-tōm). A cutting instrument used in bronchotomy.

Bronchot'omy. Surgical cutting of the trachea or of a bronchus.

Bronchotra'cheal. Pertaining to the bronchi or trachea.

Bronchovesic'ular. Bronchial and vesicular.

Bron'chus (brong'kus). Either one of the two main branches of the trachea; the trachea itself.

Bronzed skin. A symptom of Addison's disease.

Brood-cell. A mother-cell containing daughter-cells.
Broom. Same as *Scoparius*.
Brow'ache. Supra-orbital neuralgia.
Brow-presentation. Presentation of brow of fetus in labor.
Brown atrophy. Atrophy with brown discoloration. **B. induration,** induration and pigmentation of lung from long-continued congestion. **B. mixture,** compound mixture of licorice.
Brown'ian movement. Oscillatory movements seen under the microscope in fine particles suspended in a liquid.
Brown-Séquard's disease or **paralysis.** Paralysis of motion on one side of the body with paralysis of sensation on the other.
Bruch's glands (brooks). Lymph-follicles of the conjunctiva of the lower eyelid. **B.'s membrane,** inner layer of the choroid coat of the eye.
Bru'cin (bru'sin). A poisonous alkaloid, $C_{23}H_{26}N_2O_4$, from nux vomica.
Bruissement (broo-ees-maw') [Fr.]. Same as *Purring tremor*.
Bruit (broo-e'). A sound or murmur, especially an abnormal one. **Aneurysmal b.,** blowing sound heard over an aneurysm. **B. d'airain,** metallic pectoral tinkling. **B. de clapotement,** splashing sound heard in dilatation of the stomach. **B. de craquement,** crackling pericardial sound. **B. de diable,** buzzing venous murmur in anemia. **B. de drapeau,** rustling sound heard in croup and laryngitis. **B. de froissement,** a clashing sound. **B. de galop,** galloping sound in mitral stenosis. **B. de lime,** a filing cardiac murmur. **B. de moulin,** water-wheel sound in certain pericardial affections. **Placental b.,** blowing sound in pregnant uterus caused by fetal circulation. **B. de pot fêlé,** cracked-pot sound, pathognomonic of certain lung-cavities. **B. de rappel,** sound of a drum, due to delayed mitral murmur. **B. de scie,** a cardiac sawing sound. **B. skodique.** Same as *Skodaic tympany*. **B. de soufflet,** a bellows sound of the heart.
Brun'ner's glands. Tubuloracemose duodenal follicles.
Bruno'nianism. The obsolete theory of J. Brown, that all diseases are due to excess or lack of stimulus.
Brush-burn. A wound produced by friction and resembling a burn.
Bryce's test. Revaccination as a test for vaccination.
Bryo'nia. Root of *Bryonia alba*: very active poison, medicinal in various diseases.
Bry'onin. Poisonous glucosid, $C_{48}H_{80}O_{19}$, from bryonia.
Bryore'tin. A resin obtainable from bryonia.
Bu'bo. Inflammatory swelling, especially of the inguinal glands. **Gonorrheal b.,** b. developing in gonorrhea. **Indolent b.,** a syphilitic b. with no tendency to break down. **Parotid b.,** parotitis. **Pestilential b.,** b. associated with plague. **Primary b.** See *Bubon d'emblée*. **Sympathetic b.,** b. due to friction and injury. **Syphilitic b.,** one due to syphilis. **Venereal b.,** one due to venereal disease.
Bubon d'emblée. Venereal bubo without preceding symptom.
Bubon'ic. Characterized by, or pertaining to, buboes. **B. plague,** the oriental plague. See *Plague*.
Bubon'ocele (bu-bon'o-sēl). Incomplete inguinal hernia.
Buc'cal (buk'al). Pertaining to the mouth.
Buccella'tion. Arrest of hemorrhage by a lint-pad.
Buccinatolabia'lis. The buccinator and orbicularis oris together.
Buc'cinator (buk'sin-a-tor). Flat muscle of the cheek.
Buc'cula. Double chin.
Bu'chu (bu'ku). The leaves of *Barosma*, having diuretic properties, and used in genito-urinary diseases.

Buck'bean. The plant *Menyanthes trifoliata:* tonic and stomachic.
Buck'eye. Popular name for various species of *Æsculus.*
Buck'horn. A fern, *Osmunda regalis:* popular remedy for rickets.
Buck'thorn. See *Rhamnus;* also *Frangula.*
Buck's extension. A variety of extension for fractured leg. **B.'s fascia,** the superficial perineal fascia.
Bucne'mia. Inflammatory disease of the leg.
Bud'ding (bud'ing). See *Germination.*
Budge's center (budj'). Genitospinal center.
Buf'fy coat. Buff-colored stratum on the surface of a blood-clot.
Bu'fidin. A poison obtainable from certain toads.
Buhl's disease (boolz). Jaundice of the new-born.
Bu'lam boil, Bulam'a boil. A chronic sore, endemic in West Africa, said to be caused by an insect larva.
Bulb. 1. Any rounded mass. 2. The oblongata. **B. of the aorta,** foremost of the divisions of the primitive embryonic cardiac vessel. **B. of corpus cavernosum,** enlarged muscular and proximal part of the cavernous body. **Dental b.,** the dentinal papilla. **B. of the eye,** the eyeball. **Gustatory b.** See *Taste-bulb.* **Hair-b.,** bulbous expansion of lower end of hair. **Olfactory b.,** the bulb-like extremity of the olfactory nerve on the under surface of each anterior lobe of the cerebrum. **Taste-b.'s,** end organs of gustatory nerve in papillæ of tongue. **B. of urethra.** the proximal part of the corpus spongiosum. **B. of vestibule.** See *Bulbus vestibuli.*
Bul'bar. Pertaining to a bulb.
Bulbocaverno'sus. The accelerator urinæ muscle.
Bulbo-ure'thral. Pertaining to the bulb of the urethra.
Bul'bous. Resembling a bulb. **B. nerves,** nerves with swollen ends in a stump. **B. urethra.** See *Urethra.*
Bul'bus arterio'sus. The bulb of the aorta. **B. vestib'uli,** the vulvovaginal gland.
Bulim'ia. Insatiable appetite.
Bulim'ic. Affected with bulimia.
Bul'la. A bleb, or cutaneous vesicle.
Bul'late (bul'āt). Inflated; bladdery.
Bulla'tion. Inflation; inflated condition.
Bull-dog forceps. Strong forceps with teeth and a clasp.
Bull'et probe. A probe for locating bullets.
Bul'lous (bul'us). Pertaining to a bulla.
Bul'piss. A parasitic, papular skin-disease peculiar to Nicaragua.
Bundle of Vicq d'Azyr. A bunch of white fibers around the base of the anterior nucleus of optic thalamus. **Respiratory b.,** the solitary fasciculus. See *Fasciculus.*
Bun'ion (bun'yun). A swelling of the bursa mucosa at the ball of the great toe.
Buphthal'mia, Buphthal'mus. Enlargement of the eye: keratoglobus.
Bur'dach's columns. Posterior and outer columns of the spinal cord. **B.'s fissure,** cleft between the lateral surface of the insula and inner surface of the operculum.
Bur'dock. Popular name of *Lappa.*
Burette (bu-ret'). A graduated tube used in chemical work.
Bur'gundy pitch. Same as *Pix Burgundica.*
Burn. A lesion caused by undue heat.
Burns's amaurosis. Dimness of sight caused by sexual excesses. **B.'s ligament,** a falciform expansion of the fascia lata.
Burnt-sponge. Sponge charred and powdered: used in goiter and tuberculosis.
Bur'rowing. The formation of passages or tracts containing pus.
Bur'sa (ber'sah), pl. *bur'sæ.* A sac or pouch. **Boyer's b.,** bursa beneath hyoid bone. **Fleischmann's b.,** the sublingual bursa.

Gluteal b., either of three bursæ beneath gluteus maximus muscle. **Luschka's b.** Same as *B. pharyngea*. **B. muco'sa,** any membranous sac which secretes synovia. **B. pharyn'gea,** a recess in the pharynx of a fetus and young infant. **Popliteal b.**, a b. in the popliteal space beneath the tendon of the semimembranosus and the tendon of the inner head of the gastrocnemius. **Prepatellar b.**, a b. over the patella. **Synovial b.** Same as *B. mucosa*.

Bur'sal. Pertaining to a bursa.

Bursa'lis. The obturator internus muscle.

Bur'sic acid. An astringent principle from *Bursa pastoris*.

Bursi'tis (ber-si'tis). Inflammation of a bursa. **Thornwaldt's b.**, catarrhal inflammation of anterior part of median recess of nasopharynx.

Bur'ton's sign. Blue line on the gums in lead-poisoning.

Bu'tane. An anesthetic hydrocarbon, C_4H_{10}.

But'ter. Oily mass procured by churning cream. **B. of antimony,** antimony trichlorid. **B. of cacao.** See *Cacao butter*. **B. of tin,** stannic chlorid. **B. of zinc,** zinc chlorid.

But'terfly patch. Lupus erythematosus of cheeks and nose.

But'terin. Artificial butter chiefly from beef-fat.

But'ternut. See *Juglans*.

But'tock. The gluteal prominence or a lateral half of the same.

But'ton anastomosis. Anastomosis between two parts with a Murphy button.

But'tonhole fracture. That in which the bone has been perforated. **B. mitral,** an advanced state of constriction of the mitral orifice of the heart. **B. operation.** See *Boutonnière operation*.

Butylam'in. A ptomain derivable from cod-liver oil: diuretic and sudorific; probably poisonous.

Butyl-chlo'ral. A substance like chloral; its use is very limited.

Bu'tylene. A gaseous hydrocarbon, C_4H_8.

Butyra'ceous. Of the consistence of butter.

Butyr'ic acid (bu-tir'ik). See *Acid*.

Bu'tyrin. A yellowish fat, $C_3H_5(C_4H_7O_2)_3$, the chief constituent of butter.

Bu'tyroid. Somewhat butyraceous.

Bux'in. An alkaloid from boxwood.

Bux'us semper'virens. The tree which furnishes boxwood: it affords a volatile oil which has been used in medicine.

Byssocau'sis. The use of the moxa; moxibustion.

Byssophthi'sis. Phthisis from inhaling dust of cotton mills.

Bys'sus (bis'us). Lint or charpie.

C.

C. Abbreviation for *carbon*, *congius* (gallon), *compound*, *centigrade*, *centimeter*, *clonus*, *closure*, etc.

Ca. Symbol of calcium.

Caballine aloes. Coarse aloes used by veterinarians.

Cacaerom'eter (kak-a-er-om'et-er). A device for estimating the impurity of the air.

Caca'in (kak-a'in). Same as *Theobromin*.

Cacan'thrax. Malignant anthrax.

Caca'o (kak-a'o). Seeds of *Theobroma cacao*, whence chocolate is made. **C. butter,** fixed oil or fat from cacao.

Cacæ'mia (kah-se'me-ah). Ill state of the blood.

Cacæsthe'sia. Disordered sensibility.

Cachec'tic. Marked by cachexia; sickly looking.

Cachet (kah-sha'). A wafer or capsule for medicines.

Cachex'ia, Cach'exy. Depraved state of nutrition. **Lymphatic c.,** Hodgkin's disease. **Malarial c.,** chronic malaria. **Miners' c.,** ankylostomiasis. **Pachydermic c.,** myxedema. **C. splenet'ica,** spleen enlargement with anemia; often with leukemia. **C. strumipri'va** or **thyreopri'va,** a disordered state which may follow removal of the thyroid body. **Thyroid c.,** exophthalmic goiter.

Cachinna'tion (kak-in-a'shun). Excessive or hysteric laughter.

Cac'odyl (kak'o-dil). Poisonous arsenical compound, $As(CH_3)_2$.

Cacodyl'ic acid. Crystalline acid, $(CH_3)_2$, AsOOH, used in psoriasis.

Cacop'athy. Severe or malignant disease.

Cacopho'nia. Disordered state of the voice.

Cacopla'sia. Formation of diseased or abnormal tissue.

Cacoplas'tic. Susceptible of imperfect organization only.

Cacos'mia. Foul odor; stench.

Cacoth'elin. Alkaloid, $C_{42}H_{22}NO_{20}$, derived from brucin.

Cacothym'ia. Depression of spirits with morbidly ill temper.

Cacot'rophy. Ill-nourished condition.

Cac'ozyme (kak'o-zim). A ferment capable of inducing a disease.

Cac'tin. Active principle of *Cactus grandiflorus.*

Cacti'na. A proprietary preparation of night-blooming cereus; said to be a heart-stimulant.

Cacu'men (kak-u'men). 1. The top of a plant. 2. Part of cerebellum below the declivis.

Cadav'er (kad-av'er). A dead body or corpse.

Cadaver'ic. Pertaining to the cadaver.

Cadav'erin. A poisonous ptomain, $C_5H_{14}N_2$, from decaying meat.

Cadav'erous. Having the aspect of a dead body.

Cade oil (kād). A tarry oil of juniper: used in skin-diseases.

Cad'mium. A tin-like metallic element: its soluble salts are poisonous, with a limited use in medicine.

Cadu'cous membrane. Same as *Decidua.*

Cæcal, Cæcitis, Cæcum, Cæsarean operation, etc. See *Cecal, Cecitis, Cecum, Cesarean operation, etc.*

Caf'fea. Same as *Coffee.*

Caffe'ic acid. See *Acid.*

Caffe'in. An alkaloid, $C_8H_{10}N_4O_2$: diuretic, stimulant.

Caf'feinism, Caf'feism. Disease induced by excessive use of coffee.

Caf'feone (kaf'e-ōn). A heart-stimulant from coffee.

Caffeoresor'cin. A proprietary preparation containing caffein and resorcin.

Cagot ear (kah-go'). Ear with no lower lobe.

Cahin'ca. Diuretic root of various species of *Chiocca,* found in tropical America.

Cahin'cic acid (kah-hin'sik). See *Acid.*

Cais'son-disease (ka'son). Paralytic disease to which those are liable who work in subaqueous caissons.

Caj'eput, Caj'uput. The *Melaleuca cajuputi,* a tree of the Spice Islands. **C. oil,** stimulating volatile oil from cajuput leaves.

Cake, Ague. See *Ague-cake.*

Cal'abar bean. The seed of physostigma, which see.

Calab'arin. Supposed alkaloid from Calabar bean.

Calage (kah-lahzh') [Fr.]. Fixation of viscera by means of pillows to relieve sea-sickness.

Cal'amin. Native zinc carbonate.

Cal'amus. Aromatic rhizome of *Ac'orus cal'amus,* or sweet flag. **C. scripto'rius,** the lowest angle of the fourth ventricle.

Calca'neal, Calca'nean. Pertaining to the calcaneum.

Calcaneotib'ial. Pertaining to the calcaneum and tibia.
Calcaneoca'vus. Club-foot combining calcaneus and cavus.
Calcanecovalgoca'vus. Club-foot combining calcaneus, valgus, and cavus.
Calca'neum (kal-ka'ne-um). The os calcis, or heel-bone.
Calca'neus. Club-foot in which only the heel reaches the ground.
Cal'car. 1. A spur. 2. Hippocampus minor. **C. femora'le,** the plate of strong tissue which strengthens the neck of the femur.
Calca'rea (kal-ka're-ah). A calcareous homeopathic remedy of several varieties: extensively used.
Calca'reous (kal-ka're-us). Containing lime.
Cal'carine (kal'kar-in). Pertaining to the calcar.
Cal'cic (kal'sik). Pertaining to lime or to calcium.
Calcico'sis (kal-sik-o'sis). Lung-disease induced by inhaling marble dust.
Calcifica'tion. Deposition of calcium-salts in the tissues.
Calcig'erous tubes (kal-sij'er-us). Dentinal tubes of dentin.
Calcina'tion. Expulsion of moisture by heat.
Cal'cium (kal'se-um). A metal, Ca, the basis of lime, which is its oxid. **C. carbonate,** chalk, $CaCO_3$.
Cal'culous (kal'ku-lus). Of the nature of a calculus.
Cal'culus (kal'ku-lus), pl. *cal'culi.* A stone-like concretion in any organ. **Arthritic c.,** a gouty concretion. **Biliary c.,** a gall-stone. **Bronchial c.,** calculus in an air-passage. **Cutaneous c.,** milium. **Fusible c.,** urinary calculus made up of phosphate of ammonium, calcium, and magnesium. **Hemic c.,** concretion of blood coagula. **Lacteal,** or **Mammary, c.,** a concretion obstructing a lactiferous duct. **Mulberry c.,** calculus resembling a mulberry in color and shape. **Prostatic c.,** one in the prostate gland. **Renal c.,** a calculus in the kidney. **Salivary c.,** one in the ducts of the salivary glands. **Serumal c.,** tartar on teeth from serum of diseased gums. **Uterine c.,** a concretion in the substance of the uterus. **Vesical c.,** stone in the bladder. **Xanthic c.,** urinary calculus composed of xanthin.
Calefa'cient (kal-e-fa'shent). Causing a sense of warmth.
Calen'dula. The marigold, *C. officinalis:* used in wounds, bruises, and ulcers.
Calen'dulin. A principle obtained from calendula.
Cal'enture. Fever of hot regions, with delirium.
Calf. The back part of the leg below the knee.
Calibra'tion. Measurement of the caliber of an opening.
Cal'ibrator. A graduated cone; an instrument for performing calibration.
Cal'ipers. Two-bladed instrument used in various kinds of measurement.
Calisa'ya (kal-is-a'yah). Yellow cinchona bark.
Calisthen'ics. Light exercise for attaining grace and elegance of movement.
Callisec'tion. Painless vivisection.
Cal'lisen's operation. Left lumbar colotomy.
Calloma'nia. Insanity in which the patient considers herself exceedingly beautiful.
Callo'sal. Pertaining to the corpus callosum.
Callos'ity. A circumscribed hardening and thickening of the skin.
Callosomar'ginal. Pertaining to the callosal and marginal convolutions.
Callo'sum (kal-o'sum). Same as *Corpus callosum.*
Callous (kal'us). Of the nature of a callus.
Cal'lus. 1. Any callosity. 2. The osseous material by which union between ends of a fractured bone is effected. At first it is cartilage-like (**Provisional c.**), but this is afterward re-absorbed and

replaced by the **Permanent c.,** forming permanent union of bones.

Cal'mant (kahm'ant). A calming or sedative medicine; sedative.

Cal'mative (kahm'at-iv). A sedative medicine; calming.

Calolac'tose. Intestinal disinfectant, consisting of a mixture of calomel, lactose, and bismuth subnitrate.

Cal'omel. Mercurous chlorid: hydrargyri chloridum mite.

Ca'lor anima'lis. The natural or normal heat of the animal body.

Cal'orie (kal'o-re). See *Calory.*

Calorifa'cient (kal-or-if-a'shent). Heat-producing; used of certain food-elements.

Calorim'eter. An instrument for estimating the amount of heat disengaged.

Cal'ory (kal'o-re). Amount of heat required to raise one kilogram of water one degree centigrade.

Calum'ba. Root of *Jateorrhiza palmata;* tonic and stomachic.

Calum'bin. A principle obtainable from calumba.

Calva'ria, Calva'rium. That part of the cranium which is above the eyes, ears, and occipital protuberance.

Calvit'ies (kal-vish'e-ēz). Lack or loss of hair; baldness.

Calx. Lime, or calcium oxid. **C. chlora'ta,** chlorinated lime; disinfectant. **C. sulphura'ta,** sulphurated lime; depilatory. **C. vi'va,** quicklime.

Caly'ciform (ka-lis'if-orm). Goblet-shaped.

Ca'lyx (ka'lix). Any one of the cup-like divisions of a renal pelvis.

Cambo'gia (kam-bo'je-ah). Same as *Gamboge.*

Cam'era. Any cavity, chamber, or ventricle. **C. aquo'sa,** anterior aqueous chamber of the eye. **C. cor'dis,** the interior of the pericardium. **C. oc'uli,** space between the cornea and lens.

Cam'isole (kam'is-ōl) [Fr.]. Straight-jacket for restraining maniacal patients.

Cam'omile (kam'o-mil). Same as *Chamomile.*

Cam'per's ligament. Deep perineal fascia.

Cam'phene. Any one of a class of volatile oils with the formula $C_{10}H_{16}$.

Cam'phoid. Pyroxylin dissolved in alcoholic solutions of camphor.

Cam'phol. A camphor and salol preparation.

Camphophénique (kam-fo-fen-ēk'). A compound containing camphor and phenol, for external use.

Cam'phor. A concrete volatile oil, $C_{10}H_{16}O_4$; also, any one of a series of substances called camphors. **C.-ice,** simple cerate nine parts, camphor one part; for toilet and slight eruptions. **C.-naphtol,** two parts camphor and one of naphtol; antiseptic.

Cam'phorated. Combined with camphor. **C. oil,** linimentum camphoris, or camphorated liniment.

Camphor'ic acid. See *Acid.*

Campim'eter (kam-pim'et-er). An instrument for measuring the field of vision.

Can'ada balsam. Oleoresin of fir; terebinthina canadensis. **C. hemp,** apocynum. **C. pitch,** pix canadense; resin of hemlock or *Abies canadensis.*

Can'adol. A local anesthetic, or freezing hydrocarbon, used as a spray.

Canal (kan-al'). Any passage or duct in the body. **Alcock's c.,** a sheath of the obturator fascia containing the internal pudic artery. **Alimentary c.,** the entire digestive tube from mouth to anus. **Arachnoid c.,** a space beneath arachnoid membrane of brain, transmitting great veins of Galen. **C. of Arantius,** the ductus venosus. **Archinephric c.,** the duct of the primitive kidney. **Bernard's c.**, the accessory duct of the pancreas. **Bichat's c.**, small subarachnoid space transmitting veins of Galen. **Bulbular c.**, the canal of Petit. **Caroticotympanic c's.**, short canals from carotid canal to the tympanum, transmitting branches of carotid plexus. **Carotid c.**, one in petrous portion of temporal bone, transmitting internal carotid artery. **Cervical c.**, the canal of the cervix uteri. **C. of Cloquet.** See *Hyaloid c.* **Cochlear c.**, the spiral cavity of the cochlea. **C. of Corti.** triangular canal enclosed between pillars of Corti and the basilar membrane. **Crural c.** Same as *Femoral c.* **C. of Cuvier**, the ductus venosus. **Dentinal c's.**, the minute canals in dentin. **Facial c.**, the aqueduct of Fallopius. **Femoral c.**, canal from femoral ring to upper part of saphenous opening. **C. of Ferrein**, the canal between the free edges of the eyelid when closed. **C's. of Fontana**, ring-shaped series of spaces in the sclerotic in front of its attachment to the iris. **C. of Gärtner**, the remains in the female of the main part of the Wolffian duct of the embryo. **Haversian c's.**, canals ramifying in the compact substance of bone and transmitting vessels and lymph to the interior. **C. of Huguier**, small canal in between squamous and petrous portions of temporal bone, transmitting chorda tympani nerve. **Hunter's c.**, a triangular canal in the adductor magnus of the thigh, transmitting femoral artery and vein and long saphenous nerve. **Huschke's c.**, canal formed by union of tubercles of tympanic ring. **Hyaloid c.**, canal running through vitreous body, transmitting hyaloid artery of fetus. **Incisor c.**, canal opening into the mouth by an opening behind the incisor teeth of upper jaw. **Infra-orbital c.**, small canal running obliquely through floor of orbit, transmitting infra-orbital artery and nerve. **Inguinal c.**, a canal between internal and external abdominal ring. **Jacobson's c.** Same as *Tympanic c.* **Lacrimal c.**, the canal lodging the lacrimal duct. **C. of Lœwenberg**, portion of cochlear canal above membrane of Corti. **Malar c.**, canal in malar bone, transmitting branch of superior maxillary nerve. **Medullary c.**, the cavity of a long bone, containing the marrow. **Nasal c.**, 1. Canal in posterior part of nasal bone, transmitting nasal nerves. 2. Same as *Lacrimal c.* **Nasopalatine c.** Same as *Incisor c.* **Neural c.**, the canal in the epiblast of the embryo forming the cerebrospinal cavity. **Neurenteric c.**, canal in embryo from medullary tube to archenteron. **C. of Nuck**, a tubular process of peritoneum projecting into inguinal canal of female fetus. **Parturient c.**, canal through which child passes in childbirth. **C. of Petit**, a small channel surrounding the lens of the eye. **Portal c.**, space in capsule of Glisson of liver, transmitting branches of hepatic artery, portal vein, and hepatic duct. **Pterygoid c.** Same as *Vidian c.* **Pterygopalatine c.**, one in sphenoid and palate bones, transmitting vessels and nerve. **C. of Rosenthal**, the spiral canal of the modiolus of the ear. **Sacral c.**, continuation of vertebral canal in the sacrum. **C. of Schlemm**, circular canal surrounding eye at sclerocorneal junction. **Semicircular c.**, long canals of the labyrinth of the ear. **Spermatic c.** Same as *Inguinal c.* **Spinal c.**, the canal through the vertebræ, transmitting the spinal cord. **Spiral c.**, the canal of the cochlea enclosing the scala vestibuli, scala media, and scala tympani. **Stilling's c.**, the hyaloid canal. **Tarsal c.**, the canal under the head of the abductor hallucis. **Temporomalar c.**, canal in malar bone from orbital to temporal surfaces, transmitting superior maxillary bone. **Tubotympanal c.**, a canal of hypoblast in the embryo, forming Eustachian tube and tympanum. **Tympanic c.**, one in petrous portion of temporal bone, transmitting Jacobson's nerve.

Uterine c., the entire cavity of the uterus. **Vertebral c.**, the canal enclosed by the vertebral arches. **Vidian c.**, one in sphenoid bone, transmitting Vidian artery and nerve. **Volkmann's c's.**, canals in subperiosteal layer of bones communicating with Haversian canals. **Vomerobasilar c.**, canal formed by junction of vomer and sphenoid bone. **Wharton's c.**, the duct of the submaxillary gland. **C. of Wirsung**, the pancreatic duct. **Zygomaticotemporal c.** Same as *Temporomalar c.*

Canalic'ular. Pertaining to a canaliculus.

Canalic'ulus. A small canal or channel.

Cana'lis. A canal or channel. **C. arterio'sus**, in a fetal blood-vessel which connects the pulmonary artery and the aorta. **C. veno'sus**, a fetal canal which connects the umbilical vein at the liver to the ascending vena cava.

Canaliza'tion. The formation of canals or perforations.

Can'cellate, Can'cellated. Having a lattice-like structure.

Cancel'li. Mesh-like or lattice-like structure in bone.

Can'cellous tissue. Spongy tissue in bone.

Can'cer (kan'ser). A malignant tumor made up chiefly of epithelial cells; carcinoma. **Adenoid c.**, malignant cancer composed of cylindrical tubes lined with epithelium. **C. aquat'icus.** Same as *Cancrum oris.* **Black c.**, melanotic cancer. **C.-cell**, the epithelial cells of cancer. **Clay-pipe c.** See *Smokers' c.* **Colloid c.**, one containing colloid matter. **Encephaloid c.** Same as *Soft c.* **C. en cuirasse**, cancer about the skin of the thorax. **Epithelial c.**, epithelioma. **Hard c.**, one made up chiefly of fibrous tissue. **C.-juice**, the milk-juice flowing from a cut cancer. **Medullary c.** Same as *Soft c.* **Melanotic c.**, a pigmented cancer. **Scirrhous c.** Same as *Hard c.* **Smokers' c.**, epithelioma of lip from irritation of a pipe. **Soft c.**, one made up chiefly of cells.

Cancera'tion. The assumption of cancerous qualities.

Can'cerin (kan'ser-in). A ptomain from urine in cancer of uterus.

Can'cerism (kan'ser-izm). Tendency to the formation of cancer; cancerous diathesis.

Can'cerous (kan'ser-us). Relating to, or of the nature of, a cancer.

Can'criform (kang'krif-ôrm). Resembling a cancer.

Can'croid (kang'kroid). 1. Cancer-like. 2. A skin-cancer of a lesser degree of malignity. **C. corpuscles**, the pearly bodies of epithelioma.

Cancro'in. Supposed alexin of cancer-poison.

Can'crum o'ris. Fetid ulceration of the mouth. **C. puden'di.** Same as *Noma.*

Can'dle-fish oil. Same as *Eulachon oil.*

Canel'la. Bark of *Canella alba;* tonic stimulant.

Cane-sugar. See *Sugar.*

Ca'nine eminence. See *Eminence.* **C. fossa.** See *Fossa.* **C. tooth.** See *Tooth.*

Cani'ties (kan-ish'e-ēz). Grayness of the hair.

Can'ker. Ulceration, especially of the mouth or lips.

Can'nabene hydrid. An oily hydrocarbon, $C_{18}H_{22}$, from cannabis; poisonous.

Can'nabin. 1. A resin from *Cannabis indica.* 2. A hypnotic alkaloid of *Cannabis indica.*

Cannab'inone. A dangerous alkaloidal resin from *Cannabis.*

Can'nabis. Hemp; a genus of plants. **C. in'dica**, an Asiatic variety of common hemp; preferred for medicinal use. **C. sati'va**, the common hemp; narcotic and antispasmodic.

Can'nabism. Habitual use of hemp-derivatives as intoxicants.

Cannabitet'anin. A powerful convulsant alkaloid from cannabis.

Can'nula. A tube for introduction into the body, often enclosing a trocar.

Canquoin's paste (kang-kwahz'). Caustic paste of equal parts zinc chlorid and flour.

Canta'ni's diet (kahn-tah'nĕz). Exclusive meat-diet in diabetes.

Can'thal. Pertaining to a canthus.

Canthar'idal. Pertaining to cantharides.

Canthar'ides (kan-thar'id-ēz). Blistering flies. See *Cantharis.*

Canthar'idin. Crystalline active principle, $C_{20}H_{24}O_8$, from cantharides.

Canthar'idism. Morbid effect of injudicious use of cantharides.

Can'tharis, pl. *canthar'ides.* A genus of beetles. **C. vesicato'ria,** the Spanish or blistering fly: vesicant, diuretic, and stimulant.

Canthec'tomy (kan-thek'to-me). Surgical removal of a canthus.

Canthi'tis (kan-thi'tis). Inflammation of a canthus.

Canthol'ysis. Surgical section of a canthus and canthal ligament.

Can'thoplasty. Operation to restore the palpebral fissure to its full length.

Canthor'rhaphy (kan-thor'af-e). Suturing of a canthus.

Canthot'omy (kan-thot'o-me). Surgical slitting of either canthus.

Can'thus. The angle at the junction of the eyelids.

Can'tus gal'li. Child-crowing; laryngismus stridulus.

Can'ula. Same as *Cannula.*

CaOC. Symbol for cathodal opening contracture.

Caou'tchouc (koo'tshuk). India-rubber or gum elastic: much used in dentistry and surgery.

Capac'ity, vital. See *Vital capacity.*

Cap'elet, Cap'ped hock. A swelling on the heel of a horse's hock.

Cap'eline bandage. A hood-like bandage applied to a stump.

Ca'piat. An instrument for removing foreign bodies from the uterus.

Capillaire (cap-il-air'). A demulcent syrup from maiden-hair fern.

Cap'illary. 1. Pertaining to a hair; hair-like. 2. Any one of the minute vessels which conduct the blood from the arteries to the veins.

Capil'liculture. Treatment for the restoration of the hair.

Capita'tum (kap-it-a'tum). The os magnum.

Capitel'lum. The rounded eminence on the humerus for the articulation of the radius.

Capit'ulum. A small boss on the surface of a bone.

Capotement (kah-pŏt-maw'). A splashing sound heard in dilatation of stomach.

Cap'reolate, Cap'reolary. Tendril-shaped, as the spermatic vessels.

Cap'ric acid. See *Acid.*

Cap'rizant. Leaping or bounding; goat-like: said of an irregular pulse.

Cap'rone. A clear, volatile oil, $C_{11}H_{22}O$, from oil of rue.

Caproylam'in. A poisonous ptomain; hexylamin.

Capryl'ic acid. An acid from butter and other oils.

Cap'sicin. Acrid resin from capsicum.

Cap'sicol. Volatile oil of capsicum.

Cap'sicum. Genus of plants; cayenne, or red pepper.

Capsi'tis. Same as *Capsulitis.*

Cap'sula. The internal capsule of the brain.

Cap'sular. Pertaining to a capsule.

Capsula'tion. The enclosure of a medicine in capsules.

Cap'sule (kap'sūl). 1. Same as *Capsular ligament.* 2. A soluble case for enclosing a dose of medicine. **Atrabiliary c.** Same as *Suprarenal c.* **Auditory c.**, capsule of cartilage in embryo developing into external ear. **Bonnet's c.**, posterior part of sheath of eyeball. **Bowman's c.** Same as *Malpighian c.* **Cartilage c.**, cavities in matrix of cartilage, containing cartilage-cells. **Glisson's c.**, sheath of connective tissue inclosing hepatic artery, hepatic duct, and portal vein. **Internal c.**, tract of nerve-fibers internal to lenticular nucleus. **C. of lens**, transparent sac enclosing lens of eye. **Malpighian c.**, the globular dilatation forming commencement of a uriniferous tubule in the kidney. **Müller's c.** Same as *Malpighian c.* **Nasal c.**, cartilage in embryo, developing into nose. **Optic c.**, capsule in embryo, developing into sclerotic. **Suprarenal c.**, small organ in front of upper part of either kidney. **C. of Tenon**, the fibrous sheath enveloping the eyeball.

Capsuli'tis. Inflammation of a capsule, as that of the lens.

Capsulocil'iary. Pertaining to the capsule of the lens and the ciliary apparatus.

Capsulolentic'ular. Pertaining to the capsule and lens.

Capsulopu'pillary. Pertaining to the capsule and pupil.

Cap'sulotome. A cutting instrument for use in capsulotomy.

Capsulot'omy. Surgical cutting of a capsule, as that of the lens.

Capta'tion (kap-t-a'shun). The first stage of hypnotism.

Cap'ut [L.]. The head; any head-like object. **C. co'li**, the head of the colon; the cecum. **C. cor'nu, C. gelatino'sum**, the expanded end of the posterior horn of the gray matter of the spinal cord. **C. gallinu'ginis**, the verumontanum, or crista urethræ; literally, wood-cock's head. **C. medu'sæ**, a congested appearance of the cutaneous veins around the navel, due to portal obstruction. **C. obsti'pum**, wry-neck or torticollis. **C. succeda'neum**, a swelling on the presenting part of the head of the fetus.

Caragheen' (kar-ag-ēn'). Irish moss. See *Chondrus.*

Carau'na. A resin from various tropical American trees: now little used.

Car'away. The plant *Carum carui*; also its aromatic seed.

Carbam'ic acid. See *Acid.*

Car'basus. Canvas; also, surgical gauze. **C. carbola'ta**, carbolized gauze. **C. iodoforma'ta**, iodoform gauze.

Car'binol. Same as *Methyl alcohol.*

Car'bo anima'lis. Animal charcoal; a deodorant and decolorizer. **C. lig'ni**, charcoal; a deodorant, absorbent and disinfectant.

Carbohe'mia (kar-bo-he'me-ah). Incomplete oxidation of the blood.

Carbohy'drate. Any compound made up of carbon in groups of six atoms, and of hydrogen and oxygen in the proportions to form water.

Carbohydratu'ria. Presence of an excess of carbohydrates in the urine.

Car'bol-fuch'sin. Staining fluid containing carbolic acid and fuchsin.

Carbol'ic acid (kar-bol'ik). See *Acid.*

Car'bolism (kar'bo-lizm). Carbolic-acid poisoning.

Car'bolize. To impregnate with carbolic acid.

Carbolu'ria. Carbolic acid in the urine.

Car'bon (kar'bon). A tetrad element found in charcoal, diamond, and graphite. **C. dioxid**, a gas, CO_2, said not to be poisonous, but to cause death by suffocation. **C. disulphid**, poisonous compound, CS_2; local anesthetic. **C. monoxid**, a gas, CO, formed by imperfect combustion; poisonous.

Carbonaphthol'ic acid. An antiseptic; called also oxynaphthoic acid.

Car'bonate. Any salt of carbonic acid.

Carbone'mia (kar-bo-ne'me-ah). Excess of carbonic acid in the blood.

Carbon'ic acid (kar-bon'ik). See *Acid.*

Car'bonize (kar'bon-īz). To convert into charcoal.

Carbonom'etry. Estimation of the amount of carbon dioxid exhaled in the breath.

Carboxyhemoglo'bin. A compound of carbon monoxid and hemoglobin found in the blood after poisoning by carbon monoxid.

Car'buncle (kar'bung-kl). A subcutaneous inflammation, often ending in a suppurating slough.

Carbun'cular. Pertaining to a carbuncle.

Carcasonne's ligament (kar-kah-zonz'). The triangular ligament of the urethra.

Carcinelco'sis. A cancerous sore.

Car'cinoid. Resembling a cancer.

Carcino'ma. Malignant tumor made up of connective tissue enclosing epithelial cells. See *Cancer.*

Carcinom'atous. Pertaining to, or of the nature of, cancer.

Carcino'sis. Development of a cancer; cancerous diathesis.

Car'damom, Cardamo'mum. Fruit of *Elettaria cardamomum;* a warm aromatic.

Cardarel'li's sign. Lateral movements of trachea, a symptom of aneurysm of aorta.

Car'dia. The upper orifice of the stomach.

Car'diac. Pertaining to the heart.

Cardiag'ra. Pain or gout in the heart.

Cardial'gia (kar-de-al'je-ah). Pain in the region of the heart, or of the cardia.

Cardiamor'phia. Deformity of the heart.

Car'diant. A medicine affecting the heart; used also adjectively.

Cardiec'tasis (kar-de-ek'tas-is). Dilatation of the heart.

Car'din. An extract of the heart of the ox; a heart tonic.

Car'dinal (kar'din-al). Of special importance. **C. points,** the two nodal and two principal points, and the anterior and posterior foci of the eye. **C. points of Capuron,** the two iliopectineal eminences and the two sacro-iliac joints of the pelvis. **C. veins,** those embryonic venous trunks which form the primitive jugular veins.

Car'diocele (kar'de-o-sēl). Hernial protrusion of the heart through the diaphragm.

Cardiocente'sis (kar-de-o-sen-te'sis). Surgical puncture of the heart.

Cardiodyn'ia. Pain in the heart or cardiac region.

Car'diogram. The trace made by a cardiograph.

Car'diograph. An instrument for recording the heart movements.

Cardio-inhib'itory. Restraining the action of the heart.

Car'diolith. A cardiac concretion or calculus.

Cardiomala'cia. Softening of the heart's substance.

Cardiop'athy. Any disease of the heart.

Cardiopericardi'tis. Inflammation of heart and pericardium.

Cardiople'gia. A paralysis of the heart.

Cardiopneumat'ic. Pertaining to the heart and breath.

Cardiopneu'mograph (kar-de-o-nu'mog-raf). A machine for registering cardiopneumatic movements.

Car'diopuncture. Same as *Cardiocentesis.*

Cardiopylor'ic. Pertaining to the cardia and pylorus.

Cardiovas'cular. Pertaining to the heart and blood-vessels.

Cardi'tis (kar-di'tis). Inflammation of the heart.

Car'dol. An irritant oil from the cashew-nut.

Car'duus benedic'tus. The blessed thistle: now seldom used as a remedy.

Car'ica. The genus which produces the true papaw. See *Papaya*.

Car'icin. The same as *Papayin*.

Ca'ries (ka're-ēz). Molecular decay of bone. **Dry c.** See *C. sicca*. **C. fungo'sa,** form of tuberculosis of bone. **Necrotic c.,** form in which pieces of the bone lie in a suppurating cavity. **C. sic'ca,** dry tubercular caries of joints and ends of bones.

Cari'esin. A medicinal preparation from carious bone.

Car'inated (kar'in-a-ted). Boat-shaped.

Ca'rious (ka're-us). Affected with caries.

Car'min. Red coloring derived from cochineal. **Borax-c.** See *Borax*.

Carmin'ative. Soothing and calming; relieving flatulence.

Carmin'ic acid. See *Acid*.

Carnau'ba (kar-na-oo'bah). A South American palm, *Corypha cerifera;* also, its medicinal root. **C. wax,** a variety of wax, largely obtainable from the above tree.

Car'neous columns. Same as *Columnæ carneæ*.

Carnifica'tion. Change of a tissue or material into flesh.

Car'nin. A leukomain, said to be somewhat poisonous.

Car'nogen (kar'no-jen). A preparation of fibrin and bone-marrow.

Ca'ro. [L.]. Flesh or muscular tissue. **C. luxu'rians,** exuberant spongy granulations.

Caro'ba. Same as *Jacaranda*.

Caro'bin. An alkaloid from jacaranda.

Caro'ta. L. name for *Carrot*.

Carot'id. Either one of the two main right and left arteries of the neck.

Caro'tin. A lipochrome or coloring matter from carrots and tomatoes.

Carpag'ra (kar-pag'rah). Pain or gout in the wrist.

Carpa'in. An alkaloid from papaw: used in heart-diseases.

Car'pal. Pertaining to the wrist or carpus.

Carpholo'gia, Carphol'ogy (kar-fo-lo'je-ah, kar-fol'o-je). Picking at the bedclothes; floccitation: usually a sign of great exhaustion.

Carpometacar'pal. Pertaining to the carpus and metacarpus.

Carpope'dal spasm. Spasm of the wrists and feet, or thumbs and toes: oftenest seen in rickety or croupy children.

Carpopto'sis. Same as *Wrist-drop*.

Car'pus. The wrist or its eight bones.

Carragheen (kar-ag-ēn'). Irish moss. See *Chondrus*.

Carreau (kar-ō'). Enlarged, hard state of the abdomen, as in tabes mesenterica.

Car'ron oil. Linseed oil and lime-water: used for burns.

Car'-sickness. The symptoms of sea-sickness induced by railway travel.

Cars'well's grapes. Pulmonary tubercles at the extremities of bronchioles like a bunch of grapes.

Cartham'in. The coloring-matter of safflower.

Car'tilage (kar'til-aj). The gristle or white elastic substance attached to articular bone-surfaces and forming parts of the skeleton. **Articular c.,** that lining the articular surfaces of bones. **Arytenoid c's.,** two cartilages of the larynx. **C.-capsules,** cavities in the matrix of cartilages containing cartilage-cells. **C.-cells, C.-corpuscles,** those connective-tissue cells which are found in the cartilage-capsules. **Costal c's.,** cartilages between true ribs and the sternum. **Cuneiform c.,** cartilage at the side of the aryteno-epiglottidean fold. **Ensiform c.,** the third or lower piece of the sternum. **Epactal c.**, nodules of cartilage on upper edge of cartilages of the nose. **Hyaline c.**, that having a granular or homogeneous matrix. **Jacobson's c.**, hyaline cartilage supporting Jacobson's organ. **Meckel's c.**, the cartilage of the first branchial arch. **Palpebral c's.** See *Tarsal c's.* **Parachordal c.**, one of the two cartilages beside the occipital part of notochord. **Reichart's c.**, cartilage of the hyoid arch of the embryo, developing into styloid process, etc. **Reticular c.**, cartilage in which the matrix consists of a network of yellow fibers. **C. of Santorini.** Same as *Corniculum laryngis.* **Sesamoid c's.**, small cartilages in the side of the wing of the nose. **Tarsal c's.** Same as *Tarsus*, second definition. **Weitbrecht's c.**, the fibrocartilage of the acromioclavicular joint. **C. of Wrisberg**, the cuneiform cartilage of the larynx. **Xiphoid c.** Same as *Ensiform c.* **Y-c.**, Y-shaped cartilage within the acetabulum, joining ilium, ischium, and pubes. **Yellow c.** Same as *Reticular c.*

Cartil'agin. A principle of cartilage changed by boiling into chondrin.

Cartilaginifica'tion. Change into cartilage.

Cartila'ginoid (kar-til-aj'in-oid). Resembling cartilage.

Cartila'ginous (kar-til-aj'in-us). Consisting of cartilage.

Cartila'go. L. for *Cartilage.*

Ca'rum. L. for *Caraway.*

Car'uncle (kar'ung-kl). A small fleshy eminence, often abnormal. **Lacrimal c.**, red eminence at inner angle of eye. **Morgagnian c.**, the middle lobe of the prostate. **Myrtiform c's.** See *Carunculæ myrtiformes.* **Urethral c.**, small, painful red growth on posterior lip of urinary meatus in women.

Carun'cula. L. for *Caruncle.* **C. mammilla'ris**, the olfactory tubercle.

Carun'culæ myrtifor'mes. Supposed relics of the ruptured hymen.

Car'vacrol. Stimulant antiseptic oil from camphor and from various volatile oils.

Car'vol. An aromatic alcohol from oil of cumin.

Caryocine'sis. Same as *Karyokinesis.*

Caryol'ysis (kar-e-ol'is-is). Same as *Karyokinesis.*

Caryom'itome. Same as *Nuclear fibril.*

Caryomito'sis. Same as *Karyokinesis.*

Caryophyl'lin. A resin or camphor from oil of cloves.

Caryophyl'lus. L. for *Clove.*

Car'yoplasm (kar'e-o-plazm). The plasma of a cell-nucleus.

Caryorrhex'is. Rupture of the envelop of cell-nucleus.

Cas'ca bark. Same as *Erythrophlœum.*

Casca'ra amar'ga. Honduras bark, from *Picramnia antidesma:* antiluetic. **C. sagra'da**, bark of *Rhamnus purshiana:* laxative.

Cascaril'la. Bark of *Croton eleuteria:* tonic, aromatic.

Cascaril'lin. A bitter crystalline principle from cascarilla.

Casea'tion. Precipitation of casein; cheesy degeneration.

Ca'sein (ka'se-in). Principal proteid of milk.

Casein'ogen. A proteid whence casein is formed.

Ca'seose. A digestion-product of casein.

Ca'seous (ka'se-us). Cheesy; cheese-like.

Case-taking. Collection of diagnostic, prognostic, or other memoranda.

Cash'ew-nut. The fruit of *Anacardium:* its oil is used in leprosy.

Cassa'va (kas-sah'vah). Jatropha-starch: identical, except in appearance, with tapioca.

Casse'rian ganglion. Same as *Gasserian ganglion.* See *Ganglion.*

Cas'sia bark, Cas'sia lig'nea. A variety of cinnamon. **C. buds**, dried cinnamon buds from China. **C. fis'tula,** the purging cassia; pods afford an aperient pulp.

Cast. A mass of moulded plastic material produced by effusion. Casts are named according to their constituents, as *Blood, epithelial, fatty, granular, hyaline, mucous, waxy*, etc. **Tube c's.,** casts of renal tubes in urine of kidney-disease.

Casta'nea. The leaves of *C. vesca* or chestnut: used in pertussis.

Cas'tor oil. Purgative oil from seeds of *Ricinus communis.*

Casto'reum. Substance like musk from the follicles of the beaver: antispasmodic stimulant.

Casto'ria. Proprietary laxative preparation.

Castra'tion. The removal of the testicles; orchectomy. **Female c.,** the removal of the ovaries; oöphorectomy.

Cas'ualty (kaz'u-al-te). An accidental or other injury; a wound.

Catabol'ic (kat-ab-ol'ik). Pertaining to catabolism.

Catab'olin. A product of catabolic change.

Catab'olism. Passage from a higher to a lower form; retrograde metabolism.

Catab'olite (kat-ab'o-līt). Same as *Catabolin.*

Catacrot'ic. Breaking the descending line of the sphygmogram.

Catac'rotism (kat-ak'ro-tizm). Interruption of the line of descent in the sphygmogram.

Catadicrot'ic. Twice breaking the descending line of the sphygmogram.

Catadi'crotism. Double interruption of the descending line of the sphygmogram.

Catadid'ymus (kat-ad-id'im-us). Joined into one, as twins, the upper parts being double.

Cat'alepsy. Neurosis marked by suspensions of sensibility and voluntary motion.

Catalep'tic. Pertaining to catalepsy.

Catalep'tiform (kat-al-ep'tif-orm). Resembling catalepsy.

Catalep'toid. Resembling catalepsy.

Catalyt'ic (kat-al-it'ik). 1. Alterative. 2. An alterative medicine.

Catame'nia. The menstrual discharge; menstruation.

Catame'nial. Pertaining to the menses.

Cat'apasm. A powder to be sprinkled upon the surface.

Catapha'sia. Speech-disorder in which the patient constantly repeats a word or phrase.

Cataph'ora. State resembling sleep, with privation of feeling and voice.

Cataphore'sis (kat-af-o-re'sis). Introduction of medicine into the system through the unbroken skin, especially by means of an electric current.

Cataphor'ic. Pertaining to cataphora or to cataphoresis.

Cat'aplasm. A poultice.

Cataplec'tic. Sudden and overwhelming; fulminant.

Cat'aract (kat'ar-akt). Opacity of the lens of the eye. **Capsular c.,** cataract from opacity of the capsule. **Cortical c.,** loss of transparency of the outer layers of the lens. **Diabetic c.,** one associated with diabetes. **Discission of c.,** operation of rupturing the capsule, so that the aqueous humor gains access to the lens. **Extraction of c.,** removal of the cataractous lens by operation. **Fluid c.,** the breaking up of an opaque lens into a milky fluid. **Green c.,** a greenish reflex seen in glaucoma; also seen when the pupil is dilated and the media are not entirely transparent. **Hard c.** See *Senile c.* **Immature c.,** only a part of the lens is cataractous. **Incipient c.,** a cataract in its early stages. **Lacteal c.** See *Fluid c.* **Lamellar c.,** one due to opacity of some of the layers between the cortex and nucleus, the remaining layers being transparent. **Lenticular c.**, one occurring in the lens proper. **Mature c.**, one in which the whole lens-substance is involved. **Morgagnian c.**, when an over-ripe c. shrinks and leaves a nucleus floating in the dissolved outer layers. **Polar c.** (anterior or posterior), the opacity is confined to one pole of the lens. **Pyramidal c.**, the opacity is at the anterior pole and is conoid, the apex extending forward. **Recurrent capsular c.**, or **Secondary c.**, capsular cataract, appearing after the extraction of the lens. **Ripe c.** See *Mature c.* **Senile c.**, the cataract of old persons. **Soft c.**, one in which the lens-matter is soft and milky. **Unripe c.** Same as *Immature c.* **Zonular c.** Same as *Lamellar c.*

Catarac'tous. Of the nature of cataract.

Cata'ria. Same as *Catnep.*

Catarrh (kat-ahr'). Inflammation of a mucous membrane with free discharge: chiefly used of the nose and pharynx and of the bladder, etc. **Epidemic c.**, influenza. **Gastric c.**, gastritis. **Intestinal c.**, enteritis. **Nasal c.**, coryza. **Pulmonary c.**, bronchitis. **Uterine c.**, endometritis. **Vesical c.**, cystitis.

Catar'rhal (kat-ahr'al). Of the nature of a catarrh.

Cat'astate (kat'as-tāt). Any one of a series of catabolic conditions or substances.

Catastat'ic. Pertaining to a catastate.

Catato'nia, Catat'ony. Insanity passing from melancholia to mania and thence to complete mental and physical decay.

Catatricrot'ic. Producing three breaks in the descending line of the sphygmogram.

Cat'echin. A crystalline principle from catechu.

Cat'echu. Astringent extract, chiefly from *Acacia catechu*, of the East Indies.

Catechu'ic acid. Same as *Catechin.*

Catelectrot'onus. Increase of nerve-irritability near the cathode.

Cat'enating ague. See *Ague.*

Cat'gut. Sheep's intestine prepared for use as a ligature.

Cathar'sis (kath-ar'sis). A purgation; a cleansing.

Cathar'tic. 1. Purgative. 2. A purgative medicine. **C. acid**, the purgative principle of senna.

Cath'eter (kath'e-ter). A tubular instrument for discharging fluids from a cavity. **Bozeman's c.**, a double-current uterine catheter. **Eustachian c.**, an instrument for distending the E. tube. **Female c.**, short catheter for female bladder. **C.-fever**, fever following the introduction of the catheter into the urethra. **Gouley's c.**, a solid, curved instrument grooved on its lower aspect, for passing over a guide, through a stricture into the bladder. **Nélaton's c.**, a catheter of soft rubber. **Schrötter's c.**, catheter of hard rubber and of varying caliber, used for dilating laryngeal strictures. **Self-retaining c.**, one that will hold itself within the bladder.

Cath'eterism, Catheteriza'tion. The employment or passage of a catheter.

Cath'odal. Pertaining to a cathode.

Cath'ode. The negative electrode or pole of an electric circuit.

Cathod'ic. 1. Pertaining to a cathode. 2. Efferent, or centrifugal.

Cat'ion (kat'e-on). An electropositive element.

Cat'lin, Cat'ling. A form of amputating knife.

Cat'nep, Cat'nip. The herb *Nepeta cataria*: diaphoretic, carminative.

Catop'tric test. Test for cataract by light reflected from the lens.

Catop'trics. The science of reflected light.

Cat's ear. A deformed ear not unlike that of a cat.

Cat's-eye pupil. A narrow, slit-like pupil.

Cat's purr. Fremissement cataire; a purring heart-sound indicative of a valvular disease.

Cat'tle plague. Contagious typhus in cattle.

Cau'da (kaw'dah). Any tail-like appendage. **C. cerebel'li,** vermiform process of cerebellum. **C. equi'na,** a bundle of nerves at the distal end of the spinal canal. **C. stria'ta,** posterior part of the caudate nucleus.

Cau'dad (kaw'dad). Toward any cauda.

Cau'dal (kaw'dal). Pertaining to the tail.

Cau'date (kaw'dāt). Having a tail.

Cauda'tum. The caudate nucleus.

Caul (kawl). Part of the amnion which sometimes envelops the child's head at birth.

Cau'liflower excrescence. A form of cancer of the cervix uteri.

Caulophyl'lin. A resinoid from *Caulophyllum thalictroides.*

Causal'gia (kaw-sal'je-ah). Neuralgia with a sense of heat.

Caus'tic (kaw'stik). Burning or escharotic. **C. arrows,** sharp points charged with a caustic material. **Lugol's c.** See *Lugol's caustic.* **Lunar c.,** silver nitrate. **Mitigated c.,** silver nitrate diluted with potassium nitrate. **C. potash,** potassium hydrate. **C. soda,** sodium hydrate.

Cau'terant (kaw'ter-ant). A caustic material or application.

Cauteriza'tion. Application of the cautery.

Cau'tery (kaw'ter-e). The application of a caustic, or burning substance or instrument. **Actual c.,** burning by a hot iron, moxa, or lens. **C. battery,** a battery used in galvanocautery. **Galvanic c.** Same as *Galvanocautery.* **Potential c.,** cauterization by means of an escharotic.

Ca'va (ka'vah). A vena cava.

Ca'val. Pertaining to a vena cava.

Cav'alry bone. Rider's bone; bony formation in the adductor magnus femoris.

Cav'ascope. An instrument for illuminating a cavity.

Caverni'tis. Inflammation of the corpus cavernosum.

Caverno'ma. A vascular tumor with sinuses.

Caverno'sum. Same as *Corpus cavernosum.*

Cav'ernous. Containing caverns or hollow spaces.

Cav'itary. 1. Forming cavities. 2. Any entozoon with a body-space or alimentary canal.

Cav'ity (kav'it-e). A hollow. **Abdominal c.,** the cavity of the peritoneum. **Amniotic c.,** the cavity of the amnion. **Cotyloid c.** Same as *Acetabulum.* **Glenoid c.,** cavity in head of scapula for articulation with humerus. **Pleuroperitoneal c.,** the body-cavity or celom. **Preperitoneal c.,** the loose subperitoneal tissue in front of the bladder. **Pulp c.,** cavity in a tooth containing the dental pulp. **Rosenmüller's c.,** depression in pharynx on either side of openings of Eustachian tube. **Serous c.,** one of the larger lymph-spaces. **Sigmoid c.,** either of two depressions in head of ulna for articulation with the humerus and the radius.

Cavoval'gus (ka-vo-val'gus). Cavus combined with valgus.

Ca'vum (ka'vum). Any hollow or cavity. **C. Ret'zii.** Same as *Preperitoneal cavity.*

Ca'vus (ka'vus). See *Talipes cavus.*

Cayenne pepper (ki-en'). Same as *Capsicum.*

Cazenave's lupus (kahz-nahvz'). Lupus erythematosus.

C.C. Cubic centimeter.

C.CCl. Cathodal closure contraction.

Cd. Symbol of *Cadmium.*

Ce. Symbol of *Cerium.*

Cebocepha'lia, Cebоceph'aly. Monkey-like deformity of the head, with eyes close together and nose flat.
Cebоceph'alus. A teratism marked by cebocephalia.
Ce'cal (se'kal). Pertaining to the cecum.
Cecec'tomy (se-sek'to-me). Surgical removal of a part of the cecum.
Ce'cum (se'kum). Proximal part of large intestine.
Ceci'tis (se-si'tis). Inflammation of the cecum.
Cecos'tomy (se-kos'to-me). Formation of artificial anus in the cecum.
Ce'dar (se'dar). See *Juniper.* **Oil of c.,** oil of *Juniperus Virginiana;* used in microscopy. See also *Cade, oil of.*
Ced'ron (sed'ron). The *Simaba cedron,* a tree of tropical America; reputed to afford useful remedies.
Cel'andine. Same as *Chelidonium.*
Cela'rium (se-la're-um). The membrane lining the celom.
-cele. An affix indicating a tumor.
Cel'ery (sel'er-e). The plant *Apium graveolens:* nerve-stimulant.
Ce'liac (se'le-ak). Pertaining to the abdomen. **C. axis.** See *Axis.*
Celiadel'phus. A double monstrosity joined at abdomen.
Celial'gia (se-le-al'je-ah). Pain in the abdomen.
Celiec'tomy (se-le-ek'to-me). Excision of an abdominal organ.
Celiohysterec'tomy (se-le-o-his-ter-ek'to-me). Excision of uterus through an abdominal incision.
Celiot'omy (se-le-ot'o-me). Same as *Laparotomy.*
Celi'tis (se-li'tis). Any abdominal inflammation.
Cell. Any one of the minute protoplasmic masses which make up organized tissue. **Acid c.** Same as *Delomorphous c.* **Adelomorphous c.,** transparent columnar cells lining the glands of the stomach · believed to secrete pepsinogen. **Air-c.,** an air-vesicle. **Ameboid c.,** a cell which is able to change its form and to move about. **Apolar c.,** a nerve-cell without processes. **Beaker-c.** Same as *Goblet-c.* **C.-body,** the portion of the cell which encloses the nucleus. **C.-capsule,** a thick strong cell-wall. **Central c.** Same as *Adelomorphous c.* **Ciliated c.,** a cell provided with cilia. **C. of Corti,** any one of the hair-cells in outer surface of organ of Corti. **Cylindrical c.,** an epithelial cell of cylindrical shape. **Daughter-c.,** a cell-formed by division of a mother-cell. **C's. of Deiters.** 1. Cells with fine processes on the basilar membrane of the cochlea. 2. Neuroglia-cells. **Delomorphous c's.,** large cells in the glands of the stomach, believed to secrete the acid of the gastric juice. **Demilune c's.,** granular protoplasmic cells in mucous glands between the mucous cells and the basement membrane. **C.-division.** Same as *Karyokinesis.* **Embryonal c's.,** small round cells composing embryonal tissue. **Endothelial c's.,** cells composing endothelium. **Epithelial c's.,** cells composing epithelium. **Fat-c's.,** connective-tissue cells filled with oil. **Fiber-c.,** a cell elongated into a fiber. **Floor-c's.,** cells of the floor of the arch of Corti. **Formative c's.** Same as *Embryonal c's.* **Ganglion-c.,** a large nerve-cell, especially one of those of the spinal ganglia. **Giant c.,** large multinucleated cell. **C's. of Gianuzzi.** Same as *Demilune c's.* **Glia-c's.,** neuroglia-c's. **Goblet-c.,** an epithelial cell bulged out like a goblet by contained mucin. **Guard-c.,** endothelial cells lining stomata of serous membranes. **Gustatory c's.,** taste-cells. **Hair-c's.,** epithelial cells with hair-like processes. **Lymphoid c's.,** a small connective-tissue cell with a large nucleus. **Marrow-c's.,** large cells characteristic of true marrow. **Mastoid c's.,** the mastoid sinuses. See *Sinus.* **Mother-c.,** a cell that divides to form new cells. **Mucous c's.,** cells which secrete mucus. **Myeloid c's.,** myeloplaxes.

C.-nests, a mass of closely packed epithelial cells surrounded by a stroma of connective tissue. **Nuclear c.**, nerve-cell consisting of a nucleus surrounded by a branching protoplasm. **Oxyntic c's.** Same as *Delomorphous c's.* **Parietal c's.** Same as *Delomorphous c's.* **Peptic c's.** Same as *Adelomorphous c's.* **Pigment c's.**, cells containing granules of pigment. **Polar c's.**, the polar bodies. See *Bodies.* **Prickle c's.**, a cell provided with delicate radiating processes which connect with similar cells. **Purkinje's c's.**, branched nerve-cells of the middle layer of the brain. **Sertoli's c's.**, cells developing into spermatoblasts. **Sperm c.** 1. A spermatozoon. 2. A spermatoblast. **Squamous c's.**, epithelial cells which are flat, like scales. **Taste-c's.**, cells in taste-buds associated with the nerves of taste. **C.-theory**, the theory that all organic matter consists of cells, and that cell-activity is the essential process of life. **Vasofactive c.**, **Vasoformative c.**, a cell that joins with other cells to form blood-vessels. **C.-wall**, the membranous investment of a cell. **Wandering c's.**, leukocytes. **Yolk-c's.**, the elements composing the yolk.

Celloi'din (sel-loi'din). A collodion prepared for use in microscopic work.

Cell'ular (sel'u-lar). Pertaining to, or composed of, cells. **C. pathology.** See *Pathology.*

Cel'lule (sel'ūl). A minute cell.

Celluli'tis (sel-u-li'tis). Inflammation of cellular or subperitoneal tissue. **Pelvic c.**, parametritis.

Cellulocuta'neous (sel-u-lo-ku-ta'ne-us). Pertaining to cellular tissue and the skin.

Cel'luloid (sel'u-loid). A substance made up of pyroxylin and camphor.

Cel'lulose (sel'u-lōs). A carbohydrate forming the framework of plant-structures.

Ce'lom (se'lom), **Celo'ma** (se-lo'mah). The body-cavity, especially of the embryo or of a simple animal organism.

Ce'loscope (se'los-kōp). An instrument for lighting up a cavity.

Celoso'mia (se-lo-so'me-ah). Protrusion of fetal viscera.

Celot'omy (se-lot'o-me). Same as *Kelotomy.*

Cement (se-ment', sem'ent). Bony crust of the roots of teeth.

Cemento'ma. A tumor made up of the cement of a tooth.

Cenesthe'sia (sen-es-the'ze-ah). The sense or feeling of consciousness.

Cent. Abbreviation for *Centimeter* and *Centigrade.*

Centaure'a (sen-taw-re'ah). Same as *Carduus benedictus, Chicus benedictus.*

Centau'rium, Cen'taury. *Erythræa centaurium*, a plant resembling gentian.

Cen'ter (sen'ter). The plexus or ganglion giving off nerves which control a function. **Accelerating c.**, a center in the medulla sending accelerating fibers to the heart. **Arm c.**, cerebral center controlling arm movements. **Association c.**, nerve-center controlling associated movements. **Auditory c.**, a center in the first temporosphenoidal convolution. **Broca's c.** See *Speech c.* **Cardio-inhibitory c.**, in the medulla, efferent impulses being carried by the vagus. **Ciliospinal c.**, a center in the lower cervical part of the cord connected with the dilatation of the pupil. **Deglutition c.**, nerve-center controlling swallowing. **Diabetic c.**, in the posterior part of the anterior half of the floor of the fourth ventricle, in the median line. **Erection c.** is in the lumbar region of the spinal cord, but is controlled from the oblongata. **Gustatory c.**, cerebral center controlling taste. **Heat-regulating** or **Temperature c.**, the center for the control of body-temperature. **Leg c.**, in the upper portion of the ascending frontal convolution. **Motor c.,** nerve-center controlling motion. **Nerve c.,** a group of ganglion cells acting together in the performance of some function. **C. of ossification,** the place in bones at which ossification begins. **Reflex c.,** brain-center at which afferent sensory impressions are converted into efferent motor ones. **Respiratory c.,** in the medulla, between the nuclei of the vagus and accessorius. **Setschenow's c's.,** reflex inhibitory centers in oblongata and cord. **Spasm c.,** in the medulla, at its junction with the pons. **Speech c.,** in the third left frontal convolution in right-handed people. **Swallowing c.,** on the floor of the fourth ventricle. **Sweat c.,** the dominating center is in the oblongata, with subordinate centers in the spinal cord. **Trophic c.,** nerve-center regulating nutrition. **Vasodilator c.,** in the medulla. **Vasomotor c.,** in the medulla. **Visual c.,** in the occipital lobe, especially in the cuneus. **Word c.,** brain-center controlling the perception of the meanings of words.

Centes'imal (sen-tes'im-al). In the proportion of 1 to 100.

Cente'sis (sen-te'sis). Perforation, as by the trocar and cannula.

Cen'tigrade thermometer (sen'tig-rād). A thermometer which is marked off into 100° between the boiling and freezing points of water.

Cen'tigram (sen'tig-ram). One-hundredth part of a gram; one-sixth of a grain.

Cen'tiliter (sen'til-e-ter). One-hundredth part of a liter; 0.6102 of a cubic inch.

Cen'timeter (sen'tim-e-ter). One-hundredth part of a meter; two-fifths of a linear inch.

Centinor'mal (sen-tin-or'mal). Of one-hundredth part of the standard strength.

Cen'trad (sen'trad). Toward a center.

Cen'tral (sen'tral). Situated at, or pertaining to, a center.

Cen'traphose (sen'tra-fōz). A subjective sensation of sight originating in the optic centers.

Cen'tre. Same as *Center.*

Cen'tric (sen'trik). Pertaining to a nerve-center.

Centric'iput (sen-tris'ip-ut). The head, excluding the occiput and sinciput.

Centrif'ugal (sen-trif'yu-gal). Moving away from a center.

Cen'trifuge (sen'trif-ūj). A machine for freeing solids from liquids by rotation.

Centrip'etal (sen-trip'e-tal). Tending toward a center.

Centrolec'ithal (sen-tro-les'ith-al). Having the yolk in the center.

Centroscleero'sis, Centrosteosclero'sis. Osteosclerosis or ossification of a bone-cavity.

Cen'trosome (sen'tro-sōm). The pole-corpuscle or attraction-sphere of a sexual cell.

Centrostal'tic (sen-tro-stal'tik). Pertaining to a center of motion.

Cen'trum (sen'trum). Any center; body of a vertebra. **C. commu'ne,** the solar plexus.

Cephae'lin (sef-a-e'lin). Alkaloid, $C_{15}H_{22}NO_2$, from ipecacuanha; nearly twice as strong as emetin.

Ceph'alad (sef'al-ad). Toward the head; not caudad.

Cephalal'gia (sef-al-al'je-ah). Headache.

Cephalede'ma (sef-al-e-de'mah). Edema of the head.

Cephalemato'ma (sef-al-em-at-o'mah). Sanguineous tumor of the head of a new-born child.

Cephale'mia. Congestion of the head or brain.

Cephalemom'eter (sef-al-e-mom'et-er). Instrument for measuring blood-pressure in the head.

Cephalhy′drocele (sef-al-hi′dro-sēl). Same as *Hydrencephalocele*.
Cephal′ic (sef-al′ik). Pertaining to the head.
Cephali′tis (sef-al-i′tis). Same as *Encephalitis*.
Cephal′ocele (sef-al′o-sēl). Protrusion of a part of the cranial contents.
Cephalocente′sis (sef-al-o-sen-te′sis). Surgical puncture of the head.
Cephalodyn′ia (sef-al-o-din′e-ah). Pain in the head.
Cephalo′ma (sef-al-o′mah). A soft or encephaloid tumor.
Cephalom′elus (sef-al-om′el-us). A double monster with a limb attached to the head.
Cephalome′nia (sef-al-o-me′ne-ah). Metastasis of the menses to the head.
Cephalomeningi′tis (sef-al-o-men-in-ji′tis). Inflammation of the meninges of the brain.
Cephalom′eter (sef-al-om′et-er). An instrument for measuring the head.
Cephalom′etry (sef-al-om′et-re). Measurement of the head.
Cephalopa′gia (sef-al-o-pa′je-ah). Union of fetuses by their heads.
Cephalop′athy (sef-al-op′ath-e). Any disease of the head.
Cephalorhachid′ian (sef-al-o-ra-kid′e-an). Pertaining to the head and spinal column.
Ceph′alotome (sef′al-o-tōm). Instrument for cutting the fetal head.
Cephalot′omy (sef-al-ot′o-me). Dissection of the fetal head.
Cephalotrac′tor (sef-al-o-trak′tor). Obstetrical forceps.
Ceph′alotribe (sef′al-o-trib). Instrument for crushing fetal head.
Ceph′alotripsy (sef′al-o-trip-se). The crushing of the fetal head.
Cephalotrype′sis (sef-al-o-tri-pe′sis). Trephination of the skull.
Ce′ra al′ba. Bleached beeswax. **C. fla′va.** unbleached beeswax.
Ceramu′ria (ser-am-u′re-ah). Same as *Phosphaturia*.
Cera′sein (se-ra′se-in). Sedative and diuretic resin from the cherry tree.
Cer′asin (ser′as-in). Substance from cherry and plum tree gums; said to be a carbohydrate charged with a lime-salt.
Cer′asus (ser-as-us). See *Cherry*.
Ce′rate (se′rāt). A salve with a basis of wax and fat. **Goulard's c.,** cerate of lead and subacetate.
Cer′atin (ser′at-in). Same as *Keratin*.
Cerati′tis (ser-at-i′tis). Same as *Keratitis*.
Cerat′ocele (ser-at′o-sēl). Protrusion of Descemet's membrane through the cornea.
Ceratocri′coid muscle (ser-at-o-kri′koid). See *Muscles, Table of*.
Ceratoglos′sus. See *Muscles, Table of*.
Ceraton′osus (ser-at-on′o-sus). Any disease of the cornea.
Cer′atoplasty (ser′at-o-plas-te). Same as *Keratoplasty*.
Cer′atoscope (ser′at-o-skōp). Same as *Keratoscope*.
Cerat′otome (se-rat′o-tōm). A knife for dividing the cornea.
Ceratot′omy (ser-at-ot′o-me). Same as *Keratotomy*.
Cera′tum (se-ra′tum). L. for *Cerate*.
Cer′berin (ser′ber-in). A poison obtained from *Cerbera odollam*, an Asiatic tree.
Cercom′onas intestina′lis. A protozoon parasitic in the human intestine.
Ce′real (se′re-al). Any edible graminaceous seed.
Cerebel′lar (ser-e-bel′lar). Pertaining to the cerebellum.
Cerebelli′tis (ser-e-bel-li′tis). Inflammation of the cerebellum.

Cerebellospi'nal (ser-e-bel-lo-spi'nal). Pertaining to cerebellum and spinal cord.

Cerebel'lum (ser-e-bel'lum). Main portion of the brain below and behind the cerebrum.

Cer'ebral (ser'e-bral). Pertaining to the cerebrum.

Cerebrasthe'nia (ser-e-bras-the'ne-ah). Asthenia complicated with brain-disorders.

Cerebra'tion (ser-e-bra'shun). Functional activity of the brain. **Unconscious c.,** mental action, of which the subject is unconscious.

Cerebrif'ugal. Conveying impulses away from the brain.

Cer'ebrin (ser'e-brin). A fatty principle from brain-tissue: also, a remedy from brain-tissue.

Cerebri'tis (ser-e-bri'tis). Inflammation of the cerebrum.

Cer'ebroid (ser'e-broid). Resembling the brain-substance.

Cerebrol'ogy (ser-e-brol'o-je). Treatise on, or science of, the brain.

Cerebro'ma (ser-e-bro'mah). Abnormal mass of brain-tissue, outside the cranium.

Cerebromala'cia (ser-e-bro-mal-a'se-ah). Abnormal softness of the brain.

Cerebrom'eter (ser-e-brom'et-er). Instrument for registering brain-movements.

Cerebrop'athy (ser-e-brop'ath-e). Any brain-disease.

Cerebrophysiol'ogy (ser-e-bro-fiz-e-ol'o-je). Physiology of the brain.

Cerebropon'tile (ser-e-bro-pon'til). Pertaining to the cerebrum and pons.

Cerebropsycho'sis. Any cerebral disorder characterized by mental aberration.

Cerebroscle'ro'sis. Abnormal hardness of the brain.

Cere'broscope (ser-e'bro-skōp). Ophthalmoscope used in diagnosing brain-disease.

Cerebroscop'ic (ser-e-bro-skop'ik). Pertaining to cerebroscopy.

Cerebros'copy (ser-e-bros'ko-pe). Diagnostic use of the cerebroscope.

Cerebro'sis (ser-e-bro'sis). Any brain-disease.

Cerebrospi'nal. Pertaining to brain and spinal cord.

Cerebrospi'nant. Any agent which affects the brain and cord.

Cer'ebrum (ser'e-brum). The anterior and larger part of the brain.

Ce'reus (se're-us). A genus of cacti affording cardiant medicines.

Cerevis'ia (ser-e-vis'e-ah). Beer, ale, or porter.

Ce'rium (se're-um). A metal whose oxalate and nitrate are used as medicines.

Cero'sis (se-ro'sis). A waxy degeneration.

Ceru'men (se-ru'men). Ear-wax, a secretion of the meatus of the ear.

Ceru'minal, Ceru'minous. Pertaining to the cerumen.

Ceruminο'sis (se-ru-min-o'sis). Excessive secretion of cerumen.

Ce'ruse (se'rūs). Basic carbonate and hydrate of soda.

Cer'vical (ser'vik-al). Pertaining to the neck or to a cervix.

Cervica'lis ascen'dens. See *Muscles, Table of.*

Cervi'ciplex (ser-vis'ip-lex). The cervical plexus.

Cervici'tis (ser-vis-i'tis). Inflammation of the cervix uteri.

Cervicofa'cial (ser-vik-o-fa'shal). Pertaining to the neck and face.

Cervicoves'ical. Relating to the cervix uteri and the bladder.

Cer'vix (ser'vix). The neck; any neck-like part. **C. u'teri,** the narrow lower end of the uterus. **C. ves'icæ,** the neck of the bladder.

Cesa'rean (Cæsa'rean) section. Delivery of fetus by abdominal incision.

Cesarot'omy. Same as *Cesarean section.*

Ce'sium, Cæ'sium. A rare metallic element: its binary compounds have a limited medicinal use.

Ces'tode, Ces'toid (ses'tōd, ses'toid). Resembling a tape-worm.

Cestoi'dea (ses-toi'de-ah). An order of platyhelmians, including the tape-worms.

Ceta'ceum (se-ta'se-um). L. for *Spermaceti.*

Cetra'ria Islan'dica. The Iceland moss: nutritious and medicinal.

Cev'adin (sev'a-din). An alkaloid from sabadilla.

Chæroma'nia (ke-ro-ma'ne-ah). Mania characterized by exaltation and cheerfulness.

Cha'gres fever (tshah'gres). A malarial fever endemic near Chagres in Colombia.

Chala'za (kal-a'zah). The spiral cord which connects each end of the yolk of a bird's egg with the outer wall.

Chala'zion (ka-la'ze-on). A tumor on the eyelid, formed by the distention of a Meibomian gland.

Chalco'sis (kal-ko'sis). The presence of copper-deposits in tissue.

Chal'ice-cells (tshal'is). Same as *Goblet-cells.*

Chalico'sis (kal-ik-o'sis). Lung-disease from the inhalation of stony particles.

Chalin'oplasty (kal-in'o-plas-te). Plastic surgery of the angle of the mouth.

Chalk (chawk). Non-crystalline form of calcium carbonate. **C.-stone,** gouty concretion of the hands and feet.

Chalyb'eate (ka-lib'e-āt). Impregnated with iron.

Cham'bers (chām'berz). The spaces of the eye. **Anterior c.,** the space between the cornea and iris. **Aqueous c.,** space between cornea and lens of eye. **Posterior c.,** the space between the iris and the lens.

Cham'ois skin (sham'me, sham'wah). A soft leather, usually of sheepskin; used in surgery.

Cham'omile (kam'o-mil). Flower-seeds of *Anthemis nobilis:* a tonic refrigerant.

Chan'cer, Chan'cre (shang'ker). Primary lesion of syphilis. **Hard, Hunterian,** or **True c.,** venereal chancer followed by constitutional syphilis. **Non-infecting, Simple,** or **Soft c.** Same as *Chancroid.*

Chan'croid (shang'kroid). A soft, non-syphilitic venereal sore. **Phagedenic c.,** chancroid with a tendency to slough. **Serpiginous c.,** phagedenic c. spreading in curved lines.

Chan'crous (shang'krus). Of the nature of chancer.

Change of life. The menopause.

Char'bon (shar'bon). Anthrax or malignant pustule.

Char'coal (char'kōl). Carbon prepared by burning organic material.

Charcot'-Neu'mann crystals (shar-ko'noi'mahn). Crystals of spermin-phosphate.

Charcot pains (shar-ko'). Rheumatism of a testicle.

Charcot'-Robin crystals (shar-ko'-ro-bang'). Crystals seen on leukemic blood.

Charcot's arthropathy (shar-kōz'). Joint-effusion in locomotor ataxia. **C.'s crystals.** Same as *Charcot-Neumann crystals.* **C.'s disease,** multiple cerebrospinal sclerosis.

Char'latan (shar'lat-an). A quack, a medicaster.

Char'latanry (shar'lat-an-re). Quackery.

Charles's law. The volume of a gas at a constant pressure varies directly with the temperature.

Char'leyhorse. Stiffness of arms and legs in baseball players.
Char'pie (shar'pe). Lint; also a preparation of spun linen used like lint.
Char'ta (kar'tah). L. for *Paper;* also medicated paper.
Char'tula (kar'tu-lah). Paper packet containing a dose of powder.
Chassaignac's tubercle (shahs-sān-yaks'). The carotid tubercle.
Chaud-pisse (shōd-pēs'). Burning sensation during micturition.
Chaulmoo'gra oil (tshawl-moo'grah). Oil from Asiatic tree *Gynocardia odorata:* used in syphilis and leprosy.
Chauvel's operation (sho-velz'). Plastic surgery of the upper lip.
Chaw'stick. Twigs and bark of *Gouania domingensis:* tonic and dentifrice.
Check-experiment. Same as *Control-experiment.*
Cheek. Side of face below the eye. **C.-bone,** the malar bone.
Chee'sy (che'ze). Cheese-like; caseous.
Cheili'tis (ki-li'tis). Inflammation of a lip.
Chei'loplasty (ki'lo-plas-te). Plastic surgery of a lip.
Cheilostomat'oplasty (ki-los-to-mat'o-plas-te). Plastic surgery of lip and mouth.
Cheiromeg'aly. Pseudo-acromegaly in which the swelling affects the hands, wrists, and ankles.
Cheiropom'pholyx (ki-ro-pom'fo-lix). A skin-disease with peculiar vesicles on the palms and soles.
Chei'rospasm (ki'ro-spasm). Same as *Writers' cramp.*
Che'ken (che'ken). Leaves of *Myrtus cheken:* used like eucalyptus.
Che'lene (ke'lēn). Proprietary local anesthetic, containing ethyl chlorid.
Chelido'nium ma'jus. Celandine; a narcotic, expectorant, and cathartic plant.
Che'loid (ke'loid). Skin-disease with growths like crab's claws.
Chelo'ne gla'bra. Balmony, a plant with tonic and aperient properties.
Chelo'nin (ke-lo'nin). A preparation from chelone; aperient, anthelmintic.
Chem'ic, Chem'ical. Pertaining to chemistry.
Chemicocau'tery (kem-ik-o-kau'ter-e). Cauterization by chemical means.
Chemiotax'is. Same as *Chemotaxis.*
Chemise (she-meez'). A muslin dressing for use in rectal and vesical surgery.
Chem'ist (kem'ist). An expert in chemistry.
Chem'istry (kem'is-tre). The science of the composition of matter.
Chemo'sis (ke-mo'sis). Edema of conjunctiva of the eye.
Chemotac'tic (kem-o-tak'tik). Pertaining to *Chemotaxis.*
Chemotax'is (kem-o-tax'is). The movement of certain cells toward or from other cells.
Chemot'ic (ke-mot'ik). Pertaining to chemosis.
Chemot'ropism (ke-mot'ro-pizm). Same as *Chemotaxis.*
Chenopo'dium ambrosio'ides. The plant which produces American wormseed and its oil: anthelmintic.
Cher'ry. See *Prunus virginiana.* **C.-lau'rel,** *Prunus laurocerasus,* an old-world cherry tree: its preparations contain hydrocyanic acid.
Chest. Same as *Thorax.*
Chest'nut. The tree *Castanea vesca;* the leaves are used in whooping-cough.
Cheyne-Stokes' respiration (chān-stōks). Respiration in which there is a rhythmical increase and decrease in respiratory

movements. **C.-S' nystagmus,** nystagmus in which the oscillations have a rhythmic increase and decrease.

Chi'an turpentine (ki'an). A turpentine from *Pistacia terebinthinus.*

Chi'asm (ki'azm). A crossing or decussation; especially the crossing of the fibers of the optic nerve.

Chiastom'eter (ki-as-tom'et-er). An instrument for ascertaining the deviation of optic axes.

Chick'en-breast. Undue prominence of the sternum.

Chick'en-fat clot. A yellowish blood-clot.

Chick'en-pox. Same as *Varicella.*

Chignon fungoid (shēn-yong'). A nodular growth on the hair.

Chigo, Chigre (tshe'gō, tshe'grā). A tropical sand-flea which often burrows in the toes and feet.

Chil'blain. Inflammation and swelling of toes and feet from cold.

Child'bed. The puerperal state or season.

Child crowing. Same as *Laryngismus stridulus.*

Chill. A rigor; cold stage, as of intermittent fever.

Chills and fever. Intermittent fever.

Chi'loplasty. See *Cheiloplasty.*

Chimaph'ila umbella'ta. The plant pipsissewa: diuretic and astringent.

Chim'ney-sweeps' cancer. Scrotal epithelioma.

Chi'na (ki'nah). Same as *Cinchona.*

Chin'-cough. Pertussis or whooping-cough.

Chin'-jerk. Reflex closure of the mouth on depressing the jaw.

Chinoi'din (ke-noi'din). An amorphous alkaloidal precipitate from cinchona; antiperiodic.

Chi'nol (ki'nol). An antipyretic and analgesic coal-tar derivative.

Chin'olin (kin'o-lin). An alkaloid, C_9H_7N: antipyretic and antiseptic.

Chi'non (ki'non). Same as *Quinone.*

Chinotox'in (ki-no-tox'in). An artificial substance with the poisonous properties of curare.

Chionablep'sia (ki-o-na-blep'se-ah). Snow-blindness.

Chionan'thin (ki-o-nan'thin). Resinoid from *Chionanthus virginica,* or fringe-tree: narcotic and aperient.

Chira'ta, Chiret'ta (ki-ra'tah, ki-ret'tah). The plant *Swertia chirata* of India: a bitter tonic.

Chirop'odist (ki-rop'o-dist). One who treats corns, bunions, etc.

Chirop'ody (ki-rop'o-de). The art or practice of a chiropodist.

Chirur'gery (ki-rur'je-re). Same as *Surgery.*

Chirur'gia (ki-rur'je-ah). L. for *Surgery.*

Chirur'gical (ki-rur'jik-al). Same as *Surgical.*

Chi'tin (ki'tin). The horny substance of the shells of crabs and lobsters, and of the shards of beetles.

Chit'inous degeneration. Amyloid degeneration.

Chloas'ma (klo-az'mah). Discoloration of the skin: sometimes due to a microsporon. **C. hepat'icum,** a kind following dyspepsia; liver spots. **C. uteri'num,** chloasma occurring during pregnancy.

Chloracet'ic acid. See *Acid.*

Chloracetiza'tion (klo-ras-set-iz-a'shun). Induction of anesthesia by chloroform and acetic acid.

Chlo'ral (klo'ral). A liquid, C_2HCl_3O; also, chloral hydrate. **C. hydrate,** hydrate of chloral; hypnotic and anodyne.

Chloralam'id (klo-ral-am'id). A hypnotic, said to be safer, but slower, than chloral hydrate.

Chloralantipy'rin (klo-ral-an-tip-i'rin). Same as *Hypnal.*

Chloralcarbam'id. A mildly hypnotic preparation.

Chloralim'id. A compound which has been used as a chloral-hydrate substitute.
Chlo'ralism (klo'ral-izm). The habitual use of chloral; also, the poisonous effect of chloral.
Chlo'ralize (klo'ral-iz). To put under the influence of chloral.
Chlo'ralose (klo'ral-ōs). A substance said to be safer and more efficient than chloral.
Chloralu'rethane (klo-ral-u'reth-ān). Same as *Ural.*
Chloram'id (klo-ram'id). Same as *Chloralamid.*
Chlorane'mia (klo-ra-ne'me-ah). Same as *Chlorosis.*
Chloran'odyne. A proprietary anodyne.
Chlo'rate (klo'rāt). Any salt of chloric acid.
Chlorcam'phor (klor-kam'for). Any chlorin and camphor compound: some have been used in medicine.
Chlore'mia (klo-re'me-ah). Decrease of hemoglobin and red corpuscles of the blood.
Chlo'ric ac'id. See *Acid.*
Chlo'rid (klo'rid). Any binary compound of chlorin.
Chlo'rin (klo'rin). A yellowish gaseous element: disinfectant and decolorizer.
Chlo'rinated (klo'rin-a-ted). Charged with chlorin.
Chlo'rite (klo'rīt). Any salt of chlorous acid: all are disinfectants and bleaching agents.
Chloroane'mia (klo-ro-a-ne'me-ah). Same as *Chlorosis.*
Chlo'robrom (klo'ro-brōm). A hypnotic mixture of potassium bromid and chloramid.
Chlo'rodyne (klo'ro-dīn). A proprietary anodyne and narcotic.
Chlo'roform (klo'ro-form). A volatile liquid, $CHCl_3$, anesthetic, soporific, and counter-irritant.
Chlo'roformism (klo'ro-form-izm). Excessive use of chloroform or ill effects thereof.
Chlo'rol (klo'rol). A non-official antiseptic solution.
Chloro'ma (klo-ro'ma). Greenish sarcoma of the pericranium.
Chlo'rophane (klo'ro-fān). A green-yellow pigment from the retina.
Chlo'rophyl. The green coloring matter of plants.
Chlorosarco'ma. Same as *Chloroma.*
Chloro'sis. Green-sickness; anemia of young women about the time of puberty.
Chlorot'ic (klo-rot'ik). Affected with chlorosis.
Chlo'rous acid (klo'rus). See *Acid.*
Chlo'rozone (klo'ro-zōn). A yellow disinfectant fluid.
Chlorphe'nol (klōr-fe'nol). A chlorin and phenol compound: antiseptic and antituberculous.
Chlorsal'ol. A salol and chlorin compound.
Chlo'rum (klo'rum). L. for *Chlorin.*
Chlo'ryl. Anesthetic containing chlorids of ethyl and methyl.
Choa'næ (ko-a'ne). The posterior nares.
Choc'olate (chok'o-let). Paste from the seeds of *Theobroma cacao.*
Choked disk. Congested and inflamed state of the optic disk.
Cho'lagogue (ko'lag-og). A medicine which promotes the discharge of bile.
Cholal'ic acid. See *Acid.*
Cholangi'tis (ko-lan-ji'tis). Inflammation of a bile-duct.
Cholecy'anin (ko-le-si'an-in). Same as *Bilicyanin.*
Cho'lecyst, Cholecys'tis. See *Gall-bladder.*
Cholecystecta'sia (ko-le-sis-tec-ta'ze-ah). Distention of the gall-bladder.
Cholecys'tectomy (ko-le-sis-tek'to-me). Excision of the gall-bladder.
Cholecystenteros'tomy (ko-le-sis-ten-ter-os'to-me). Surgical formation of a passage from the gall-bladder to the intestine.

Cholecysti'tis (ko-le-sis-ti'tis). Inflammation of the gall-bladder.

Cholecystocolos'tomy (ko-le-sis-to-ko-los'to-me). Surgical formation of a passage from gall-bladder to colon.

Cholecystocolot'omy (ko-le-sis-to-ko-lot'o-me). Incision of the gall-bladder and colon.

Cholecystoduodenos'tomy. Formation of a communication between gall-bladder and duodenum.

Cholecystolith'otripsy (ko-le-sis-to-lith'o-trip-se). Crushing of a gall-stone in the cholecyst.

Cholecystor'rhaphy (ko-le-sis-tor'raf-e). Suturing of the gall-bladder.

Cholecystos'tomy (ko-le-sis-tos'to-me). Surgical formation of an opening into the cholecyst.

Cholecystot'omy. Incision of the gall-bladder.

Choledochoduodenos'tomy. Surgical formation of an opening between the bile-duct and duodenum.

Choledochoenteros'tomy. Surgical creation of a passage from gall-duct to intestine.

Choledocholith'otripsy. Crushing of a gall-stone in the bile-duct.

Choledochos'tomy. Formation of an opening into bile-duct.

Choledochot'omy. Surgical incision of the bile-duct.

Cholehe'mia (ko-le-he'me-ah). Presence of bile in the blood.

Chole'ic (ko-le'ik). Pertaining to the bile.

Cholelithi'asis. The formation of gall-stones.

Cholelithot'omy (ko-le-lith-ot'o-me). Surgical incision for the removal of a gall-stone.

Cholelithot'rity (ko-le-lith-ot'rit-e). Crushing of a gall-stone.

Chole'mia (ko-le'me-ah). Presence of bile or bile-pigment in the blood.

Cholepyr'rhin (ko-le-pir'in). Same as *Biliphein*.

Chol'era (kol'e-rah). A disease characterized by vomiting, purging, spasms, and griping pains. **Asiatic c.,** epidemic and markedly severe form of cholera. **Chicken-c.,** fatal epidemic disease of fowls, with inflammation of lymphatic glands and digestive organs. **Hog-c.,** infectious disease of swine, with ulceration of bowels, congestion of lungs, and red patches on the skin. **C. infan'tum,** a summer-cholera of young children. **Malignant c.,** Asiatic c. **C. mor'bus,** acute gastro-enteritis, with diarrhea, cramp, and vomiting. **C. nos'tras.** Same as *C. morbus*. **C.-red,** a red pigment obtainable from cholera spirillum. **C.-spirillum,** the comma bacillus, the pathogenic organism of epidemic cholera. **Summer c.,** cholera morbus.

Cholera'ic (kol-er-a'ik). Pertaining to cholera.

Choler'iform (ko-ler'if-orm). Resembling cholera.

Chol'erine (kol'er-in). A relatively mild form of cholera.

Cholerapho'bia (kol-er-o-fo'be-ah). Morbid fear of cholera.

Choler'ythrin (ko-ler'ith-rin). Same as *Bilirubin*.

Cholesteato'ma. Tumor containing fat-like materials.

Cholestere'mia (ko-les-ter-e'me-ah). Excess of cholesterin in the blood.

Choles'terin (ko-les'ter-in). A crystalline fat from bile, gall-stones, and nerve-tissue.

Cholete'lin (ko-let-e'lin). A yellow coloring matter from bilirubin.

Cholether'apy. Use of bile as a medicine.

Choleu'ria (ko-lu're-ah). Presence of bile in urine.

Cholever'din (ko-le-ver'din). The same as *Bilicyanin*.

Cho'lic acid (ko'lik). See *Acid*.

Cho'lin (ko'lin). A poisonous ptomain, $C_5H_{15}NO_2$, from brain-substance, bile, etc.

Chol'olith (kol'o-lith). A gall-stone.

Cholu'ria (ko-lu're-ah). Presence of bile in the urine.
Chon'dral (kon'dral). Pertaining to cartilage.
Chondral'gia (kon-dral'je-ah). Pain in a cartilage.
Chondrec'tomy (kon-drek'to-me). Surgical removal of a cartilage.
Chondrifica'tion (kon-drif-ik-a'shun). Development of cartilage.
Chon'drin (kon'drin). A cartilage proteid.
Chondri'tis (kon-dri'tis). Inflammation of a cartilage.
Chon'droblast (kon'dro-blast). Cell forming cartilage.
Chon'droclast (kon'dro-klast). A giant cell concerned in the absorption and removal of cartilage.
Chondrocos'tal (kon-dro-kos'tal). Pertaining to ribs and costal cartilages.
Chondrocra'nium (kon-dro-kra'ne-um). The cartilaginous embryonic cranium.
Chondrodyn'ia (kon-dro-din'i-a). Pain in a cartilage.
Chondrodystro'phia. Rickets in the fetus. See *Achondroplasia.*
Chondrofibro'ma (kon-dro-fib-ro'mah). Chondroma with fibrous elements.
Chon'drogen (kon'dro-jen). The base of cartilage.
Chondrogen'esis (kon-dro-jen'es-is). Formation of cartilage.
Chon'droid (kon'droid). Resembling cartilage.
Chondrol'ogy (kon-drol'o-je). The science or study of cartilages.
Chondro'ma (kon-dro'mah). A cartilaginous tumor.
Chondromala'cia (kon-dro-mal-a'she-ah). Preternatural softness of cartilage.
Chondromalaco'sis (kon-dro-mal-ak-o'sis). Same as *Chondromalacia.*
Chondromyo'ma (kon-dro-mi-o'mah). Myoma with cartilaginous elements.
Chondromyxo'ma (kon-dro-mix-o'mah). Myxoma with cartilaginous elements.
Chondroporo'sis (kon-dro-po-ro'sis). The formation of sinuses or spaces in cartilage.
Chondrosarco'ma (kon-dro-sar-ko'mah). Sarcoma with cartilaginous elements.
Chon'drotome (kon'dro-tōm). An instrument for dividing cartilage.
Chondrot'omy (kon-drot'o-me). The surgical division of a cartilage.
Chondroxi'phoid (kon-dro-zi'phoid). Pertaining to the ensiform cartilage.
Chon'drus (kon'drus). Pharmacopeial name for caragheen.
Chopart's amputation (sho-parz'). Removal of the foot at the mediotarsal articulation.
Chor'da (kor'dah). Any cord or sinew. **C. dorsa'lis.** Same as *Notochord.* **C. saliva.** saliva produced by stimulation of the chorda tympani. **C. tym'pani,** a branch of the facial nerve going to the tongue and submaxillary gland. **C. umbilica'lis,** the umbilical cord. **C. vertebra'lis.** Same as *Notochord.* **C. voca'lis,** vocal cord.
Chor'dæ tendin'eæ (kor'de ten-din'e-e). The tendinous strings joining the papillary muscles of the heart with the valves.
Chor'dæ Willis'ii (kor'de wil-lis'e-i). See *Willis's cords.*
Chor'dal (kor'dal). Pertaining to a chorda.
Chor'dee (kor'de). Painful deflection of the penis in gonorrhea.
Chordi'tis (kor-di'tis). Inflammation of the vocal or spermatic cords.
Chordoskel'eton (kor-do-skel'et-on). That part of the skeleton which is formed about the notochord.

Chordurethri'tis (kor-du-re-thri'tis). Same as *Chordee*.

Chore'a (ko-re'ah). A nervous disease with involuntary and irregular movements; St. Vitus's dance. **Chronic c.** See *Huntingdon's c.* **Electric c.** See *Dubini's disease*. **Epidemic c.**, dancing mania. **Habit c.** See *Spasm*. **Hereditary c.** See *Huntingdon's c.* **Huntingdon's c.**, an hereditary affection of adult life, marked by irregular movements, speech disturbance, and dementia. **Hysteric c.** See *C. major*. **C. insan'iens**, a grave form of chorea, associated with mania, and usually ending fatally. **C. ma'jor**, hysteria in which there are continual regular oscillatory movements. **Maniacal c.** See *C. insaniens*. **Mimetic c.**, that which is caused by imitation. **C. mi'nor**, simple chorea. **Posthemiplegic c.**, **Postparalytic c.**, involuntary movement seen in patients after an attack of hemiplegia. **Rhythmical c.**, chorea in which the movements occur at regular intervals. **School-made c.**, chorea from over-stimulation of children at school. **Senile c.**, a choreiform affection coming on in old age. **Sydenham's c.**, ordinary chorea.

Chore'al (ko-re'al). Pertaining to chorea.

Chore'ic (ko-re'ik). Of the nature of chorea.

Chore'iform (ko-re'if-orm). Resembling chorea.

Choreoma'nia (ko-re-o-ma'ne-ah). Dancing mania.

Choriocapilla'ris. The second or capillary layer of the choroid coat.

Cho'rioid (ko're-oid). Same as *Choroid*.

Chorioidi'tis (ko-re-oid-i'tis). Same as *Choroiditis*.

Cho'rion (ko're-on). The outermost of the fetal membranes. **C. frondo'sum**, the part of c. covered by villi. **C. læ've**, the smooth, membranous part of the chorion. **Shaggy c.** Same as *C. frondosum*.

Chorion'ic villi (ko-re-on'ik). The vascular tufts which cover the chorion in early pregnancy.

Chorioni'tis (ko-re-on-i'tis). Same as *Scleroderma*.

Chorioretini'tis. Inflammation of the choroid and retina.

Cho'roid (ko'roid). The vascular coat of the eye, between the sclerotic and retina.

Choroidere'mia (ko-roi-de-re'me-ah). Absence of the choroid.

Choroidi'tis (ko-roi-di'tis). Inflammation of the choroid. It may be **anterior**, when the points of exudation are at the periphery of the choroid; **areolar**, when it starts around the macula lutea and spreads toward the periphery; **central**, when in the region of the macula lutea; **diffuse** or **disseminated**, characterized by spots scattered over the fundus; **exudative**, when there are patches of inflammation scattered over the choroid; **metastatic**, when due to embolism; and **suppurative**, when proceeding to suppuration. **C. sero'sa.** Same as *Glaucoma*.

Choroidocycli'tis. Inflammation of the choroid and ciliary processes.

Choroidoiri'tis (ko-roi-do-i-ri'tis). Inflammation of the choroid and iris.

Choroidoretini'tis. Inflammation of the choroid and the retina.

Choroma'nia (ko-ro-ma'ne-ah). Epidemic dancing mania.

Chris'tison's formula. See *Trapp's formula*.

Chro'atol (kro'a-tol). Green, oily liquid used in skin-diseases.

Chro'mate (kro'māt). Any salt of chromic acid.

Chromat'ic (kro-mat'ik). Pertaining to color.

Chro'matin (kro'mat-in). The more stainable portion of cell-nucleus.

Chromatodysso'pia (kro-mat-o-dis-o'pe-ah). Color-blindness.

Chromatog'enous (kro-mat-oj'en-us). Producing color or coloring matter.

Chromatom'eter (kro-mat-om'et-er). Instrument for measuring color or color-perception.

Chromatop'sia (kro-mat-op'se-ah). Colored vision.

Chromatoptom'etry (kro-mat-op-tom'et-re). Measurement of the power of color-perception.

Chromato'sis (kro-mat-o'sis). Abnormal pigmentation of the skin.

Chromatu'ria (kro-mat-u're-ah). Abnormal coloration of the urine.

Chromesthe'sia (kro-mes-the'zhe-ah). Association of color-sensations with sensations of taste, hearing, and smell.

Chro'mic ac'id (kro'mik). See *Acid*. **C. anhydrid**, chromium trioxid, C_2O_3: caustic.

Chro'micized. Treated with a chromium-compound.

Chromidro'sis (kro-mid-ro'sis). Coloration of the sweat.

Chro'mium (kro'me-um). A metal whose compounds have a limited use in medicine.

Chro'mocyte (kro'mo-sit). Any colored cell.

Chromocytom'eter (kro-mo-si-tom'et-er). An instrument for measuring the hemoglobin of the red blood-corpuscles.

Chro'mogen (kro'mo-jen). Any principle which may give origin to a coloring matter.

Chro'momere (kro'mo-mēr). Any one of the granules of a chromosome.

Chromom'eter (kro-mom'et-er). Instrument for measuring coloring matter present.

Chromom'etry (kro-mom'et-re). The measurement of coloring matter.

Chro'mophane (kro'mo-fān). Any retinal pigment.

Chro'mophil (kro'mo-phil). Any easily stainable structure; used also adjectively.

Chromophil'ic (kro-mo-fil'ik), **Chromoph'ilous** (kro-moph'il-us). Readily stained.

Chro'mophose (krō'mo-fōz). A subjective sensation of color.

Chromophyto'sis. Skin-discoloration due to a vegetable parasite.

Chromoplas'tid. A protoplasmic pigment granule.

Chromop'sia. Same as *Chromatopsia*.

Chromoptom'eter (kro-mop-tom'et-er). Instrument for measuring color-perception.

Chro'mosome (kro'mo-sōm). Any chromatin fiber formed in the process of karyokinesis.

Chron'ic (kron'ik). Not acute; long-continued.

Chroni'city (kro-nis'it-e). Quality of being chronic.

Chron'ograph (kron'o-graf). An instrument for recording small intervals of time.

Chrysaro'bin (kris-ar-o'bin). A principle derived from Goa powder; used in skin-diseases.

Chrysokreat'inin (kris-o-kre-at'in-in). A leucomain from muscle.

Chrysophan'ic acid. See *Acid*.

Chthonopha'gia (thon-o-fa'je-ah). The eating of clay or earth; geophagy.

Chvos'tek's sign (kvos'teks). Spasm of one cheek following a tap in cases of tetany.

Chylangio'ma (ki-lan-je-o'mah). Tumors made up of intestinal lymph-vessels filled with chyle.

Chyle (kil). The milky liquid found in the lacteals after digestion.

Chyle'mia (ki-le'me-ah). The presence of chylous material in the blood.

Chylifac'tion (ki-lif-ak'shun). The formation of chyle.
Chylifac'tive (ki-lif-ak'tiv). Forming chyle.
Chylif'erous (ki-lif'er-us). Conveying the chyle.
Chylifica'tion (ki-lif-ik-a'shun). The formation of chyle.
Chylopericar'dium (ki-lo-per-e-kar'de-um). The presence of chyle in the pericardium.
Chylopoie'sis (ki-lo-poi-e'sis). Same as *Chylification*.
Chylopoiet'ic (ki-lo-poi-et'ik). Pertaining to the formation of chyle.
Chylotho'rax. Presence of chyle in pleural cavities.
Chy'lous (ki'lus). Of the nature of chyle.
Chylu'ria (ki-lu're-ah). The presence of fat in the blood.
Chyme (kim). Food which has undergone gastric digestion.
Chymifica'tion. Conversion of food into chyme.
Cibis'itome (sib-is-it-ōm). Instrument for incising the capsule of the lens.
Cicatri'cial (sik-at-rish'al). Pertaining to a cicatrix.
Cicat'rix (sik-at'rix). A scar; mark left by a sore or wound.
Cicat'rizant (sik-kat'riz-ant). Promoting or causing cicatrization.
Cicatriza'tion. Healing process which leaves a cicatrix.
Cic'atrize (sik'at-riz). To heal and be replaced by a cicatrix.
Cicu'ta (si-ku'tah). A genus of poisonous plants; water parsnip; cowbane.
Cicutox'in. A poisonous principle from cicuta.
Cil'ia (sil'e-ah). 1. Eyelashes. 2. Minute lash-like processes.
Ciliar'iscope. Instrument for examining ciliary region of eye.
Cil'iary (sil'e-a-re). Pertaining to, or like, the eyelashes.
Cil'iated (sil'e-a-ted). Provided with cilia.
Ciliospi'nal center (sil-e-o-spi'nal). The center in the spinal cord which controls movements of the iris.
Cil'ium (sil'e-um). 1. An eyelash. 2. A minute lash-like process.
Ci'mex lectula'rius (si'mex lek-tyu-la're-us). The bedbug: used homeopathically.
Cimicif'uga racemo'sa. Black snakeroot; a valuable antispasmodic and tonic.
Ci'na (si'nah). The plant *Artemisia santonica* and its seed; wormseed.
Cincham'idin (sin-kam'id-in). A cinchona alkaloid.
Cincho'na (sin-ko'nah). Genus of trees furnishing Peruvian bark, which yields quinin.
Cinchonam'in (sin-ko-nam'in). A powerful alkaloid from cuprea bark.
Cinchon'icin (sin-kon'is-in). An alkaloid from cinchona.
Cinchon'idin (sin-kon'id-in). One of the cinchona alkaloids.
Cincho'nin (sin-ko'nin). One of the cinchona alkaloids.
Cin'chonism (sin'ko-nizm). Morbid effect of injudicious use of cinchona bark or its alkaloids.
Cin'chonize (sin'ko-niz). To bring under the influence of cinchona alkaloids.
Cinc'ture feeling or **sensation** (sink'tūr). Same as *Zonesthesia*.
Cine'rea (sin-e're-ah). The gray matter of the nervous system.
Cineri'tious (sin-e-rish'us). Ash-colored, as the gray nervous matter.
Cinesi-. See under *Kinesi-*.
Cin'gulum (sin'gu-lum). Part of gyrus fornicatus near the corpus callosum.
Cin'nabar (sin'nab-ar). Red bisulphid of mercury.
Cin'namene (sin'nam-ēn). Same as *Styrol*.
Cinnam'ic aldehyd. An oil nearly identical with oil of cinnamon.

Cinnamo'mum, Cin'namon. Bark of various species of *Cinnamomum:* carminative and stimulant.

Cionec'tomy (si-o-nek'to-me). Removal of the uvula.

Cioni'tis, Cion'otome, Cionot'omy. See *Uvulitis, Uvulotome, Uvulotomy.*

Cir'cle of diffusion. Same as *Diffusion circle.*

Circle of Willis. A loop of vessels near the base of the brain.

Circles of Haller. Venous and arterial circles of the eye.

Cir'cuit (ser'kit). The course of an electric current.

Cir'cular amputation. See *Amputation.* **C. insanity.** See *Insanity.*

Cir'culating albu'min. See *Albumin.*

Circula'tion (ser-ku-la'shun). Movement in a circle, as c. of the blood. **Allantoic c.,** circulation in fetus through the umbilical vessels. **Collateral c.,** that carried on through secondary channels after stoppage of the principal course. **Fetal c.,** that of the fetus, through the placenta and umbilical cord. **First or Primitive c.,** that carrying nutriment and oxygen to the embryo. **Placental c.,** the fetal circulation. **Portal c.,** the passage of the blood from the gastro-intestinal tract and spleen through the liver, and out by the hepatic vein. **Pulmonary c.,** the circulation of blood through the lungs for purpose of oxygenation. **Systemic c.,** the general circulation, as distinguished from the pulmonary circulation. **Vitelline c.,** first or primitive circulation.

Cir'culatory. Pertaining to circulation.

Circum-. A prefix signifying around.

Circumcis'ion (ser-kum-sizh'un). Removal of a part or all of the foreskin.

Circumclu'sion (ser-kum-klu'zhun). Compression of an artery by a wire and pin.

Circumduc'tion (sur-kum-duk'shun). Circular movement of a limb.

Cir'cumflex (ser'kum-flex). Having winding course or direction.

Circumpolariza'tion. The rotation of polarized light.

Cir'cumscribed. Confined to a limited space.

Circumval'late papillæ. Papillæ near the base of tongue, arranged in a V-shaped row.

Cir'cus movements (ser'kus). Certain involuntary movements due to nervous lesions.

Cirrho'sis (sir-ro'sis). Interstitial inflammation of an organ, particularly the liver. **Atrophic c.** is marked by shrivelling and shrinkage in size. **Bil'iary c.,** c. of liver from chronic retention of bile. **Fatty c.,** form in which liver-cells become infiltrated with fat. **Hypertrophic c.** is marked by enlargement.

Cirrhot'ic (sir-rot'ik). Of the nature of cirrhosis.

Cir'socele (sir'so-sēl). The same as *Varicocele.*

Cir'soid (ser'soid). Resembling a varix.

Cirsom'phalos (ser-som'fal-os). Varicose state of navel.

Cir'sotome (ser'so-tōm). Cutting instrument for operations on varicose veins.

Cirsot'omy (ser-sot'o-me). Excision of a varicosity.

Cissam'pelos (sis-sam'pe-los). See *Pareira.*

Cis'tern (sis'tern). A name of various lymph-spaces, etc. **C. of Pecquet** (pek-ka'). The receptaculum chyli.

Cit'rate (sit'rāt). Any salt of citric acid.

Cit'ric acid (sit'rik). See *Acid.*

Cit'rine ointment (sit'rin). Ointment of mercuric nitrate.

Citronel'la oil. Fragrant oil of *Andropogon nardus:* antirheumatic.

Cit'rophene (sit'ro-fēn). An antipyretic containing phenetidin and nitric acid.

Cl. Symbol of chlorin.

Clad'othrix Fœr'steri. A schizomycete from lacrimal canaliculi.

Clamp. Surgical device for compression.

Clang-tint. A delicate quality of tone.

Clap. Same as *Gonorrhea.* **C.-threads,** slimy, stringy matter in gonorrheal urine.

Clapotement (klah-pŏt-maw'). Any splashing sound, as in succussion.

Clap'ton's lines. Green lines on the gums or teeth in lead-poisoning.

Clar'et-stain. Same as *Nævus.*

Clarif'icant (klar-if'ik-ant). A substance which clears a liquid of turbidity.

Clar'ifying agent. See *Clearing agent.*

Clarke's bodies. Certain intranuclear bodies from alveolar sarcoma of breast. **C.'s column.** 1. The anterior pyramidal tract of the spinal cord. 2. Same as *Vesicular column.*

Clasmat'ocyte (klas-mat'o-sīt). A large cell tending to break up into fragments.

Clasmatocyto'sis (klas-mat-o-si-to'sis). The division of a clasmatocyte.

Clasp-knife rigidity. Spastic extension of leg with a spring like that of a clasp-knife.

Clas'tic (klas'tik). Undergoing, or causing, a division into parts.

Clathrocys'tis (klath-ro-sis'tis). A genus of schizomycetes: some are found on fish.

Claudica'tion (klaw-dik-a'shun). Limping; lameness.

Clau'dius's cells (klaw'de-us). Large cells near the organ of Corti.

Claustropho'bia (klaw-stro-fo'be-ah). Dread of being in an enclosed place.

Claus'trum (klaw'strum). A thin gray or cinereous layer outside the external capsule of the brain.

Cla'va (kla'vah). An enlargement of the funiculus gracilis in the oblongata.

Cla'vate nucleus (kla'vāt). A double group of cells within the clava.

Clav'iceps purpu'rea. The fungus which produces ergot.

Clav'icle (klav'ik-el). The collar-bone.

Clavic'ular (kla-vik'u-lar). Pertaining to the clavicle.

Cla'vus (kla'vus). A corn; any tubercle of the skin. **C. hyster'icus,** a sensation as if a nail were being driven into the head.

Claw-foot. Atrophy and distortion of foot.

Claw-hand. Flexion and atrophy of hand and fingers.

Clay-pipe cancer. Epithelioma of the lip.

Clear'ing agent. Agent for rendering microscopic objects more transparent.

Clea'vage-nucleus (kle'vej). Segmentation-nucleus.

Cleft palate. Congenital fissure of palate and roof of the mouth. **C. sternum,** congenital fissure of the sternum.

Cleido-. A prefix indicating connection with the clavicle.

Cleidomastoide'us. See *Muscles, Table of.*

Cleptoma'nia (klep-to-ma'ne-ah). Insane desire to steal.

Cler'gyman's sore throat. Pharyngitis with dysphonia.

Clev'enger's fissure. The inferior occipital fissure.

Climacter'ic (kli-mak-ter'ik). The turn of life; especially the menopause. **Grand c.,** the 63d year.

Climatol'ogy (kli-mat-ol'o-je). The science or study of climates.

Climatother'apy (kli-mat-o-ther'ap-e). Treatment of disease by change of climate.

Clin'ic (klin'ik). Instruction at the bedside.

Clin'ical (klin'ik-al). Pertaining to a clinic, or to the bedside.

Clini'cian, Clin'icist. An expert clinical teacher.

Cli'noid (kli'noid). Bed-shaped. **C. processes,** three pairs of processes of the sphenoid bone.

Cliscom'eter (klis-e-om'et-er). Instrument for measuring the angles between the axis of the body and that of the pelvis.

Clit'ion (klit'e-on). The mid-point of the anterior border of the clivus.

Clitoridec'tomy (klit-or-id-ek'to-me). Surgical removal of the clitoris.

Clit'oris (klit'o-ris). A female organ homologous with the penis. **C. crises.** See *Crisis.*

Clit'orism (klit'o-rizm). Hypertrophy of the clitoris.

Clitori'tis (klit-o-ri'tis). Inflammation of the clitoris.

Cli'vus Blumenbach'ii. The bony surface sloping down from the pituitary fossa.

Cloa'ca (klo-a'kah). 1. Common fetal opening of urogenital tract and anus. 2. Opening in the involucrum of necrosed bone.

Clon'ic (klon'ik). Of the nature of clonus.

Clo'nus (klo'nus). Spasm in which rigidity and relaxation succeed each other. Varieties are named from the parts affected, as, *ankle, foot, jaw,* etc.

Cloquet's canal (klo-káz'). The hyaloid canal of the eye. **C.'s fascia,** the septum crurale, which closes the femoral ring. **C.'s hernia,** a variety of femoral hernia.

Close skein. A knot of chromatin fibrils in indirect cell-division.

Clostrid'ium (klos-trid'e-um). A genus of microbes.

Clot. A soft mass of semisolidified liquid: coagulum.

Clothes-louse. The body-louse, *Pediculus corporis.*

Clou'dy swelling. Degeneration in which the tissues swell and become cloudy.

Clove. The aromatic dried flower-bud of the tree *Eugenia aromatica.* **C. hitch,** a knot formed by a double loop: used in forcible extension and traction.

Clo'ven spine. The *Spina bifida.*

Clown'ism. The hysterical performance of grotesque actions.

Club'bed fingers. Deformed fingers with knotty ends.

Club-foot. See *Talipes.* **C.-hand,** deformity of the hand like club-foot.

Clys'ter (klis'ter). Enema; rectal injection.

Cm. Abbreviation for *Centimeter.*

Cne'mial (ne'me-al). Pertaining to the tibia, or shin.

Co. Symbol for cobalt.

Coagula'tion (ko-ag-u-la'shun). Formation of a clot.

Coag'ulative (ko-ag'u-la-tiv). Associated with coagulation. **C. necrosis.** See *Necrosis.*

Coag'ulum (ko-ag'u-lum). A clot.

Coales'cence, Coali'tion. Fusion of parts; a growing together.

Coal-tar. Viscid semisolid product of the distillation of coal.

Coapta'tion (ko-ap-ta'shun). A fitting together or adjustment of parts.

Coarc'tate ret'ina (ko-ark'tāt). Funnel-shaped condition of the retina.

Coarcta'tion. Condition of stricture.

Coarctot'omy. The cutting of a stricture.

Coarse lesion. Same as *Macroscopic lesion.*

Coat, buffy. See *Buffy coat.*

Coat-sleeve amputation. See *Amputation.*

Co'balt (ko'bawlt). A metal whose salts afford pigments: very seldom used as medicines.

Co'ca (ko'kah). The plant *Erythroxylon coca* and its leaves.

Coca'in (ko-ka'in). An alkaloid, $C_{17}H_{21}NO_4$, from coca: local anesthetic and mydriatic.

Coca'inism (ko-ka'in-izm). Morbid result of the misuse of cocain.

Coca'inize (ko-ka'in-īz). To treat or affect with cocain.

Cocainoma'nia (ko-ka-in-o-ma'ne-ah). The habit of using cocain as an intoxicant.

Coccidio'sis (kok-sid-e-o'sis). Ill-health caused by coccidia.

Coccid'ium (kok-sid'e-um). A genus of protozoans. **C. ova'le** has been found in the liver and intestinal epithelium. **C. sarkol'ytus,** a supposed parasite of carcinoma.

Coccinel'la (kok-sin-nel'ah). L. for *Cochineal.*

Coccobacte'ria. Spheroidal or rod-like bacteria.

Coc'culus in'dicus. The poisonous berry of *Anamirta cocculus.*

Coc'cus (kok'us). A spheroidal bacterial cell-form, such as macrococcus, micrococcus, streptococcus, gonococcus, etc.

Coccyal'gia (kok-se-al'je-ah). Pain in the coccyx.

Coccydyn'ia (kok-se-din'e-ah). Same as *Coccygodynia.*

Coccyg'eal (kok-sij'e-al). Pertaining to the coccyx. **C. gland,** a small gland near the point of the coccyx; Luschka's gland.

Coccygec'tomy (kok-se-jek'to-me). Excision of the coccyx.

Coccyg'eus (kok-sij'e-us). See *Muscles, Table of.*

Coccygodyn'ia (kok-sig-o-din'e-ah). Pain in the coccyx.

Coccygot'omy (kok-sig-ot'o-me). Surgical removal of the coccyx.

Coc'cyx (kok'six). Small bone below the sacrum.

Co'chia pills (ko'ke-ah, ko'che-ah). Pills of aloes and colocynth.

Cochineal' (coch-in-ēl'). Dried insect, *Coccus cacti,* from tropical America.

Coch'lea (kok'le-ah). Spiral cavity of the internal ear.

Coch'lear (kok'le-ar). Relating to the cochlea. **C. canal,** space between the membrane of Reissner and the basilar membrane.

Cochlea're (kok-le-a're). L. for *Spoonful.*

Cochlea'ria (kok-le-a're-ah). Genus of plants including horseradish and scurvy-grass.

Cochlear'iform (kok-le-ar'if-orm). Spoon-shaped.

Cochlei'tis (kok-le-i'tis). Inflammation of the cochlea.

Cocilla'na (ko-sil-yah'nah). Bark of *Sycocarpus Rusbyi,* a tree of tropical America: emetic; serviceable in diseases of the air-passages.

Cock'roach. See *Blatta.*

COCL. Abbreviation for cathodal opening contraction.

Co'coa (ko'ko). See *Cacao.* **C.-nut oil,** the oil of cocoa-nut, *Cocos nucifera.*

Co'dein (ko'de-in). An opium alkaloid, $C_{18}H_{21}NO_3$, milder than morphin.

Cod-liver oil. Oil from the liver of codfish, *Gadus morrhua.*

Cœliac, Cœliotomy, Cœnesthesis, etc. See *Celiac, Celiotomy, Cenesthesis,* etc.

Cof'fee. The dried seeds of *Coffea Arabica* and the decoction of the same. **C.-ground vomit,** vomits of gastric juice mixed with blood and stomach-contents in cancer of stomach.

Coffe'inism (kof-fe'in-ism). Habitual excess in the use of coffee.

Coffeu'rin (kof-fe-u'rin). A substance said to exist in urine after free use of coffee.

Cof'fin bone. The third phalanx of the horse's hoof.

Cognac (kon'yahk). A variety of French brandy.

Cog-wheel respiration. A variety of interrupted respiration.

Cohe'sion. The force which holds together the particles of a body.

Cohn'heim's areas or **field** (kōn'hīmz). Dark spaces seen on cross-section of a muscle, bounded by bright lines of sarcoplasm. **C.'s theory,** theory that true tumors are due to faulty development in embryo.

Cohoba'tion (ko-ho-ba'shun). Repeated distillation of a fluid from the same material.

Co'hosh (ko'hosh). See *Actæa, Caulophyllum, Cimicifuga.*

Coil. A spiral. **C.-gland.** See convoluted portion of sweat-gland. **Induction-c.,** coil for producing electricity by induction. **Leiter's c.** See *Leiter's coil.* **Resistance c.,** coil of wire placed in electric circuit to produce additional resistance.

Coin-test. See *Bell-metal resonance.*

Coit'ion (ko-ish'un). See *Coitus.*

Coitopho'bia (ko-it-o-fo'be-ah). Morbid fear of coitus.

Co'itus (ko'it-us). Sexual connection or intercourse.

Co'ko disease. A kind of yaws in Fiji Islands.

Co'la (ko'lah). Same as *Kola.*

Cola'tion (ko-la'shun). The process of straining.

Col'chicin (kol'kis-in). Alkaloid from colchicum.

Col'chicum autumna'le (kol'ki-kum, kol'tschi-kum). Plant useful in gout and rheumatism; poisonous.

Cold. Catarrhal disorder from exposure. **C. abscess.** See *Abscess.* **Rose c.,** hay fever occurring at the time of roses.

Colec'tomy (ko-lek'to-me). Excision of a part of the colon.

Col'ic (kol'ik). Acute abdominal pain. **Biliary c., Hepatic c.,** that caused by gall-stones. **Lead c.,** intestinal colic from lead-poisoning. **Menstrual c.,** the pain of menstruation. **Renal c.,** colic caused by calculus. **Uterine c.,** colicky pains of a paroxysmal character at the menstrual period.

Col'ica pic'tonum. Lead colic.

Co'li-infection. Infection with bacillus coli communis.

Coli'tis (ko-li'tis). Inflammation of the colon.

Col'lagen (kol'laj-en). A leading constituent of the bones and flesh.

Collapse (kol-laps'). State of extreme depression or prostration.

Collap'sing pulse. Corrigan's pulse.

Col'lar-bone. See *Clavicle.*

Collat'eral circulation. See *Circulation.*

Collec'ting plates. The electronegative element of a galvanic battery. **C. tubes,** direct uriniferous tubules of the kidney.

Col'les's fascia (kol'lis). Superficial perineal fascia. **C.'s fracture,** fracture near distal end of radius.

Collic'ulus semina'lis. The verumontanum.

Col'lidin (kol'lid-in). A ptomain, $C_8H_{11}N$, from decaying flesh.

Col'lier's lung. Same as *Anthracosis.*

Collilon'gus. The longus coli muscle.

Colliqua'tion (kol-lik-wa'shun). Liquefactive degeneration of tissue.

Colliq'uative. Characterized by excessive liquid discharge, or by liquefaction of tissue.

Collo'dion (kol-lo'de-on). Solution of gun-cotton in ether and alcohol: useful in burns and wounds. **Cantharidal c.** See *Collodium cantharidatum.* **Styptic c.,** a preparation of tannic acid, alcohol, ether, and collodion.

Collo'dium. L. for *Collodion.* **C. cantharida'tum,** a blistering varnish of collodion and cantharides.

Col'loid. 1. Resembling glue. 2. Any substance not a crystalloid. **C. cancer,** carcinoma in which the cells assume a glue-like aspect. **C. cyst,** cyst with jelly-like contents. **C. degeneration.** See *Degeneration.*

Colloi'din (kol-loi'din). A jelly-like principle produced in colloid degeneration.

Collo'ma (kol-o'mah). Colloid cancer.

Collox'ylin (kol-lox'il-in). A variety of soluble gun-cotton.

Col'lum. Neck or neck-like organ. **C. distor'tum.** Same as *Torticollis.*

Col'lutory (kol'lu-to-re). Mouth-wash or gargle.
Collyr'ium (ko-lir'e-um). An eye-lotion.
Colobo'ma. A fissure or gap in the eyeball.
Colocente'sis (kol-o-sen-te'sis). Surgical puncture of the colon.
Col'ocynth (kol'o-sinth). The fruit of *Citrullus colocynthis;* cathartic.
Colocyn'thin (kol-o-sin'thin). Strongly purgative principle from colocynth.
Colo-enteri'tis. Inflammation of small and large intestines.
Colom'ba (ko-lom'bah). Same as *Calumba.*
Co'lon (ko'lon). That part of the large intestine which extends from the cecum to the rectum.
Colon'ic (ko-lon'ik). Pertaining to the colon.
Colon'oscope. Speculum for the lower part of the intestine.
Colonos'copy. Examination of lower intestine with colonoscope.
Col'ony. A collection of bacteria in a culture.
Colopexot'omy. Fixation and incision of the colon.
Col'opexy (kol'o-pek-se). Fixation of the sigmoid flexure to the abdominal wall.
Coloph'ony (ko-lof'o ne). Rosin; ordinary resin of pine.
Colopto'sis (ko-lop-to'sis). Prolapse of the colon.
Col'or-blindness. Inability to perceive differences of color. **C.-gustation.** Same as *Pseudogeusesthesia.* **C.-hearing.** Same as *Pseudochromesthesia.*
Colorectos'tomy (ko-lo-rek-tos'to-me). Surgical formation of passage between the colon and rectum.
Colorim'eter. An instrument for measuring pigments present.
Colos'tomy. Formation of a permanent colonic fistula.
Colos'trum (ko-los'trum). First milk after childbirth. **C.-corpuscles.** large cells found in colostrum.
Colot'omy (ko-lot'o-me). Surgical incision of the colon. It is termed *abdominal, lateral, lumbar, iliac,* or *inguinal,* according to the region of incision. **Littre's c.,** inguinal colotomy.
Col'peurynter (kol'pu-rin-ter). A form of vaginal dilator.
Colpeu'rysis (kol-pu'ris-is). Operative dilatation of vagina.
Colpi'tis (kol-pi'tis). Inflammation of the vagina.
Col'pocele (kol'po-sēl). Vaginal hernia.
Colpoclei'sis (kol-po-kli'sis). Surgical closure of vagina.
Colpocysti'tis. Inflammation of the vagina and bladder.
Colpocys'tocele (kol-po-sis'to-sēl). Protrusion of a fold of the vagina into bladder.
Colpocystot'omy. Incision of the bladder through the vagina.
Colpodesmorrha'phia. The suturing of vaginal sphincter.
Colpohysterec'tomy. Removal of the uterus through a vaginal incision.
Colpohysterot'omy. Surgical incision of the vagina and uterus.
Colpomyomec'tomy. Removal of a myoma through a vaginal incision.
Colpomyomot'omy. Same as *Colpomyomectomy.*
Colpomyot'omy. Same as *Colpomyomectomy.*
Colpoperine'oplasty (kol-po-per-in-e'o-plas-te). Plastic surgery upon the vagina and perineum.
Colpoperinor'rhaphy. Suturing of the vagina and perineum.
Col'poplasty (kol'po-plas-te). Plastic surgery upon the vagina.
Colpopto'sis (kol-pop-to'sis). Prolapse of the vagina.
Colpor'rhaphy. Narrowing of the vagina by a suture.
Colpot'omy. Surgical cutting operation upon the vagina.
Colt's-foot. See *Tussilago.*
Colum'bin (ko-lum'bin). Active principle of calumba.
Colum'bo (ko-lum'bo). Same as *Calumba.*
Columel'la. Central axis of the cochlea of the ear. **C. na'si,** the septum of the nose.

Col'umn (kol'um). A supporting part. **Anterior c.**, layer of white matter in either half of spinal cord between the anterior horn and the anterior median fissure. **C. of Burdach.** See *Postero-external c.* **C. of Clarke**, a column of gray matter to the outer and posterior side of the central canal of the spinal cord, at the base of the posterior cornu. **Direct cerebellar c.**, a tract outside of the lateral pyramidal tract. **C. of Goll**, posteromedian column of the spinal cord. **C. of Gowers**, a mass of fibers in front of the direct cerebellar tract. **Lateral c.**, layer of white matter in either half of the spinal cord between the posterior horn and nerve-roots and the anterior horn and nerve-roots. **C. of Morgagni**, folds of mucous membrane seen at the junction of the rectum with the anus. **Posterior c.**, a mass of white matter in the spinal cord on either side between the posterior horns and the posterior median fissure. **Postero-external c.**, the outer wider portion of the posterior column of the cord. **Posteromedian c.**, the middle portion of the posterior column of the cord. **Posterovesicular c.** See *C. of Clarke*. **Respiratory c.**, the solitary fasciculus. **C. of Sertoli**, an elongated cell in the seminiferous tubule supporting spermatogenic cells. **C. of Spitzka-Lissauer**, a group of nerve-fibers of cord in front of and behind the posterior horns. **C. of Türck**, the anterior or direct pyramidal tract. **Vesicular c.**, column of nerve-cells in posterior gray horn of cord.

Colum'na (ko-lum'nah). A pillar or column. **C. adipo'sa.** Same as *Fat-column.* **C. Berti'ni**, cortical part of kidney separating any two pyramids. **C. car'nea**, any one of the muscular projections within the ventricles of the heart. **C. na'si**, the septum of the nose.

Colum'næ papilla'res. Same as *Musculi papillares.* **C. vagi'næ**, rugosities within the vagina.

Colum'nar layer. The rod-and-cone layer of the retina.

Col'umning (kol'um-ing). Support of the prolapsed uterus by means of tampons.

Co'ma (ko'mah). Profound stupor in sickness or after severe injury. **Alcoholic c.**, coma from alcoholism. **Apoplectic c.**, that due to apoplexy. **Diabetic c.**, peculiar coma seen in fatal diabetes. **Kussmaul's c.**, coma with acetone in urine from diabetes. **Uremic c.**, that due to uremia. **C. vigil**, stupor with wakefulness, low delirium, and semi-consciousness.

Co'matose (ko'mat-ōs). Pertaining to, or affected with, coma.

Combus'tion. Burning; rapid oxidation, with emission of heat.

Com'edo (kom'e-do). 1. Disease due to the presence of comedones. 2. Singular of comedones; a blackhead.

Comedo'nes (kom-e-do'nēz). Blackheads; plugs of dried sebum in the excretory ducts of the skin.

Co'mes (ko'mēz). A companion; an artery which accompanies a nerve-trunk.

Com'ma bacillus. The spirillum of epidemic cholera. **C. tract**, a comma-shaped tract in the dorso-external column of the cord.

Commeli'na. Any one of several plants of Mexico having styptic properties.

Commen'sal. An organism living on or within another, but not as a parasite; used also adjectively.

Com'minuted frac'ture. A crushed bone.

Comminu'tion. A breaking into small fragments.

Commissu'ra bre'vis. The posterior part of the inferior vermiform process of the cerebellum. **C. mag'na.** Same as *Corpus callosum.* **C. sim'plex**, a lobule on the superior cerebellar vermiform process.

Com'missure (kom'is-ūr). Tissue linking corresponding right and left parts of brain or cord. **Anterior c.**, a cord of white fibers in front of crura of fornix. **Arcuate c.**, the posterior optic c. **Gray c.**, band of gray matter joining the lateral masses of gray matter of the spinal cord. **Meynert's c.**, c. of nerve-fibers extending from floor of third ventricle through optic tracts to subthalamic body. **Middle c.**, band of gray matter joining optic thalami. **Optic c.**, the crossing of the two optic nerves. **Posterior c.**, a white band joining the optic thalami posteriorly.

Commo'tio (kom-mo'she-o). A concussion; shock from a violent shaking.

Commu'nicans. A communicating nerve. **C. hypoglos'si, C. no'ni**, nerves joining the cervical plexus to the descendens noni. **C. perone'i**, a nerve which joins the external popliteal and short saphenous nerves. **C. Willis'ii**, the posterior communicans artery of the brain.

Com'mutator (kom'mū-ta-ter). A device for reversing electric currents.

Compact' tissue. The hard, external portion of bone.

Compar'ative anat'omy. See *Anatomy*.

Compatibil'ity. Suitableness for administration with another specified medicine.

Com'pensating operation. Tenotomy of an ocular muscle when its antagonist is paralyzed.

Compensa'tion. The counterbalancing of defect of structure or function.

Complement'al air. See *Air*.

Complemen'tary colors. Those which when blended produce a white.

Com'plex of symptoms. The sum of signs of any morbid condition.

Complex'us. See *Muscles, Table of*.

Com'plicated fracture. See *Fracture*.

Complica'tion (kom-ple-ka'shun). A disease or diseases concurrent with another disease.

Com'pos men'tis. Of sound mind.

Composi'tion powder. Compound powder of bayberry.

Com'pound astigmatism. See *Astigmatism*. **C. cathartic pills**, pills of colocynth, jalap, calomel, and gamboge. **C. fracture.** See *Fracture*. **C. microscope**, one with two lenses, the eye-piece, and objective.

Com'press. Folded cloth for applying pressure. **Graduated c.**, a compress consisting of layers of gradually decreasing size.

Compres'sion (kom-presh'un). Act of pressing together; state of being pressed together. **C.-atrophy.** See *Atrophy*. **C. of the brain**, abnormal pressure upon the brain, as by abscess, tumor, fracture, congestion, or effusion. **Digital c.**, compression of an artery by the fingers. **C.-myelitis.** See *Myelitis*.

Compres'sor. Instrument or muscle for compressing. See *Muscles, Table of*.

Compul'sory movements. Co-ordinated movements due to injury of a nerve-center.

Cona'rium (ko-na're-um). The pineal gland.

Conca'to's disease (kon-kah'tōz). Progressive inflammation of serous membranes.

Con'cave (kon'kāv). Having a depressed or hollow surface.

Concav'ity. A depression or hollowed surface.

Concavocon'cave. Concave on either side.

Concavocon'vex. Having one concave and one convex side.

Concentra'tion (kon-sen-tra'shun). 1. Increase in strength by evaporation. 2. Medicine which has been strengthened by evaporating its non-active parts.

Concep'tion (kon-sep'shun). The fecundation of the ovum. **Imperative c.**, a false idea dominating a person's actions.

Con'cha (kong'kah). The hollow of the external ear. **C. labyryn'thi.** Same as *Cochlea.*

Conchi'nin. Same as *Quinidin.*

Conchi'tis (kong-ki'tis). Inflammation of the concha.

Con'choscope (kong'ko-skōp). A nasal speculum.

Concom'itant squint. See under *Strabismus.* **C. symptoms.** See *Symptoms.*

Con'crete (kon'krēt). Condensed or solidified.

Concre'tion. 1. Calculus. 2. Abnormal union of parts adjacent.

Concus'sion. Violent shock or jarring. **C. of the brain,** effect of severe head-injury. **C. of the labyrinth,** deafness, vertigo, and tinnitus from head-injury. **C.-myelitis.** See *Myelitis.* **Spinal c.,** result of shocks or blows affecting the myelon.

Condensa'tion. Pathologic hardening of a part, with or without shrinkage.

Conden'ser. 1. Device for illuminating microscopic objects. 2. Worm, or corresponding part, of apparatus for distillation.

Conden'sing ostei'tis. Same as *Osteosclerosis.*

Con'dom. A capote or sheath for the penis.

Conduc'tion (kon-duk'shun). Transference of heat, sound, nerve-impulse, or electricity. **Aerial c.,** conduction of sound-waves to the ear through the air. **Aerotympanal c.,** conduction of sound to the ear through the air and the tympanum. **C.-aphasia.** See *Aphasia.* **Bone-c.,** conduction of sound through the bones of the skull.

Conductiv'ity. Capacity for conduction; ability to convey.

Conduc'tor. 1. A substance or part which possesses conductivity. 2. A guide for the surgeon's knife.

Conduran'go (kon-du-rang'go). Bark of *Gonolobus condurango* of Peru; a bitter stimulant and reputed alterative.

Con'dylar (kon'dil-ar). Pertaining to a condyle.

Condylarthro'sis. Articulation in which a bony eminence is lodged in a joint-cavity.

Con'dyle (kon'dil). Rounded eminence at articular end of bone.

Condylec'tomy (con-dil-ek'to-me). Removal of a condyle.

Condyl'ion (kon-dil'e-on). Point at lateral tip of the mandibular condyle.

Con'dyloid (kon'dil-oid). Resembling a condyle or knuckle.

Condylo'ma (kon-dil-o'mah). Wart-like growth about the vulva or anus. **C. la'tum,** a wide, flat condyloma with yellowish discharge.

Condylo'matous (kon-dil-o'mat-us). Of the nature of a condyloma.

Condylot'omy (kon-dil-ot'o-me). Excision, or division, of a condyle.

Con'dy's fluid. A disinfectant solution of sodium or potassium permanganate.

Cone of light. Triangular light-reflex on the membrana tympani. **Retinal c's.,** minute percipient organs near the outermost layer of the retina.

Confec'tion. A medicated sweetmeat, conserve, or electuary.

Confec'tioners' disease. Finger-nail disease peculiar to confectioners.

Confine'ment (kon-fīn'ment). Childbirth; the puerperal state or condition.

Con'fluent. Running together; becoming merged in one. **C. articulation.** See *Articulation.* **C. smallpox,** smallpox in which the pustules become more or less blended.

Con'formator. Instrument for determining outlines of skull.

Confronta'tion (kon-frun-ta'shun). The bringing of two patients together for diagnostic purposes.

Congela'tion (kon-je-la'shun). Frostbite or freezing.

Congen'erous muscles (kon-jen'er-us). Those which act together as one organ.

Congen'ital (kon-jen'it-al). Existing at or before birth.

Conges'ted (kon-jes'ted). Hyperemic; overloaded with blood.

Conges'tion (kon-jes'chun). Abnormal accumulation of blood in a part.

Conges'tive (kon-jes'tiv). Associated with congestion. **C. fever,** a form of malarial fever.

Con'gius (kon'je-us). L. for *Gallon.*

Conglom'erate gland. A gland made up of several lobes.

Conglu'tin (kon-glu'tin). A proteid from the lupines, peas, beans, and almonds.

Conglu'tinant. Promoting union, as of the lips of a wound.

Conglutina'tion. Abnormal adherence of parts to each other.

Con'go-red. Red pigment, turned blue by HCl: used in the study of gastric juice.

Co'ni vasculo'si. Conical masses in globus major of epididymis.

Con'ical cor'nea. See *Keratoconus.*

Co'niin, Con'in. Liquid alkaloid of conium, $C_8H_{17}N$.

Coni'um (ko-ni'um). Fruit of *Conium maculatum,* poison hemlock: sedative and narcotic.

Con'jugal diabetes. See *Diabetes.*

Con'jugate deviation. Deviation of both eyes to right or left. **C. diameter,** sacro-pubic diameter of superior strait of pelvis.

Conjuga'tion (kon-ju-ga'shun). Reproduction by the union of one organism with another. **C.-nucleus.** Same as *Segmentation nucleus.*

Conjuncti'va (kon-junk-ti'vah). Delicate membrane which lines the lids and covers the eyeball.

Conjunctivi'tis (kon-junk-tiv-i'tis). Inflammation of the conjunctiva. **Catarrhal c.,** mild form resulting from cold or irritation. **Croupous c.,** associated with the formation of a whitish-gray membrane. **Diphtheric c.,** purulent form due to the Klebs-Löffler bacillus. **Egyptian c.** See *Trachoma.* **Follicular c.,** a form marked by round, pinkish bodies in the retrotarsal fold. **Gonorrheal c.,** a severe form caused by infection with gonococci. **Granular c.,** trachoma. **Phlyctenular c.,** one marked by small vesicles surrounded by a reddened zone. **Purulent c.,** one characterized by a creamy discharge. **Spring c., Vernal c.,** c. coming on with the spring.

Connec'tive tissue. The tissue which binds together and is the basis of the various parts and organs of the body.

Co'noid. Cone-shaped or conical. **C. ligament,** inner portion of the coracoclavicular ligament. **C. tubercle,** eminence on lower surface of clavicle for attachment of c. ligament.

Consanguin'ity. Blood-relationship; kinship.

Consen'sual motion. That excited by reflex stimulation.

Conser'vancy. The sum of hygienic and preservative legislation; care of things which restore and maintain public health.

Conserv'ative. Aiming at a preservation and repair of parts.

Con'serve. A confection, electuary, or medicated sweetmeat.

Consolida'tion. Solidification, as of a lung in pneumonia.

Con'stant battery, C. cell. A galvanic battery or cell which affords a fairly constant and uniform current. **C. current,** unbroken or uninterrupted electric current.

Con'stipated. Affected with constipation; costive.

Constipa'tion. Infrequent and difficult evacuation of the feces.

Constitu'tion. The make-up or functional habit of the body.

Constitu'tional. Affecting the whole body; not local.

Constric'tor muscles. See *Muscles, Table of.*

Construct'ive metabolism. Anabolic change or process.

Consult'ant. A consulting physician or surgeon.

Consulta'tion. A deliberation of two or more physicians with respect to the diagnosis or treatment of a particular case.

Consump'tion. Wasting of the body; pulmonary tuberculosis.

Con'tact breaker. Instrument for breaking a galvanic current.

Conta'gion (kon-ta'jun). Communication of disease through mediate or immediate contact. **Psychic c.,** transfer of nervous disease by imitation.

Contagios'ity. The quality of being contagious.

Contagious (kon-ta'jus). Communicable by direct or indirect contact.

Conta'gium (kon-ta'je-um). Virus or morbific matter which may spread disease. **C. vi'vum,** a living organism that causes disease.

Contigu'ity (kon-tig-u'it-e). Contact or proximity. **Amputation in the c.,** amputation at a joint. **Solution of c.,** dislocation, luxation, or displacement.

Contin'ued current. See *Current.* **C. fever.** See *Fever.*

Continu'ity (kon-tin-u'it-e). The quality of being continuous. **Amputation in the c.,** amputation by cutting through a bone. **Solution of c.,** fracture, rupture, or division of a bone or other tissue.

Contrac'tile. Contracting under the proper stimulus.

Contractil'ity. Ability to contract with a suitable stimulus.

Contrac'tion (kon-trak'shun). A drawing together; a shortening or shrinkage. **Anodal, Closing** or **Opening c.,** the contraction at the anode on closing or opening the circuit. **Carpopedal c.,** a kind of tetany in infants, with flexing of the fingers, toes, elbows, and knees, and a general tendency to convulsions. **Closing c.,** muscular contraction at the instant that the electric current is closed. **Dupuytren's c.,** a contraction of palmar fascia causing flexing of the fingers. **Front-tap c.,** contraction of gastrocnemius on tapping muscles of front of leg. The foot is placed at a right angle to the leg, and the muscles of the front of the leg are tapped, the foot is extended. **Hour-glass c.,** contraction of an organ, as the stomach or uterus, at the middle. **Idiomuscular c.,** contraction produced by direct stimulation of the muscle. **Opening c.,** muscular contraction produced by opening or breaking the circuit. **Paradoxic c.,** contraction of a muscle, caused by the passive approximation of its extremities. **C.-remainder,** the contraction persisting in a muscle after withdrawal of the stimulus. **C.-ring,** the boundary between the upper and lower segments of the parturient uterus. **Tonic c.,** tonic spasm.

Contrac'ture (kon-trak'tūr). Shortening and distortion; *permanent*, as from the shrinkage of muscles, or *spasmodic*, as from electric or sudden stimulus.

Contraindica'tion. A condition which forbids any particular course of treatment.

Contralat'eral muscle. A muscle which acts in harmony with a muscle on the other side of the body.

Contrecoup' (kon-ter-koo'). Injury resulting from a blow on a remote part.

Control' (kon-trōl'). An experiment, or other standard, by which to test the correctness of observations. **C.-animal.** an animal not immune which is exposed to the effects of a virus, an immune animal being submitted to the same treatment at the same time. **C.-experiment,** any experiment made under standard conditions by which to test the correctness of other observations.

Contuse' (kon-tūz'). To bruise: to wound by beating.

Contu'sion (kon-tū'zhun). A bruise; the act of bruising. **C.-pneumonia,** pneumonia from traumatism.

Co'nus (ko'nus). 1. A cone. 2. Posterior staphyloma of the myopic eye. **C. arterio'sus,** the upper anterior angle of the right ventricle of the heart. **C. medulla'ris,** the lower and conical end of the spinal cord. **C. termina'lis,** same as *Conus medullaris.*

Convales'cence. The stage of recovery following an illness.

Convallam'arin. A glucosid from convallaria: emetic, diuretic.

Convalla'ria maja'lis. Lily of the valley: cardiac stimulant, diuretic.

Convalla'rin. A purgative glucosid from convallaria.

Conver'gence (kon-ver'jens). The fact or point of converging.

Conver'gent (kon-ver'jent). Tending toward the same point. **C. strabismus.** See *Strabismus.*

Con'vex. Having a rounded and somewhat elevated surface.

Convexocon'cave. Same as *Concavoconvex.*

Convexocon'vex. Convex on each of the two faces.

Convolu'tion (kon-vo-lu'shun). The elevated part of the brain-surface more or less marked off by fissures. **Angular c.,** the posterior part of a convolution between the intraparietal fissure and the horizontal limb of the Sylvian fissure. **Annectant c.,** small convolutions connecting the occipital with the temporo-sphenoidal and parietal lobes. **Ascending frontal c.,** convolution in front of fissure of Rolando. **Ascending parietal c.,** convolution just behind fissure of Rolando. **Broca's c.,** the inferior or third frontal convolution. **Dentate c.,** a cerebral c. in the hippocampal fissure. **Fornicate c.,** a long convolution on mesial surface of the brain above corpus callosum. **Frontal c.,** the convolutions of the frontal lobe. **Hippocampal c.,** the part of the fornicate convolution winding around the splenium of the corpus callosum. **Inframarginal c.,** the superior temporal c. **Insular c.,** small convolutions composing the island of Reil. **Marginal c.,** mesial surface of the first frontal convolution. **Occipital c.,** the convolutions making up the occipital lobe. **Paracentral c.,** a convolution on mesial surface of the brain, representing the junction of the upper ends of the ascending frontal and ascending parietal convolutions. **Parietal c.,** the convolutions of the parietal lobe. **Supramarginal c.** See *Angular c.* **Temporal c.,** the convolutions of the temporal lobe. **Uncinate c.,** the hook-like end of the fornicate convolution.

Convol'vulin. Purgative glucosid, $C_{31}H_{50}O_{16}$, from jalap.

Convul'sion. An involuntary spasm or contraction of muscle. **Epileptiform c.,** convulsion marked by loss of consciousness. **Hysteric c.,** one due to hysteria. **Mimetic c.,** c. of facial muscles. **Puerperal c.,** c. just before or after childbirth. **Tetanic c.,** tonic convulsion without loss of consciousness. **Uremic c.,** one due to retention in the blood of matters that should be eliminated by the kidney.

Convul'sive. Pertaining to a convulsion; of the nature of a convulsion. **C. tic,** spasm of those parts of the face supplied by the seventh nerve.

Coör'dinate cramps. Same as *Circus movements.*

Coördina'tion. Harmonious working together of parts and normal sequence of functions.

Copa'iba (ko-pa'ib-ah). Resinous and diuretic juice of various trees, as *Copaifera officinalis:* used in gonorrhea and catarrhal diseases.

Copio'pia (ko-pe-o'pe-ah). Eye-strain; worn-out state of the eyes.

Cop'per. A metal with poisonous salts. **C. acetate,** verdigris; now sparingly used, mainly in ointments. **C. aceto-arsenite,** Paris-green: highly poisonous. **C. sulphate,** blue vitriol; bluestone: astringent, emetic.

Cop'peras. Ferrous sulphate: deodorizer, tonic, and astringent.

Copre'mia (ko-pre'me-ah). General blood-poisoning from chronic constipation.

Coprola'lia. Insane utterance of obscene words.

Cop'rolith (kop'ro-lith). Hard fecal concretion in the intestine.

Coproph'agy (kop-rof'aj-e). The eating of ordure.

Copros'tasis (kop-ros'tas-is). The impaction of feces in scybalous masses.

Cop'tis trifolia'ta. Gold thread, a plant: bitter tonic.

Copula'tion (kop-u-la'shun). Sexual congress.

Cor. L. for *Heart.* **C. adipo'sum.** fatty heart. **C. bovi'num,** "ox-heart;" greatly enlarged heart. **C. hirsu'tum, C. tomento'sum.** Same as *Hairy heart.*

Coraco-acro'mial. Pertaining to acromion and coracoid process.

Coracobrachia'lis. See *Muscles, Table of.*

Cor'acoid (kor'ak-oid). Like a crow's beak. **C. ligament** extends across the coracoid notch. **C. notch.** a notch in upper border of the shoulder-blade. **C. process.** a projection from the anterior and superior edge of shoulder-blade.

Cor'dial (kor'jal). A strong aromatic alcoholic liqueur.

Cor'diform. Heart-shaped.

Corec'tome (ko-rek'tōm). Cutting instrument for iridectomy.

Corectomedial'ysis. Same as *Coredialysis.*

Corec'tomy (ko-rek'to-me). Same as *Iridectomy.*

Corecto'pia (kor-ek-to'pe-ah). Displacement of pupil.

Coredial'ysis (ko-re-di-al'is-is). Artificial detachment of the iris from the ciliary ligament for new pupil.

Corel'ysis (ko-rel'is-is). Detachment of adhesions of iris to cornea or lens.

Coremorpho'sis. Creation of an artificial pupil.

Coreom'eter (ko-re-om'et-er). Device for use in measuring the pupil.

Coreom'etry. Measurement of the pupil.

Co'reoplasty (ko're-o-plas-te). Creation of an artificial pupil.

Coret'omy (ko-ret'o-me). Same as *Iridotomy.*

Corian'der. The *Coriandrum sativum;* a plant whose fruit is aromatic and stimulant.

Co'rium (ko're-um). The true skin; derma or cutis vera.

Corn. Horny induration of skin from pressure; clavus. **C. silk.** See *Stigmata maydis.*

Cor'nea (kor'ne-ah). The transparent anterior part of the eye. **Conic c.** Same as *Keratoglobus.*

Cor'neal. Pertaining to the cornea. **C. corpuscles.** See *Corpuscles.* **C. spaces.** star-shaped lacunæ between the laminæ of the cornea.

Cornei'tis (kor-ne-i'tis). Inflammation of the cornea.

Corneo-iri'tis. Inflammation of the cornea and iris.

Corneoscle'ra. The cornea and sclera regarded as one organ.

Cor'neous (kor'ne-us). Horny; horn-like. **C. layer.** Same as *Stratum corneum.*

Cor'niculum laryn'gis. Cartilaginous nodule on the arytenoid cartilage.

Cornifica'tion. The process of becoming horny.

Cor'nu. L. for *Horn.* **C. ammo'nis.** Same as *Hippocampus major.* **C. cer'vi.** deer's or stag's horn. **C. cuta'neum, C. huma'num,** horny excrescence on the skin.

Cor'nual. Pertaining to the horns of the spinal cord. **C. myeli'tis.** See *Myelitis.*

Cor'nus. The tree *Cornus florida;* dogwood: root-bark is antiperiodic and tonic.

Cornu'tin (kor-nu'tin). An alkaloid of ergot.

Coro'na. A crown. **C. den'tis.** the crown of a tooth. **C. glan'-**

dis, rim around proximal part of glans penis. **C. radia'ta,** fibers which radiate from the optic thalamus. **C. Ven'eris,** zone of syphilitic sores on the forehead.

Cor'onal suture. The suture between parietal and frontal bones.

Cor'onary. Encircling, in the manner of a crown.

Cor'oner. Officer who holds inquests over violent and sudden deaths.

Cor'onoid fossa. Hollow in the humerus which receives coronoid process of the ulna. **C. process,** a process of the ulna; also one of the lower jaw.

Coros'copy (ko-ros'ko-pe). Same as *Skiascopy.*

Cor'pora. Pl. of *Corpus.* **C. albican'tia,** two small protuberances at the base of the brain. **C. amyla'cea,** masses like starch in neuroglia, prostate, etc. **C. oliva'ria,** two oval masses behind the pyramid of the medulla.

Cor'pulency (korp'u-len-se). Undue fatness; obesity.

Cor'pus. Pl. *cor'pora.* L. for *Body.* **C. alie'num,** a foreign body. **C. annula're.** Same as *Pons Varolii.* **C. Aran'tii.** Same as *Arantius' body.* **C. bigem'inum.** Same as *Optic lobe.* **C. callo'sum,** the great commissure of the cerebrum. **C. cavernosum,** either one of the two erectile columns of the dorsum of the penis or clitoris. **C. cilia're.** Same as *Ciliary body.* **C. denta'le.** Same as *Corpus dentatum.* **C. denta'tum,** a layer of gray substance in the white matter of the cerebellum. **C. fimbria'tum,** band of white matter bordering the lateral edge of the lower cornu of the lateral ventricle. **C. genicula'tum,** one pair of tubercles on the lower part of the optic thalami. **C. Highmoria'num.** Same as *Mediastinum testis.* **C. lu'teum,** yellow mass in the ovary in the place of an ovisac which has discharged its ovum. **C. pyramida'le,** pyramid of the medulla. **C. quadrigem'inum,** organ made up of four oval bodies behind the third ventricle. **C. restifor'me,** either of the two columns of the oblongata extending to the cerebrum and the cord. **C. spongio'sum,** erectile rod in the lower part of the penis. **C. stria'tum,** a gray mass on the floor of either lateral ventricle. **C. subthalam'icum.** Same as *Subthalamus.* **C. vit'reum,** the vitreous body of the eye. **C. Wolffia'num.** Same as *Wolffian body.*

Cor'puscle (kor'pus'l). Any small mass, organ, or body. **Amylaceous c's.** See *Corpora amylacea.* **Bizzozero's c's.** See *Blood-platelets.* **Cartilage-c's.** See *Cartilage.* **Colostrum-c's.,** large granular cells in colostrum. **Corneal c's.,** star-shaped c's. within the corneal spaces. **C. of Donne.** See *Colostrum corpuscles.* **Genital c's.,** special nerve-endings in the external genitals. **Gluge's c's.,** granular corpuscles in diseased nervous matter. **Hassal's c's.,** nucleated cells in the thymus gland. **Krause's c's.,** round bodies constituting nerve-endings in mucous membrane of mouth, nose, eyes, and genitals. **Lostorfer's c's.,** granular bodies from the blood in syphilis. **Lymph-c's.,** corpuscular matter of lymph. **Malpighian c.** 1. The lymphoid nodules of the spleen. 2. The tuft of blood-vessels surrounded by the expanded portion of the uriniferous tubule of the kidney. **Meissner's c's.,** tactile corpuscles. **Norris's c's.,** colorless, transparent disks, invisible in the blood-serum. **Pacinian c's.,** small corpuscles in the subcutaneous cellular tissue of the fingers and toes, surrounding the termination of a sensory nerve. **Phantom c.,** a decolorized red blood-corpuscle. **Red blood-c's.,** biconcave circular disks containing hemoglobin. The red corpuscles of man are about $\frac{1}{3200}$ in. in diameter and $\frac{1}{12400}$ in. thick, and their number is about five millions to each cubic millimeter of blood. **Tactile c's. of Wagner,** the small, oval bodies in the papillæ of the skin surrounded by nerve-fibers. **C's. of Vater.** Same as *Pacinian c's.* **White** or **colorless blood-c's.,** flattened cells, about $\frac{1}{2500}$ in. in diameter.

Corpus'cular. Pertaining to corpuscles.

Correc'tant, Correc'tive. An ingredient which modifies the action of another.

Cor'rigan's disease. Incompetence of aortic valves. **C's. pulse.** Same as *Water-hammer pulse.*

Corro'sion-anatomy. The removal of tissue by a corrosive process.

Corro'sive (kor-ro'siv). Having a caustic and locally destructive effect. **C. sublimate,** Mercuric chlorid, $HgCl_2$: disinfectant, poisonous.

Corruga'tor supercil'ii. See *Muscles, Table of.*

Cor'tex. Outer layer or bark. **C. cer'ebri,** external layer of the brain, composed of gray matter.

Cor'tical (kor'tik-al). Pertaining to the cortex. **C. cataract,** opacity in the cortex of the lens. **C. paralysis,** paralysis from lesion of cerebral cortex.

Corti's arches (kor'tēz). Arches made up of Corti's rods. **C.'s canal,** passage made by the arches of Corti. **C.'s cells,** hair-cells in Corti's organ. **C.'s membrane,** lamina which covers Corti's organ. **C.'s rods,** double row of pillars which form Corti's arches. **C.'s teeth.** See *Auditory teeth.* **C.'s tunnel.** Same as *Corti's canal.*

Co'ryl (ko'ril). Mixture of ethyl and methyl chlorids: used as local anesthetic.

Coryleur (ko-ril-er'). Apparatus for applying a spray of coryl.

Cory'za (ko-ri'zah). Acute nasal catarrh or cold in the head.

Cosmet'ic (koz-met'ik). A substance used for improving the complexion. **C. operation,** operation for correcting an unsightly defect.

Cos'moline (koz'mo-lin). Petrolatum or vaselin.

Cos'ta. L. for *Rib.*

Cos'tal (kos'tal). Pertaining to a rib. **C. arch,** the arch of the ribs. **C. cartilages,** cartilages which prolong the ribs anteriorly. **C. respiration.** See *Respiration.*

Cos'tive. Affected with constipation; constipated.

Cos'tiveness. Constipation of the bowels.

Costochon'dral. Pertaining to a rib and its cartilage.

Costoclavicu'lar. Pertaining to ribs and clavicle.

Costocor'acoid. Pertaining to ribs and coracoid process.

Costoster'nal. Pertaining to a rib and to the sternum.

Cos'totome (kos'to-tōm). Knife for dividing costal cartilages.

Costotransverse'. Lying between the ribs and transverse processes of the vertebræ.

Costover'tebral. Pertaining to a rib and a vertebra.

Co'to (ko'to). An aromatic astringent bark from Bolivia.

Coto'in (ko-to'in). Active principle, $C_{22}H_{18}O_6$, from coto.

Cot'ton. Hair of seeds of various species of *Gossypium.* **Absorbent c.,** cotton so prepared as to absorb liquids. **C.-root,** bark of root of cotton-plant; emmenagogue and oxytocic. **Styptic c.,** cotton impregnated with styptic.

Cot'tonseed oil. Fixed oil from seeds of cotton-plant.

Cotun'nius's fluid or **liquor.** Same as *Perilymph.* **C.'s nerve.** The nasopalatine nerve.

Cotyle'don. Any subdivision of the uterine surface of the placenta.

Cot'yloid (kot'il-oid). Cup-shaped. **C. cavity,** the acetabulum. **C. foramen.** See *Foramen.* **C. ligament,** the fibro-cartilaginous rim of the acetabulum. **C. notch,** notch on lower border of the acetabulum.

Couch-grass. See *Triticum.*

Couch'ing (kow'ching). Displacement of the lens in cataract.

Cough. Sudden noisy expulsion of air from lungs. It is **dry,** when without expectoration; or **wet,** when attended by expectoration. **Ear-c.,** reflex cough produced by disease of the ear. **Reflex c.,** cough due to irritation of some remote organ. **Stomach-c.,** cough caused by reflex irritation from stomach disorder.

Cough'ing taxis (kawf'ing). Manipulation for reduction of hernia while the patient coughs.

Cou'lomb (koo'lom). The unit of electrical quantity.

Cou'marin (koo'ma-rin). An aromatic principle, $C_9H_6O_2$, from sweet clover, Tonka bean, etc.

Counterexten'sion (kown-ter-ex-ten'shun). Traction in a proximal direction coincident with traction in opposition to it.

Counterir'ritant. Producing a counterirritation; an agent which produces a counterirritation.

Counterirrita'tion. Superficial irritation which is intended to relieve some other irritation.

Countero'pening. A second opening, as in an abscess, sometimes made to facilitate drainage.

Coun'terpoison. A poison given to counteract another poison.

Coun'terpuncture. A second puncture made opposite to another.

Coup de soleil (koo-da-so'lāl). Sunstroke.

Cour'ses (kōr'siz). Menses, or woman's monthly illness.

Court'-plaster. Silken plaster spread with isinglass.

Cous'so. Same as *Kousso.*

Couveuse (koo-vuhz'). Same as *Incubator.*

Cov'er-glass. Thin glass plate to cover a mounted microscopical object.

Cow'age. See *Mucuna.*

Cowperi'tis. Inflammation of Cowper's glands.

Cow'per's glands. Two glands below membranous urethra, near bulb of spongy body.

Cow'pox. Same as *Vaccinia.*

Cox'a. The hip or hip-joint. **C. va'ra,** bending of neck of femur without hip-joint disease.

Cox'algia (kok-sal'je-ah). Hip-joint disease.

Coxi'tis (kok-si'tis). Inflammation of the hip-joint.

Coxofem'oral. Pertaining to the hip and thigh.

C. P. Abbreviation for *Chemically pure.*

Crab's eyes, C's. stones, concretions from the stomach of craw-fish.

Crab-louse. A louse that infests the pubic region, *Phthirius inguinalis.*

Crachotement (krah-shôt-maw'). Inability to spit, even with a strong desire to do so.

Cracked-pot sound. Percussion sound indicative of a pulmonary cavity into which the breath may pass.

Cra'din (kra'din). Peptic ferment from twigs and leaves of the fig-tree.

Cra'dle. Frame for keeping bed-clothes from a wounded limb.

Cramp. A painful spasmodic muscular contraction. **Intermittent c.,** tetany. **Professional c.,** spasm of a group of muscles from excessive use in one's daily occupation. **Seamstresses' c.,** neurosis of seamstresses resembling writers' cramp. **Telegraphers' c.,** neurosis resembling writers' cramp, seen in telegraphers. **Watchmakers' c.,** spasm of finger-muscles in watchmakers.

Cram-stunt. Mental defect from overstudy.

Cra'nial (kra'ne-al). Pertaining to the cranium.

Craniec'tomy. Surgical removal of strips of cranial bone.
Craniocer'ebral. Pertaining to skull and brain.
Cra'nioclast. Instrument for crushing fetal skull.
Cra'nioclasty. The crushing of the fetal head.
Craniol'ogy (kra-ne-ol'o-je). The scientific study of skulls.
Craniom'eter. Instrument for measuring the head.
Craniomet'rical points. Any one of a set of points established for use in craniometry.
Craniom'etry (kra-ne-om'et-re). Measurement of skull or head.
Craniop'agus (kra-ne-op'ag-us). Twin monster joined by the head.
Cra'nioplasty (kra'ne-o-plas-te). Plastic surgery of the skull.
Craniorrhachis'chisis (kra-ne-o-rak-is'kis-is). Congenital fissure of skull and spinal column.
Craniosto'sis (kra-ne-os-to'sis). Congenital ossification of the cranial sutures.
Craniota'bes (kra-ne-o-ta'bēz). Thinning in spots of the infantile skull in rickets.
Cra'niotome. Cutting instrument used in craniotomy.
Craniot'omy. The cutting up of the fetal head to effect delivery.
Craniotonos'copy. An osculatory percussion of the cranium.
Craniotympan'ic. Pertaining to skull and tympanum.
Cra'nium (kra'ne-um). The skull or brain-pan.
Crap'ulent. Due to excess in eating and drinking.
Crassamen'tum. A clot, as of blood.
Cravat' (krav-at'). A form of triangular handkerchief dressing.
Craw-craw. An African sore, perhaps same as Bulam boil.
Cream. The oily and lightest ingredient of milk. **C. of tartar,** potassium bitartrate.
Crease (krēs). A fold. **Gluteofemoral c., Ileofemoral c.,** the crease that bounds the buttocks below.
Cre'asol (kre'as-ol). See *Creosol.*
Cre'asote (kre'as-ōt). Same as *Creosote.*
Cre'atin (kre'at-in). A crystallizable nitrogenous principle from muscle-juice, etc.
Creatine'mia (kre-a-tin-e'me-ah). Excess of creatin in the blood.
Creat'inin (kre-at'in-in). A basic principle, creatin anhydrid, from urine.
Crede's method (krēdz). Method of expelling placenta by kneading and pressing down the uterus.
Cremas'ter (kre-mas'ter). The muscle by which the testicle is supported.
Cremaster'ic. Pertaining to the cremaster. **C. fascia,** thin envelop of the spermatic cord. **C. reflex.** See *Reflex.*
Crema'tion (kre-ma'shun). The burning of dead bodies; incineration.
Cre'mor. L. for *Cream.* **C. tar'tari,** cream of tartar.
Cre'nate (kre'nāt). Notched or scalloped.
Crena'tion (kre-na'shun). Notched appearance of the margins of red blood-corpuscles.
Cren'othrix (kren'o-thrix). A genus of schizomycete fungi.
Cre'olin (kre'o-lin). Antiseptic and hemostatic coal-tar product.
Cre'osol (kre'o-sol). An oily liquid, $C_8H_{10}O_2$, from creosote.
Creoso'tal. Creosote carbonate; milder than creosote.
Creo'sote (kre'o-sōt). An oily distillate from wood-tar: antiseptic, anesthetic, and escharotic.
Crep'itant rale. Dry crackling sound which marks the early stage of pneumonia. See *Râles, Table of.*
Crepita'tion (krep-it-a'shun). 1. The grating of the ends of fractured bones. 2. Crepitant râle.
Crep'itus (krep'it-us). Crepitation; a crepitant râle. **C. re'dux,**

the return of crepitus which announces the approach of recovery in pneumonia.

Cresal'ol. Cresol salicylate, an internal antiseptic.

Crescen'tic (kres-en'tik). Shaped like the new moon.

Cres'cents of Gianuzzi. See *Gianuzzi's crescents.* **Myopic c.** Same as *Conus*, second definition.

Cre'sin (kre'sin). Compound of cresol with sodium cresoxylacetate: antiseptic.

Cres'ochin. Disinfectant compound of tricresol sulphate and quinolin with tricresol.

Cre'sol (kre'sol). A compound, C_7H_8O, from coal-tar or wood-tar.

Cresolsulphur'ic acid. See *Acid.*

Crest. A ridge upon a bone. **Frontal c.,** a ridge in the middle line of internal surface of the frontal bone. **C. of ilium,** the thickened upper border of the ilium. **Lacrimal c.,** a vertical ridge on the external surface of the lacrimal bone. **Nasal c.,** a crest on the internal border of the nasal bone. **Occipital c.,** a vertical ridge on the external surface of the occipital bone. **C. of pubes,** a crest from the spine to the inner extremity. **Supramastoid c.,** ridge on temporal bone above auditory meatus. **Temporal c.,** a ridge on the frontal bone. **C. of tibia,** the prominent ridge on the front of the tibia. **Turbinated c.,** a horizontal ridge on the internal surface of the palate bone.

Cresyl'ic acid. Same as *Cresol.*

Cre'ta. L. for *Chalk.* **C. præpara'ta,** prepared chalk, U. S. P.; chalk powdered and washed.

Cre'tin (kre'tin). One who is affected with cretinism.

Cre'tinism. Endemic idiocy, with deformity, stunted growth, and often with goiter. **Sporadic c.,** congenital form of myxedema.

Cre'tinoid (kre'tin-oid). Resembling a cretin.

Cre'tinous (kre'tin-us). Affected with cretinism.

Cribra'tion (kri-bra'shun). The quality of being cribriform.

Crib'riform (crib'rif-orm). Perforated like a sieve. **C. fascia,** part of deep superficial fascia of the thigh which closes the saphenous opening. **C. plate,** the upper perforated plate of the ethmoid bone.

Cri'co-aryte'noid. Pertaining to the cricoid and arytenoid cartilages. **C.-arytenoid'eus.** See *Muscles, Table of.*

Cri'coid cartilage. The lowest cartilage of the larynx.

Cricothy'roid membrane. Ligamentous membrane between cricoid and thyroid cartilages. **C. muscle.** See *Muscles, Table of.*

Cricot'omy. The cutting of the cricoid cartilage.

Cricotracheot'omy. Incision through the cricoid and trachea.

Crim'inal abortion. See under *Abortion.*

Cri'sis (kri'sis). Pl. *cri'ses.* The turning point of a disease. **Bronchial c.,** paroxysms of dyspnea in locomotor ataxia. **Clitoris c.,** attacks of sexual excitement in women with tabes dorsalis. **Gastric c.,** paroxysms of intense pain in abdomen in locomotor ataxia. **Rectal c.,** severe seizures of pain in rectum in locomotor ataxia. **Vesical c.,** paroxysms of pain in bladder in locomotor ataxia.

Cris'ta. Same as *Crest.* **C. acus'tica,** the ridge on the inner side of the semicircular canals of the ear. **C. gal'li,** a ridge on the ethmoid bone to which the falx cerebri is attached. **C. hel'icis,** a projection on the helix, above the external meatus of the ear. **C. il'ii,** the crest of the ilium. **C. spira'lis,** a ridge on the spiral lamina of the cochlea. **C. vestib'uli,** a ridge on the floor of the vestibule between the vestibular aqueduct and fossa hemisphærica.

Crit'ical (krit'ik-al). Of the nature of a crisis.

Cro'cated. Tinctured with or containing saffron.

Cro'cus. The dried stigmas of *Crocus sativus*, or true saffron.

Crookes's tube. The vacuum tube used in skiagraphy.

Cross-birth. Abnormal presentation of fetus, requiring a version.

Cross-knee. Same as *Genu valgum.*

Crossed amblyopia. See *Amblyopia.* **C. anesthesia.** See *Anesthesia.* **C. hemiplegia.** See *Hemiplegia.* **C.-leg progression,** a gait in which one foot is placed before the other.

Crot'alus (krot'al-us). The rattlesnake; also its virus.

Crota'phion (kro-ta'fe-on). Cranial point at tip of great wing of sphenoid bone.

Crot'chet (krot'chet). A hook used in delivering the fetus after craniotomy.

Cro'ton. A genus of trees which affords cascarilla and croton oil. **C. chloral.** Same as *Butyl chloral.* **C. oil,** drastic purgative oil from *Croton tiglium.*

Croup. Disease with laryngeal spasm, dyspnea, difficult respiration, and often with a local membranous deposit. **Catarrhal c.,** simple inflammation of larynx with formation of membrane. **False c., Spasmodic c.,** spasm of laryngeal muscles with slight inflammation.

Crou'pous (kroo'pus). Of the nature of croup. **C. membrane,** the false membrane characteristic of croup.

Crown of a tooth. The exposed or enamelled part of a tooth.

Cru'cial (kroo'shal). 1. Cross-shaped; as a crucial incision, or crucial ligament. 2. Decisive; as a crucial test.

Cru'cible. A vessel for melting refractory substances.

Cru'ciform (kroo'sif-orm). Shaped like a cross.

Crude (krood). Raw or unrefined.

Cru'ra. The plural of *crus,* q. v. **C. cerebel'li,** peduncles of cerebellum. **C. cer'ebri,** pair of bands which join the pons and medulla with the cerebrum. **C. of diaphragm,** two pillars which connect the diaphragm to the spinal column. **C. of the fornix,** arches formed by division of the extremities of the fornix.

Crure'us (kroo-re'us). See *Muscles, Table of.*

Cru'ral (kroo'ral). Pertaining to the leg. **C. arch,** the femoral arch. **C. canal.** See *Canal.* **C. hernia,** femoral hernia. **C. sheath.** Same as *Femoral sheath.*

Crure'us (kroo-re'us). See *Muscles, Table of.*

Crus. Pl. *cru'ra.* A leg or structure like a leg.

Crusocreat'inin. Same as *Chrysokreatinin.*

Crus'ta. 1. Any crust. 2. Part of crus cerebri below the substantia nigra. **C. lac'tea,** seborrhea of the scalp of a nursing infant. **C. petro'sa,** the cement of a tooth. **C. phlogis'tica.** Same as *Buffy coat.*

Crutch paralysis. Arm-palsy from pressure of crutch-head.

Cruveilhier's disease (kroo-väl-e-äz'). 1. Simple ulcer of stomach. 2. Progressive muscular atrophy.

Cryalge'sia (kri-al-je'zhe-ah). Pain on application of cold.

Cryesthe'sia (kri-es-the'zhe-ah). Abnormal sensitiveness to chill.

Cry'osate. Antiseptic mixture of camphor, carbolic acid, and saponin with minute quantity of oil of turpentine.

Crypt. A follicle or pit. **C.'s of Lieberkühn.** See *Lieberkühn.*

Crypti'tis (krip-ti'tis). Inflammation of a crypt or crypts.

Cryptoceph'alus. A monster with an inconspicuous head.

Cryptodid'ymus. The enclosure of one fetus within another.

Cryptogen'ic (krip-to-jen'ik). Of obscure or doubtful origin.

Cryptophthal'mus. Complete adhesion of eyelids.

Cryp'topin. A hypnotic alkaloid from opium.

Cryptor'chid (krip-tor'kid). A person with testicles not descended.

Cryptor'chidism. Concealment of the testicles.
Cryptor'chis (krip-tor'kis). Same as *Cryptorchid.*
Cryp'toscope (krip'to-skōp). The fluoroscope.
Crys'tal. A naturally-produced angular solid of definite form. **Blood c's.**, hematoidin crystals in the blood. **Böttcher's c's.**, microscopic crystals seen on adding a drop of solution of ammonium phosphate to a drop of prostatic fluid. **Charcot-Leyden c's.**, minute crystals in sputa of asthma and bronchitis. **Charcot-Neumann c's.**, minute crystals of spermin phosphate. **Charcot-Robin c's.**, crystals formed in blood of leukemic patients. **Hedgehog c's.**, wedge-shaped shiny crystals of uric acid. **Knife-rest c's.**, peculiar notched crystals of triple phosphate in urine. **Teichmann's c's.**, hemin crystals.
Crys'tallin (kris'tal-lin). Globulin from the lens of the eye.
Crys'talline (kris'tal-lēn). Resembling a crystal; clear like crystal. **C. humor. C. lens,** the lens of the eye.
Crystalliza'tion. Formation of crystals.
Crys'talloid. Resembling a crystal; a non-colloid substance.
Cs. Symbol for *Cæsium.*
Cu. Symbol for *Copper.*
Cu'beb. Dried fruit of *Piper cubeba:* diuretic and stimulant.
Cube'bic acid. Diuretic and cathartic resin, $C_{13}H_{14}O_7$, from cubebs.
Cu'bital (ku'bit-al). Pertaining to the forearm.
Cu'bitus (ku'bit-us). The forearm.
Cu'boid. Bone on outside of foot in front of the calcaneum.
Cuirass can'cer (kwe-rahs'). Cancer on front and sides of the chest.
Cul-de-sac (kul-deh-sahk'). A cecum, sac, or blind pouch. **Douglas's c.**, pouch between anterior wall of rectum and posterior wall of uterus.
Cu'lex. A genus of insects; the mosquitos and gnats.
Culic'ifuge (ku-lis'if-ūj). An application to prevent mosquito-bites.
Cul'men. The anterior and upper part of monticulus.
Cultiva'tion. Artificial propagation of micro-organisms.
Cul'tural (kul'tu-ral). Pertaining to cultures.
Cul'ture. 1. Propagation of any organism. 2. A medium for propagating micro-organisms. **Bouillon c's.**, cultures of bacteria in bouillon. **Gelatin c.**, a bacterial culture on gelatin. **Hanging-drop c.**, a culture in which the bacterium is inoculated into a drop of fluid on a cover-glass. **C.-media,** substances used for cultivating bacteria, as bouillon, milk, gelatin, agar-agar, blood-serum, and potato. **Nail c.**, a bacterial culture resembling a nail in shape. **Plate c.**, a culture on a medium spread upon a flat plate. **Pure c.**, a culture of a single micro-organism. **Stab c.**, one in which the medium is inoculated by means of a needle inserted deeply into the medium. **Streak c.**, bacterial culture in which the matter is sown in streaks.
Cu'mene (ku'mēn). Same as *Cumol.*
Cu'mol (ku'mol). Colorless, oily compound, C_9H_{12}, used for sterilizing catgut.
Cu'mulative action or **effect.** A sudden marked effect after the administration of a number of ineffective doses.
Cundurau'go. Same as *Condurango.*
Cu'neate (ku'ne-āt). Wedge-shaped. **C. fasciculus. C. funiculus,** extension of oblongata into the vertebral canal. **C. nucleus,** gray matter at upper end of the cuneate fasciculus.
Cune'iform (ku-ne'if-orm). Wedge-shaped; cuneate. **C. bones,** three bones of the foot; pyramidal bone of wrist. **C. cartilage,** cartilage at side of arytenoid bone. **C. hysterectomy,** removal of a wedge of uterine tissue.

Cuneocu'boid. Pertaining to the cuboid and cuneiform bones.

Cu'neus. Wedge-shaped lobule of the brain.

Cunic'ulus. Burrow in the skin made by the itch-mite.

Cunniling'uist. A pervert who licks the vulva.

Cun'nus. The vulva; female pudenda.

Cup. A cupping-glass. **Favus c.**, depression in a favus scale around a hair. **Glaucomatous c.**, depression of optic papilla in glaucoma. **Physiological c.**, the normal depression of the optic papilla.

Cu'pola. The dome at the end of the cochlear canal. **C.-space**, the attic of the tympanum.

Cup'ped disk. A depressed eye-fundus.

Cup'ping. Application of the cupping-glass. **Dry c.**, drawing of blood to the surface without abstraction. **C.-glass**, cup for drawing blood, or for local stimulation. **Wet c.**, cupping with scarification and withdrawal of blood.

Cu'prum. L. for *Copper.*

Curacoa (koo-ras-o'). A strong cordial or liqueur.

Curare (koo-rah're). A South American arrow-poison; used in tetanus and in physiologic experiments.

Cur'cas (ker'kas). See under *Jatropha.*

Cur'cin (ker'sin). Poisonous principle from *Jatropha curcas.*

Cur'cuma (ker'ku-mah). See *Turmeric.*

Curd. Coagulated milk.

Cure. 1. Care and treatment of patients. 2. Successful treatment.

Curet (ku-ret'). See *Curette.*

Curettage (ku-ret'ej). Application of a curette.

Curette (ku-ret'). A scoop or scraper for cleansing a diseased surface.

Curette'ment (ku-ret'ment). Same as *Curettage.*

Cur'rant-jelly clot. Soft, red, post-mortem clot in heart and vessels.

Cur'rent. That which flows; electric transmission in a circuit. **After-c.**, a current produced in muscle and nerve when a current which has been flowing through it has stopped. **Alternating c.**, a current which is alternately direct and reversed. **Ascending c.**, an electric current passing toward a nerve-center. **Axial c.**, the central colored part of the blood-current. **Centrifugal c.** Same as *Descending c.* **Centripetal c.** Same as *Ascending c.* **Constant c.**, **Continuous c.**, an uninterrupted galvanic current. **Descending c.**, a current passed through a nerve from its origin toward its termination. **Direct c.**, a current whose direction is always the same. **Faradic c.**, a current of induced electricity. **Galvanic c.**, a current of galvanic electricity. **Induced c.** Same as *Secondary c.* **Interrupted c.**, a current that is alternately opened and closed. **Labile c.**, a current applied to the body with electrodes moving over the surface. **Reversed c.**, a current produced by changing the poles. **Secondary c.**, a current of induced electricity. **Stabile c.**, a current applied to the body with both electrodes stationary.

Curric'ulum (kur-rik'u-lum). An established course of study.

Cursch'mann's spirals (koorsh'mahnz). Coiled fibrils of mucin in sputum of asthma, etc.

Curtom'eter. Instrument for measuring curved surfaces.

Cur'vature, spinal. Abnormal curvature of spinal column. See *Kyphosis, Lordosis, Scoliosis.*

Curve of Carus. The normal axis of the pelvic outlet.

Cuscam'idin (kus-kam'id-in). A cinchona alkaloid.

Cus'co bark. A variety of cinchona.

Cus'conin (kus'ko-nin). An alkaloid from cinchona.

Cus'co's spec'ulum. A vaginal speculum with two blades worked by a screw.

Cusp. A pointed projection, such as the crown of a tooth or a segment of a cardiac valve.

Cus'pidate (kus'pid-āt). Provided with cusps.

Cus'so. Same as *Kousso.*

Cu'tal. Disinfecting astringent solution of aluminum borotannate.

Cuta'neous (ku-ta'ne-us). Pertaining to the skin. **C. reflex,** a reflex produced by stimulating the skin. **C. respiration,** normal passage of gases and vapors through the skin.

Cu'ticle. The outer layer of the skin; epidermis. **Enamel c.,** the tough membrane covering an enamel rod.

Cutic'ula den'tis. Same as *Nasmyth's membrane.*

Cuticulariza'tion. The formation of skin upon a sore or wound.

Cu'tis. The true skin or derma. **C. anseri'na,** goose-flesh; erection of the papillæ of the skin, as from cold or shock. **C. pen'dula,** abnormal flabbiness of the skin. **C. testa'cea,** a general seborrhea. **C. unctuo'sa,** seborrhea. **C. vera,** the true skin, derma, or corium.

Cu'tisector. An instrument for removing bits of skin.

Cuti'tis (ku-ti'tis). Skin-inflammation; dermatitis.

Cutiza'tion (ku-tiz-a'shun). Change into skin.

Cu'tol (ku'tol). Antiseptic compound of tannic and boric acids with an aluminum salt for skin-diseases.

Cuvier's sinuses (ku-ve-āz'). Two venous organs of the embryo.

Cy. Symbol of *Cyanogen.*

Cyanhidro'sis (si-an-id-dro'sis). Exudation of bluish sweat.

Cyan'ic acid (si-an'ik). See *Acid.*

Cy'anid (si'an-id). Any binary compound of cyanogen.

Cyan'ogen (si-an'o-jen). The halogen radical CN; also C_2N_2 (dicyanogen), the latter a poisonous gas.

Cyanop'athy (si-an-op'ath-e). Same as *Cyanosis.*

Cyano'pia. Cyanop'sia (si-an-o'pe-ah, si-an-op'se-ah). Vision in which all objects seem to be blue.

Cyano'sis (si-an-o'sis). Blueness of skin, often from cardiac malformation.

Cyanot'ic (si-an-ot'ik). Affected with, or pertaining to, cyanosis.

Cyclarthro'sis (si-klar-thro'sis). A pivot joint; joint which permits rotation.

Cy'cle (si'kl). A succession or round of symptoms. **Aberrant c.,** development of a communication between the pulmonary and bronchial vessels resulting from excessive congestion from mitral stenosis. **Cardiac c.,** a complete cardiac movement; a heart-beat.

Cyclenceph'alus (si-klen-sef'al-us). A monster with one eye at the median line.

Cyc'lic (sik'lik). Occurring in a definite course. **C. albuminuria.** See *Albuminuria.*

Cycli'tis (sik-li'tis). Inflammation of the ciliary body.

Cyclooceph'alus (si-klo-sef'al-us). Same as *Cyclencephalus.*

Cyclochoroidi'tis. Inflammation of ciliary body and choroid.

Cyclo'pia (si-klo'pe-ah). Monstrosity in which there is but one eye.

Cyclople'gia (si-klo-ple'je-ah). Paralysis of the ciliary structure of the eye.

Cy'clops (si'klops). A monster born with but one eye.

Cyclot'omy (si-klot'o-me). Surgical incision of ciliary muscle.

Cydo'nium (si-do'ne-um). Quince; quince seed.

Cyesiol'ogy (si-e-ze-ol'o-je). The science of pregnancy.

Cye'sis (si-e'sis). Pregnancy.

Cyet'ic (si-et'ik). Pertaining to pregnancy.

Cylicot'omy (sil-ik-ot'o-me). Same as *Cyclotomy.*

Cylin'droid. 1. Shaped somewhat like a cylinder. 2. So-called mucous, or spurious, cast in urine.

Cylindro'ma. Malignant tumor, especially about the face.
Cylindru'ria. The presence of cylindroids in the urine.
Cymbocephal'ic (sim-bo-sef-al'ik). Having a boat-shaped head.
Cynan'che (si-nan'ke). Severe sore throat with threatened suffocation. **C. malig'na**, putrid sore throat, diphtheritic or scarlatinal. **C. tonsilla'ris.** Same as *Quinsy*.
Cynan'thropy. Insanity in which the patient considers himself, or behaves like, a dog.
Cyn'ic spasm. Same as *Sardonic laugh*.
Cyn'obex (sin'o-bex). Dry cough of early youth.
Cynopho'bia (sin-o-fo'be-ah). Spurious hydrophobia.
Cynuren'ic acid (sin-u-ren'ik). An acid from dog's urine.
Cyoph'orin (si-of'o-rin). Same as *Gravidin*.
Cype'rus (si-pe'rus). A genus of sedges, *C. articulatus* (adrue) of tropical America; anti-emetic and tonic.
Cypho'sis (si-fo'sis). Same as *Kyphosis*.
Cyphot'ic (si-fot'ik). Same as *Kyphotic*.
Cypripe'dium. Genus of orchids; root of *C. pubescens* and others, reputed to be nervine.
Cypripho'bia (sip-rif-o'be-ah). Morbid fear of coitus.
Cyrtom'eter (sir-tom'et-er). An instrument for measuring curved surfaces.
Cyrto'sis (sir-to'sis). Backward curvature of the spine.
Cyst (sist). Any sac containing a liquid. **Blood-c.** See *Hematoma*. **Boyer's c.**, cyst of the subhyoid bursa. **Colloid c.**, a cyst with jelly-like contents. **Daughter-c.**, small cyst developed from the walls of a large cyst. **Dentigerous c.**, one containing teeth. **Dermoid c.**, a cyst containing bone, hair, teeth, etc. **Echinococcus-c.**, a cyst formed by the larva of the tænia echinococcus of the dog, taken into the stomach. **Extravasation-c.**, a cyst formed by a hemorrhage into the tissues. **Follicular c.**, one due to the occlusion of the duct of a small follicle or gland. **Hydatid c.** Same as *Echinococcus c.* **Mucous c.**, a retention-cyst containing mucus. **Retention-c.**, one due to the retention of the secretion of a gland. **Sebaceous c.**, a retention-cyst of a sebaceous gland. **Seminal c.**, a cyst containing semen. **Sublingual c.** See *Ranula*. **Unilocular c.**, a cyst having only a single cavity.
Cystadeno'ma (sis-tad-en-o'mah). Cystoma blended with adenoma.
Cystal'gia (sis-tal'je-ah). Pain in the bladder.
Cystatro'phia. Atrophy of the bladder.
Cystauchenot'omy. Surgical incision of the neck of the bladder.
Cystenceph'alus. Monstrosity with a brain like a membranous bag.
Cyster'ethism. Irritability of the bladder.
Cysthypersarco'sis. Thickening of muscular coat of the bladder.
Cys'tic (sis'tik). 1. Pertaining to cysts. 2. Relating to the urinary bladder. **C. degeneration.** See *Degeneration*. **C. duct**, duct of the gall-bladder. **C. tumor**, tumor made up of cysts.
Cysticer'cus (sis-tis-er'kus). A larval form of tape-worms.
Cysticot'omy (sis-tik-ot'o-me). Same as *Choledochotomy*.
Cystidolaparot'omy. Incision into bladder through abdomen.
Cystidotrachelot'omy. Same as *Cystauchenotomy*.
Cystifellot'omy. Same as *Cholecystotomy*.
Cys'tin (sis'tin). A crystalline principle from urine.
Cystinu'ria (sis-tin-u're-ah). The presence of cystin in the urine.
Cysti'tis (sis-ti'tis). Inflammation of the bladder.
Cys'titome (sis'tit-ōm). Instrument for opening sac of crystalline lens.

Cystocarcino'ma. Cystoma blended with carcinoma.
Cys'tocele (sis'to-sēl). Protrusion of a knuckle of the bladder.
Cystodyn'ia (sis-to-din'e-ah). Pain in the bladder.
Cystofibro'ma. Fibroma blended with cystoma.
Cys'toid (sis'toid). Like a cyst.
Cystolu'tein (sis-to-lu'te-in). Yellow pigment from ovarian cysts.
Cysto'ma (sis-to'mah). A cystic tumor.
Cystomyxo-adeno'ma. Cystomyxoma blended with adenoma.
Cystomyxo'ma. Myxoma with cystic degeneration.
Cystoneural'gia. Neuralgia of the bladder.
Cystoparaly'sis. Paralysis of the bladder.
Cys'topexy. Fixation of bladder to abdominal wall.
Cystophotog'raphy. Photography of the interior of bladder.
Cys'toplasty (sis'to-plas-te). Plastic surgery of the bladder.
Cystople'gia (sis-to-ple'je-ah). Paralysis of the bladder.
Cystopto'sis (sis-top-to'sis). Prolapse of a portion of the bladder into the urethra.
Cystopyeli'tis (sis-to-py-e-li'tis). Cystitis blended with pyelitis.
Cystorectos'tomy. The making of a passage from the bladder to the rectum.
Cystor'rhaphy (sis-tor'raf-e). Suture of the bladder.
Cystorrhe'a (sis-tor-rhe'ah). Catarrh of the bladder.
Cystosarco'ma. Sarcoma with contained cysts.
Cys'toscope (sis'to-skōp). An endoscope for examining the bladder.
Cystos'copy (sis-tos'ko-pe). Examination by means of the cystoscope.
Cystospermi'tis. Inflammation of the seminal vesicles.
Cystos'tomy (sis-tos'to-me). Formation of an opening into the bladder.
Cys'totome (sis'to-tōm). A cutting instrument for bladder-operations.
Cystot'omy (sis-tot'o-me). Surgical incision of the bladder.
Cystotrachelot'omy. Same as *Cystauchenotomy.*
Cyst-worm. Same as *Cysticercus.*
Cyt'isin (sit'is-in). Alkaloid from *Cytisus laburnum.*
Cyti'tis (sit-i'tis). Same as *Dermatitis.*
Cy'toblast (si'to-blast). The cell-nucleus.
Cytoblaste'ma. Supposed mother-liquid of cells.
Cytochem'ism (si-to-kem'izm). Reaction of body-cells to injections of antitoxin, producing in the organism specific antitoxic substances.
Cy'tochrome. A nerve-cell deficient in cell-protoplasm.
Cytochyle'ma. The more fluid part of cell-protoplasm.
Cy'tode (si'tōd). A non-nucleated cell or cell-element.
Cytogen'esis (si-to-jen'es-is). Development of the cell.
Cytog'enous (si-toj'en-us). Producing cells.
Cytoglo'bin. A proteid from white blood-corpuscles.
Cytohyal'oplasm. Reticular substance of cell-protoplasm.
Cy'toid (si'toid). Resembling a cell.
Cytol'ogy (si-tol'o-je). Sum of what is known regarding cells.
Cy'tolymph (si'to-limf). Same as *Cytochylema.*
Cytol'ysis (si-tol'is-is). The dissolution of cells.
Cytom'eter. Device for counting and measuring cells.
Cytomi'erosome. A microsome of chromatin found in cytohyaloplasm.
Cytom'itome. A fibril, or fibrillar network, of spongioplasm.
Cytoph'agous (si-tof'ag-us). Devouring or consuming cells.
Cytoph'agy (si-tof'aj-e). Absorption of cells by other cells.
Cy'toplasm (si'to-plazm). Protoplasm of the cell-body.
Cytoretic'ulum. A fibrillar network of spongioplasm.
Cy'tosome (si'to-sōm). The body of a cell apart from its nucleus.

Cytozo'on (si-to-zo'on). A protozoic parasite inhabiting a cell or having the structure of a simple cell.

Czer'mak's spa'ces (chär'mahks). The interglobular spaces.

Czerny-Lembert suture (chär-ne-law-bair'). A suture for intestinal surgery; one row of Lembert stitches, and another row which includes the muscular and peritoneal coats.

D.

D. Abbreviation for *diopter*, for *dexter* (right), and for *dose;* and symbol for closed circuit.

DaCos'ta's disease. See *Disease.*

Dacryadenal'gia. Pain in a lacrimal gland.

Dacryadeni'tis. Inflammation of a lacrimal gland.

Dacryadenoscir'rhus. Scirrhus of a lacrimal gland.

Dac'ryagogue (dak're-ag-og). 1. Causing a flow of tears. 2. A medicine which provokes a flow of tears.

Dacryoadeni'tis (dak-ro-ad-en-i'tis). Same as *Dacryadenitis.*

Dacryoblennorrhe'a. Mucous flow from the tear-apparatus.

Dac'ryocele (dak're-o-sēl). Hernia of the lacrimal sac.

Dac'ryocyst (dak're-o-sist). The tear-sac.

Dacryocystal'gia (dak-re-o-sis-tal'je-ah). Pain in the lacrimal sac.

Dacryocysti'tis. Inflammation of the dacryocyst.

Dacryocystoblennorrhe'a. Blennorrhea of the lacrimal sac.

Dacryocys'totome. Knife for cutting the lacrimal sac.

Dacryocystot'omy. Surgical puncture of the lacrimal sac.

Dacryohemorrhe'a. The discharge of bloody tears.

Dac'ryolin. An albuminous substance from tears.

Dac'ryolite, Dac'ryolith. A lacrimal calculus.

Dacryo'ma. 1. A lacrimal tumor. 2. Closure of a punctum lacrimale.

Dac'ryon (dak're-on). The lacrimal point; the point where the lacrimal, frontal, and upper maxillary bones meet.

Dac'ryops (dak're-ops). Distention of a tear-duct.

Dacryopyorrhe'a. Discharge of purulent tears.

Dacryorrhe'a. Excessive morbid flow of tears.

Dac'tyl (dak'til). A finger or toe; a digit.

Dactyl'ion. Union of the fingers; webbed fingers or toes.

Dactyli'tis (dak-til-i'tis). Inflammation of a finger or toe.

Dactylogrypo'sis. Permanent bending of the fingers.

Dactylol'ogy. Conversation by means of the fingers.

Dactylol'ysis (dak-til-ol'is-is). Same as *Ainhum.*

Dæmonomania. See *Demonomania.*

Dak'ryon, etc. See *Dacryon.*

Dal'tonism (dawl'ton-izm). See *Color-blindness.*

Dam. See *Rubber-dam.*

Damal'ic acid. An acid, C_7H_8O, reported as occurring in urine.

Damalu'ric acid. An acid, $C_7H_{12}O_2$, found in the urine.

Damia'na (dah-me-ah'nah). The leaves of three or more Mexican plants, alleged to be aphrodisiac.

Dam'mar. A resin of many varieties used for plasters and in microscopic work.

Dance, St. Vitus'. See *Chorea.*

Dan'ce's sign. Depression in the right iliac region in intussusception.

Dan'cing disease. See *Tarantism.* **D. mania.** See *Choromania.*

Dan'delion. See *Taraxacum.*

Dan'druff. Scaly scurf from or on the scalp.

Dan'dy fever (dan'de). Same as *Dengue.*

Daph'ne (daf'ne). See *Mezereon.*

Daph'nin (daf'nin). Active principle, $C_{15}H_{16}O_9+2H_2O$, from barks of species of *Daphne*.

Darier's disease (dar-yāz'). Same as *Keratosis follicularis*.

Dar'toid (dar'toid). Resembling the dartos.

Dar'tos. The contractile tissue under the skin of the scrotum.

Dar'tre (dar'tr). See *Herpes*.

Dar'trous. Pertaining to herpes; herpetic.

Darwin'ian tubercle. An eminence sometimes seen on the edge of the helix of the ear.

Dar'winism. The theory of evolution, as propounded by C. R. Darwin.

Datu'ra (da-tu'rah). A plant genus. See *Stramonium*.

Datu'ria. An alkaloid like atropin, from stramonium.

Datu'rism (da-tu'rizm). Stramonium-poisoning.

Daugh'ter-cell (daw'ter). See *Cell*. **D.-cyst.** See *Cyst*. **D.-nucleus,** a new nucleus formed in karyokinesis by the diaster. **D.-star.** Same as *Amphiaster*. **D.-wreath,** the d.-star viewed from its surface.

Day-blind'ness. Partial blindness by day, with better vision at night.

Deaf-mu'tism. The condition of being deaf and dumb.

Deaf'ness (def'nes). The state of being deaf or dull of hearing. **Base d.,** deafness to certain low tones. **Boilermakers' d.,** deafness from working among machinery, marked by inability to hear ordinary conversation, while hearing is increased amidst loud noise. **Cerebral d.,** that due to a brain-lesion. **Cortical d.,** that due to disease of the cortical centers. **Mind d.** Same as *Psychic d.* **Paradoxical d.,** state in which hearing is best during a loud sound. **Psychic d.,** inability to comprehend spoken language. **Tone d.,** sensory amnesia. **Word d.** Same as *Psychic d.*

Death. Cessation of life. **Black d.,** the plague. **Molar d.,** death in mass, as gangrene or necrosis. **Molecular d.,** death of cellular elements, as by ulceration. **D.-rate,** the proportion of those who die to those who survive. **D. rattle,** the rattling sound in the throat of a dying person. **Somatic d.,** death of the whole body.

Debil'itant. 1. Inducing weakness. 2. A remedy which allays excitement.

Debove's membrane (de-bōvz'). Layer of connective-tissue cells between the epithelium and tunica propria of bronchial, vesicular, and intestinal mucous membrane.

Débridement (da-brēd-maw'). [Fr.] Surgical division of constricting bands or tissue.

Dec'agram (dek'ag-ram). Ten grams or 154.34 grains.

Decalcifica'tion. Removal or diminution of calcareous matter from tissues.

Decal'cify. To deprive of calcium or its salts.

Dec'aliter (dek'a-le-ter). Ten liters; 610.28 cubic inches.

Decal'vant (de-kal'vant). Removing or destroying hair.

Dec'ameter. Ten meters; 393.71 cubic inches.

Decanta'tion. The pouring off a clear liquid from a sediment.

Decapita'tion. Removal of the head, as of the fetus or of a bone.

Decentra'tion. The act of removing from a center.

Decerebra'tion. The removal of the brain in craniotomy or in vivisection.

Decid'ua (de-sid'u-ah). The membranous structure formed during gestation and thrown off after childbirth. **D. reflex'a,** that which surrounds the ovum. **D. serot'ina,** that which intervenes between the placenta and the uterine wall. **D. ve'ra,** that which lines the interior of the uterus.

Deciduo'ma (de-sid-u-o'mah). Intra-uterine tumor derived from a retained decidua.

Decid'uous (de-sid'u-us). Falling off; caducous. **D. teeth**, the first or temporary teeth.

De'cigram (des'ig-ram). One-tenth of a gram.

De'ciliter (des'il-e-ter). One-tenth of a liter; 6.1 cubic inches; about 3.4 fluidounces.

De'cimeter (des'im-e-ter). One-tenth of a meter; 3.9 linear inches.

Decinor'mal. Being of one-tenth the normal strength.

Dec'linator. An instrument for holding aside a part during surgical operation.

Decline' (de-klin'). Progressive decrease, whether of disease or of the strength or health.

Decli'vis cerebel'li. Sloping posterior surface of the superior vermis of the cerebellum.

Decoc'tion. 1. The process of boiling. 2. A preparation made by boiling.

Decolla'tion. Same as *Decapitation*.

Decolla'tor. An instrument for removing the head of the fetus.

Decolora'tion. The removal of color; bleaching.

Decomposi'tion (de-kom-po-zish'un). 1. Putrefactive decay. 2. Chemical separation into component elements or simpler compounds.

Decompres'sion. The removal of compressive force, as of the air.

Decortica'tion. The removal of bark or cortex.

Decrep'itate. To explode with a crackling noise.

Decrepita'tion. A crackling noise, as of material thrown into a fire.

Decu'bital. Pertaining to a bed-sore or to decubitus.

Decu'bitus. 1. Posture in bed. 2. Act of lying down. 3. A bed-sore. **D. acu'tus**, bed-sore seen in connection with cerebral lesions.

Decus'sate. 1. To cross in the form of an x. 2. Crossed like the letter x.

Decussa'tion. 1. The position of one part athwart another and similar part. 2. The point of crossing; chiasma. **D. of the pyramids**, the crossing of the fibers of the pyramids of the oblongata from one pyramid to the other.

Deep reflex. Reflex induced by stimulation of deep parts.

Defeca'tion (def-ek-a'shun). Discharge of the feces.

Defen'sive proteid. Any alexin, toxin, or phylaxin.

Def'erent. Conveying anything away or downward. Cf. *Afferent*, *efferent*. **D. duct.** Same as *Vas deferens*.

Deferen'tial (def-er-en'shal). Pertaining to the vas deferens.

Deferenti'tis. Inflammation of the deferent duct.

Deferred' shock. Same as *Delayed symptoms*.

Deferves'cence (def-er-ves'ens). The period during which fever heat is declining to the normal standard.

Defibrina'tion, Defibriniza'tion. Deprival of fibrin.

Defi'ning power, Defini'tion. The power of a lens to give a clear outline.

Defin'itive. Permanent; not temporary; clear and final.

Deflagra'tion. Sudden, rapid combustion with slight explosion.

Deflu'vium capillo'rum. The rapid or sudden loss of the hair.

Deflux'ion (de-fluk'shun). A flowing down; copious discharge or loss of any kind.

Deforma'tion, Deform'ity. Distortion or malformation, congenital or acquired.

Defor'ming arthritis, osteitis. See *Arthritis*, *Osteitis*.

Defunctionaliza'tion. The act of destroying a function.

Degan'glionate. To remove a ganglion or ganglia.

Degenera'tion. Alteration of tissue from a higher to a lower form. **Adipose d.** See *Fatty d.* **Albuminoid d., Amyloid d.,** d. with the formation of an albuminous matter. **Ascending d.,** degeneration of nerve-fibers progressing from the original lesion toward the brain. **Bacony d.** Same as *Amyloid d.* **Calcareous d.,** d. with the deposit of calcium carbonate. **Caseous** or **Cheesy d.,** caseation. **Colloid d.,** the change of the protoplasm of epithelial cells into a substance resembling mucus. **Cystic d.,** d. with formation of cysts. **Descending d.,** a degeneration of nerve-fibers extending from the original lesion toward the periphery. **Fatty d.,** a change of tissues into fat. **Fibroid d.,** degeneration into fibrous tissue. **Gray d.,** gray atrophy. See *Atrophy.* **Hyaline d.,** a degeneration affecting the walls of blood-vessels, and forming a substance resembling amyloid matter. **Lardaceous d.** Same as *Albuminoid d.* **Mucoid d., Myxomatous d.,** degeneration of tissue into a jelly-like substance containing mucin. **Parenchymatous d.** See *Cloudy swelling.* **Secondary d.** Same as *Wallerian d.* **Vitreous d.** Same as *Hyaline d.* **Wallerian d.,** degeneration of nerve-fibers after separation from their nutritive centers. **Waxy d.** 1. Amyloid d. 2. Hyaline d. **Zenker's d.,** peculiar glassy degeneration of muscle.

Degen'erative. Associated with or pertaining to degeneration.

Deglutl'tion (deg-lu-tish'un). The act or process of swallowing. **D. center.** See *Center.* **D. pneumonia.** See *Pneumonia.*

Degote' (de-göt'). Oil of birch, used in skin-diseases.

Dehis'cence (de-his'ens). The formation of a fissure.

Dehu'manized virus. Vaccine virus modified by retrovaccination.

Dehydra'tion. The removal of water from a substance.

Dei'ters's cells (dī'terz). 1. Specialized cells associated with the cells of Corti in the inner ear. 2. Branching cells constituting the reticulum of neuroglia. **D.'s nucleus,** the external auditory nucleus. **D.'s process,** any axis-cylinder process.

Dejec'tion (de-jek'shun). 1. Discharge of feces; fecal matter. 2. Depression of spirits.

Delacta'tion (de-lak-ta'shun). 1. Weaning. 2. Cessation of lactation.

Delamina'tion. The division of a blastoderm into layers.

Delayed symptoms. Symptoms, as of shock, which are slow in making their appearance.

Del'hi boil or **sore** (del'le). Same as *Furunculus orientalis.*

Deliga'tion (del-ig-a'shun). 1. Ligation. 2. Bandaging.

Delimita'tion. The act or process of limiting, or becoming limited; the determination of limits.

Deliques'cence (del-ik-wes'ens). The act or process of becoming liquid by the absorption of water from the air.

Deliques'cent (del-ik-wes'ent). Having a tendency to become liquid by absorbing moisture from the air.

Delir'iant. Delirifa'cient. Any medicine which produces delirium.

Delir'ium (de-lir'e-um). Disordered mental state with excitement and illusions. **Alcoholic d.** Same as *D. tremens.* **D. cor'dis,** violent, tremulous beating of the heart. **Febrile d.,** delirium of fever. **D. of grandeur,** d. in which patient has exaggerated ideas of his importance or power. **Lingual d.,** utterance of meaningless words and sentences. **D. of negation,** that in which patient thinks he has lost some part of his body. **D. of persecution,** d. in which patient thinks he is being persecuted. **Toxic d.,** delirium produced by poisons.

Traumatic d., that occurring after the shock which follows an injury. **D. tre'mens**, delirium from the excessive use of alcoholics.

Delites'cence (del-it-es'ens). Sudden disappearance of symptoms or of a tumor; latency of a poison or morbid agent.

Deliv'er. 1. To aid in childbirth. 2. To remove, as a fetus, placenta, or lens of the eye.

Deliv'ery. The act of freeing from the contents of the gravid uterus; removal, as from the uterus.

Delomor'phous cells (de-lo-mor'fus). See *Cells*.

Del'phinin (del'fin-in). A poisonous alkaloid from staphysagria.

Del'ta for'nicis. Same as *Lyra fornicis*.

Del'toid (del'toid). See *Muscles, Table of*. **D. ligament**, the internal lateral ligament of the ankle. **D. ridge**, a ridge on the humerus to which the deltoid muscle is attached.

De lunat'ico inquiren'do. [L.] A commission or jury for investigating the mental status of persons whose sanity is questioned.

Delu'sion (de-lu'zhun). An insanely erroneous belief or fancy.

Delu'sional. Pertaining to a delusion.

Dement'. A person who has lost his intellect.

Demen'ted (de-men'ted). Deprived of reason.

Demen'tia (de-men'she-ah). Insanity characterized by more or less complete loss of intellect. **Paralytic d.**, general paralysis of the insane. **Primary d.**, d. independent of other forms of insanity. **Secondary d.**, that following another kind of insanity. **Terminal d.**, that coming on near the end of other kinds of insanity.

Dem'ibain. [Fr.] A hip-bath or sitz-bath.

Dem'ilune cells. Crescentic cells, such as Gianuzzi's crescents (**D.'s of Heidenhain**).

Dem'odex folliculo'rum. The pimple-mite.

Demog'raphy. That branch of anthropology which deals with social statistics, including questions of health, disease, births, and mortality.

Demonoma'nia. Insanity characterized by the patient's belief that he is possessed by demons.

Dem'onstrator. A practical instructor who does not rank as a professor.

Demorphiniza'tion. The gradual withdrawal of morphin from one addicted to its misuse.

Demours's membrane (de-moorz'). Same as *Descemet's membrane*.

Demul'cent (de-mul'sent). Soothing; bland; a soothing mucilaginous medicine.

Demutiza'tion. The instruction of deaf-mutes in the utterance of speech, or in the use of sign-language.

Denar'cotize. To deprive of narcotin or of narcotic properties.

Den'dric. Pertaining to or having a dendron.

Den'driform (den'drif-orm). Tree-shaped.

Den'drite (den'drit). Same as *Dendron*.

Dendrit'ic, Den'droid. Tree-like in appearance or form.

Den'dron. A branching protoplasmic process from a nerve-cell.

Den'gue (deng'ge). The so-called break-bone fever of hot climates.

Denida'tion. The supposed disintegration and removal, during menstruation, of certain epithelial elements, potentially the nidus of an embryo.

Dens (denz), pl. *den'tes*. [L.] A tooth.

Dentag'ra. 1. Tooth-ache. 2. A form of forceps or key for pulling teeth.

Den'tal. Pertaining to teeth. **D. arch.** Same as *Alveolar pro-*

cess. **D. engine,** a machine for use in dentistry and general surgery.

Den'taphone (den'taf-ōn). An audiphone by which sounds are rendered perceptible through the medium of the teeth.

Denta'ta. The second cervical vertebra or axis.

Den'tate (den'tāt). Notched; tooth-shaped.

Den'tes sapien'tiæ. [L.] Wisdom teeth.

Dentic'ulate body. Same as *Corpus dentatum.*

Den'tifrice (den'tif-ris). A tooth-powder or tooth-wash.

Dentig'erous (den-tij'er-us). Containing or producing teeth.

Dentila'bial. Pertaining to the teeth and lips.

Dentilin'gual. Pertaining to the teeth and tongue.

Den'tin. The bone-like material which forms the body, neck, and roots of the teeth.

Den'tinal (den'tin-al). Pertaining to dentin.

Dentinifica'tion. The formation of dentin.

Dentini'tis. Inflammation of the dentin.

Den'tinoid. A tumor composed of dentin.

Dentin-os'teoid. A tumor composed of dentin and bone.

Den'tist (den'tist). A dental surgeon.

Den'tistry. The professional care of the teeth; dental surgery.

Denti'tion (den-tish'un). 1. The process or time of cutting the teeth. 2. The kind, number, and arrangement of the teeth.

Den'ture (den'tūr). 1. A set or partial set of artificial teeth. 2. The normal arrangement of the teeth.

Denu'cleated (de-nu'kle-a-ted). Deprived of the nucleus.

Denuda'tion. The stripping or laying bare of any part; the surgical or pathologic removal of an integument.

Denutri'tion (den-u-trish'un). Lack or failure of nutrition.

Deob'struent. A medicine which removes obstructions.

De'odar. The noble tree, *Cedrus deodara* of the Himalaya: its turpentine is medicinal.

Deod'orant. Destroying odors; a deodorizing agent.

Deo'dorize (de-o'dor-īz). To deprive of odor.

Deodo'rizer (de-o'dor-i-zer). A deodorizing agent.

Deontol'ogy (de-on-tol'o-je). The science of duty; medical ethics.

Deoppila'tion. The removal of obstructions.

Deor'sum. [L.] Downward. **D. ver'gens,** turning or directed downward.

Deorsumduc'tion. The downward turning or drawing of a part.

Deox'idate, Deox'idize, Deox'ygenate, Deox'ygenize. To deprive of oxygen.

Deoxida'tion, Deoxidiza'tion, Deoxygena'tion. The removal of oxygen.

Deox'idizer (de-ok'sid-ī-zer). A deoxidizing agent.

Dep'ilate (dep'il-āt). To remove the hair from.

Depila'tion (dep-il-a'shun). The process of removing hair.

Depil'atory. 1. Having the power of removing the hair. 2. An agent which destroys or removes the hair.

Deplete' (de-plēt'). To empty; to unload; to cause depletion.

Deple'tion (de-ple'shun). The act or process of depleting; removal of congestion or plethora; the state of being depleted.

Depluma'tion (de-plu-ma'shun). Loss of eyelashes by disease.

Depolariza'tion. Destruction or loss of polarity.

Depos'it (de-poz'it). 1. Sediment or dregs. 2. Extraneous inorganic matter collected in the tissues or in a viscus.

Deprava'tion. Change for the worse; deterioration.

Depraved (de-prāvd'). Vitiated or perverted; as a depraved appetite.

Depres'sant. An agent which retards any function; an active sedative.

Depressed (de-prest'). Flattened from above.

Depres'sion (de-presh'un). 1. Reduction of vital or functional activity. 2. A hollow or fossa, normal, pathological, or other.

Depressomo'tor. Diminishing motor action.

Depres'sor. An instrument like a spatula, for depressing a part. **D. a'læ na'si,** the muscle which draws down the nostrils. See *Muscles, Table of.* **D. la'bii inferio'ris,** the depressor muscle of the lower lip. See *Muscles, Table of.* **D. nerve.** any nerve whose stimulation lowers the vasomotor tension.

Dep'rimens oc'uli. The rectus inferior muscle.

Depri'val, Depriva'tion, Deprive'ment. Loss or absence of organs, parts, or powers.

Dep'urant. 1. Removing impurities. 2. A purifying medicine.

Depura'tion. Act or process of purifying.

Dep'urative. Same as *Depurant.*

Depura'tor. 1. A purifying medicine. 2. An emunctory organ.

Deradel'phus. A twin monster with one neck and head.

Deradeni'tis. Inflammation of the glands of the neck.

Deradenon'cus. Swelling of a gland of the neck.

Derange'ment (de-rānj'ment). Insanity; disorder of the reason.

Der'byshire neck. Goiter or bronchocele.

Derencephal'ocele. Protrusion of brain-substance through a slit in one of the cervical vertebræ.

Derenceph'alus. A monster with no cranium, the cervical vertebræ containing the relics of a brain.

Der'ic (der'ik). Pertaining to ectoderm.

Der'ivant. 1. Derivative. 2. A derivative medicine.

Deriva'tion (der-iv-a'shun). Revulsive treatment; alleged suctional action of the heart.

Deriv'ative. Revulsive; a counterirritant.

Derm, Der'ma. The skin, or true skin.

Der'mad. Toward the skin; inward.

Dermag'ra (der-mag'rah). Same as *Pellagra.*

Der'mal. Pertaining to the derm or skin. **D. muscle.** a muscle which acts upon the skin.

Dermalax'ia. Morbid softness of the skin.

Dermal'gia (der-mal'je-ah). Neuralgia of the skin.

Derman'oplasty (der-man'o-plas-te). Skin-grafting.

Dermapos'tasis. A skin-disease with abscess formation.

Dermatag'ra (der-mat-ag'rah). Pellagra.

Dermatal'gia (der-mat-al'je-ah). Same as *Dermalgia.*

Dermatatro'phia. Atrophy of the skin.

Dermati'tis (der-mat-i'tis). Inflammation of the skin. **D. congelatio'nis.** Same as *Frostbite.* **D. contusifor'mis.** erythema nodosum. **D. exfoliati'va.** inflammation of the skin, in which the epidermis is shed in scales. See *Pityriasis rubra.* **D. gangræno'sa.** sphaceloderma; gangrenous inflammation of the skin. **D. herpetifor'mis,** an inflammatory skin-disease of an herpetic character, the various lesions showing a tendency to group. **D. medicamento'sa.** a drug-eruption. **D. papilla'ris capillit'ii,** a chronic skin-disease of the neck and adjacent parts, marked by minute red papules, which occasionally suppurate, and from which hairs protrude. **D. venena'ta.** that caused by the local action of irritant substances. **X-ray d.,** inflammation of skin due to exposure to *x*-rays.

Dermato-au'toplasty. Grafting of skin taken from the patient's own body. See *Dermatoheteroplasty.*

Dermatocelluli'tis. Inflammation of the skin and subcutaneous cellular tissue.

Der'matocyst (der'mat-o-sist). A cyst of the skin.

Dermatog'raphy. A description or account of the skin.

Dermatohet'eroplasty. Grafting of skin from the body of another person or from an animal.

Der'matoid (der'mat-oid). Skin-like.
Dermatokelido'sis. A spotted condition of the skin.
Der'matol. Bismuth-subgallate: antiseptic and astringent.
Dermatol'ogist. An expert in dermatology.
Dermatol'ogy. The science of the skin.
Dermatol'ysis. A relaxed and pendulous state of the skin.
Dermato'ma. An abnormal growth of skin-tissue.
Der'matome (der'mat-ōm). Instrument for cutting the skin.
Dermatomyco'sis. Any skin-disease due to parasitic vegetation.
Dermatomyo'ma. Myoma involving the skin.
Dermatomyosi'tis. Inflammation of the skin and muscles.
Dermatoneuro'sis. Neurosis of the skin.
Der'matophyte (der'mat-o-fīt). A vegetable skin-parasite.
Dermatoplas'tic. Pertaining to dermatoplasty.
Der'matoplasty. Plastic surgery of the skin.
Dermatorrhe'a (der-mat-or-re'ah). Morbid excess of sweat.
Dermatosclero'sis. Same as *Scleroderma.*
Dermato'sis (der-mat-o'sis). Any disorder of the skin.
Der'matosome. Portion of the equatorial plate in karyokinesis.
Dermatoxera'sia (der-mat-o-ze-ra'zhe-ah). Same as *Xeroderma.*
Dermatozo'on. Any animal parasite on the skin.
Dermatro'phia (der-mat-ro'fe-ah). Atrophy of the skin.
Dermen'chysis. Hypodermic exhibition of medicines.
Der'mic (der'mik). Pertaining to the skin.
Der'mis (der'mis). The skin; true skin.
Dermi'tis. Inflammation of the skin.
Der'moblast. Part of mesoblast, developing into the true skin.
Dermocy'ma, Dermocy'mus. A monstrosity in which one twin is contained within another.
Dermogra'phia, Dermog'raphism, Dermog'raphy. Same as *Autographism.*
Der'moid (der'moid). Same as *Dermatoid.*
Der'mol. Compound, $Bi(C_{15}H_9O_4)_2Bi_2O_3$, used in dermatology.
Dermomyco'sis. A skin-disease produced by a fungus.
Dermoneuro'sis. Same as *Dermatoneurosis.*
Dermonosol'ogy. The pathology of skin-diseases.
Dermop'athy (der-mop'ath-e). Any skin-disease.
Dermophlebi'tis (der-mo-fle-bi'tis). Inflammation of the veins of the skin.
Der'moplasty (der'mo-plas-te). Same as *Dermatoplasty.*
Dermorrha'gia. Hemorrhage from the skin.
Dermoskel'eton. The external and visible investments of the body; skin, teeth, hair, and nails.
Dermosteno'sis (der-mo-sten-o'sis). Contraction of the skin.
Dermosyphilop'athy. A syphilitic skin-disease.
Derodid'ymus. A monster with one body, two necks, and two heads.
Der'rid. A poisonous resin from *Derris elliptica*, a tree of southern Asia.
Desanima'nia. Amentia; mindless insanity.
Desault's bandage (de-zōz'). See *Bandage.*
Descemeti'tis (des-em-et-i'tis). Inflammation of Descemet's membrane.
Descemet'ocele (des-se-met'o-sēl). Hernia of Descemet's membrane.
Descemet's membrane (des-māz'). Posterior living membrane of the cornu.
Descen'dens no'ni. Fibers from the cervical nerves forming a portion of the ansa hypoglossi.
Descend'ing aorta. See *Aorta.* **D. degeneration.** See *Degeneration.*
Descrip'tive anatomy. See *Anatomy.*

Des'iccant (des'ik-ant). Promoting dryness.
Desicca'tion (des-ik-a'shun). The act of drying.
Desic'cative (des-sik'at-iv). Drying or lessening moisture.
Desmi'tis (des-mi'tis). Inflammation of a ligament.
Desmobacte'rium. A bacterium of a filiform shape.
Desmodyn'ia. Pain in a ligament or in ligaments.
Desmog'raphy. A description of ligaments.
Des'moid (des'moid). A hard fibrous tumor.
Desmol'ogy (des-mol'o-ge). Science of ligaments.
Desmo'ma (des-mo'mah). Same as *Fibroma.*
Desmone'oplasm. A connective-tissue neoplasm.
Desmop'athy (des-mop'ath-e). Any disease of the ligaments.
Desmot'omy. The anatomy, dissection, or cutting of ligaments.
Despuma'tion. Removal of froth or scum from a liquid.
Desquama'tion. Separation of scales or laminæ from any surface.
Detan'nate (de-tan'nāt). To deprive of tannin.
Deter'gent (de-ter'jent). Cleansing; a cleansing medicine or lotion.
Determina'tion. A flow, as of blood, to the head or other part.
Detona'tion. Explosive combustion.
Detri'tion (de-trish'un). The wearing away, as of teeth, by friction.
Detri'tus. Residual debris; granular remains of a broken-down tissue.
Detrunca'tion (de-trung-ka'shun). Decollation; decapitation.
Detru'sor uri'næ. Muscular coat of bladder.
Deutenceph'alon. Same as *Thalamencephalon.*
Deutero-al'bumose. An albumose soluble in water and in saline solutions.
Deutero-elas'tose. A material formed in the digestion of elastin.
Deuteromyo'sinose. A substance formed in digestion of myosin.
Deuteropathi'a, Deuterop'athy. A secondary or sympathetic affection.
Deu'teroplasm. The nutritive portion of the yolk of ovum.
Deu'toplasm (du'to-plazm). Same as *Deuteroplasm.*
Deutosco'lex. Secondary scolex; hydatid form of a tænia.
Developmen'tal (de-vel-op-men'tal). Pertaining to development.
Devia'tion (de-ve-a'shun). A turning aside, as in strabismus. **Conjugate d.,** deviation of both eyes to the same side. **Minimum d.,** the smallest deviation of a ray that a given prism can produce.
Devisceration (de-vis-er-a'shun). Removal of viscera.
Devitaliza'tion. Deprival or loss of vitality.
Devolu'tion. The reverse of evolution; catabolic change.
Devor'ative capsule. A capsule to be filled with medicine and swallowed.
Dewees's carminative. Mixture of magnesium carbonate, tincture of asafetida, and tincture of opium.
Dew'lap. A fold resembling the dewlap of the ox, sometimes seen under the human chin.
Dew'-point. That temperature at which dew begins to be deposited. **D.-cure.** See *Kneippism.*
Dexiocar'dia. Presence of heart in right side of thorax.
Dex'ter (dex'ter). On the right side.
Dex'trad (dex'trad). Toward the right side.
Dex'tral (dex'tral). Pertaining to the right side.
Dex'tran. A gummy substance formed in milk by the action of bacteria.

Dex'trin. A substance prepared from starch and used in making mucilage.

Dextrocar'dia (dex-tro-kar'de-ah). Same as *Dexiocardia.*

Dextrococa'in. An artificial cocain substitute.

Dex'trogyre, Dextroro'tatory. Turning plane of polarization to right.

Dextromen'thol. An oxidation product of menthol.

Dex'trose (deks'trōs). Ordinary glucose.

Dextrosinis'tral. Extending from right to left.

Dextrotartar'ic acid. Ordinary or dextrorotatory tartaric acid.

Dextrover'sion. Displacement toward the right side.

Dezym'otize (de-zim'o-tiz). To deprive of ferments or germs.

Diabe'tes (di-ab-e'tēs). Inordinate and persistent increase in the urinary secretion. **Biliary d.**, hypertrophic cirrhosis of liver with jaundice. **Conjugal d.**, diabetes affecting both husband and wife. **D. deceip'iens**, diabetes mellitus without polyuria or polydipsia. **D. insip'idus**, that which is not characterized by an increase in the sugar normally present in the urine. **D. melli'tus**, that which is associated with chronic glycosuria. **Pancreatic d.**, glycosuria associated with disease of pancreas. **Phloridzin-d.**, that produced by administration of phloridzin. **Phosphatic d.**, a variety in which there is excess of phosphates in urine. **Puncture d.**, diabetes produced by puncturing the oblongata.

Diabet'ic (di-ab-et'ik). Pertaining to diabetes. **D. center.** See *Center.* **D. ear**, otitis media diabetica. **D. neuritis**, multiple neuritis of diabetes. **D. sugar**, glucose found in the sugar of the urine of diabetes.

Diabe'tide. A cutaneous manifestation of diabetes.

Diabe'tin. Proprietary name for levulose for use in diabetes.

Diabetom'eter. A polariscope for use in estimating the percentage of sugar in urine.

Diabolep'tic. An insane person who believes himself beset by the devil.

Diabrot'ic. 1. Ulcerative; caustic. 2. A corrosive or escharotic.

Di'acele (di'ah-sēl). The third ventricle of the brain.

Diacetan'ilid. A derivative of acetanilid, having similar but stronger action.

Diac'etate (di-as'et-āt). A salt of diacetic acid.

Diace'tic acid. See *Acid.*

Diace'tin (di-as-e'tin). Same as *Acetidin.*

Diacetu'ria (di-as-e-tu're-ah). The presence of diacetic acid in urine.

Diach'ylon, Diach'ylum. Lead-plaster.

Diac'id. Having an acidity of two.

Diacla'sia, Diacla'sis. A fracture; especially one made for surgical purposes.

Di'aclast (di'ak-last). An instrument used in breaking up the fetal head.

Diacœle, Diacœlia (di-a-si'le-ah). Same as *Diacele.*

Diac'risis (di-ak'ri-sis). 1. A disease characterized by change in the secretions. 2. A secretion or excretion. 3. Diagnosis.

Diacrit'ic, Diacrit'ical. Diagnostic; pathognomonic.

Di'ad (di'ad). A bivalent element or radical.

Di'aderm. Blastoderm during that stage in which it consists of ectoderm and entoderm.

Diagnose', Diagnos'ticate. To make a diagnosis; to ascertain or recognize a disease.

Diagno'sis. The art or process of determining the nature of an attack of disease. **Differential d.**, the distinguishing between two similar diseases by comparing their symptoms. **D. by exclusion**, the determination of a disease by excluding all other conditions. **Physical d.,** the determination of disease by external examination.

Diagnos'tic. Pertaining to a diagnosis; distinctive; pathognomonic.

Diagnosti'cian, Di'agnost. One who is expert in diagnosis.

Di'agram. A figure or outline; especially one which illustrates a truth or principle, but does not attempt an exact representation of nature.

Diagrammat'ic. Of the nature of a diagram.

Di'agraph (di'a-graph). An instrument for recording outlines, as in craniometry.

Dial'ysate (di-al'is-āt). A liquid that has been dialysed.

Di'alysed iron. A preparation of iron obtained by dialysis.

Dial'ysis (di-al'is-is). 1. The separation of crystalloids from colloids by diffusion through a membrane. 2. Weakness. 3. Solution of continuity.

Di'alyzer (di'al-iz-er). An apparatus for performing dialysis.

Diamagnet'ic. Repelled by the magnet.

Diam'eter (di-am'et-er). A straight line joining opposite points of a figure. **Craniometric d's.,** imaginary lines connecting points on opposite surfaces of the cranium. The most important are: **biparietal,** one joining the parietal eminences; **bitemporal,** one joining the extremities of the coronal sutures; **occipitofrontal,** one joining the root of the nose and the most prominent point of the occiput; **occipitomental,** one between external occipital protuberance and the chin; **trachelobregmatic,** one between the anterior fontanel and the junction of the neck with the floor of the mouth. **D. of the pelvis.** Of these the most important are: **anteroposterior** (of inlet), that between the sacrovertebral angle and the pubic symphysis; **anteroposterior** (of outlet), that between the tip of the coccyx and the subpubic ligament; **conjugate,** the anteroposterior d. of the inlet; **diagonal conjugate,** that joining the sacrovertebral angle and the subpubic ligament; **external conjugate,** that joining the depression above the spine of the first sacral vertebra and the middle of the upper border of the pubic symphysis; **true conjugate,** that joining the sacrovertebral angle and the most prominent portion of the posterior aspect of pubic symphysis; **transverse** (of inlet), that joining the two most widely separated points of inlet of pelvis; **transverse** (of outlet), that between the ischial tuberosities.

Diam'id, Diam'ide (di-am'id). A double amid.

Diam'in (di-am'in). A double amin.

Diapa'son. A tuning-fork: employed in diagnosis of ear-troubles.

Diapede'sis. The oozing out of blood; the passage of blood-corpuscles through vessel-walls.

Diapen'te. An old tonic electuary, made of aristolochia, myrrh, laurel-berries, ivory, and gentian.

Di'aphane (di'af-ān). The investing membrane of a cell.

Diaphanom'eter. A device for testing milk, alcohol, or urine, by means of transmitted light.

Diaphan'oscope. A device for examining closed cavities by means of transmitted light.

Diaphanos'copy. Examination by the diaphanoscope.

Diaphemet'ric (di-af-e-met'rik). Pertaining to the measurement of tactile sensibility.

Diaphore'sis (di-af-or-e'sis). Profuse perspiration.

Diaphoret'ic. 1. Causing perspiration. 2. A sudorific medicine.

Di'aphragm (di'af-ram). 1. The midriff, or septum between the thorax and abdomen. 2. Any thin septum which divides a cavity. **D.-phenomenon,** Litten's sign. See under *Sign*.

Diaphragmal'gia. Neuralgia of the diaphragm.

Diaphragmati'tis, Diaphragmi'tis. Inflammation of the diaphragm.

Diaphragmat'ocele (di-af-rag-mat'o-sēl). Diaphragmatic hernia.

Diaphragmodyn'ia. Pain in the diaphragm.

Diaph'therin. Oxyquinaseptol; an antiseptic powder.

Diaph'thol (di-af'thol). An antiseptic remedy, quinaseptol.

Diaph'ysis. The shaft of a long bone between the epiphyses.

Diaphysi'tis. Inflammation of a diaphysis.

Di'aplex, Diaplex'us. The choroid plexus of third ventricle.

Diapoph'ysis. An upper transverse process of a vertebra.

Diapye'sis (di-ap-i-e'sis). Suppuration.

Diapyet'ic (di-ap-i-et'ik). Promoting suppuration.

Diarrhe'a, Diarrhœa (di-ar-e'ah). Frequent discharge of loose alvine evacuations. **Choleraic d.**, severe, acute diarrhea with serous stools, and accompanied by vomiting and collapse. **Critical d.**, d. occurring at the crisis of a disease or producing a crisis. **Lienteric d.**, diarrhea marked by fluid stools containing undigested food. **Mucous d.**, that marked by the presence of mucus in the stools. **Summer d.**, acute d. in children during the intense heat of summer.

Diarthro'sis. A joint characterized by mobility in any direction. **D. rotato'ria**, a pivot joint.

Diastal'tic. Performed reflexly through the medium of the spinal cord.

Di'astase (di'as-tās). An important ferment derivable from germinating seeds and from malt.

Dias'tasis (di-as'tas-is). 1. Separation of bones without fracture. 2. Fracture of a bone at the junction of an epiphysis.

Diastematocra'nia. Longitudinal congenital fissure of the cranium.

Diastematomye'lia. Congenital separation of the lateral halves of the spinal cord.

Diastematopye'lia. Congenital median slit of the pelvis.

Dias'ter. Daughter-star; double-star figure in karyokinesis.

Dias'tole (di-as'to-le). The expansion of the heart: opposed to systole.

Diastol'ic (di-as-tol'ik). Pertaining to diastole.

Diastre'phia. Insanity with extreme cruelty and moral perversion.

Diate'la, Diate'le (di-ah-te'lah, di-ah-te'le). The roof of the third ventricle.

Diater'ma. Part of the floor of the third ventricle.

Diather'mal (di-ath-er'mal). Permeable by heat.

Diather'manous. Permeable by heat.

Diather'many, Diatherman'sis. Permeability to heat.

Diath'esis. Predisposition to a disease. **Aneurysmal d.**, constitutional predisposition to aneurysms. **Furuncular d.** See *Furunculosis*. **Hemorrhagic d.**, hemophilia. **Lithic d.**, a tendency to lithemia. **Rheumatic d.**, constitutional predisposition to rheumatism. **Uratic d.**, a tendency toward gout.

Diathet'ic (di-ath-et'ik). Pertaining to diathesis.

Di'atom. A unicellular microscopic plant.

Diatom'ic. 1. Containing two atoms. 2. Bivalent.

Dia'zo-reaction. A deep-red color in urine produced in certain diseased conditions by $C_6H_4N_2S.O_3$.

Diba'sic. Doubly basic.

Diblas'tula. A blastule in which the ectoderm and entoderm are present.

Dical'cic orthophosphate. A salt, $Ca_2H_2(PO_4)_2$, often found in urinary deposits.

Diceph'alous (di-sef'al-us). Two-headed.

Diceph'alus (di-sef'al-us). A teratic fetus with two heads.
Dichloralantipy'rin. A production of trituration of antipyrin with chloral hydrate.
Dichro'ic (di-kro'ik). Characterized by dichroism.
Di'chroism(di'kro-izm). The showing one color by reflected and another by transmitted light.
Dicrot'ic, Dic'rotous (di-krot'ik, dik'ro-tus). Having a double pulsation.
Dic'rotism (dik'ro-tizm). The quality of being dicrotic.
Didac'tylism. The congenital quality of having only two digits on one hand or foot.
Didymal'gia (did-im-al'je-ah). Pain in a testis.
Did'ymin. A preparation from epididymis of ox.
Didymi'tis (did-im-i'tis). Inflammation of a testis.
Didymodyn'ia. Pain in a testis.
Did'ymous (did'im-us). Twin; occurring in pairs.
Diencephalon. Same as *Thalamencephalon.*
Di'et (di'et). The regulation of food to the requirements of the body. **Diabetic d.,** diet of meats and green vegetables, sugars and starches being excluded. **Fever d.,** a nutritious, light, easily-digested diet. **Gouty d.,** simple, nutritious diet without wines, fats, pastry, or much meat.
Di'etary (di'et-a-re). A course or system of diet.
Dietet'ic (di-et-et'ik). Pertaining to a diet.
Dietet'ics (di-et-et'iks). The science of questions of diet.
Diethylam'in. A harmless ptomain from fish.
Differen'tial diagnosis (dif-er-en'shal). Discrimination between similar diseases.
Differentia'tion. Acquirement of special organs and functions.
Dif'fusate (dif'fu-sāt). Same as *Dialysate.*
Diffuse (dif-fūs'). Widely spread; not definitely limited. **D. inflammation,** that which affects parenchyma and interstitial tissue.
Diffu'sible (dif-fu'zib-l). Capable of rapid diffusion.
Digas'tric (di-gas'trik). Having two bellies. **D. muscle.** See *Muscles, Table of.* **D. nerve.** See *Nerves, Table of.*
Digest'ant (di-jest'ant). 1. Aiding digestion. 2. A remedy which aids digestion.
Diges'tion (di-jes'chun). The conversion of food into assimilable matter. **Artificial d.,** digestion carried on outside of the body. **Gastric d.,** digestion by the action of the gastric juice. **Intestinal d.,** digestion by the action of the intestinal juices. **Pancreatic d.,** digestion by the action of the pancreatic juice. **Peptic d.** See *Gastric d.* **Primary d.,** gastro-intestinal digestion. **Salivary d.,** digestion by the saliva. **Secondary d.,** the assimilation by the body-cells of their nutritious matter.
Diges'tive (di-jes'tiv). Pertaining to digestion.
Digit (did'jit). A finger or toe; a dactyl.
Dig'ital (did'jit-al). Pertaining to a digit.
Digita'lin. An active glucosid of digitis; poisonous.
Digita'lis (did-jit-a'lis). The leaves of *Digitalis purpurea,* foxglove: narcotic, cardiant, diuretic.
Dig'itate (dij'it-āt). Branched like digits.
Digita'tion (dij-it-a'shun). A finger-like slit or process.
Digitox'in. A poisonous principle from digitalis.
Diglos'sia (di-glos'se-ah). Double tongue, or bifid tongue.
Digna'thus (dig-na'thus). A teratism with two lower jaws.
Dihydrocol'lidin. Oily liquid ptomain, $C_8H_{13}N.H_2$.
Dihydroresor'cin. Antiseptic product of action of resorcin or sodium amalgam.
Diiod'oform (di-i-od'o-form). Compound, C_2I_4, used like iodoform.

Diiodosalicyl'ic acid. An antipyretic, antiseptic, and analgesic.

Diiodosal'ol. A preparation used in dermatology.

Dilacera'tion (di-las-er-a'shun). The rending asunder of a part or organ.

Dila'tant. An agent or medicine that causes dilation.

Dilata'tion (di-la-ta'shun). The expansion of any orifice or canal. **D. of heart,** increase in size of one or more of the heart-cavities from weakness or relaxation.

Dilata'tor, Dila'tor. A muscle or instrument which effects a dilatation. **Barnes's d.,** a rubber bag which is inserted into the cervix uteri and distended with water. **D. ir'idis,** the set of fibers which dilate the pupil. **D. na'ris.** See *Muscles, Table of.* **D. tu'bæ.** Same as *Tensor palati.*

Dil'uent (dil'u-ent). Diluting; an agent that dilutes or renders fluid.

Dilu'tion (di-lu'shun). 1. The act of attenuating by admixture of a neutral agent. 2. An attenuated substance.

Dilu'tionist. One who advocates the attenuation of medicines.

Dimethylam'in. A non-toxic base, $(CH_3)_2NH$.

Dime'tria (di-me'tre-ah). Double uterus.

Dimor'phous. Having two distinct forms.

Dineu'ric (di-nu'rik). Having two nerve-cells.

Din'ical (din'ik-al). Pertaining to dizziness; relieving dizziness.

Din'ner-pill. A pill to take with the meals.

Dinoma'nia (di-no-ma'ne-ah). Dancing mania.

Diopsim'eter. A device for measuring the field of vision.

Diop'ter. The power of a lens with the focal length of one meter.

Dioptom'eter. An instrument for testing ocular refraction.

Dioptom'etry. The measurement of ocular accommodation and refraction.

Diop'tral (di-op'tral). Pertaining to a diopter.

Diop'tric (di-op'trik). 1. Pertaining to refracted light. 2. A diopter.

Diop'trics. The science of refracted light.

Diop'try (di-op'tre). Same as *Diopter.*

Diosco'rea villo'sa. Wild yam; antirheumatic, antispasmodic, and diaphoretic.

Diosco'rein. A medicinal resinoid from dioscorea.

Diox'id. Oxid with two oxygen atoms and one of base.

Diphthe'ria (dif-the're-ah). An infectious disease, characterized by the formation of false membranes, especially in the throat. **Bretonneau's d.,** true d. of the pharynx. **Surgical** or **Wound d.,** formation of diphtheritic membrane on wounds.

Diph'therin (dif'the-rin). The poison generated by *Bacillus diphtheriæ.*

Diphtherit'ic (dif-ther-it'ik). Pertaining to diphtheria.

Diphtheri'tis (dif-ther-i'tis). Same as *Diphtheria.*

Diphtherotox'in. Toxalbumin from cultures of diphtheria bacillus.

Diphthon'gia (dif-thon'je-ah). The utterance at the same time of two vocal sounds of the same pitch.

Diplacu'sis. Diplaku'sis. The hearing of one sound as two.

Diple'gia (di-ple'je-ah). Paralysis of like parts on either side of the body.

Diplobacte'rium. A bacterium made up of two distinct cylinders.

Diploblas'tic (dip-lo-blas'tik). Having two germ-layers.

Diplococ'cus, pl. *diplococ'ci.* A schizomycete made up of cocci joined in twos. **D. al'bicans am'plus,** non-pathogenic species from the mucus of healthy vagina. **D. al'bicans tardis'simus,** non-pathogenic species resembling gonococcus. **D. al'bicans tar'dus,** non-pathogenic species found in eczema.

D. cory'zæ, non-pathogenic species from nasal secretions in acute nasal catarrh. **D. fla'vus liquefa'ciens tar'dus,** non-pathogenic d. from the skin in seborrhea. **D. intercellula'ris meningit'idis,** pathogenic d. from the cells of the exudate of cerebrospinal meningitis. **D. lac'teus faviformis,** non-pathogenic species from vaginal secretions. **D. pneumo'niæ.** the pathogenic species of croupous pneumonia. **D. pyo'genes ure'æ,** a species found in purulent urine. **D. ro'seus,** non-pathogenic d. found in the air, and producing a pink pigment. **D. ure'æ.** Same as *D. pyogenes ureæ.* **D. ure'æ trifolia'tus,** a species found in purulent urine.

Diploco'ria (dip-lo-ko're-ah). Double pupil.

Dip'loë (dip'lo-e). Cellular bony tissue between the two tables of the skull.

Diploët'ic, Diplo'ic. Pertaining to the diploë.

Diplogen'esis. Duplication of a part.

Diplomye'lia (dip-lo-mi-e'le-ah). Lengthwise fissure of the spinal cord.

Diplopho'nia (dip-lo-fo'ne-ah). Same as *Diphthongia.*

Diplo'pia (dip-lo'pe-ah). The seeing of single objects as double. **Binocular d.,** due to a derangement of the muscular balance, the images of the object being thrown upon non-identical points of the retinæ. **Crossed** or **Heteronymous d.,** that in which the image of the right eye appears upon the left side, and that of the left eye upon the right side. **Direct** or **Homonymous d.,** the reverse of crossed d. **Monocular d.,** diplopia with a single eye.

Diplopiom'eter. An instrument for measuring diplopia.

Dip'pel's oil (dip'pelz). An oily liquid made by distilling animal substances.

Dip'ping. Palpation of the liver by sudden and forcible pressure.

Diproso'pus. A monster with a more or less double face.

Dipsoma'nia. Insane thirst for alcoholic drink.

Dipsop'athy. Thirst-cure; limitation of drink for purposes of cure.

Dipso'sis (dip-so'sis). Morbid thirst.

Dipy'gus (di-pi'gus). A monstrosity with a more or less double pelvis.

Direct' current. See *Current.* **D. illumination,** that which is made from in front. **D. murmur,** that which is due to obstruction of the blood-current.

Direc'tor. A grooved instrument for guiding a bistoury.

Dirigomo'tor. Controlling muscular activity.

Disarticula'tion. Amputation at a joint.

Disassimila'tion. Catabolic change.

Disc. See *Disk.*

Discharge (dis-charj'). 1. The outflow of any substance. 2. A substance evacuated.

Dischar'ger. An instrument for liberating electricity.

Dischar'ging lesion. A lesion of nerve-center marked by sudden discharges of force.

Discis'sion (dis-sizh'un). Rupture of lens-capsule in operating on cataract.

Discoblas'tic. Showing vitelline discoid segmentation.

Dis'coid or **Discoid'al placenta.** Placenta of a flat, cake-like form.

Discoplacen'ta. A discoid placenta.

Discrete' (dis-krēt'). Distinct; not confluent.

Dis'cus prolig'erus. The cellular envelop of the ripe ovum within the Graafian vesicle.

Discuss'. To promote the resolution of; to scatter, as a tumor.

Discus'sion (dis-kush'un). The scattering or dispersal of a swelling.

Discu'tient (dis-ku'shent). A scattering or dispersing remedy.

Disdi'aclast. A small doubly-refracting element found in the contractile substance of muscle.

Disease (diz-ēz'). Deviation from a state of health. **Acute d.**, a disease characterized by rapid onset and short course. **Addison's d.**, disease marked by bronzing of the skin, anemia, and exhaustion, from tuberculosis of suprarenal capsules. **Albert's d., Anserine d.**, disease marked by emaciation of extremities, making the hands and feet resemble a goose's. **Aran-Duchenne's d.**, progressive muscular atrophy. **Bael's d.**, small ulcerating papules of labial mucous membrane. **Barlow's d.**, infantile scurvy. **Basedow's d.**, exophthalmic goiter. **Bazin's d.**, psoriasis of the mucous membrane of the cheek. **Begbie's d.** 1. Same as *Graves's d.* 2. Same as *Bergeron's d.* **Beigel's d.** Same as *Bergeron's d.* **Bell's d.**, acute peri-encephalitis. **Bergeron's d.**, hysterical chorea. **Bleeder's d.**, hemophilia. **Blue d.** Same as *Cyanosis.* **Bouillard's d.**, endocarditis. **Bright's d.**, kidney-disease with albuminuria. **Brodie's d.**, chronic synovitis producing a pulpy state of the tissues. **Brown-Séquard's d.**, paralysis of motion on one side of the body with paralysis of sensation on the other. **Buhl's d.**, jaundice of the new-born. **Chabert's d.**, symptomatic anthrax. **Charcot's d.**, multiple cerebrospinal sclerosis. **Chronic d.**, a disease that is slow in its course. **Concato's d.**, malignant inflammation of serous membranes. **Constitutional d.**, one in which the whole of the body or an entire system of organs is affected. **Corrigan's d.**, insufficiency of the aortic valves. **Cruveilhier's d.**, simple ulcer of the stomach. **DaCosta's d.**, retrocedent gout; lithemia. **Dancing d.** See *Tarantism.* **Darier's d.**, skin-disease, with formation of papules which contain scab-like scales. **Devergie's d.**, pityriasis rubra. **Dressler's d.**, intermittent hemoglobinuria. **Dubini's d.**, electrical chorea. **Duchenne's d.** 1. Bulbar paralysis. 2. Electrical chorea. **Duhring's d.**, dermatitis herpetiformis. **Eichstedt's d.**, pityriasis versicolor. **Erb's d.**, idiopathic muscular atrophy. **Erichsen's d.**, traumatic hysteria. **Fauchard's d.**, alveolar pyorrhea. **Fish-skin d.** See *Ichthyosis.* **Flajani's d.**, exophthalmic goiter. **Flaxdresser's d.**, pneumonia from inhaling particles of flax. **Focal d.**, a localized disease. **Fothergill's d.**, facial neuralgia. **Friedreich's d.** 1. Hereditary ataxia. 2. Same as *Paramyoclonus multiplex.* **Functional d.**, a disease without apparent organic lesion. **Gerlier's d.**, disease marked by pains in neck and head, vertigo and paralysis. **Glénard's d.**, enteroptosis. **Gourand's d.**, inguinal intestinal hernia. **Graves's d.**, exophthalmic goiter. **Hall's d.**, spurious hydrocephalus. **Halstern's d.**, endemic syphilis. **Hammond's d.**, posthemiplegic chorea. **Hanot's d.**, hypertrophic cirrhosis of liver. **Heberden's d.**, rheumatic arthritis. **Heubner's d.**, syphilitic endocarditis. **Hodgkin's d.**, pseudoleukemia. **Hodgson's d.**, dilatation of the first portion of the aorta. **Huguier's d.**, fibromyoma of the uterus. **Hydrocephaloid d.**, a condition resembling hydrocephalus, but with depressed fontanels, caused by severe diarrhea. **Idiopathic d.**, one that exists without any connection with any other disease. **Intercurrent d.**, a disease occurring during the course of another disease with which it has no connection. **Kaposi's d.**, xeroderma pigmentosum. **Krishaber's d.**, nervous disease with hyperesthesia, vertigo, and delusions of sense. **Kussmaul's d.**, acute atrophic spinal paralysis. **Leber's d.**, hereditary atrophy of the optic nerve. **Legal's d.**, headache in tympanic region due to inflammation.

Little's d., spasmodic paraplegia of infants. **Malassez's d.**, cyst of the testicle. **Marie's d.**, acromegaly. **Ménière's d.**, vertigo due to disease of the labyrinth of the ear. **Mitral d.**, disease of the mitral valves. **Morand's d.**, paresis of the extremities. **Morvan's d.**, paresis of upper extremity, with analgesia and ulceration of the digits. **Occupation d.**, nervous disease due to exhaustion from the habitual performance of some occupation. **Organic d.**, one due to structural changes. **Paget's d.** 1. Hypertrophic deforming osteitis. 2. Inflammation of the nipple, with a tendency to formation of cancer. **Parasitic d.**, one due to parasites. **Parkinson's d.**, paralysis agitans. **Parrot's d.**, syphilitic pseudoparalysis. **Pavy's d.**, recurrent albuminuria. **Paxton's d.**, tinea nodosa. **Pott's d.**, caries of the vertebræ. **Quincke's d.**, angioneurotic edema. **Quinquaud's d.**, folliculitis decalvans. **Rag-sorters' d.**, febrile disease, with headache and cough, in rag-sorters of paper-mills. **Raynaud's d.** 1. Symmetric gangrene of the extremities. 2. Paralysis of throat-muscles secondary to parotitis. **Reclus's d.**, cystic disease of the mammary gland. **Riga's d.**, cachectic aphthæ. **Riggs's d.**, pyorrhea affecting the alveolar processes of the gums. **Ritter's d.**, dermatitis exfoliativa of infants. **Rivolta's d.**, actinomycosis. **Rokitansky's d.**, acute yellow atrophy of the liver. **Roosbach's d.**, hyperchlorhydria. **Scythian d.**, atrophy of testicles and penis from sexual perversion. **Septic d.**, one caused by putrefactive organisms within the body. **Specific d.**, one caused by a specific virus or poison. **Stokes's d.** Same as *Graves's d.* **Structural d.**, a disease with anatomical changes in tissue. **Strümpell's d.**, polioencephalitis. **System d.**, disease affecting a number of tissues which perform a common function. **Thomsen's d.**, hereditary disease, with rigidity of muscles of arms and legs. **Thornwaldt's d.**, suppurative inflammation of Luschka's tonsil. **Tourette's d.**, nervous disease marked by inco-ordination, convulsions, and speech disorders. **Tricuspid d.**, disease of the tricuspid valves. **Vagabond's d.**, discoloration of the skin from lice. **Van Buren's d.**, chronic inflammation of corpora cavernosa of penis. **Venereal d.**, one acquired in sexual intercourse. **Voltolini's d.**, acute suppurative inflammation of the internal ear, with fever and delirium. **Wardrop's d.**, malignant onychitis. **Weil's d.**, acute infectious jaundice. **Werlhoff's d.**, purpura hæmorrhagica. **Willis's d.**, diabetes. **Wilson's d.**, universal exfoliative dermatitis. **Winckel's d.**, fatty degeneration of the organs of newborn infants, with cyanosis, bloody urine, etc. **Woillez's d.**, severe congestion of the lungs. **Wool-sorter's d.**, anthrax in those who handle wool. **Zymotic d.**, a disease produced by some living germ within the body.

Disengage'ment (dis-en-gāj'ment). The liberation of a fetus, or part thereof, from the vaginal canal.

Disinfect' (dis-in-fekt'). To free from infection.

Disinfec'tant. Destroying infection; a disinfecting agent.

Disinfec'tin. Disinfectant compound of residue from distillation of naphtha and one part of concentrated sulphuric acid.

Disk. A lamella charged with some active medicine. **Blood-d.**, a blood-corpuscle. **Bowman's d.**, one of the segments making up a muscle-fiber. **Choked d.** See *Papillitis.* **D. diameter**, the diameter of the optic disk. **Germinal d.**, the small disk of the blastoderm in which the first traces of the embryo appear. **Hensen's d.**, pale line running transversely through a sarcous element. **Optic d.**, circular area in the retina representing the termination of the optic nerve.

Disloca'tion. Displacement of a part. **Complete d.**, one in which the surfaces are entirely separated. **Compound d.**, one in which the joint communicates with the air through a wound. **Consecutive d.**, one in which the displaced bone is not in the same position as when dislocated. **Old d.**, one in which inflammatory changes have occurred. **Partial** or **Incomplete d.**, one in which the surfaces remain in partial contact. **Pathologic d.**, one due to disease of the joint or to paralysis of the muscles. **Primitive d.**, one in which the bones remain as originally displaced. **Recent d.**, one in which no inflammatory changes have occurred. **Simple d.**, one in which there is no communication with the air through a wound.

Disorganiza'tion. Loss or destruction of organic tissue.

Dis'parate points (dis'par-āt). Points on the two retinæ upon which light does not produce the same impression.

Dispen'sary. Place for free dispensation of medical treatment.

Dispen'satory. A book which describes medicines and their preparation.

Dispense' (dis-pens'). To deliver medicines to those who are to receive them.

Disper'sing lens. Same as *Concave lens*.

Dispi'rem (di-spi'rem). The karyokinetic figure which follows the diaster.

Disrup'tive discharge. Electrical discharge with sound and heat.

Dissect' (dis-sekt'). To perform dissection upon.

Dissect'ing aneurysm. See *Aneurysm*.

Dissec'tion (dis-sek'shun). Cutting up an organism for study. **D. tubercle**, warty growth on hands of dissectors, due to poisonous fluids of cadaver.

Dissem'inated. Disposed in separate patches.

Dissimila'tion. Same as *Disassimilation*.

Dissipa'tion (dis-ip-a'shun). Dispersion of morbid matters.

Dissocia'tion (dis-so-se-a'shun). Separation into parts or elements. **D.-symptom**, anesthesia to pain and to heat or cold, but with tactile sensibility: seen in syringomyelia.

Dissolu'tion. Death; resolution into elements.

Dissolve' (diz-olv'). To liquefy by means of a solvent.

Dissol'vent (diz-ol'vent). A solvent medium.

Dis'tad (dis'tad). Toward the distal part.

Dis'tal (dis'tal). Situated toward the end; not proximal.

Distichia'sis, Distich'ia (dis-te-ki'a-sis, dis-tik'e-ah). Presence of two rows of eyelashes.

Distil'late (dis-til'āt). A product, or educt, of distillation.

Distilla'tion (dis-til-a'shun). The separation of the more volatile parts by heat. **Destructive d.**, decomposition of a substance in a closed vessel so as to obtain liquid products. **Dry d.**, distillation of solids without the addition of liquids. **Fractional d.**, separation of substances from each other by distilling the compound containing them at gradually increasing temperature.

Dis'toma, Dis'tomum. A genus of trematode entozoa; flukes.

Disto'mia. The condition of having two mouths.

Distomi'asis. Disease due to the presence of distomata.

Dis'trix. The splitting of the hairs at the end.

Disuse-amblyopia. See *Amblyopia*.

Di'ta bark (de'tah). The bark of *Alstonia scholaris*: antiperiodic.

Dit'ain (dit'ah-in). A poisonous alkaloid from dita bark.

Ditam'in. An alkaloid from dita bark.

Dith'ion. Sodium dithiosalicylate: used as antiseptic.

Dithiosalicyl'ic acid. A salicylic-acid derivative, $C_{14}H_{10}O_6S_2$: its sodium salt is antirheumatic and antiseptic.

Dithy'mol-dii'odid. Same as *Aristol*.

Dito'çia (di-to'se-ah). Birth of twins.

Dit'trick's plugs (dit'ricks). Plugs in bronchial tubes in cases of gangrene of lungs.

Diure'sis (di-u-re'sis). Increased flow of urine.

Diuret'ic. 1. Causing diuresis. 2. A medicine which stimulates the flow of urine. **Alterative d.**, one used for its local action on the surfaces over which it passes. **Hydragogue d.**, one that increases the flow of water from the kidneys. **Refrigerant d.**, one that renders the urine less irritating.

Diure'tin. Theobromin sodiosalicylate; diuretic.

Diurn'ule (di-urn'ūl). A capsule containing the maximum diurnal dose.

Divaga'tion. The use of incoherent or wandering speech.

Diver'gence (di-ver'jens). Limit of possible outward rolling of ocular axes.

Diver'gent strabismus. Wall-eye. See *Strabismus.*

Di'vers' paralysis. Same as *Caisson disease.*

Divertic'ular hernia. Hernia containing a knuckle of intestine.

Diverticuli'tis. Inflammation of a diverticulum.

Divertic'ulum. A cecum; cul-de-sac. **Meckel's d.**, an occasional appendix to the ileum near the cecum. **Nuck's d.**, the canal of Nuck. See *Canal.*

Divul'sion (di-vul'shun). Forcible separation of parts.

Divul'sor. Instrument for forcible dilatation.

Do'bell's solution (do'belz). An antiseptic cleansing fluid.

Dochmi'asis, Dochmio'sis. State induced by infestation with *Dochmius.*

Doch'mius (dok'me-us). Same as *Ankylostoma.*

Docima'sia (dos-e-ma'se-ah). Assay or examination; official test.

Docimas'tic (dos-im-as'tik). Pertaining to docimasia.

Dodecadactyli'tis. Inflammation of duodenum.

Dodecadac'tylon (do-dek-ad-ak'til-on). The duodenum.

Dog'wood. See *Cornus, Rhus, Jamaica dogwood.*

Dolichocephal'ic (dol-e-ko-sef-al'ik). With a long head.

Dolichoceph'alism, Dolichoceph'aly. The quality or fact of being dolichocephalic.

Dolichohier'ic. Having a narrow sacrum.

Dolichopel'lic, Dolichopel'vic. Having an abnormally narrow pelvis.

Doll's-head anesthesia. Anesthesia of the chest, neck, and head.

Do'lor (do'lor). L. for *Pain.*

Dolorif'ic (dol-o-rif'ik). Inducing pain.

Domatopho'bia (dom-at-o-fo'be-ah). Insane dread of being in a house.

Donné's corpuscles (don-nāz'). The colostrum corpuscles. **D.'s test**, for pus in urine; made by adding liquor potassæ.

Don'ovan's solution. Liquor arseni et hydrargyri iodidi.

Dor'sad (dor'sad). Toward the dorsal aspect.

Dor'sal (dor'sal). Pertaining to the back.

Dor'siduct (dor'sid-ukt). To draw toward the back.

Dorsiduc'tion. The act of drawing toward the back.

Dor'siflect (dor'sif-lekt). To bend backward.

Dorsiflex'ion. The act of bending a part backward.

Dorsimu'esad. Toward the dorsimeson.

Dorsim'eson. The median lengthwise line of the back.

Dorsispi'nal veins. Veins which ramify in the parts around the vertebræ.

Dorsoceph'alad. Toward the back of the head.

Dor'sum. 1. The back. 2. An upper surface.

Do'sage (do'sāj). A determination or system of doses.

Dose. A portion of medicine to be taken at one time. [See *Table of Doses*, pp. 506 519.] **Divided d.,** a relatively small dose taken at short intervals. **Lethal d.,** a dose sufficient to kill. **Maximum d.,** the largest dose consistent with safety. **Minimum d.,** the smallest dose that will produce an effect.

Dosim'eter. Instrument for measuring minute doses.

Dosimet'ric system (do-sim-et'rik). A system of exact or determinate dosage.

Dosim'etry (do-sim'et-re). Measurement of doses; dosimetric system.

Dos'sil. A pledget of lint, cotton, or wool.

Do'tage. Senile decay or second childhood.

Dothienenteri'tis. The enteritis of typhoid fever.

Double consciousness. The presence of two or more distinct mental states. **D. touch,** exploration with a finger in one cavity and thumb in another. **D. uterus.** Same as *Dihysteria*. **D. vision.** Same as *Diplopia*.

Doubt'ing insanity (dowt'ing). Insanity marked by doubt or suspicion.

Douche (doosh). [Fr.] A stream of water or other liquid directed against a part. **Air-d.,** a current of air directed against a part for therapeutic purposes.

Douglas's cul-de-sac (dug'las-ez). The rectovaginal pouch.

Do'ver's powder. Pulvis ipecacuanhae et opii.

Doyère's eminence (dwah-yärz'). The papilla where a nerve-filament enters a muscle-fiber.

D. P. Proper direction.

Dr. Dram or drachm.

D. R. Reaction of degeneration.

Drachm (dram). Same as *Dram*.

Draconti'asis. Disease produced by dracunculus.

Dracon'tium. The skunk-cabbage, *Symplocarpus fœtidus*; antispasmodic and nervine.

Dracun'culus. The *Filaria medinensis*, or guinea-worm.

Draft, Draught (drahft). A copious liquid potion or dose.

Dragee (drah-zha'). [Fr.] A sugared pill; medicated sweetmeat.

Drag'on's blood. Resin of various origin; little used in medicine.

Drain (drān). A device to promote the escape of fluids from a sore.

Drain'age. The escape of purulent or sanious fluids from a sore or wound. **Capill'ary d.,** drainage by capillary attraction, as by wisps of hair, threads, etc. **Funnel d.,** drainage by glass funnels. **D.-tube,** a tube giving vent to peccant fluids.

Dram, Drachm (dram). 1. Three scruples, or 60 grains; 3.8 grams. 2. A fluid-dram.

Dram'atism. Dramatic behavior and speech in insanity.

Drapetoma'nia. Insane desire to wander away from home.

Dras'tic (dras'tik). Violently purgative.

Draught. See *Draft*.

Drench. In veterinary medicine. Same as *Draft*.

Dres'sing. Application of a bandage or remedy; also, the thing so applied.

Drom'ograph (drom'o-graf). The recording hemodromometer.

Drop. 1. Same as *Gutta*. 2. Less correctly, a minim. **Ague d.,** solution of potassium arsenite. **Black d.,** vinegar of opium. **D.-culture,** a bacterial culture made in a drop of culture material.

Dropped-beat pulse. An intermittent pulse.

Dropped feet. Paraplegia of the anterior tibial muscles. **D. hand or wrist.** Same as *Wrist-drop*. **D. lid.** Same as *Ptosis*.

Drop'per. A pipette or tube for emitting drops.

Drop'sical (drop'sik-al). Affected with dropsy.

Drop'sy. The accumulation of serous fluid in a cavity or in the tissues. **D. of belly**, ascites. **Cardiac d.**, that due to heart-disease. **D. of chest**, hydrothorax. **Ovarian d.**, ovarian cyst. **D. of peritoneum**, hydroperitoneum or ascites.

Dros'erin. Antiseptic ferment from sun-dew.

Drug. Any medicinal substance.

Drum. The tympanum of the ear. **D.-belly**, tympanites.

Dru'min. An alkaloid from *Euphorbia Drummondii*, a local anesthetic.

Drum'stick bacillus. The bacillus putrificus coli.

Druse (drūs). Rupture of tissues with no superficial lesion.

Dry amputation. See *Amputation*. **D. cupping.** See *Cupping*. **D. gangrene**, that with little free moisture.

Drys'dale's corpuscles. Microscopic cells in the fluid of ovarian cysts.

Dubi'ni's disease (doo-be'nēz). Electric chorea, or myelitis convulsiva.

Duboi'sia. A genus of toxic plants.

Duboi'sin (du-boi'sin). Alkaloid, $C_{17}H_{23}NO_3$; same as hyoscyamin, from *Duboisia myoporoides:* acts much like atropin.

Duchenne's disease (deh-shenz'). 1. Locomotor ataxia. 2. Pseudohypertrophy of muscles. **D.'s paralysis**, progressive bulbar paralysis. **D.'s trocar**, trocar for procuring minute samples of deep-seated tissues.

Duct. A canal or passage for fluids. **Alimentary d.** Same as *Thoracic d.* **D. of Bartholin**, the larger and longer of the sublingual ducts. **Botallo's d.** Same as *Ductus arteriosus*. **Common bile d.**, a duct formed by the union of the cystic and hepatic ducts. **D. of Cuvier**, two short venous trunks in the fetus, opening into the auricle of the heart; the right one becomes the superior vena cava. **Cystic d.**, the excretory duct of the gall-bladder. **Ejaculatory d.**, the duct carrying the semen into the urethra. **Endolymphatic d.**, a tubular process of the membranous labyrinth of the ear. **Galactophorous d.**, one of the milk-ducts of the mammary gland. **Hepatic d.**, a duct of the liver. **D. of Müller**, a duct in the embryo, developing into the oviducts, uterus, and vagina. **Nasal d.**, duct that conveys tears from lacrimal sac into the nose. **Omphalomesenteric d.** Same as *Umbilical d.* **Parotid d.**, duct by which parotid gland empties into the mouth. **Prostatic d.**, any one of the ducts conveying the prostatic secretion into the urethra. **D. of Rivini**, one of the ducts of the sublingual gland. **Salivary d's.**, the ducts of the salivary glands. **Santorini's d.**, the accessory d. of the pancreas. **Segmental d.**, a tube, on either side of the body of the embryo, opening anteriorly into the body-cavity, and posteriorly into the cloaca. **Spermatic d.**, the vas deferens. **D. of Steno, D. of Stenson**, the duct of the parotid gland. **Thoracic d.**, a duct beginning in the receptaculum chyli and emptying into the left subclavian vein. **Umbilical d.**, duct between umbilical vesicle and intestinal cavity of embryo. **Urogenital d's.**, the d. of Müller and the Wolffian d. **Vitelline d.** Same as *Umbilical d.* **D. of Wharton**, the duct of the submaxillary salivary gland. **D. of Wirsung**, the main duct of the pancreas. **Wolffian d.**, the duct of the Wolffian body.

Duct'less. Having no efferent duct.

Duc'tule (duk'tūl). A minute duct.

Duc'tus. [L.] Same as *Duct*. **D. arterio'sus**, fetal blood-vessel which joins the aorta and pulmonary artery. **D. veno'sus**, a fetal vessel which connects the umbilical vein and the vena cava ascendens.

Du'gong oil. Oil of *Halicore dugong*, a sirenian mammal: used like cod-liver oil.

Duhr'ing's disease. Same as *Dermatitis herpetiformis.*

Duip'ara. A woman pregnant for the second time.

Dulcama'ra. The plant *Solanum dulcamara*, or bittersweet: used in skin-diseases.

Dul'cin (dul'sin). A synonym of sucrol and of dulcite.

Dul'cite, Dul'citol (dul'sīt, dul'sit-ol). An extremely sweet hexatomic alcohol, $C_6H_{14}O_6$.

Dull. Not resonant on percussion.

Dul'ness (dul'nes). Lack of normal resonance.

Dumb. Mute, or aphasiac. **D. ague,** malaria with slight fever or chill.

Dumb'-bell crystals. See *Crystals.*

Dumb'ness. Muteness; aphasia.

Duod'enal. Pertaining to the duodenum.

Duodeni'tis. Inflammation of the duodenum.

Duodenocholecystos'tomy. Formation by surgical means of a communication between the duodenum and gall-cyst.

Duodenoenteros'tomy. Formation by surgical means of a communication from the duodenum to some other part of the small intestine.

Duodenostenos'tomy. The surgical formation of an opening through the walls of the abdomen into the duodenum.

Duodenos'tomy. The surgical creation of a permanent opening through the wall of the abdomen into the duodenum.

Duodenot'omy. Surgical incision of the duodenum.

Duode'num. The first or proximal portion of the small intestine.

Du'otal (du'o-tal). Guaiacol carbonate.

Duplica'tion, Du'plicature. The teratic doubling or folding of a part.

Dupuytren's contraction (du-pwē-tronz'). Contracted state of the palm and fingers. **D.'s fracture.** See *Fracture.*

Du'ra, Du'ra ma'ter. The outermost membrane of the brain and spinal cord.

Du'ral (du'ral). Pertaining to the dura.

Durémato'ma (du-re-mat-o'mah). Hematoma of the dura.

Duri'tis (du-ri'tis). Inflammation of the dura.

Duro-arachni'tis. Inflammation of the dura and arachnoid.

Duro'lenm. A petrolate resembling vaselin.

Duroziez's murmur (du-ro-ze-āz'). Double murmur over the femoral artery.

Dust'ing powder. An absorbent, antiseptic, astringent, or soothing powder for external use.

Dutch liquid. Ethylene dichlorid.

Dwarf. An undersized person. **D. pelvis,** an æquabiliter justo minor pelvis.

Dwar'fishness. Same as *Nanism.*

Dy'ad (di'ad). See *Diad.*

Dyna'mia (di-na'me-ah). Vital energy or force.

Dynam'ic (di-nam'ik). Pertaining to strength or vital force.

Dynam'ics. The science of motion and of forces.

Dynamiza'tion (di-nam-iz-a'shun). The hypothetical increase of medicinal effectiveness by dilution and trituration.

Dynamogen'ic. Pertaining to, or caused by, an increase of strength.

Dynam'ograph. An instrument for recording muscular power.

Dynamom'eter. An instrument for testing muscular power.

Dynam'oscope. A device for the auscultation of muscles.

Dynamos'copy (di-nam-os'ko-pe). Auscultation of muscles.

Dyne (dīn). The unit of force.

Dysacou'sis, Dysacous'ma. Impaired hearing.

Dysæ'mia, Dyse'mia. Blood-poisoning.
Dysæsthesia. See *Dysesthesia.*
Dysal'bumose. An insoluble variety of albumose.
Dysa'phia (dis-a'fe-ah). Impairment of the sense of touch.
Dysar'thria (dis-ar'thre-ah). Imperfect articulation or utterance.
Dysba'sia (dis-ba'se-ah). Impairment of the power of walking.
Dysbu'lia (dis-bu'le-ah). Weakness or perversion of will.
Dyscho'lia (dis-ko'le-ah). Depraved condition of the bile.
Dyschromatop'sia. Imperfect discrimination of colors.
Dyscine'sia (dis-sin-e'ze-ah). Impairment of the power of motion.
Dysco'ria. Abnormality in shape of the pupil.
Dyscra'sia, Dys'crasy. Morbid state of the constitution.
Dysenter'ic (dis-en-ter'ik). Pertaining to dysentery.
Dys'entery. Inflammation of the large intestine, with bloody and loose evacuations and tenesmus. **Amebic d.**, d. of tropics caused by amœba coli.
Dysesthe'sia. 1. Dulness of sensation. 2. Hyperesthesia. **Auditory d.** Same as *Dysacusis.*
Dysgeu'sia (dis-gu'ze-ah). Perversion of the sense of taste.
Dysgra'phia (dis-gra'fe-ah). Loss or impairment of the power of writing.
Dyshidro'sis (dis-hid-ro'sis). Disordered state of the perspiration.
Dyskine'sia. Imperfect voluntary movement.
Dysla'lia (dis-la'le-ah). Difficulty in speaking due to deformity.
Dyslex'ia (dis-lek'se-ah). Impairment of the power of reading due to a central lesion.
Dyslo'gia (dis-lo'je-ah). Impairment of the power of speaking and reasoning.
Dys'lysin (dis'lis-in). A resinous ingredient, $C_{24}H_{36}O_3$, of bilin.
Dysmenorrhe'a. Painful menstruation. **Congestive d.**, that due to congestion of pelvic viscera. **Inflammatory d.**, that due to inflammation. **Mechanic d.** Same as *Obstructive d.* **Membranous d.**, severe d. with discharge of shreds of membrane. **Obstructive d.**, that due to mechanic obstruction to the discharge of menstrual fluid. **Spasmodic d.**, that due to spasmodic uterine contraction.
Dysmim'ia (dis-mim'e-ah). Impairment of the power of expression by signs.
Dysneu'ria (dis-nu're-ah). Impairment of the nervous power.
Dyso'pia, Dysop'sia (dis-o'pe-ah, dis-op'se-ah). Defective vision.
Dysos'mia, Dysosphre'sia. Impairment of the sense of smell.
Dyspareu'nia (dis-par-eu'ne-ah). Painful coitus.
Dyspep'sia (dis-pep'she-ah). Indigestion; difficulty of digestion. **Acid d.**, d. with excessive formation of acid. **Atonic d.**, that due to deficient quantity or quality of the gastric juice, or to defective action of the gastric muscles. **Catarrhal d.**, that due to inflammation of the stomach. **Intestinal d.**, that due to imperfect action of the intestinal juices. **Nervous d.**, a form marked by gastric pains and by various reflex nervous phenomena.
Dyspep'tic (dis-pep'tik). Affected with dyspepsia.
Dyspep'tone (dis-pep'tōn). An insoluble peptone.
Dysperma'sia. Dysper'matism. Dysper'mia. Impairment of the semen.
Dyspha'gia (dis-fa'je-ah). A difficulty in swallowing.
Dyspha'sia (dis-fa'zhe-ah). Difficulty in utterance.
Dyspho'nia (dis-fo'ne-ah). Difficulty in uttering vocalized words.
Dyspho'ria (dis-fo're-ah). Disquiet; restlessness.
Dysphra'sia (dis-fra'zhe-ah). Difficulty in speaking due to mental defect.

Dyspne'a, Dyspnœ'a (disp-ne'ah). Labored or difficult breathing.
Dyspne'ic (disp-ne'ik). Affected with dyspnea.
Dysta'sia. Difficulty in standing.
Dystax'ia (dis-tax'e-ah). Incomplete ataxia.
Dysteliol'ogy. The science of rudimentary organs.
Dysthym'ia (dis-thim'e-ah). Mental distress; melancholia.
Dysto'cia (dis-to'se-ah). Difficult parturition. **Fetal d.,** that due to malformation, abnormal position, or size of fetus. **Maternal d.,** that due to small or malformed pelvis of mother.
Dysto'pia, Dys'topy. Malposition; displacement.
Dystro'phia, Dys'trophy. Faulty nutrition.
Dystrophodex'trin. A starchy material said to exist in normal blood.
Dystrophoneuro'sis. Defective nutrition, leading to nervous disease; nervous disease due to malnutrition.
Dysu'ria. Dys'ury (dis-u're-ah, dis'u-re). Painful micturition.
Dysu'riac. One who is affected with dysuria.

E.

E. Abbreviation for *Electromotive force* and for *Emmetropia*.
Ear (ēr). Organ of hearing. **E.-ache,** pain in the ear. **E.-cough,** a reflex cough in diseases of the ear. **E.-mould.** See *Otomycosis*. **E.-trumpet,** instrument devised to aid the hearing. **E.-wax,** cerumen.
Earth-eating. See *Geophagism*.
Eas'ton's syrup. A syrup of quinin, iron, and strychnin phosphate.
Eb'ner's glands. A set of mucous glands of the tongue.
Ebullit'ion (eb-ul-ish'un). The state of boiling.
Eburna'tion. Degeneration of bone into a hard and ivory-like mass.
Ebur'neous (e-bur'ne-us). Like ivory.
Ecau'date (e-kaw'dāt). Tailless.
Ecbal'ium. See *Elaterium*.
Ecbol'ic (ek-bol'ik). Hastening labor; oxytocic.
Eccen'tric (ek-sen'trik). Away from a center; peripheral. **E. atrophy,** atrophy combined with dilatation. **E. hypertrophy.** See *Hypertrophy*. **E. limitation,** limitation of the visual field, more marked at some points of the periphery than at others.
Ecchondro'ma. Ecchondro'sis. Homologous chondroma; cartilaginous tumor of a cartilage.
Ecchon'drotome. A knife for cutting cartilage.
Ecchymo'ma. Swelling due to blood-extravasation.
Ecchymo'sis (ek-im-o'sis). Extravasation of blood, or discoloration due to it.
Ecchymot'ic. Pertaining to, or resembling, ecchymosis.
Ec'crisis. The expulsion of waste-products.
Eccrit'ic. A drug promoting excretion.
Eccye'sis (ek-si-e'sis). Extra-uterine pregnancy.
Ecdemoma'nia. Insane desire to wander.
Ec'deron (ek'der-on). Epidermis; surface epithelium.
Echinococ'cus. Larval stage of *Tænia echinococcus*. **E.-cyst.** Same as *Hydatid*.
Ech'o, amphor'ic (ek'o). Amphoric sound which re-echoes a vocal sound.
Ech'o sign. Repetition of last word of a sentence in insanity.
Echokine'sia (ek-o-kin-e'ze-ah). Involuntary imitation of movements seen.

Echola'lia, Echo-speech (ek-o-la'le-ah). Insane repetition of words heard.
Echom'atism. The reverse of automatism.
Echophot'ony (ek-o-fot'o ne). Association of color sensations with sounds heard.
Ecla'bium (ek-la'be-um). Eversion of a lip, or of both lips.
Eclamp'sia (ek-lamp'se-ah). Convulsive attack of peripheral origin. **Infantile e.,** reflex convulsions in children. **Puerperal e.,** that occurring after or during childbirth. **Uremic e.,** due to uremia.
Eclamp'tic (ek-lamp'tik). Pertaining to, or of the nature of, eclampsia.
Eclec'tic (ek-lek'tik). Pertaining to eclecticism.
Eclec'ticism (ek-lek'tis-izm). A school of medicine purporting to select what is best from other schools.
E'coid (e'koid). The colorless framework of a red blood-corpuscle.
Écouvillonnage (a-koo-ve-on-nahzh'). The scrubbing of a sore or cavity.
Ecphyadec'tomy. Excision of vermiform appendix.
Ecphyadi'tis. Inflammation of vermiform appendix.
Écraseur (e-krah-zer'). Instrument with a loop of chain or wire for removing parts.
Ec'stasy (ek'sta-se). A state of exaltation, exhilaration, or trance.
Ec'strophy (ek'stro-fe). Same as *Extrophy.*
Ec'tad. Outward in direction or situation; externally.
Ec'tal. Superficial; external.
Ecta'sia, Ec'tasis. Expansion; dilatation; slight swelling.
Ec'tasin. A vasomotor dilator isolated from tuberculin.
Ectat'ic. Distended or stretched.
Ecten'tal. Pertaining to the ectoderm and the entoderm.
Ecteth'moids. Lateral masses of the ethmoid bones.
Ecthy'ma (ek-thi'mah). Eruption of pustules with hard bases and areolæ. **E. syphilit'icum,** an eruption of pustules in tertiary syphilis.
Ecthyreo'sis. Absence of the thyroid gland.
Ecti'ris (ek-ti'ris). The retinal or external portion of the iris.
Ec'toblast (ek'to-blast). The ectoderm, or epiblast.
Ectocar'dia. Displacement of the heart.
Ectochoroi'dea. Outer layer of the choroid coat.
Ectocor'nea (ek-to-kor'ne-ah). Outer layer of the cornea.
Ec'toderm. The epiblast; outer primitive layer of the embryo.
Ectoder'mal. Pertaining to the ectoderm.
Ectocu'tad. Proceeding from without inward.
Ectog'enous (ek-toj'en-us). Originating outside the body.
Ectop'agus. A twin monstrosity united at the thorax.
Ectopar'asite. Any external parasite, animal or vegetable.
Ectoperitoni'tis. Inflammation of external or attached side of the peritoneum.
Ec'tophyte (ek'to-fit). Any vegetable ectoparasite.
Ecto'pia, Ec'topy. Displacement; abnormal situation.
Ectop'ic. Displaced; not in the normal place. **E. gestation,** extra-uterine pregnancy.
Ec'toplasm. The outer layer of the protoplasm of the cell.
Ec'topy (ek'to-pe). Same as *Ectopia.*
Ectoret'ina. Outermost layer of the retina.
Ectosto'sis. Ossification beginning underneath the perichondria.
Ectotoxe'mia. Toxemia produced by a substance introduced from outside the body.
Ectozo'on. Any animal ectoparasite.
Ectrodactyl'ia. Congenital absence of digits.
Ectrom'elus. A fetus with rudimentary arms and legs.

Ectro'pion, Ectro'pium. Eversion, as of the edge of an eyelid.

Ectro'pionize. To put into a state of eversion; to evert.

Ec'zema (ek'ze-mah). A skin-disease, with itching, redness, and infiltration. **E. erythemato'sum,** a mild form with reddened skin. **E. fis'sum,** a form with painful cracks over the joints. **E. hypertroph'icum,** a form with permanent enlargement of the skin-papillæ. **E. mad'idans, E. ru'brum,** a form with moist raw surfaces with red points. **E. margina'tum,** a kind due to ringworm. **E. papulo'sum,** a variety associated with itching papules of a deep red color. **E. pustulo'sum,** eczema marked by pustular eruption. **E. seborrhe'icum.** Same as *Seborrhea.* **E. so'lare,** a form due to a scalding from the sun's rays. **E. squamo'sum,** a form characterized by adherent scales of epithelium. **E. vesiculo'sum,** eczema marked by the presence of vesicles.

Eczem'atoid. Resembling eczema.

Eczemato'sis. An eczematous skin-affection.

Eczem'atous. Of the nature of eczema.

Ede'a. The genitalia.

Edei'tis (e-de-i'tis). Inflammation of the genitals.

Ede'ma (e-de'mah). Swelling due to effusion into connective tissue. **Angioneurotic e.** See *Angioneurotic.* **Blue e.,** puffed, bluish state of a limb in hysteric paralysis. **Inflammatory e.,** edema due to inflammation. **Malignant e.,** edema marked by rapid extension, quick destruction of tissue, and the formation of gas. **Purulent e.,** fluid, purulent effusion.

Edem'atous. Pertaining to, or affected by, edema.

E'dentate, Eden'tulous. Without teeth.

Edenta'tion. A deprivation of teeth.

Edeol'ogy. A treatise on the genitalia.

Edeopto'sis. Genital prolapse.

Ef'ferent. Tending away from the center. **E. nerves,** those which convey impulses from the center.

Efferves'cent. Bubbling; sparkling; foaming. **E. powders,** Same as *Seidlitz powders.*

Effleurage (ef-flur-ahzh'). Centripetal stroking movement in massage.

Efflores'cence (ef-lor-es'ens). 1. Quality of being efflorescent. 2. A form of eruption in skin-disease.

Efflores'cent (ef-lor-es'ent). Becoming powdery by losing the water of crystallization.

Efflu'vium. A foul or mephitic exhalation.

Effu'sion (ef-fu'zhun). The escape of a fluid into a part; also effused material.

Eges'ta (e-jes'tah). The excretions, or discharges.

Egg. An ovum; chiefly an ovum that is hatched outside the body.

Eglan'dulous (e-glan'du-lus). Having no glands.

Egobronchoph'ony (e-go-brong-kof'o-ne). Peculiar bleating sound; a sign of pleuropneumonia.

Egoph'ony (e-gof'o-ne). Auscultation-sound like the bleat of a goat.

Egyp'tian chlorosis. Same as *Ankylostomiasis.* **E. ophthalmia,** trachoma.

Eh'renritter's ganglion. The jugular ganglion of the glossopharyngeal nerve.

Ehr'lich's solution. Solution of basic anilin dye in anilin oil and water.

Eich'horst's corpuscles. Microcytes in the blood of pernicious anemia.

Ei'loid tumor (i'loid). A tumor of a coiled shape.

Eisan'thema. An exanthem on a mucosa.

Eisod'ic (i-sod'ik). Afferent; centripetal.
Ejacula'tion. Forcible, sudden expulsion.
Ejac'ulatory duct. Duct which conveys semen to the urethra.
Ejec'ta (e-jek'tah). Refuse.
Elæomyen'chysis (e-le-o-mi-en'kis-is). The injection of non-irritating oil into a muscle.
Elæosac'charum. Sugar charged with a volatile oil.
Ela'idin (e-la'id-in). A fat, $C_{57}H_{104}O_6$, from various fixed oils.
Ela'in (e-la'in). The liquid principle of fats.
Elas'tic. Returning to its proper shape after stretching or compression. **E. bandage**, an india-rubber bandage for exerting continuous pressure. **E. lamina.** Same as *Descemet's membrane.* **E. tissue**, connective tissue composed of yellow elastic fibers.
Elas'ticin (e-las'tis-in). Same as *Elastin.*
Elastic'ity (e-las-tis'it-e). The quality of resuming the normal size after compression or stretching.
Elas'tin. The main albuminoid of yellow elastic tissue.
Elastom'eter. An instrument for determining elasticity of the tissues.
Elat'erin. Purgative principle, $C_{20}H_{28}O_5$, from elaterium.
Elate'rium. Hydragogue cathartic from the juice of *Ecbalium elaterium.*
El'bow. The joint of the arm and forearm. **E.-jerk**, involuntary bending of elbow on striking the tendon of the biceps or triceps muscle.
Elco'sis (el-ko'sis). Fetid ulceration.
El'der (el'der). See *Sambucus.*
Elecampane (el-e-kam-pān'). The plant *Inula helenium* and its stimulant root.
Elec'tric, Elec'trical. Pertaining to electricity.
Electric'ity (e-lek-tris'it-e). A force rendered manifest by friction, chemical action, or magnetism. **Faradic e.** 1. Electricity produced by induction. 2. Electricity in intermittent currents. **Franklinic e.**, static or frictional electricity. **Galvanic e.**, that generated by chemical action. **Induced e.**, electricity produced in a body by proximity to an electrified body. **Magnetic e.**, that which is developed by means of a magnet. **Static e.**, that which is generated by friction. **Voltaic e.** Same as *Galvanic e.*
Electriza'tion. The act of charging with electricity.
Electro-anesthesia. Anesthesia produced by electricity.
Electrobiol'ogy. Science of relations of electricity to living organisms.
Electrobios'copy. Electric test applied to determine whether life is extinct or not.
Electrocau'tery. Same as *Galvanocautery.*
Electrochem'istry. Science of the relations of electricity to chemistry.
Electrocystos'copy. Use of the electric light in cystoscopy.
Elec'trode (e-lek'trōd). End-piece attached to the conducting wires of an electric battery or machine.
Electrodiagno'sis. Diagnosis by means of electricity.
Electrodynamom'eter. Instrument to measure the faradic current.
Electrog'raphy. Same as *Skiagraphy.*
Elec'trolizer. Instrument for reducing stricture by electricity.
Electrol'ysis. Decomposition by means of electricity.
Electrolyt'ic. Pertaining to electrolysis.
Electromag'netism. Magnetism developed by the electric current.
Electromassage'. Massage combined with electrization.
Electrom'eter. An instrument for measuring electricity.
Electromo'tive force. Force of a moving electric current.

Electroneg'ative. Going to the positive pole in electrolysis.

Electropathol'ogy. Use of electricity in pathologic research.

Electrophysiol'ogy. Observation of the effects of electricity upon the body in health.

Electropos'itive. Going to the negative pole in electrolysis.

Electroprogno'sis. Prognosis by means of an electric test.

Elec'tropuncture. Electrization by means of needles thrust into the tissues.

Elec'troscope. An instrument for detecting the presence of static electricity.

Electrostat'ics. The science of static or frictional electricity.

Electrosur'gery. The employment of electricity in surgery.

Electrotherapeu'tics, Electrother'apy. The treatment of disease by electricity.

Electrot'onus. The change effected in a nerve or muscle by an electric current or shock.

Elec'tuary (e-lek'tu-a-re). A soft medicated confection. **E. of senna**, senna prepared with cassia pulp, tamarind, coriander, and syrup.

Ele'idin (el-e'id-in). A principle in the granular layer of the skin.

El'ement. An ultimate chemical constituent.

El'emi. A resin of various origin: now little used.

Eleop'tene. The liquid part of a volatile oil.

Elephanti'asis, Elephanti'asis Ara'bum. Chronic disease marked by lymphangitis and hypertrophy of the skin. **E. Græco'rum**, true leprosy. **E. telangiecto'des**, elephantiasis with great increase of blood-vessels.

El'ephant-leg. Same as *Elephantiasis*.

El'evator. An instrument for lifting up a part.

Elimina'tion. An act of expulsion or exclusion.

Elix'ir (e-lik'ser). A sweet, aromatic, excipient liquid.

El'koplasty (el'ko-plas-te). See *Helkoplasty*.

Elm. See *Ulmus*.

Elutria'tion. The separation of insoluble particles by water.

Elytri'tis (el-e-tri'tis). Same as *Kolpitis* or *Vaginitis*.

El'ytrocele. See *Kolpocele*.

El'ytroplasty. Plastic surgery of the vagina.

Elytropto'sis. Prolapse or inversion of the vagina.

Elytror'rhaphy. Suturing of the vaginal wall.

Elytrot'omy. Incision of the vaginal walls.

Emacia'tion (e-ma-se-a'shun). A wasted, lean habit of body.

Emana'tion. An effluvium.

Eman'sio men'sium. Retention or non-discharge of menses.

Emascula'tion (e-mas-ku-la'shun). Removal of the testicles.

Embalm'ing (em-bahm'ing). Prevention of the natural decay of the dead body.

Embed'ding. Fixation in a firm medium before cutting microscopic sections.

Embola'lia. Insane use of meaningless language.

Em'bole (em'bo-le). Same as *Emboly*.

Embol'ic. Pertaining to embolism or an embolus.

Embol'iform nucleus. One of the cerebellar nuclei.

Em'bolism. Obstruction of a vessel by an embolus. **Air e.**, obstruction by an air-bubble. **Fat e.**, obstruction by fat-globules. **Infective e.**, that in which emboli contain bacteria or septic poison. **Miliary e.**, embolism affecting many small blood-vessels.

Embolophra'sia. Same as *Embolalia*.

Em'bolus. A clot or plug which obstructs a blood-vessel.

Em'boly. Origination of the gastrula from invagination of the blastula.

Embroca'tion. A liniment or medicine for outward application.

Embryec'tomy (em-bre-ek'to-me). Excision of an extra-uterine fetus.

Em'bryo (em'bre-o). The fetus before end of third month.

Embryocar'dia. State in which the heart or its pulsation is like that of the fetus.

Embryoc'tomy. Destruction of the fetus *in utero.*

Embryogenet'ic, Embryogen'ic. Pertaining to the origin of the embryo.

Embryo'geny. The development of the embryo.

Embryog'raphy. A description of the embryo.

Embryol'ogy. The science of the development of the embryo.

Embry'onal, Embryon'ic. Pertaining to the embryo.

Em'bryotome (em'bre-o-tōm). Cutting instrument used in embryotomy.

Embryot'omy. The cutting up of the fetus to effect its delivery.

Embryot'rophy. Nourishment of the fetus.

Eme'sia, Em'esis. The act of vomiting.

Emet'ic. Causing vomiting: a medicine that causes vomiting. **Direct** or **Mechanic e.,** one that acts on the nerves of the stomach. **Indirect** or **Systemic e.,** one that acts through the blood.

Em'etin. Alkaloid, $C_{15}H_{22}NO_2$, derived from ipecac.

Emetocathar'tic. Both emetic and cathartic.

Emetol'ogy. Sum of knowledge regarding emetics.

E. M. F. Abbreviation for *Electromotive force.*

Emic'tion (e-mik'shun). Micturition.

Emigra'tion. Passage of leukocytes through the walls of capillaries and veins.

Em'inence. A projection or boss. **Canine e.,** prominence on outer side of upper jaw-bone. **Collateral e.,** a projection in lateral ventricle of brain between posterior and middle horns. **E. of Doyère.** Same as *Doyère's eminence.* **Frontal e.,** either of two eminences on frontal bones above superciliary ridges. **Nasal e.,** the prominence above the root of the nose. **Parietal e.,** the eminence of the parietal bone.

Eminen'tia (em-in-en'she-ah). L. for *Eminence.* **E. articula'ris,** rounded prominence on temporal bone. **E. collatera'lis,** a ridge on the inferior cornu of the lateral ventricle.

Em'issary veins. Veins which connect the sinuses within and the veins without the skull.

Emis'sion (e-mish'un). Discharge, especially of the semen.

Emmen'agogue (em-en'ag-og). A drug that promotes the menstrual flow; used also adjectively. **Direct e.,** one that acts directly on the organs. **Indirect e.,** one that acts by relieving some causative condition, as anemia.

Emme'nia. The menses.

Emmenol'ogy. Sum of what is known about menstruation.

Em'metrope (em'et-rōp). A person with perfect vision.

Emmetro'pia. Perfect visual refraction.

Emmetrop'ic. Having normal vision.

Em'met's operation. Trachelorrhaphy; suturing of the uterine neck.

E'mol (e'mol). A mineral substance which softens the skin.

Emol'lient. Soothing and softening; a soothing medicine. **E. cataplasm, species,** or **tea,** a mixture of herbs for infusion or for cataplasm.

Emo'tional insanity. Perversion of the emotions.

Em'phlysis (em'flis-is). A vesicular eruption.

Emphrac'tic (em-frak'tik). Clogging or obstructive.

Emphyse'ma. Air or gas abnormally present in the tissues. **Atrophic e.,** senile emphysema with wasting of lung-substance.

Cutaneous e., air or gas in the connective tissues under the skin. **Gangrenous e.**, malignant edema of microbic origin. **Interstitial e.**, gas in the connective tissue of the lung or of any other part. **E. of lungs, Pulmonary e.**, dilatation of air-vesicles with loss of normal elasticity of lung-substance. **Substantial e.** Same as *Pulmonary e.* **Surgical e.** Same as *Aërodermectasia.* **Vesicular e.**, dilatation of the air-vesicles.

Empir'ic. Charlatan whose skill is derived solely from experience.

Empir'icism (em-peer'is-izm). Skill or knowledge from mere experience.

Emplas'tic (em-plas'tik). A constipating medicine.

Emplas'trum. L. for *Plaster.*

Emprosthot'onos. Tetanic forward flexure of the body.

Empty'sis. Pulmonary hemorrhage.

Empu'sa. A genus of parasitic plants which infest insects.

Empye'ma (em-pi-e'mah). Pus in a cavity, as the chest. **E. necessita'tis**, empyema in which the pus can make a spontaneous escape. **Pulsating e.**, one which transmits the heart-pulsations to the chest-wall.

Empye'sis. A pustular eruption.

Empy'ocele. A purulent tumor of the scrotum.

Emul'gent (e-mul'jent). Draining out. **E. vessels**, renal blood-vessels.

Emul'sin (e-mul'sin). An albuminoid ferment from bitter almonds.

Emul'sion (e-mul'shun). An oily, resinous, or other medicine rubbed up with water and a mucilage.

Emul'sum. An emulsion.

Emunc'tory. Excretory or cleansing; an excretory organ.

Emunda'tion. Rectification; garbling of drugs.

Enam'el. The white investment of the crown of a tooth. **E. cuticle**, the membrane which ensheaths each enamel rod. **E. organ**, organ in gums of embryo which develops into the enamel. **E. rods**, prismatic fibers which make up the enamel.

Enan'thesis. A skin-eruption from an internal disease.

En'anthropes (en'an-thrōps). Sources of disease originating within the body.

Enarky'ochrome. A nerve-cell with a readily staining cell-body.

Enarthro'sis. Ball-and-socket joint.

Encan'this. A minute tumor of a lacrimal caruncle.

Encapsula'tion. Act of surrounding with a capsule.

Encephalal'gia. Cephalalgia, *q. v.*

Encephalasthe'nia. Lack of brain power.

Encephal'ic. Of, or pertaining to, the brain.

Enceph'alin. A nitrogenous glucosid from the brain.

Encephali'tis (en-sef-al-i'tis). Inflammation of the brain.

Enceph'alocele (en-sef'al-o-sēl). Protrusion of the brain through the skull.

Enceph'aloid. 1. Like the brain. 2. Encephaloma. **E. cancer**, malignant tumor of brain-like consistence.

Encephalol'ogy. A description of the encephalon.

Encephalo'ma. Encephaloid sarcoma, or cancer.

Encephalomala'cia. Softening of the brain.

Encephalomeningi'tis. Inflammation of the brain and its meninges.

Encephalomenin'gocele. Protrusion of the membranes and brain-substance through the skull.

Encephalomyelop'athy. Any disease of the brain and spinal cord.

Enceph'alon. The brain; all the cranial contents.

Encephalop'athy. Any disorder of the brain.
Encephalorrha'gia. Cerebral hemorrhage.
Encephalospi'nal axis. Same as *Cerebrospinal axis.*
Encephalot'omy. Cutting up of fetal brain to promote delivery.
Enchondro'ma. Tumor of cartilage-tissue; chondroma.
Enchondrosarco'ma. Sarcoma containing cartilaginous tissue.
Enchyle'ma (en-ki-le'mah). Same as *Cytochylema.*
Enciente (on-se-ahnt'). With child; pregnant.
Encys'ted (en-sis'ted). Enclosed in a sac or cyst.
Endan'gium (en-dan'je-um). Membrane which lines blood-vessels.
Endarteri'tis. Inflammation of the arterial intima. **E. oblit'erans,** variety in which the lumen of the vessel becomes obliterated.
End-artery. One which does not make part of an anastomosis. **E.-bud, E.-bulb,** a form of ovoid ending of sensitive nerves in mucous membrane. **E.-organ,** any distal end-structure of a nerve-branch. **E.-plate,** discoid terminal expansion of motor nerve-branches.
Endem'ic. Occurring frequently in a certain district. **E. neuritis.** See *Beriberi.*
Endemo-epidem'ic. Endemic, but occasionally becoming epidemic.
Endermat'ic, Ender'mic. Performed, or administered, by the medium of the skin.
Endo-appendici'tis. Inflammation of mucous membrane of the appendix vermiformis.
Endo-arteri'tis. Same as *Endarteritis.*
Endo-ausculta'tion. Auscultation by means of an esophageal tube introduced into the stomach.
En'doblast. The cell-nucleus.
Endobronchi'tis. Inflammation of the lining membrane of the bronchia.
Endocar'diac, Endocar'dial. Pertaining to the interior of the heart.
Endocardi'tis (en-do-kar-di'tis). Inflammation of the lining membrane of the heart. **Malignant,** or **Ulcerative e.,** rapidly fatal form with high fever and great prostration.
Endocar'dium. Lining membrane of the heart.
Endocervici'tis (en-do-ser-vis-i'tis). Inflammation in the canal of the cervix uteri.
Endochon'dral. Developed within cartilage.
Endocho'rion. The inner chorion.
Endocolpi'tis. Inflammation of vaginal mucous membrane.
Endocrani'tis. Inflammation of endocranium; cranial duritis.
Endocra'nium. The cranial dura mater.
En'doderm (en'do-derm). The hypoblast or entoderm.
Endodonti'tis. Inflammation of the dentinal pulp.
Endo-enteri'tis. Inflammation of the intestinal mucosa.
Endogastri'tis. Inflammation of the gastric mucosa.
Endo'genous (en-doj'en-us). Originating within the organism.
Endoglob'ular. Within the blood-corpuscles.
Endolaryn'geal. In the larynx.
En'dolymph (en'do-limf). The fluid within the inner ear.
Endomastoidi'tis. Inflammation of interior of mastoid cavity and cells.
Endometri'tis. Inflammation of the endometrium. **Cervical e.** Same as *Endocervicitis.* **Fungous e.,** hypertrophy of the endometrium with bleeding granulations. **Septic e.,** a variety originating from septic poisoning. **Simple e.,** catarrhal inflammation of endometrium.
Endome'trium. The mucous membrane which lines the uterus.

Endomys'ium. Connective tissue between the fibers of a fasciculus of muscle.
Endoneu'rium (en-do-nu're-um). The connective tissue amongst the fibers of a fasciculus of a nerve.
Endopar'asite (en-do-par'as-it). Any internal parasite.
Endop'athy (en-dop'ath-e). Any endogenous disease.
Endopericardi'tis. Endocarditis blended with pericarditis.
Endoperimyocardi'tis. Inflammation of the endocardium, pericardium, and myocardium.
Endoperitoni'tis. Inflammation of serous lining of peritoneal cavity.
Endophlebi'tis. Inflammation of the intima of a vein.
En'doplast (en'do-plast). Nucleus of a cell.
En'doscope. Instrument for inspecting interior of a hollow organ.
Endos'copy (en-dos'ko-pe). The use of the endoscope.
Endosep'sis. Septicemia not of extraneous origin.
Endoskel'eton. Internal bony framework.
Endosmom'eter. Instrument for measurement of endosmosis.
Endos'mose, Endosmo'sis. Inward osmosis; inward passage of liquid through a diaphragm.
En'dospore. A spore formed by cell-formation.
Endostei'tis, Endosti'tis. Inflammation of the endosteum.
Endos'teum (en-dos'te-um). Lining membrane of a hollow bone.
Endosto'ma. A bony tumor within a bone.
Endosto'sis. The formation of an endostoma.
Endothe'lial. Pertaining to endothelium.
Endothelio-ino'ma. Fibrous tumor arising from endothelium.
Endothelio'ma. Any endothelial tumor.
Endotheliomyo'ma. Leiomyoma arising from endothelium.
Endotheliomyxo'ma. Myxoma arising from endothelium.
Endothe'lium (en-do-the'le-um). Membrane which lines a serous or other closed cavity.
En'ema (en'em-ah). A clyster or rectal injection.
Enepider'mic. Applied to, or injected into, the skin.
En'ergy (en'er-je). Force applicable to overcome resistance. **Kinetic e.**, energy in action. **Potential e.**, energy that may be put in action.
Enerva'tion (en-er-va'shun). Lack of nervous energy.
English sweating fever. See *Anglicus sudor*.
Engorge'ment (en-gorj'ment). Vascular congestion.
Enoma'nia. Periodic craving for strong drink; also, delirium tremens.
Enophthal'mus. Deep-seated state of the eyes.
Enosto'sis. Bony growth in the hollow of a bone.
En'siform. Shaped like a sword.
Ensister'num. The lowest piece of the sternum.
Ensom'phalus. A double monster with bodies in part united.
En'strophe (en'stro-fe). Inversion; a turning inward.
En'tad. Toward a center; inwardly.
En'tal. Inner; central.
Enta'sia (en-ta'se-ah). A constrictive spasm.
Enteral'gia (en-ter-al'je-ah). Pain in the intestine.
Enterec'tomy. Excision of a piece of intestine.
Enterepip'locele (en-ter-ep-ip'lo-sēl). Hernia of bowel and omentum.
Enter'ic. Of, or pertaining to, the intestine.
Enteri'tis. Inflammation of the intestine.
Entero-anasto'mosis. The joining together of two parts of an intestine.
Enterobro'sia. Intestinal perforation.
En'terocele (en'ter-o-sēl). Intestinal hernia.
Enterochirur'gia. Intestinal surgery.

Enterocholecystot'omy. Incision of the gall-bladder and intestine.
Enteroc'lysis (en-ter-ok'lis-is). The injection of nutrient liquids into the intestine.
En'teroclysm. An intestinal injection.
Enterocoli'tis. Inflammation of large and small intestines.
Enterocysto'ma. Cystic tumor of the intestine.
Enterodyn'ia. Pain in the intestine.
Entero-enteros'tomy. Formation of a passage between two parts of the intestine.
Entero-epip'locele. Hernia of intestine and omentum.
Enterogastri'tis. Combination of enteritis and gastritis.
Enterog'raphy. A description of the intestines.
Enterohy'drocele (en-ter-o-hi'dro-sēl). Hernia with hydrocele.
En'terol. Brownish liquid, a combination of various cresols, used as intestinal antiseptic.
En'terolite, En'terolith. Intestinal concretion or calculus.
Enterolithi'asis. The formation of enterolites.
Enterol'ogy. Sum of what is known about the intestines.
Enteromyco'sis. Bacterial disease of the intestine.
En'teron (en'ter-on). The intestine.
Enterop'athy (en-ter-op'ath-e). Any disease of the intestine.
En'teropexy (en'ter-o-pek-se). Surgical fixation of the intestine.
En'teroplasty (en'ter-o-plas-te). Plastic surgery of intestine.
En'teroplex. Device for joining edges of a divided intestine.
En'teroplexy. Union of parts of intestine by the enteroplex.
Enteropto'sis. Prolapse of the intestine.
Enterorrha'gia (en-ter-or-a'je-ah). Intestinal hemorrhage.
Enteror'rhaphy. The stitching of a rent in the intestine.
En'teroscope (en'ter-os-kōp). Instrument for inspecting the inside of the intestine.
Enterosep'sis. Sepsis developed from the intestinal contents.
En'terospasm (en'ter-o-spazm). Intestinal colic.
Enterosteno'sis. Narrowing or stricture of the intestine.
Enteros'tomy. Formation of artificial intestinal fistula.
En'terotome (en'ter-ot-ōm). Instrument for cutting intestine.
Enterot'omy. Surgical incision of the intestine.
Enterozo'on. Any internal animal parasite.
Entheoma'nia (en-the-o-ma'ne-ah). Religious insanity.
Enthet'ic (en-thet'ik). Brought in from outside.
En'toblast (en'to-blast). The entoderm or hypoblast.
En'tocele (en'to-sēl). Internal hernia.
Entochoroi'dea. The inner layer of the choroid.
Entocor'nea. Descemet's membrane.
En'tocyte (en'to-sīt). The cell-contents.
En'toderm. The hypoblast or entoblast.
Ento-ec'tad. From within outward.
En'tome. Cutting instrument for urethral stricture.
Ento'mion. Tip of mastoid angle of parietal bone.
En'tophyte (en'to-fīt). Any plant parasite within the body.
Entop'tic. Situated or originated within the eye.
Entoptos'copy. Inspection of the interior of the eye.
Entoret'ina. The nervous or inner layer of the retina.
Entos'thoblast. The nucleus of the nucleolus.
Entot'ic. Situated or generated within the ear.
Entozo'on (en-to-zo'on). Any internal animal parasite.
En'trails. Bowels or intestines.
Entro'pion, Entro'pium. Inversion or turning in, chiefly of an eyelid or of eyelashes.
Entro'pionize. To correct, as an ectropion, by turning in.
Enuclea'tion (e-nu-kle-a'shun). Removal from an envelop.

Enure'sis. Incontinence of urine. **E. noctur'na,** passage of urine in bed.

Envi'ronment. External surroundings or influences.

En'zyme (en'zīm). Any chemical ferment formed in the body.

Enzymo'sis. Fermentation induced by an enzyme.

E'osin (e'o-sin). A red coloring matter from coal-tar.

Eosin'ophile. Eosinoph'ilous. 1. Stainable by eosin. 2. A structure stainable by eosin.

Eosinophil'ia. Accumulation of unusual number of eosinophile cells.

E'osote. Valerianate of creosote, used like creosote.

Epac'tal. 1. Supernumerary. 2. Any Wormian bone.

Epenceph'alon. Embryonic structure whence arise the pons and cerebellum.

Epen'dyma. Membrane lining a cerebral ventricle.

Ependymi'tis. Inflammation of the ependyma.

Eph'edra (ef'e-drah). Genus of plants; said to be antiluetic.

Eph'edrin. Mydriatic alkaloid from *Ephedra vulgaris.*

Eph'elis (ef'e-lis). A freckle.

Ephem'eral. Temporary; lasting but a day.

Ephidro'sis. Profuse perspiration. **E. cruen'ta,** bloody sweat.

Ep'iblast. The outermost blastodermic layer or ectoderm: from it the nervous and epidermal tissues are derived.

Epiblas'tic (ep-e-blas'tik). Pertaining to the epiblast.

Epib'oly. Differentiation of epiblast from the hypoblast.

Epican'thus. A fold of skin projected over the inner canthus.

Epicar'dium. The innermost layer of the pericardium.

Ep'icele. The fourth ventricle of the brain.

Epico'me. Monster with double head joined at summit.

Epicon'dyle (ep-e-kon'dil). A bony eminence above a condyle.

Epicra'nens. The occipitofrontal muscle.

Epicra'nium. Structures collectively which cover the skull.

Epic'risis. A secondary or supplementary crisis.

Epicysti'tis. Inflammation above the bladder.

Epicystot'omy. Cystotomy by the suprapubic method.

Ep'icyte (ep'e-sit). The wall or envelop of a cell.

Epidem'ic. A disease which attacks many patients in the same region at the same time; used also adjectively.

Epidemiog'raphy. Literature of epidemic diseases.

Epidemiol'ogy. Sum of the knowledge of epidemic diseases.

Epider'mal. Epider'mic. Pertaining to the epidermis.

Epidermidiliza'tion. Development of epidermic cells (stratified epithelium) from mucous cells (columnar epithelium).

Epidermido'sis. Any epidermal disease.

Epider'min. A cerate used as a base for ointments.

Epider'mis. The cuticle, or outermost layer of the skin.

Epidermiza'tion (ep-e-der-miz-a'shun). Skin-grafting.

Epidermol'ysis (ep-e-der-mol'is-is). A loose state of the skin. **E. bullo'sa,** a variety with formation of deep-seated bullæ, which appear after irritation.

Epidid'ymis. An oblong organ attached to the testicle.

Epididymi'tis. Inflammation of the epididymis.

Epidu'ral space. Space external to the spinal dura.

Epigas'ter. Same as *Hind-gut.*

Epigastral'gia. Pain in epigastrium.

Epigas'tric. Of, or pertaining to, the epigastrium.

Epigas'trium. Abdominal surface in front of the stomach.

Epigas'trius. Double monster in which one twin is better developed than the other.

Epigas'trocele (ep-e-gas'tro-sēl). Epigastric hernia.

Epigen'esis. Generation by successive formations.

Epiglottid'ean. Pertaining to the epiglottis.

Epiglottidi'tis. Inflammation of the epiglottis.
Epiglot'tis. Cartilaginous lid of the larynx.
Epiglotti'tis (ep-e-glot-ti'tis). Same as *Epiglottiditis*.
Epig'nathus. Double monster in which the parasite is attached to the autosite's jaw.
Epihy'al. A bone replaced in man by the stylohyoid ligament.
Ep'ilating forceps. Nippers for pulling out hairs.
Epila'tion (ep-il-a'shun). Removal of hair; depilation.
Epil'atory. Removing hair, or an agent so doing.
Ep'ilepsy (ep'il-ep-se). Nervous disease marked by seizures with convulsions and loss of consciousness. **Cardiac e.,** e. with profound disturbance of heart's action, probably due to disease of the heart or of its nerves. **Cortical e., Focal e., Jacksonian e,** localized epileptiform spasm on one side without loss of consciousness. **Idiopathic e.,** true or typical epilepsy. **Nocturnal e.,** that in which the attack comes on during sleep. **Procursive e.,** that in which at the beginning of the attack the patient runs swiftly. **Reflex e.,** a form due to peripheral irritation. **Spinal e.,** clonic spasm of the legs in paraplegia. **Toxemic e.,** that due to a toxic influence.
Epilep'tic. 1. Of, or pertaining to, epilepsy. 2. A patient subject to epileptic attacks.
Epilep'tiform. Resembling epilepsy.
Epileptogen'ic, Epileptog'enous. Giving rise to epilepsy. **E. zone,** superficial area, stimulation of which provokes an epileptic seizure.
Epilep'toid. Resembling epilepsy; epileptiform.
Epimys'ium (ep-e-mis'e-um). The fibrous sheath of a muscle; also, the material of such a sheath.
Epinephri'tis. Inflammation of a suprarenal capsule.
Epineu'rium. The sheath of an entire nerve.
Epionych'ium. Same as *Eponichium*.
Epiot'ic center. The ossification-center of the mastoid part of the temporal bone.
Epipas'tic. Intended for sprinkling upon a part.
Epiphenom'enon. An exceptional and non-essential phenomenon.
Epiph'ora. Overflow of tears from obstruction of lacrimal duct.
Epiphys'eal (ep-e-fiz'e-al). Pertaining to an epiphysis.
Epiphyseol'ysis. Detachment of an epiphysis.
Epiph'ysis (ep-if'is-is). Portion of a bone which in early life is distinct from the shaft. **E. cer'ebri,** the pineal body.
Epiphysi'tis. Inflammation of the cartilage which joins infantile epiphysis to a shaft.
Ep'iphyte (ep'e-fit). An externally parasitic plant organism.
Epipi'al (ep-e-pi'al). Situated upon the pia mater.
Epip'locele (ep-ip'lo-sēl). Omental hernia.
Epiplo'ic. Pertaining to the epiploön. **E. appendages.** Same as *Appendices epiploicæ*.
Epiploi'tis (ep ip-lo-i'tis). Inflammation of the epiploön.
Epip'loön (ep-ip'lo-on). The great or gastrocolic omentum.
Epipy'gus. Same as *Pygomelus*.
Episcle'ral. Situated over the sclera of the eye.
Episcleri'tis. Inflammation of the outer layers of the sclera.
Episior'rhaphy. The suturing of a lacerated perineum.
Episiosteno'sis. A contraction of the vulvar slit.
Episiot'omy. Surgical incision of the perineum.
Epispa'dias. Opening of urethra on dorsum of the penis.
Epispas'tic (ep-e-spas'tik). Vesicant; blistering.
Episplení'tis. Inflammation of the capsule of the spleen.
Epistax'is. Nose-bleed; hemorrhage from the nose.
Epister'nal. Situated upon the sternum.

Epister'num. The manubrium or upper piece of the sternum.
Epite'la. The thin tissue of Vieussens's valve.
Epithe'lia. Cells of the epithelium.
Epithe'lial. Pertaining to epithelium. **E. cancer.** Same as *Epithelioma*.
Epithe'lioid. Resembling or like epithelium.
Epithelio'ma. Cancer composed largely of epithelial cells.
Epithe'lium. Cellular substance of the skin and mucous membrane. **Ciliated e.,** that which is provided with cilia. **Columnar e.,** that which is made up of pillar-shaped cells. **Glandular e.,** that whose cells take part in a secretory process. **Neuro-e.,** specialized epithelium in which the nerves of special sense end. **Pavement e.,** a variety composed of flattened cells. **Pigmented e.,** that whose cells contain melanin or other pigment. **Rod e.,** peculiarly striated e. of certain glands. **Squamous e.** is made up of flattened plate-like cells. **Stratified e.,** that in which the cells are disposed in more than one layer. **Transitional e.,** that which is partly stratified.
Epitrich'ium (ep-e-trik'e-um). Superficial layer of the epidermis of the fetus and embryo.
Epitroch'lea. Inner condyle of the humerus.
Epizo'ön. An externally parasitic animal organism.
Epizoöt'ic. A disease occurring epidemically among animals; used also adjectively.
Eponych'ium (ep-o-nik'e-um). The horny embryonic membrane whence the nail is developed.
Eponym'ic. Named from some person.
Epoöphorec'tomy. Surgical removal of the parovarium.
Epoöph'oron (ep-o-of'o-ron). The parovarium.
Ep'som salts. Magnesium sulphate.
Epu'lis (ep-u'lis). A fibrous tumor of the gum. **Malignant e.,** giant-celled sarcoma of jaw.
Equa'tor of a cell. The plane at which a cell is divided. **E. of the eye,** the circle or plane which divides the eye into anterior and posterior halves.
Equato'rial plate. In karyokinesis, the equator of the nuclear spindle.
Equil'ibrating operation. Tenotomy of the muscle which antagonizes a paralyzed muscle of the eye.
Equilib'rium. A state of balance or equipoise.
Equina'tion. Inoculation with horse-pox virus.
Equin'ia (e-kwin'e-ah). L. for *Glanders*.
Equinova'rus. A blending of pes equinus with pes varus.
Equiv'alence (e-kwiv'al-ens). Quality of being equivalent.
Equiv'alent (e-kwiv'al-ent). 1. Of equal force, power, or value. 2. The unvarying quantity of one body which is requisite to replace a fixed weight of another body.
Er., E. R. Abbreviation for *external resistance*.
Era'sion (e-ra'zhun). Removal by abrasion or scraping.
Er'bium. A rare metallic element; symbol Er.
Erb's paralysis. Paralysis due to cerebral hemorrhage at birth. **E.'s point,** the supraclavicular point.
Erec'tile tissue. Tissue that may be erected or made turgescent. **E. tumor,** tumor composed of erectile tissue.
Erec'tion (e-rek'shun). State of being upright and turgid.
Erec'tor muscles. See *Muscles, Table of*.
Erecto'res pi'li. See *Arrectores pilorum*.
Eremacau'sis. Slow oxidation and decay of organic matter.
Er'ethin (er'eth-in). Poisonous principle of tuberculin.
Er'ethism (er'eth-izm). Morbid excitability.
Erethis'tic. Characterized by erethism.
Erg. The unit of work.

Er'gograph (er'go-graf). Instrument for measuring work done in muscular action.

Er'got. A fungus growing on rye: hemostatic and ecbolic.

Er'gotin. 1. Commercial precipitate from ergot. 2. An alkaloid from ergot. **Bonjeau's e.,** a purified extract of ergot.

Ergot'inin. Alkaloid from ergot.

Er'gotism (er'go-tizm). Chronic ergot-poisoning.

Er'gotized (er'go-tīzd). Diseased by the ergot-fungus.

Erig'eron (e-rij'er-on). Genus of plants, fleabanes: diuretic and refrigerant.

Eriodic'tyon Califor'nica. Yerba santa: useful in bronchitis.

Ero'dent. A caustic drug.

Ero'sion. Disintegration of structure; an eating away.

Ero'sive (e-ro'siv). Producing erosion.

Erot'ic (e-rot'ik). Pertaining to sexual appetite.

Er'otism (er'o-tizm). Sexual instinct.

Erotoma'nia. Insanity with intense sexual excitement.

Erotopath'ia. Perverted sexual instinct.

Errat'ic. Roving; wandering; also odd and eccentric.

Er'rhine (er'in). Causing sneezing and secretion from the nose.

Eructa'tion. Belching of wind from the stomach.

Erup'tion (e-rup'shun). A rash or discoloration of the skin.

Erup'tive. Attended with a breaking out or rash.

Erysip'elas. A febrile disease characterized by inflammation and redness of skin, mucous membranes, etc. **Ambulant e., Wandering e.,** erysipelatous process which repeatedly disappears to reappear at another point. **Facial e.,** variety which is mainly seated on the face. **Idiopathic e.,** that which does not follow a wound or injury. **Phlegmonous e.,** erysipelas in which pus is formed. **Surgical e., Traumatic e.,** that which invades wounds.

Erysipel'atous. Of the nature of erysipelas.

Erysip'eloid. A disease which simulates erysipelas.

Erythe'ma (er-ith-e'mah). Redness of skin or rose rash; of many varieties. **E. annula're,** a form of e. with rounded lesions, each with a raised margin. **E. congesti'vum,** simple e. with congestion of the skin. **E. multifor'me,** an acute variety with variously formed papules, tubercles, and macules. **E. nodo'sum,** inflammatory form marked by tender red nodules. **Symptomatic e.,** skin hyperemia in non-elevated patches: it may be idiopathic or truly symptomatic. **E. venena'tum,** that which is due to a poison.

Erythemat'ic, Erythem'atous. Of the nature of erythema.

Erythemomegalal'gia. See *Erythmomelalgia.*

Erythras'ma. Skin-disease marked by patches in groin or axilla.

Er'ythrite (er'ith-rit). A crystalline alcohol from various algæ and lichens.

Eryth'roblast. The rudimentary red blood-corpuscle.

Erythrochloro'pia. Color-blindness in which red and green only are recognized.

Eryth'rocyte (er-ith'ro-sit). A red blood-corpuscle.

Erythrocytom'eter. A device for counting red blood-corpuscles.

Erythrodex'trin. A dextrin stained red by iodin.

Erythrogran'ulose. A form of granulose stained red by iodin.

Er'ythrol (er'ith-rol). Same as *Erythrite.*

Erythromelal'gia. Neuritis marked by burning pain and redness of one or more of the extremities.

Eryth'rophage (er-ith'ro-fāj). A phagocyte which absorbs blood-pigments and destroys red corpuscles.

Eryth'rophile, Erythroph'ilous. Easily staining red.

Erythrophle'in. A poisonous alkaloid from casca bark.

Erythrophle'um guineen'se. An African tree, affords casca bark: poisonous cardiant.
Erythrop'ia, Erythrop'sia. State in which objects appear to have a red tinge.
Erythrop'sin. Same as *Visual purple.*
Erythrox'ylin. Cocain; also, a proprietary precipitate from coca.
Erythrox'ylon co'ca. South American plant which affords coca leaves.
Es'char (es'kar). Slough produced by burning or by a caustic.
Escharot'ic (es-kar-ot'ik). Producing a slough; caustic.
Eschrola'lia, Æschrola'lia. Same as *Coprolalia.*
Es'culin. Glucosid from horse-chestnut bark.
Eser'idin. An alkaloid of Calabar bean.
Es'erin. Same as *Physostigmin.*
Es'march, Es'march's bandage (es'mark). Caoutchouc bandage for use in bloodless surgery.
Esod'ic (es-od'ik). Centripetal or afferent.
Eso-ethmoidi'tis. Inflammation of the ethmoid sinuses.
Esogastri'tis. Inflammation of the gastric mucosa.
Esopha'geal (e-sof-a'je-al). Pertaining to the esophagus.
Esophagis'mus (e-sof-aj-is'mus). Spasm of the esophagus.
Esophagi'tis (e-sof-aj-i'tis). Inflammation of the esophagus.
Esophag'ocele (e-sof-ag'o-sēl). Esophageal hernia.
Esophagomyco'sis. Microbic disease of the esophagus.
Esophag'oscope. Speculum for seeing inside of esophagus.
Esoph'agospasm. Spasm of the esophagus.
Esophagosteno'sis. Stricture of the esophagus.
Esophagos'tomy. Creation of an artificial fistula of the esophagus.
Esophag'otome (e-sof-ag'ot-ōm). Cutting instrument used in esophagotomy.
Esophagot'omy. Surgical incision of the esophagus.
Esoph'agus (e-sof'ag-us). Part of alimentary canal between pharynx and stomach.
Esopho'ria (es-o-fo're-ah). Inward tending of the visual lines.
Esosphenoidi'tis. Osteomyelitis of the sphenoid.
Esoter'ic (es-o-ter'ik). Arising within the organism.
Esothy'ropexy. Treatment of goiter by drawing out the thyroid gland and fixing it.
Esotro'pia. Convergent strabismus, or cross-eye.
Es'sence. 1. The distinctive or individual principle of anything. 2. Mixture of alcohol with a volatile oil.
Essen'tial. Pertaining to, or of the nature of, an essence. **E. oil,** any volatile oil of vegetable origin; an attar. **E. resistance,** resistance to conductivity within an electric battery.
Es'ter. Any compound ether which has an acid and an alcohol radical.
Esthe'sioblast. A ganglioblast; embryonic cell of a spinal ganglion.
Esthesioma'nia. Insanity with perverted moral sense.
Esthesiom'ene (es-the-ze-om'en-e). Tubercular ulceration of vulva.
Esthesiom'eter. An instrument for measuring tactile sensibility.
Esthesioneuro'sis. Any disease of the sensory nerves.
Esthesiophysiol'ogy. Physiology of the perceptive faculties.
Esthesod'ic. Conveying sense impressions.
Esthiome'nus. Malignant disease of the skin.
Est'lander's operation. Resection of ribs in empyema.
Es'trual. Pertaining to the rutting of animals.
Estrua'tion. Sexual ardor of animals at season of copulation.
Es'trum, Œs'trum (es'trum). Crisis of venereal excitement.

Etat mamelloné (a-taht' mah-ma-yo-na'). Condition of stomach with small elevations of the mucous membrane.

Eth'ene chlorid. Same as *Ethylidene chlorid.*

E'ther. 1. The subtle fluid believed to fill all space. 2. Ethyl oxid, $(C_2H_5)_2O$, volatile liquid used as an anesthetic, stimulant, anodyne, and solvent. **Acetic e.,** colorless liquid, ethyl acetate: anesthetic, stimulant, and irritant. **Chloric e.,** strong solution of chloroform in alcohol. **E.-coat,** a device used in anesthetization by ether. **E.-drunkenness,** intoxication from drinking ether.

Ethe'real (e-the're-al). Pertaining to ether. **E. oil,** any volatile oil.

E'therism. More or less complete anesthesia produced by ether.

Etheriza'tion. Induction of anesthesia by means of ether.

E'therize. To anesthetize by inhalation of ether.

Etheroma'nia. Habitual use of ether as an intoxicant.

Ethiopifica'tion. Blackening of skin by silver or other metallic medicine.

Ethmoceph'alus. A monster with defective nose, and eye-orbits partly fused.

Eth'moid. Sieve-like; cribriform; also, the ethmoid bone. **E. bone,** a cribriform bone of the nose and base of skull.

Ethmoi'dal. Pertaining to the ethmoid bone.

Ethmoidi'tis. Inflammation of the ethmoid bone.

Ethnog'raphy. The science of the human race.

Ethnol'ogy. The science of races of mankind.

Ethnyphi'tis (eth-ne-fi'tis). Cellulitis.

Ethoxycaf'fein. A crystalline, diuretic, and narcotic derivative, $C_{10}H_{14}N_4O_3$, from caffein.

Eth'yl (eth'il). The radical, C_2H_5. **E. acetate.** See *Acetic ether.* **E. alcohol,** ordinary alcohol. **E. bromid,** an anesthetic, C_2H_5B. **E. chlorid,** a local anesthetic, C_2H_5Cl. **E. formate,** an antispasmodic and anesthetic liquid. **E. hydrate,** ordinary alcohol, C_2H_5OH. **E. iodid,** a liquid, C_2H_5I, used by inhalation.

Ethylam'in. Ptomain, $C_2H_5NH_2$, from decaying plant-tissue.

Ethylchloralu'rethan. Same as *Somnal.*

Eth'ylen bichlorid. An oily substance, C_2H_4Cl: anesthetic. **E. bromid,** an oily substance, $C_2H_4Br_2$: useful in epilepsy.

Ethylendiam'in. Ptomain, $C_2H_8N_2$: not poisonous.

Ethyl'iden chlorid. An anesthetic, CH_3CHCl_2. **E. diam'in,** harmful ptomain, $C_2H_8N_2$, from fish.

Ethylphenylurethane. Same as *Euphorin.*

Ethylthal'lin. An antipyretic, $C_{12}H_{17}NO$.

Etiolog'ical (e-te-o-loj'ik-al). Pertaining to etiology.

Etiol'ogy (e-te-ol'oj-e). Scientific view of causes of disease.

Euca'in (u-ka'in). Artificial alkaloid believed to be a valuable local anesthetic.

Eucalyp'teol. A white compound used as intestinal antiseptic and in pulmonary diseases.

Eucalyp'tol. Fragrant colorless liquid from oil of eucalyptus: antiseptic, expectorant, etc.

Eucalyptoresor'cin. Antiseptic combination of eucalyptol and resorcin.

Eucalyp'tus glob'ulus. Tree which affords eucalyptol and oil of eucalyptus.

Euca'sin. A proprietary diuretic casein-ammonia compound.

Euchin'in. Product of action of ethylchlorocarbonate on quinin, having properties like quinin without its disagreeable symptoms.

Euchlorhyd'ria. Normal amount of acid in the gastric juice.

Euchlo'rin. Chlorin protoxid; antiseptic in its solution.

Eudiom'eter. An instrument for analyzing air.

Eudox'in (u-dox'in). A red antiseptic powder.

Eu'genol (u'jen-ol). Derivative, $C_{10}H_{12}O_2$, from clove oil: antiseptic and local anesthetic.
Eulyp'tol (u-lip'tol). A proprietary antiseptic.
Eu'nuch (u'nuk). A male deprived of testicles.
Euon'ymin. A cholagogue aperient from euonymus.
Euon'ymus atropurpu'reus. A shrub, wahoo: cholagogue and purgative.
Eupato'rin. A diaphoretic and tonic substance from *Eupatorium perfoliatum.*
Eupato'rium perfolia'tum. Boneset: a tonic and diaphoretic herb.
Euphor'bia (u-for'be-ah). A large genus of plants; generally acrid poisons.
Euphor'bium (u-for'be-um). Gum-resin of *Euphorbia officinarum,* etc.: purgative and vesicant.
Eupho'ria (u-fo're-ah). Sound health; physical well-being.
Eu'phorin (u'fo-rin). White powder, $C_9H_{11}O_2$: antipyretic, analgesic, antiseptic.
Euplas'tic. Forming sound and healthy tissues.
Eupnœ'a (u-pne'ah). Easy or normal respiration.
Eu'rophen (u'ro-fen). A yellow powder used like iodoform.
Euro'tium malig'num. A mould occasionally found in ear.
Eu'ryon (u're-on). Either end of bilateral diameter of head.
Eu'rythrol. Thick, honey-like extract of the spleen: used for chlorosis and malaria.
Eusta'chian catheter. Instrument for dilating Eustachian tube. **E. tube,** canal leading from the tympanum to the pharynx. **E. valve,** fold of membrane in the right auricle.
Euthana'sia (u-than-a'ze-ah). An easy death.
Euto'cia (u-to'she-ah). Natural or normal parturition.
Evac'uant (e-vak'u-ant). Purgative or cathartic.
Evacua'tion (e-vak-u-a'shun). Discharge from the bowels.
Evac'uator. Instrument for washing out the bladder.
Evapora'tion. Assumption of the form of a vapor.
Eventra'tion. Protrusion of the bowels from the abdomen.
Ever'sion (e-ver'shun). A turning out, or inside out; ectropion.
Eviscera'tion. Removal of the viscera, or of inner parts. **E. of eye** or **of orbit,** removal of the eye-contents, the sclera being left in its place.
Evolu'tion. Development with increase of complexity and of specialization. **Spontaneous e.,** unaided birth of a transverse fetal presentation.
Evul'sion (e-vul'shun). Forcible tearing away of a part.
Ex. L. for *out, away from.*
Exacerba'tion. Paroxysmal increase in severity.
Exal'gin. Methyl acetanilid, $C_9H_{11}NO$: antipyretic and analgesic.
Exan'them, Exan'thema. An eruption or rash on the skin.
Exanthem'ata. Eruptive diseases or fevers.
Exanthem'atous. Characterized by an eruption or rash.
Ex'anthropes (eks'an-thrōps). Sources of disease originating outside the body.
Exarteri'tis. Inflammation of the outer arterial coat.
Exarticula'tion. Amputation at a joint.
Excava'tion. A hollow, depression, or basin. **E. of optic nerve,** cupping or hollow of the optic disk.
Excen'tric (eks-sen'trik). Out of, or away from, a center.
Excerebra'tion. Removal of the brain.
Excip'ient. An inert substance added to a medicine to give it the proper form; a vehicle.
Excis'ion (eks-sizh'un). A cutting out or off.
Excitabil'ity. Susceptibility of being stimulated.
Exci'table area. The motor area of the cerebral cortex.

Exci'tant. A medicine which arouses functional activity.

Excita'tion. Act of stimulation or irritation. **Direct e.,** stimulation of a muscle by means of an electrode on the muscle-substance. **Indirect e.,** stimulation of a muscle by means of its nerve.

Exci'ting cause. The immediate or direct cause of an attack of disease.

Excitomo'tor. Arousing muscular activity.

Ex'clave (eks'klāv). Detached part, as of the ovary or pancreas.

Exclu'sion, diagnosis by. See *Diagnosis.*

Excochlea'tion (ex-kok-le-a'shun). Operation of curetting a cavity.

Excoria'tion. Removal of a piece, or pieces, of the skin.

Ex'crement (eks'kre-ment). Any excreted or fecal matter.

Excrementit'ious. Pertaining to excrement.

Excres'cence (eks-kres'ens). Any abnormal outgrowth.

Excre'ta. Excretions or excremental matters.

Excrete' (eks-krēt'). To separate and expel useless matter.

Ex'cretin. A principle, $C_{20}H_{36}O$, in human feces.

Excre'tion. Matter excreted; also, the process of excreting.

Excretol'ic acid. Fatty acid derivable from feces.

Ex'cretory. Pertaining to excretion.

Excur'sion. Wandering of eyes from midposition.

Excurva'tion. Humpback or kyphosis.

Exenceph'alus. Monster with brain outside, or partly outside, the cranium.

Exentera'tion. Evisceration in either sense.

Ex'ercise bone. Bony growth in muscle due to exercise or pressure.

Exfeta'tion (eks-fe-ta'shun). Extra-uterine pregnancy.

Exfolia'tion. Separation of pieces of dead bone or of skin in form of scales.

Exhala'tion. Escape in form of vapor; also the vapor itself.

Exhaus'tion. Loss of vital power.

Exhib'it. To administer as a remedy.

Exhibit'ionism. Insane exposure of the genital organs.

Exhil'arant. A medicine which cheers the mind.

Exhuma'tion. The digging up of a buried body.

Ex'ner's plexus. A mesh of medullated fibers in the cerebral cortex.

Exocar'dial. Pertaining to, or situated on, outside of heart.

Exocoli'tis. Inflammation of outer coat of the colon.

Exod'ic (ek-sod'ik). Centrifugal or efferent.

Ex'odyne (ek'so-dīn). An antipyretic and anodyne mixture.

Exogen'ic, Exog'enous. Derived from without the body.

Exom'phalos. Undue prominence of the navel.

Exopath'ic. Originating outside the body.

Exopho'ria. Tendency of eyes to turn outward.

Exophthal'mia. Same as *Exophthalmos.*

Exophthal'mic goiter. Disease characterized by protrusion of the eyes, anemia, and enlarged thyroid.

Exophthal'mos. Abnormal protrusion of the eye.

Exor'bitism. Protrusion of the eyeball.

Exor'mia (ex-or'me-ah). A papular skin-eruption.

Exosep'sis. Septic poison originating outside the body.

Exoskel'eton. The dermoskeleton.

Exosmo'sis. Osmosis or diffusion from within outward.

Exosto'sis. Abnormal bony outgrowth from the surface of a bone.

Exoter'ic. Developed or generated without the organism.

Exothy'reopexy, Exothy'ropexy. Surgical exposure of the thyroid and fixation of the gland outside.

Exotro'pia. Divergent strabismus; wall-eye.

Expan'sion (eks-pan'shun). Increase of volume or bulk.

Expec'tant. Waiting; watching. **E. treatment,** treatment which leaves the cure to nature, attempting only the relief of untoward symptoms.

Expecta'tion of life. Probable future duration of any life.

Expec'torant. A medicine that aids expectoration; used also adjectively.

Expectora'tion. The coughing up of sputum from the air-passages; also, matter expectorated. **Prune-juice e.,** sputum stained with blood and blood-pigments in various severe and grave diseases of the lungs. **Rusty e.,** blood-stained sputum of lobar pneumonia.

Expira'tion. Expulsion of air in breathing.

Ex'piratory. Pertaining to expiration.

Explora'tion. An act of investigation or search; a probing.

Explo'ratory. Subserving an exploration.

Explor'ing needle. A needle used in exploratory puncture.

Explo'sive speech. Sudden and forcible utterance.

Expres'sion. 1. The act of squeezing out. 2. Manifestation of subjective feeling by facial lineaments.

Expul'sive. Tending to expel or extrude.

Exsan'guinate. To deprive of blood.

Exsanguina'tion. Forcible expulsion of blood from a part.

Exsan'guine. Very pale; of bloodless aspect.

Exsec'tion. An excision or cutting out.

Exsicca'tion. A thorough drying by heat.

Exsic'cative. Causing dryness; also, a drying application.

Ex'strophy. The turning inside out of an organ, as the bladder.

Extempora'neous. Prepared and dispensed, or taken, at once.

Exten'sion. 1. The straightening of a flexed limb. 2. Traction on a fractured or dislocated limb. **Buck's e.,** extension of fractured leg by weights, the foot of the bed being raised so that the body makes counterextension.

Exten'sor. Any muscle which antagonizes a flexor.

Exte'rior. 1. Pertaining to the outside; outer. 2. The outside.

Exter'nal. Pertaining to the outside.

Extirpa'tion. Complete removal, or eradication.

Extra-artic'ular. Situated outside a joint.

Extracap'sular. Outside a capsule or capsular ligament.

Ex'tract. A preparation made by treating a drug with a solvent and evaporating the solution. **Alcoholic e.,** one prepared by the use of alcohol as a solvent. **Aqueous e.,** one prepared by the use of water as a solvent. **Aromatic fluid e.,** fluid extract from aromatic powder. **Compound e.,** one which is prepared from more than one drug. **Ethereal e.,** one for which ether is the menstruum. **Fluid e.,** a solution of the medicinal principles of a vegetable drug. **Powdered e.,** a dried and pulverized extract. **Soft e.,** one which is of pilular consistence. **Solid e.,** one prepared by evaporating a solution of the active part of a drug.

Extrac'tion. Act of pulling out; process of making an extract.

Extrac'tive. A substance separated by a process of extraction.

Extrac'tor. An instrument for extracting bullets, etc.

Extrac'tum. L. for *Extract.*

Extradu'ral. Situated outside the dura mater.

Extramedul'lary. Situated outside the medulla oblongata.

Extra'neous (eks-tra'ne-us). Not proper to the organism.

Extranu'clear. Situated outside a nucleus.

Extrapo'lar. Outside or beyond the poles.

Extra-u'terine pregnancy. See *Pregnancy.*

Extravasa'tion. The escape or effusion of any fluid from its proper vessel into the tissues.

Extravas'cular. Situated or occurring outside a vessel.
Extrem'ital. Pertaining to, or situated at, an extremity.
Extrin'sic. From without; of exterior origin. **E. muscles,** those on the outside of an organ.
Extrover'sion. Same as *Exstrophy.*
Extuba'tion. The removal of a laryngeal tube.
Ex'udate (eks'u-dāt). Substance that has oozed into the tissues.
Exuda'tion. Filtration of serum into the tissue; also, the resulting exudate.
Ex'udative. Of the nature of exudation.
Exumbilica'tion. Marked protrusion of navel.
Exu'viæ (eks-u'vc-e). Cast-off epidermis; slough.
Eye (ī). The organ of vision. **E.-ball,** the ball or globe of the eye. **E.-brow,** hairy ridge above the eye; supercilium. **E.-glass,** a lens for aiding the sight. **E.-ground,** the fundus of the eye. **E.-lashes,** hairy fringe of an eyelid; cilia. **E.-lids,** pair of folds which protect the eye. **E.-piece,** the lens of a microscope next the eye; the ocular. **E.-speculum,** an instrument for holding the eye open. **E.-strain,** weariness of the eye from overuse, or from uncorrected defect of form in the eye. **E.-teeth,** the canine teeth of the upper jaw.

F.

F. Abbreviation of *Fahrenheit* and *Fluorin.*
Fabel'la. A sesamoid fibrocartilage in the gastrocnemius.
Face. The anterior aspect of the head. **F. presentation,** presentation of the child's face in labor.
Fac'et (fas'et). A small nearly plane area on a bone or other hard surface.
Fa'cial (fa'shal). Pertaining to the face. **F. angle.** See *Angle.* **F. center,** center in frontal convolutions for face-movements. **F. hemiplegia.** See under *Hemiplegia.* **F. nerve.** See *Nerves, Table of.*
Facies (fa'she-ēz). 1. L. for *Face.* 2. Facial expression. **F. Hippocrat'ica,** facial appearance indicating impending death. **F. leoni'na.** Same as *Leontiasis.* **F. ovari'na,** anxious look indicative of ovarian disease.
Faciolin'gual. Affecting the face and the tongue.
Fac'ultative. Capable of assuming a part.
Fac'ulty. A normal power or function, especially a mental one.
Fæcal, Fæces. See *Fecal, Feces,* etc.
Fa'gin (fa'jin). Narcotic principle from husks of beech-nuts.
Fah'renheit's thermometer (fah'ren-hītz). One with the boiling point of water at 212°, melting point of ice at 32°.
Faint. Same as *Syncope.*
Fal'ciform. Shaped like a sickle. **F. ligament,** the broad ligament of the liver. **F. process.** 1. Process of fascia lata around saphenous opening. 2. Same as *Falx cerebri.*
Fall'ing sickness. Same as *Epilepsy.* **F. of the womb,** prolapse of the uterus; procidentia uteri.
Fallo'pian canal. The aqueduct of Fallopius. **F. ligament,** the round ligament of the womb. **F. tubes,** the oviducts.
False. (For phrases see the nouns.)
Falx. The sickle-shaped fold of the dura between the cerebral hemispheres (**F. cer'ebri**) and the cerebellar hemispheres (**F. cerebel'li**).
Famil'ial. Affecting different members of a family.
Fam'ine fever. See *Fever.*
Fang. The root of a tooth.
Far'ad. The unit of electric capacity; capacity to hold one coulomb with a potential of one volt.

Farada'ic or **Farad'ic electricity.** Induced electricity.

Far'adism. 1. Faradization. 2. Faradic electricity.

Faradiza'tion. Therapeutic use of induced currents.

Farcino'ma (far-sin-o'mah). A glanderous tumor.

Farcy. A form of glanders affecting especially the skin and lymphatics. **F.-bud,** a farcinoma.

Fari'na (far-i'nah). Meal or flour; also, a form of maize starch.

Farina'ceous (far-in-a'shus). Prepared from flour; also, starchy.

Far-point. The remotest point at which an object is clearly seen when the eye is at rest.

Farre's tubercles (farz). Nodules on the surface of a carcinomatous liver.

Far-sight'ed. Same as *Hypermetropic.*

Fascia (fash'e-ah). A band or sheet of tissue investing and connecting muscles. **Anal f.,** the ischiorectal fascia. **Buck's f.,** continuation of Colles's fascia upon the penis. **Cervical f., deep,** one which invests the muscles, vessels, and nerves of the neck. **Cervical f., superficial,** a thin lamina external to the platysma myoides. **Cloquet's f.,** areolar tissue closing femoral ring. **Colles's f.,** deep layer of the superficial perineal fascia. **Cremasteric f.,** the cremaster muscle. **Cribriform f.,** that part of the superficial fascia of the thigh which covers the saphenous opening. **F. denta'ta,** a serrated band under the hippocampus minor. **Infundibuliform f.,** a process of the transversalis fascia over the spermatic cord. **Intercolumnar f.,** the pouch which covers the spermatic cord and testis. **Ischiorectal f.,** that which covers the perineal side of the levator ani. **F. la'ta,** wide dense sheath of the thigh muscles. **Transversalis f.,** that fascia which lies between the transversalis muscle and the peritoneum.

Fas'cial (fash'e-al). Pertaining to a fascia.

Fascic'ulus (fas-ik'u-lus). A bundle or cluster. **Cuneate f.,** a continuation of the dorsolateral column of spinal cord into the oblongata. **Fundamental f.,** a part of the anterior column extending into the oblongata. **F. gra'cilis,** a continuation into the oblongata of the dorsomedian column of the spinal cord. **Olivary f.,** a fillet beneath the olivary body. **Posterolongitudinal f.,** fibers which extend from the nuclei of the fourth and sixth nerves to the corpora quadrigemina. **Pyramidal f., direct. F. of Türck,** a part of the anterior column of the cord extending to the pyramid. **F. of Rolando,** the enlarged head of the posterior cornu of gray matter in the oblongata. **Solitary f.,** f. which connects the internal capsule and lenticular nucleus with parts beneath. **F. subcallo'sus,** a tract of long fibers beneath the callosum. **F. te'res.** Same as *Funiculus teres.* **F. uncifor'mis,** the fibers which connect the frontal and temporosphenoid lobes.

Fasciot'omy. Surgical incision or division of a fascia.

Fasci'tis (fas-i'tis). Inflammation of a fascia.

Fastig'ium (fas-tij'e-um). The acme; the highest point.

Fat. The oily material that covers the connective tissue of an animal. **F.-columns,** columns of adipose tissue extending from subcutaneous tissue to the hair-follicles and sweat-glands.

Fatigue' disease, F. fever. Febrile attack due to over-exertion. **F. stuff,** toxic material due to tissue-disintegration after excessive fatigue.

Fat'ty series. Methane and its derivatives and homologous hydrocarbons.

Fau'ces (faw'sēz). The passage between throat and pharynx.

Fau'cial (faw'she-al). Pertaining to the fauces.

Fa'vus. Skin-disease with honeycomb crusts due to a fungus.

Fe. A symbol of iron.

Febric'ula (fe-brik'u-lah). A slight or insignificant fever.
Febrifa'cient (feb-rif-a'shent). Producing fever.
Febrif'ugal (feb-rif'u-gal). Good against fever.
Feb'rifuge (feb'rif-ûj). A remedy that dispels fever.
Feb'rile (feb'ril). Pertaining to fever; feverish.
Feb'rinol. A proprietary antipyretic and analgesic.
Fe'bris (fe'bris). L. for *Fever*. **F. enter'ica,** typhoid fever.
Fe'cal. Pertaining to, or of the nature of, feces.
Fec'aloid (fek'al-oid). Resembling fecal matter.
Fe'ces (fe'sēz). Excrement discharged from the bowels.
Fech'ner's law (fek'nerz). The sensation produced by a given stimulus varies as the logarithm of the stimulus.
Fec'ula. 1. Lees or sediment. 2. Starch.
Fec'ulent (fek'u-lent). Having sediment.
Fecunda'tion. Fertilization; impregnation. **Artificial f.,** fecundation by mechanical injection of semen into uterus.
Fecun'dity (fe-kun'dit-e). Fruitfulness.
Feh'ling's solution (fā'lingz). Aqueous solution of cupric sulphate with potassio-sodic tartrate and a potassic hydrate solution for testing for sugar in urine.
Fel bo'vis. The bile of the ox; ox-gall.
Fel'lic acid. A constituent of bile, $C_{23}H_{40}O_4$.
Fel'on. Same as *Paronychia*.
Fe'male. Pertaining to a woman. **F. blade,** the blade of a forceps which has a slot. **F. catheter.** See *Catheter*.
Fem'oral (fem'o-ral). Pertaining to the thigh.
Fem'orocele. Femoral hernia.
Femorotib'ial. Pertaining to the femur and tibia.
Fe'mur. The thigh bone; also the thigh itself.
Fenes'tra ova'lis. An oval opening in the inner wall of the middle ear. **F. rotun'da,** round opening in the inner wall of the middle ear.
Fen'estrated. Pierced with one or more openings. **F. membrane,** the thickest and outermost layer of the arterial intima.
Fenestra'tion. The act of perforating; condition of being pierced with openings.
Fen'nel. The plant *Fœniculum vulgare:* its seeds and oil are stimulant and carminative.
Fen'ugreek. The plant *Trigonella fœnum-græcum:* the seed is demulcent.
Fer'ment. A substance which causes fermentation in other substances with which it comes in contact. **Organized f.,** a living plant or animal ferment, as a microbe. **Unorganized f.,** a chemical ferment.
Fermenta'tion. Physical or chemical change induced by a ferment. **Acetic f.,** the conversion of weak alcoholic solutions into acetic acid or vinegar. **Alcoholic f.,** the formation of ethylic alcohol from carbohydrates. **Ammoniacal f.,** formation of ammonia and carbon dioxid from urea. **Butyric f.,** change of carbohydrates, milk, etc., into butyric acid. **Caseous f.,** the coagulation of soluble casein under the influence of rennet ferment. **Diastatic f.,** the change of starch into glucose, under the influence of ptyalin, the glycolytic ferment of the liver, etc. **Lactic f.,** the souring of milk, due to various bacilli. **F.-test,** test for glucose in the urine made with yeast. **Viscous f.,** production of gummy substances, as in wine, milk, or urine, under the influence of various bacilli.
Fermente'mia. The presence of a ferment in the blood.
Fermen'tum (fer-men'tum). L. for *Yeast*.
Fern, female. See *Asplenium*. **Male f.** See *Aspidium*.
Ferra'lia. Medicinal iron preparations; chalybeates.
Fer'ratin. Proprietary preparation of iron from blood.

Fer'rein's pyramids (fer'rinz). Conical masses in the cortex of kidney, each containing straight tubules surrounded by convoluted ones. **F.'s tubule,** cortical portion of a uriniferous tubule.
Fer'ric. Containing iron in its higher valency.
Ferricy'anid. A compound containing $Fe_2(CN)_6$, or ferric cyanid.
Ferricyan'ogen. A tetravalent radical, $Fe(CN)_6$.
Ferrocy'anid. A compound containing $Fe(CN)_2$, or ferrous cyanid.
Ferrocyan'ogen. A hexad radical, $(FeC_6N_6)_2$.
Ferropy'rin. Compound of antipyrin and ferric chlorid: used in anemia and neuralgia and as an external astringent.
Ferrostyp'tin. An antiseptic and styptic iron preparation.
Fer'rous. Containing iron in its lower valency.
Ferru'ginous (fer-ru'jin-us). Containing iron; chalybeate.
Fer'rum. L. for *Iron.*
Fer'tile. Able to produce offspring; not sterile.
Fertiliza'tion. Impregnation; fecundation.
Fer'ula. Genus of plants. See *Asafetida, Galbanum, Sumbul, Sagapenum.*
Fes'ter. A small superficial ulcer or sore.
Festina'tion. A gait in which the patient takes quicker and quicker steps, as in paralysis agitans.
Fe'tal. Pertaining to a fetus. **F. abortion.** See under *Abortion.*
Feta'tion. 1. Development of the fetus. 2. Pregnancy.
Fet'icide (fet'is-id). The killing of a fetus *in utero.*
Fe'tid. Having a rank, disagreeable smell.
Fe'tor. Stench or offensive odor.
Fe'tus. The unborn child after end of the third month.
Fe'ver. 1. Abnormally high bodily temperature; pyrexia. 2. Disease marked by increase of temperature. **Asthenic f.,** one in which there is nervous depression, feeble pulse, and a clammy skin. **Bilious f.,** one with apparent liver complications. **Blackwater fever,** dangerous tropical bilious fever. **Brain f.,** cerebral meningitis or cerebritis. **Breakbone f.** See *Dengue.* **Catheter f.,** fever that may follow misuse of a catheter. **Cerebrospinal f.** See *Meningitis, cerebrospinal.* **Chagres f.,** a malignant type of malarial fever. **Childbed f.** Same as *Puerperal fever.* **Continued f.,** one which is neither intermittent nor remittent. **Dandy f.** Same as *Dengue.* **Enteric f.** Same as *Typhoid fever.* **Eruptive f., Exanthematous f.,** any fever accompanied by an eruption on the skin. **Famine f.** Same as *Relapsing fever.* **Fracture f.,** fever following fracture of a bone. **Gastric f.,** any acute abdominal attack with gastric disturbances. **Hay f., Hay asthma,** acute catarrh of conjunctiva and nasal mucous membrane, of annual recurrence. **Hectic f.,** daily recurring fever with profound sweating, chills, and flushed countenance; associated with tuberculosis and septic poisoning. **Low f.** Same as *Asthenic fever.* **Lung f.,** croupous pneumonia. **Mediterranean f.,** a fever of bacterial origin in the Mediterranean region. **Milk f.** 1. Mild form of puerperal septicemia. 2. Fever said to attend the establishment of lactation after delivery. 3. Endemic fever said to be caused by the use of unwholesome cow's milk. **Puerperal f.,** septic poisoning occurring in childbed. **Relapsing f.,** a contagious bacterial fever often associated with famine and poverty. **Remittent f.,** a malarial fever with exacerbations and remissions, but no intermissions. **Rheumatic f.,** acute inflammatory rheumatism. **Scarlet f.** Same as *Scarlatina.* **Septic f.,** one due to the entrance of septic poisons into the blood. **Simple continued f.,** a non-contagious fever with neither remissions nor intermissions. **Spirillum f.** Same as *Relapsing fever.* **Splenic f.,** true anthrax. **Sthenic f.,** fever characterized by a full strong pulse, hot and

dry skin, high temperature, thirst, and active delirium. **Traumatic f.**, that which follows injury or wounds. **Typhoid f.**, a specific eruptive communicable fever with lesions of the spleen and Peyer's patches. **Typhus f.**, a contagious eruptive fever with no characteristic lesions, but with great prostration. **Urethral f.**, fever following the use of catheter, sound, or bougie. **Yellow f.**, an infectious fever, chiefly of tropical America, with intense pains, jaundice, and the vomiting of blackened blood.

Fe'verfew. See *Matricaria.*

Fi'at, pl. **Fi'ant.** L. for *let there be made.*

Fi'ber. An elongated thread-like structure of organic tissue. **Arciform** or **Arcuate f.**, bow-shaped fibers crossing the anterior aspect of the medulla. **Axial f.**, the axis-cylinder of a nerve-fiber. **Beale's f.**, a spiral nerve-fiber. **Bühlmann's f.**, peculiar lines in carious teeth caused by bacteria. **F. cell**, any one of the elongated cells of which a fiber is composed, especially if still nuclear. **Corti's f's.**, rods of Corti. **Gottstein's f's.**, nerve-fibers of auditory nerve in cochlea. **Müller's f's.**, supporting fibers of neuroglia in retina. **F's. of Remak**, non-medullated nerve-fibers. **Sharpey's f's.**, fibers joining together the lamellæ of bone. **Tomes's f's.**, branching processes of odontoblasts in dentinal canals.

Fi'bril. Fibril'la. A minute fiber or filament.

Fibril'lar. Fib'rillary. Pertaining to, or made up of, fibrils.

Fibrilla'tion. 1. Quality of being fibrillar. 2. Muscular tremor.

Fi'brin (fi'brin). A whitish proteid of the blood and of serous fluids. **F.-ferment**, a principle believed to convert fibrinogen into fibrin.

Fibrina'tion (fib-rin-a'shun). Excess of fibrin in the blood.

Fibrin'ogen. A globulin from which fibrin is mainly derived.

Fibrinoplas'tin. Same as *Paraglobulin.*

Fibrino'sis. Condition marked by excess of fibrin in the blood.

Fib'rinous (fib'rin-us). Pertaining to, or of the nature of, fibrin.

Fibrinu'ria. Discharge of fibrin in the urine.

Fibro-adeno'ma. Adenoma containing fibrous tissue.

Fibro-are'olar (fi-bro-ar-e'o-lar). Both fibrous and areolar.

Fi'broblast. Any cell-element from which fibers are developed.

Fibrocar'tilage. A cartilage containing fibrous elements.

Fibrocel'lular. Partly fibrous and partly cellular.

Fibrochondri'tis. Inflammation of a fibrocartilage.

Fi'brocyst. Fibroma that has suffered cystic degeneration.

Fibrocys'tic (fi-bro-sis'tik). Partly fibrous and partly cystic.

Fibrocysto'ma. Fibroma blended with cystoma.

Fi'brogen. The forerunner of fibrin.

Fibroglio'ma. Glioma containing fibrous elements.

Fi'broid (fi'broid). 1. Resembling fiber, or a fibrous structure. 2. Same as *Fibroma.*

Fibro'in. White albuminoid, $C_{15}H_{23}N_5O_6$, from spiders' webs and cocoons of insects.

Fibrolipo'ma. Tumor that is both fibroid and fatty.

Fibro'ma. A tumor composed of connective tissue.

Fibromato'sis. A tendency to develop fibromata.

Fibromyi'tis. Inflammation of muscle with fibrous degeneration.

Fibromyo'ma. Fibroma blended with myoma.

Fibromyxo'ma. Tumor that is both fibrous and mucous.

Fibroneuro'ma. A neuroma blended with fibroma.

Fibroplas'tic. Giving origin to fibrous tissue. **F. tumor**, a variety of spindle-celled sarcoma.

Fibrosarco'ma. Sarcoma blended with fibroma.

Fibro'sis. Formation of fibrous tissue; fibroid degeneration. **Arteriocapillary f.** See *Arteriocapillary.*

Fi'brous (fi'brus). Composed of, or containing, fibers.

Fib'ula. Outer bone of the leg below the knee.

Fi'cus (fi'kus). L. for *Fig.*

Field of vision. The area or space which the fixed eye can see.

Fifth nerve. See *Trifacial* in *Nerves, Table of.* **F. ventricle.** See *Ventricle.*

Fig. Fruit of *Ficus carica:* used as a laxative and digestant. **F.-wart.** Same as *Verruca acuminata.*

Fila'ceous (fil-a'she-us). Composed of filaments.

Fil'ament. A delicate fiber or thread.

Fila'ria. A genus of nematode parasitic worms. **F. medinen'sis.** See *Guinea worms.* **F. san'guinis hom'inis,** a parasite found in the blood-vessels, lymphatics, etc.

Filari'asis. Disease due to *Filaria.*

Filic'ic acid. A substance, $C_{14}H_{18}O_5$, from male fern.

Fil'iform. Shaped like a thread. **F. bougie.** See *Bougie.* **F. papillæ,** the smallest variety of papillæ on the tongue.

Fil'ipuncture. Insertion of wire or thread in aneurysm.

Fi'lix (fi'lix). Male fern.

Fil'let. 1. A loop-shaped bandage. 2. White band on outer side of superior cerebellar peduncles. **Olivary f.,** nerve-fasciculus surrounding olivary body.

Fil'mogen. Solution of nitrated cellulose in acetone: used in applying drugs to the skin.

Fi'lopressure. Compression of a blood-vessel by a thread.

Fil'ter. A device for straining liquids. **F.-paper,** coarse paper used in filtration.

Fil'trate. A liquor which has passed through a filter.

Filtra'tion. The operation of straining a liquid.

Fi'lum termina'le. The slender inferior end of spinal cord.

Fim'bria. A fringe; especially, fringe-like end of oviduct.

Fim'briate. Fringed. **F. body,** the corpus fimbriatum.

Fin'ger (fing'ger). Either one of the five extremities of a hand. **Morse f.,** deformity of finger due to constant use of Morse telegraph key. **F.-stall,** a cap for an injured or sore finger.

First inten'tion. See under *Healing.* **F. nerve,** the olfactory nerve.

Fish'er's murmur. A head murmur in the systole heard in rickety children.

Fish-skin disease. Same as *Ichthyosis.* **F.-slime disease,** septicemia from punctured wounds by fish-spines.

Fis'sion (fish'un). Division of a cell into parts; segmentation.

Fissip'arous. Propagated by fission.

Fissu'ra. L. for *Fissure.*

Fis'sure (fis'yur). A narrow slit or cleft. **Anal f.,** painful lineal ulcer at margin of anus. **Auricular f.,** a fissure in the petrous bone. **F. of Bichat,** transverse fissure between the fornix and upper surface of cerebellum. **Broca's f.,** the fissure which surrounds the third left frontal convolution. **Burdach's f.,** fissure between lateral surface of insula and inner surface of operculum. **Calcarine f.,** fissure between the cuneate lobe and the lingual lobule on the mesial aspect of the cerebrum. **Callosomarginal f.,** fissure on the median surface of each cerebral hemisphere midway between the callosum and the margin of the surface. **Central f.,** the fissure of Rolando. **Clevenger's f.,** the inferior occipital fissure. **Longitudinal f.,** the deep fissure between the cerebral hemispheres. **Occipital f.,** a deep fissure between the parietal and occipital lobes of the cerebrum. **Palpebral f.,** the slit or opening between the eyelids. **Portal f.,** the transverse fissure of the liver. **Precentral f.,** a fissure parallel to the fissure of Rolando and anterior to it. **Rolando's f.,** the fissure between the parietal and frontal lobes. **Sphenoidal f.,** a cleft in the wings and body of sphenoid and orbital plate of frontal bone for various nerves and vessels. **F. of Sylvius,** fissure which separates the anterior and middle lobes of the cerebrum. **Transverse f.** 1. Fissure crossing transversely the under surface of the right lobe of the liver. 2. Horseshoe-shaped fissure from the descending cornu of the cerebrum on one side to that on the other. **Umbilical f.,** the anterior part of the longitudinal fissure of the liver.

Fis'tula (fis'tu-lah). A deep sinuous ulcer, often leading to an internal hollow organ. **Anal f.,** a fistula near the anus which may or may not communicate with the rectum. **Blind f.,** one which is open at one end only. It may open upon the skin (*external, blind f.*) or upon a mucous surface (*internal, blind f.*). **Branchial f.,** an unclosed branchial cleft. **Complete f.,** one which opens upon the skin and upon an internal cavity. **Fecal f.,** one which communicates with the intestine. **Vesicovag'inal f.,** an opening from the bladder to the vagina.

Fis'tulatome (fist'u-lat-ōm). Same as *Syringotome*.

Fis'tulous. Pertaining to, or of the nature of, a fistula.

Fit. A convulsion; a paroxysm; a sudden attack.

Fixa'tion. The act of holding or fastening in a fixed position. **F.-forceps,** forceps for holding a part during an operation. **F. point,** point for which accommodation of the eye is adjusted, and where vision is clearest.

Fix'ing. Speedy killing of tissues in such a way that their normal form is preserved.

Fl. Symbol of *Fluorin*.

Flabel'lum. A set of radiating white fibers in corpus striatum.

Flac'cid (flak'sid). Weak, lax, and soft.

Flag. See *Calamus* and *Iris*.

Flagel'late cell. Cell with long cilia for propulsion.

Flagel'lum (fla-jel'lum). A slender lash-like cilium.

Flail-joint. Abnormal mobility of a joint after resection.

Flank. The part of the body between ribs and ilium.

Flap. A mass of tissue partly detached by the knife. **F. amputation.** See *Amputation*. **F. extraction,** removal of cataract by making a flap in the cornea.

Flat-bones. Bones that have a flat shape. **F.-foot,** a foot with a flat sole and sunken tarsus.

Flat'ness. Resonance heard on percussing a part that is abnormally solid.

Flat'ulence (flat'u-lens). Excessive formation of gases in the stomach or intestine.

Flat'ulent (flat'u-lent). Characterized by flatulence.

Fla'tus. Gas or air in the stomach or intestine.

Flax-dressers' disease. Phthisis or pneumonia due to inhalation of dust in dressing flax.

Flax'seed. Same as *Linseed*.

Fldr. Abbreviation of *Fluidram*.

Flea (flē). An insect of the genus *Pulex*: in part parasitic.

Flea'bane (flē'bān). See *Erigeron*.

Fleam (flēm). A lancet for venesection.

Flech'sig's tract. The anterior or fundamental ground bundle of the spinal cord.

Fleece of Stilling. The lacework of white fibers that surrounds the dentate nucleus.

Fleischmann's bursa (flish'manz). The bursa sublingualis.

Flesh. The muscles and other soft parts of animals. **Proud f.,** excessive granulation-tissue.

Flex. To bend or put in a state of flexion.

Flexibil'itas ce'rea. Cataleptic state in which the limbs retain the position in which they are placed.

Flex'ible, Flex'ile. Readily bent without danger of breaking.

Flex'ion (flek'shun). Act of bending; condition of being bent.

Flex'or. A muscle that flexes a joint. See *Muscles, Table of.*

Flexu'ra. L. for *Flexure.*

Flex'ure (flek'shur). A bend or fold; a curvation. **Caudal f.,** bend at the aboral end of the embryo. **Cephalic f., Cranial f.,** curve at the cephalic end of the embryo. **Sigmoid f.,** part of colon between descending colon and rectum.

Flint disease. Chalicosis.

Floating albumin, F. proteid. See *Albumin.* **F. ribs.** See *Ribs.*

Floccilla'tion. Floccita'tion. Same as *Carphology.*

Floc'culent (flok'u-lent). Containing downy or flaky shreds.

Floc'culus. Small lobe on anterior part of under surface of each cerebellar hemisphere.

Flood'ing. Copious uterine hemorrhage.

Flood's ligament. One of the three glenohumeral ligaments.

Floor cells. The cells of the floor of the arch of Corti.

Flourens's doctrine (floo-ronz'). The opinion that the entire cerebrum takes a part in every mental process.

Flow. To menstruate copiously.

Flow'ers of sulphur. Sublimed sulphur.

Fluctua'tion. A wave-like motion, as of a fluid in a cavity of the body after succussion.

Fluid. A liquid or a gas. **Allantoic f.,** the fluid contained in the allantois. **Amniotic f.,** the liquor amnii. **Cerebrospinal f.,** fluid contained in cerebral ventricles, subarachnoid spaces, and central canal of cord. **Condy's f.,** disinfecting solution of sodium or potassium permanganate. **F. extract,** a strong liquid solution of a vegetable medicine. **Labyrinthine f.,** the perilymph. **Subarachnoid f.** Same as *Cerebrospinal f.*

Flu'idounce. Eight fluidrams.

Flu'idram. Measure equal to 56.96 grains of distilled water.

Fluke. A parasitic trematode worm. See *Distoma, Bilharzia.*

Flu'or al'bus. Same as *Leucorrhea.*

Fluores'cein, Fluores'cin. A coal-tar derivative, $C_{20}H_{12}O_5$, used in observing motions of eye-fluids.

Fluores'cence (flu-or-es'ens). The property of certain bodies to emit a gleam when exposed to violet rays. **F. screen,** a plate in the fluoroscope coated with crystals of calcium tunstate.

Flu'orid (flu'or-id). Any binary compound of fluorin.

Flu'orin (flu'or-in). A halogen element, not unlike chlorin.

Flu'orol (flu'or-ol). Sodium fluorid, NaF: a germicide.

Fluor'oscope (flu-or'os-kōp). A device used in skiagraphy.

Flux. 1. An excessive discharge. 2. Matter discharged. **Alvine f.,** diarrhea. **Bloody f.,** dysentery.

Fly-blis'ter. A blister prepared from cantharides.

Fly'ing-blister. A blister to be moved from place to place.

F. M. = *fi'at mistu'ra,* "make a mixture."

Fo'cal. Pertaining to a focus. **F. depth,** penetrating power of a lens. **F. distance,** distance of center of lens from its principal focus. **F. lesion,** a central lesion of definite limits.

Fo'cus (fo'kus). 1. The point of convergence of light-rays or of sound-waves. 2. Chief center of a morbid process.

Fœnic'ulum. Same as *Fennel.*

Fœtus, etc. See *Fetus,* etc. **F. papyra'ceus,** a dead fetus flattened out by its living twin.

Fo'lia. L. for *Leaves.*

Fo'lian pro'cess. The processus gracilis of the malleus.

Fol'licle (fol'ik-l). A very small excretory or secretory sac or gland. **Graafian f.,** any one of the small spherical ovarian bodies each of which contains an ovum. **Hair-f.,** the depression from which each hair grows. **Lieberkuhn, f's. of,** little tubular pits on the mucous membrane of the small intestine. **Lymph-f.**, an aggregation of adenoid substance: chiefly found on mucous surfaces. **Sebaceous f.**, a sebaceous gland of the skin. **Solitary f.**, any discrete lymph-follicle on the mucous membrane of the intestine.

Follic'ular. Of or pertaining to a follicle or follicles. **F. tumor**, a sebaceous cyst; a dilated sebaceous follicle.

Follicull'tis. Inflammation of a follicle or follicles. **F. bar'bæ**, inflammation of the hair-follicles of the beard. **F. decal'vans**, chronic f. of scalp, leading to cicatricial alopecia.

Follic'ulose (fol-ik'u-lōs). Full of follicles.

Fomenta'tion. A warm application, usually moist.

Fo'mes, pl. *fo'mites*. A porous substance absorbing contagium.

Fonta'na's canal or **spaces** (fon-tah'nahz). A ring of spaces at the junction of cornea, iris, and sclera. **F.'s markings**, minute transverse fold seen on a divided nerve-trunk.

Fon'tanel, Fontanelle (fon-tan-el'). Any one of the unossified spots on the cranium of a young infant.

Fontic'ulus (fon-tik'u-lus). A fontanel.

Food. Anything that serves to nourish; aliment.

Foot. The terminal organ of the leg. **F.-clonus**, same as *Ankle-clonus*. **F.-fungus**, the fungus that produces mycetoma or madura foot. **F.-phenomenon, F.-reflex.** Same as *Ankle-clonus*. **F.-plate**, plate that forms the base of the stapes. **F.-pound**, the energy needful to raise a pound one foot.

Foot-and-mouth-disease. Contagious epizoötic aphthæ.

Foot'ling presentation. Presentation of the feet in labor.

Fora'men. A perforation or hole. **Aortic f.**, the hindmost of the openings of the diaphragm. **Arachnoid f.** Same as *F. of Magendie*. **Auditory f., external**, the external meatus of auditory canal. **Auditory f., internal**, passage for auditory and facial nerves in petrous bone. **Bichat's f.**, a canal from subarachnoid space to third ventricle. **Botallo's f.** connects the auricles of the fetal heart. **F. cæ'cum, Cecal f.** 1. Foramen between the frontal bone and crista galli. 2. A canal over the root and dorsum of the tongue. 3. In the mucous membrane of the posterior wall of the pharynx. **Condyloid f., anterior**, passage in occipital bone for hypoglossal nerve. **Condyloid f., posterior**, a fossa behind either occipital condyle. **Cotyloid f.**, passage between the margin of acetabulum and transverse ligament. **Dental f., inferior**, the outer aperture of the inferior d. canal in the ramus of the lower jaw. **Esophageal f.**, passage for esophagus through the diaphragm. **Ethmoid f., anterior**, a canal formed by the ethmoid and frontal bones. **Frontal f.**, the supra-orbital notch. **Incisor f.**, the aperture for anterior palatine artery in the alveolar margin. **Infra-orbital f.**, passage for infra-orbital nerve and artery. **Intervertebral f., anterior**, passage for spinal nerves and vessels between laminæ of adjacent vertebræ. **Intervertebral f., posterior**, space between the articular processes of adjacent vertebræ. **Jugular f.** Same as *F. lacerum posterius*. **F. la'cerum ante'rius.** Same as *Sphenoidal fissure*. **F. la'cerum me'dium**, a cleft in petrous bone and great wing of sphenoid for carotid artery, etc. **F. la'cerum poste'rius**, space made by jugular notches of the temporal and occipital bones. **Magendie's f.**, orifice in the pia of the roof of fourth ventricle. **F. mag'num**, great orifice in occipital bone through which the brain and spinal cord are connected. **Mastoid f.**, small hole behind mastoid process. **Medullary f., Nutrient f.**, passage which admits the nutrient vessels to the medullary cavity of a bone. **Mental f.**, foramen of lower jaw for mental nerve and vessels. **F. of Monro**, passage from third to lateral ventricle of brain. **Nutrient f.** Same as *Medullary f.* **Obturator f.**, the large opening between os pubis and ischium. **Olfactory foramina**, many openings of the cribriform plate of ethmoid bone. **Optic f.**, passage for optic nerve and ophthalmic artery at apex of orbit. **F. ova'le.** 1. Fetal opening between the heart's auricles. 2. Aperture in great wing of sphenoid for vessels and nerves. **Palatine f., anterior**, an orifice in anterior part of roof of mouth for a nerve and artery. **Palatine f., posterior**, orifice in hard palate for descending palatine canal. **Parietal f.**, passage in parietal bone for vessels. **Pterygopalatine f.**, passage for p. vessels and nerve. **Quadrate f.**, passage for postcava in the diaphragm. **F. rotun'dum**, a round opening in great wing of sphenoid for the superior maxillary nerve. **Sacral f., anterior**, eight passages for anterior branches of sacral nerves. **Sacral f., posterior**, eight passages for posterior branches of sacral nerves. **Sacrosciatic f., great**, oval space between the innominate bone and lesser sacrosciatic ligament. **Sacrosciatic f., smaller**, space between the greater and lesser s. ligaments and innominate bone. **Scarpa's f.**, apertures in roof of mouth for nasopalatine nerve. **Sömmering's f.** Same as *Fovea centralis.* **Sphenopalatine f.**, space between the orbital and sphenoidal processes of palate bone. **F. spino'sum**, hole in great wing of sphenoid for middle meningeal artery. **Supra-orbital f.**, notch of frontal bone for supra-orbital vessels and nerve. **Thebesius's foramina.** Same as *Venæ Thebesii;* also, the orifices of the same in right auricle. **Thyroid f.** Same as *Obturator f.* **Vertebral f.**, space between body and arch of a vertebra and the spinal cord and its meninges. **Vertebro-arterial f.**, foramen in transverse process of a cervical vertebra for vertebral vessels. **F. of Vesalius**, opening at inner side of *f. ovale* of the sphenoid. **F. of Winslow**, the aperture between the greater and lesser peritoneal cavities.

Forced feeding. The administration of food by force. **F. movements.** Same as *Compulsory movements.*

For'ceps. 1. A two-pronged instrument for grasping or seizing. 2. Any forcipate organ or part.

For'cipate (for'sip-āt). Shaped like a forceps.

For'cipressure. Pressure by a forceps to check hemorrhage.

Fore'arm (fōr'arm). The part of arm between elbow and wrist.

Fore'brain (fōr'brān). Same as *Prosencephalon.*

Fore'finger. The first or index finger.

Fore'gut. Embryonic organ whence pharynx, esophagus, stomach, and duodenum are formed.

Fore'head (for'ed). Part of face above the eyes.

For'eign body. Any substance in a place where it does not belong.

Foren'sic medicine. Same as *Medical Jurisprudence.*

Fore'skin. The prepuce.

For'mal. A somnifacient anesthetic, $CH_2,(OCH_3)_2$.

Formal'dehyd. A powerfully disinfectant gas, CH_2O; formic aldehyd. **F.-ca'sein**, a mildly antiseptic preparation. **F.-gel'atin**, an antiseptic for dressing wounds.

For'malin. Wood-alcohol containing 40 per cent. of formaldehyd.

For'malith. A solid preparation of formaldehyd.

Formam'id. The amid, $CHO(NH_2)$.

Forman'ilid. An antipyretic and local anesthetic substance, $C_6H_5NH(HCO)$.

For'mate (for'māt). Any salt of formic acid.

Forma'tio reticula'ris. The interlacing fibers of the anterior columns of the oblongata.

For'mative cells. The embryonic cells. **F. yolk**, that part of the ovum whence the embryo is developed.

For'mic acid. See *Acid.* **F. aldehyd.** Same as *Formaldehyd.*
Formica'tion. Sensation as if ants were creeping on the body.
For'min (for'min). Urotropin.
For'mol. An antiseptic solution of formic aldehyd.
Formopy'rin. Combination of antipyrin and formaldehyd: said to be antipyretic and antiseptic.
For'mula. 1. A union of symbols to express a chemical combination. 2. A recipe to prepare a medicine.
Form'ulary. A collection or book of recipes and formulæ.
For'nicate convolution. Same as *Gyrus fornicatus.*
For'nix. A band of white substance under the callosum extending from the fimbria to the corpora mammillaria.
Fortifica'tion spectrum. Same as *Teichopsia.*
Fos'sa. A pit, depression, trench, fovea, or hollow. **Acetabular f.** See *Acetabulum.* **Canine f.,** depression on external surface of superior maxilla. **Cranial f.,** either one of three hollows in base of cranium for lobes of the brain. **Digastric f.,** groove on inner aspect of mastoid process. **Digital f.,** a depression at base of inner surface of mastoid process. **Glenoid f.,** fossa in the temporal bone for condyle of lower jaw. **F. hemiellip'tica,** the uppermost of two recesses in fore part of vestibule. **F. hemisphæ'rica.** one of the recesses of the anterior part of vestibule. **Hyaloid f.** Same as *Patellar f.* **Iliac f., external,** the wide depression on outer surface of ilium. **Iliac f., internal,** wide depression on inner surface of ilium. **Ischiorectal f.,** triangular space between rectum and tuberosity of the ischium. **Lacrimal f.,** in roof of orbit, lodges the lacrimal gland. **F. navicula'ris.** Same as *Navicular fossa.* **F. ova'lis,** fovea in right auricle of heart; remains of fetal forामen ovale. **F. patella'ris,** depression in front of vitreous body which lodges the lens. **Pituitary f.,** depression in the sphenoid which lodges the pituitary gland. **F. of Rosenmüller.** See *Cavity of Rosenmüller.* **Sublingual f.,** space on inside of lower jaw which lodges the sublingual gland. **Submaxillary f.,** depression on the inner surface of inferior maxillary bone for the submaxillary gland. **Trochanteric f.** Same as *Digital f.* **Zygomatic f.,** cavity below and within the zygoma.
Fossette' (fos-et'). 1. A small depression. 2. A small, deep, corneal ulcer.
Foudroyant (foo-drwah-yong') Same as *Fulminant.*
Fourchet, Fourchette (foor-shet'). Posterior junction of labia majora.
Fourth nerve. The trochlear nerve. **F. ventricle,** the space between the cerebellum, pons, and oblongata.
Fo'vea (fo've-ah). A pit, fossa, or cup. **F. centra'lis,** pit in middle of macula lutea. **F. hemisphæ'rica, F. hemiellip'tica.** See *Fossa hemisphærica, Fossa hemielliptica.* **F. pharyngis,** abnormal fossa in middle line of pharynx. **F. trochlea'ris,** notch in frontal bone for the trochlea of the superior oblique muscle.
Fo'veate (fo've-āt). Pitted.
Fow'ler's operation. Hysterorrhaphy. **F.'s solution,** solution of potassium arsenite: antiperiodic.
Fox'glove. Same as *Digitalis.*
Frac'tional culture. The obtaining of a micro-organism or a single species from a culture containing more than one. **F. distillation,** separation of the component parts of a substance by distilling.
Fract'ure (frakt'yur). The breaking of a bone. **Barton's f.,** fracture of distal end of radius. **F.-bed,** a bed constructed for the use of patients with fractured bones. **F.-box,** a box to support a broken limb. **Colles's f.,** fracture of lower third of

radius. **Comminuted f.**, one in which the bone is crushed or splintered. **Complete f.**, one in which the bone is entirely broken across. **Complicated f.**, fracture with injury of adjacent parts. **Compound f.**, fracture with external wound leading into the bone. **F. by contrecoup**, fracture of skull at a distance from the point struck. **Depressed f.**, fracture of skull in which a fracture is depressed below the surface. **Double f.**, fracture of a bone at two places. **Dupuytren's f.** Same as *Pott's f.* **F. fever.** See *Fever.* **Greenstick f.**, fracture in which one side of a bone is broken, the other being bent. **Impacted f.**, fracture in which one fragment is firmly driven into the other. **Interperiosteal f.**, greenstick fracture. **Pott's f.**, fracture of lower part of fibula with serious injury of the lower tibial articulation. **Simple f.**, one in which the overlying integument is intact. **Smith's f.**, fracture of lower end of radius near its articular surface. **Spiral f.**, one in which the bone has been twisted apart. **Spontaneous f.**, one occurring as a result of disease of the bone or from some undiscoverable cause, and not due to violence. **Trophic f.**, one due to a trophic disturbance. **Ununited f.**, one not followed by a bony reunion.

Fræn'ulum, Fræ'num. See *Frenulum, Frenum.*

Fragil'itas crin'ium. Brittle state of the hair. **F. os'sium**, abnormal brittleness of the bones.

Fragmenta'tion. A division into fragments.

Frambe'sia, Frambœ'sia. A contagious disease of hot regions, marked by raspberry-like tumors; yaws.

Fran'gula. Bark of *Rhamnus frangula*, a species of buckthorn: purgative.

Fran'gulin. A purgative extract, $C_{20}H_{20}O_{10}$, from frangula.

Frank'enhäuser's ganglion (frank'en-hoi-zerz). A ganglion near the cervix uteri.

Frank'incense. Same as *Olibanum.*

Frank'lin glasses. Bifocal spectacles.

Franklin'ic electricity. Frictional or static electricity.

Franklinization. Therapeutic use of static electricity.

Fra'serin. Tonic and stimulant preparation from the root of *Frasera Walteri.*

Fraun'hofer lines (frawn'ho-fer). Dark lines on solar spectrum.

Freck'le (frek'kl). See *Lentigo.*

Freez'ing microtome. A microtome for cutting frozen objects. **F. mixture**, a mixture for producing artificial cold. **F.-point**, the temperature at which any substance becomes frozen.

Frem'itus. A thrill; especially one that is perceptible on palpation. **Friction f.**, thrill caused by the rubbing together of two dry surfaces. **Hydatid f.**, tremulous impulse felt in palpation over a hydatid cyst. **Rhonchal f.**, vibrations produced by the passage of air through a large bronchial tube loaded with mucus. **Tactile f.**, a thrill, as in the chest-wall, which may be felt by a person speaking. **Tussive f.**, thrill felt on chest while patient coughs. **Vocal f.**, thrill caused by speaking and perceived by the ear of the auscultator.

Fren'ulum. 1. A frenum. 2. A ridge on the upper part of the valve of Vieussens.

Fre'num (fre'num). Any part that serves as a curb or check. **F. puden'di.** Same as *Fourchette.*

Fre'tum of Haller. A constriction between the auricles and ventricles of the fetal heart.

Freund's operation (froyndz). Same as *Laparohysterectomy.*

Fri'able. Broken easily into small pieces.

Fri'ar's balsam. Compound tincture of benzoin.

Fric'tion (frik'shun). The act of rubbing. **F.-murmur, F.-sound**, an auscultatory rubbing sound in pleurisy.

Fric'tional electricity. Static or Franklinic electricity.

Fried'rich's ataxia, F.'s disease (freed'rix). Same as *Hereditary ataxia.* **F.'s sign,** diastolic collapse of the cervical veins caused by an adhering pericardium.

Frigorif'ic. Producing coldness. **F. nerve,** the sympathetic, stimulation of which lowers the temperature.

Frigother'apy. Treatment of disease by cold.

Frog-belly. Tympanitic state of a child's belly. **F.-face,** flatness of the face due to intranasal disease.

Fröhde's (froe'dez) **reagent.** A test for alkaloids; 1 part of sodium molybdate in 100 parts of sulphuric acid.

From'mann's lines (from'mahnz). Black lines developed on axis-cylinders by silver nitrate.

Fron's test (fronz). Double iodid of potassium and bismuth: used in testing for alkaloids and for sugar.

Fron'tad. Toward a front, or frontal aspect.

Fron'tal (fron'tal). Pertaining to the forehead. **F. bone,** the bone of the forehead. **F. sinuses,** two air-cavities in the lower border of the frontal bone.

Frontoma'lar. Pertaining to the frontal and malar bones.

Frontomax'illary. Pertaining to the frontal bone and the upper jaw-bone.

Frontopari'etal. Pertaining to the frontal and parietal bones.

Frontotem'poral. Pertaining to frontal and temporal bones.

Front-tap contraction. Contraction of gastrocnemius on tapping the muscles on the front of the leg.

Frost-bite. Lesion produced by freezing of a part. **F.-itch,** pruritus hiemalis.

Fruc'tose. Levulose, or fruit-sugar.

Ft. Abbreviation of L. *fiat*, or *fiant*, let there be made.

Fuch'sin (fook'sin). Rosanilin hydrochlorid or rosanilin acetate: used as a dye and as a medicine.

Fuchsin'ophile, Fuchsinoph'ilous (fook-sin-of'il-us). Readily stained by fuchsin.

Fu'cus cris'pus. Same as *Chondrus.* **F. vesiculo'sus,** a seaweed with resolvent and deobstruent properties.

Fu'gitive (fu'jit-iv). Wandering; also transient.

Ful'gurating. Coming and going like a flash of lightning: used chiefly of pains.

Ful'minant, Ful'minating. Coming on suddenly with intense severity; foudroyant.

Fumiga'tion. Exposure to disinfecting fumes.

Fum'ing (fūm'ing). Smoking; emitting a visible vapor.

Func'tion. The special action or office of any organ.

Func'tional. Of, or pertaining to, a function. **F. disease,** any disease that affects the functions, but not the structure.

Fun'dal (fun'dal). Of, or pertaining to, a fundus.

Fund'ament. The anus and parts adjacent to it.

Fun'dus. The base or part remotest from the mouth of a hollow organ. **F. glands.** Same as *Delomorphous cells.*

Fun'giform papillæ (fun'jif-orm). Papillæ of the tongue more red than, and next in size to, the conical papillæ.

Fun'goid (fung'oid). Resembling a fungus. **Chignon f.,** a nodular growth on the hair.

Fungos'ity. A fungoid growth or excrescence.

Fun'gous. Of the nature of or like a fungus.

Fun'gus. Any plant of the class to which mushrooms and moulds belong. **F.-foot.** Same as *Madura foot.* **F. hæmato'des,** a bleeding and vascular malignant tumor.

Fu'nic (fu'nik). Pertaining to the funis.

Fu'nicle. Same as *Funiculus.*

Funic'ular (fu-nik'u-lar). Of, or pertaining to, a funiculus.

Funiculi'tis. Inflammation of a funiculus, or of the spermatic cord.

Funic'ulus. The umbilical or spermatic cord; also, any bundle of nerve-fibers. **F. cunea'tus,** an extension of a posterior lateral column of the spinal cord into the oblongata. **F. gra'cilis,** an extension of the posterior median column of the cord into the oblongata. **F. of Rolando,** longitudinal prominence on each side of lower part of medulla oblongata. **F. te'res,** prominent column on floor of fourth ventricle on each side of median furrow.

Fu'nis. A cord; but chiefly the umbilical cord.

Fun'nel-drainage. The draining of diseased parts by glass funnels. **F.-breast,** condition in which the thorax is narrowed toward the abdomen.

Fur. The coating of the tongue seen in various diseases.

Fur'culum. United clavicles of a bird.

Furfura'ceous (fur-fu-ra'shus). Like dandruff or bran; branny.

Fur'furol. An oily substance, $C_5H_7O_2$, from bran, etc.

Fu'runcle (fu'rung-kl). A boil; a painful cutaneous sore enclosing a core or slough.

Furun'cular diathesis. Condition of the system that leads to the appearance of boils.

Furun'culoid (fu-rung'ku-loid). Same as *Furunculous.*

Furunculo'sis. Diseased condition that accompanies the appearance of a crop of boils.

Furun'culous. Of the nature of a boil.

Furun'culus orienta'lis. Aleppo boil, Biscara button, and other similar affections.

Fus'cin (fus'sin). A brown pigment of the retinal epithelium.

Fu'sel oil (fu'sel). A poisonous oil obtained from the distillation of whiskey; amyl alcohol.

Fu'sible (fu'zib-l). That may be melted.

Fu'siform (fu'sif-orm). Spindle-shaped.

Fu'sion (fu'zhun). Act of melting or state of being melted.

Fusocel'lular. Having spindle-shaped cells.

Fustiga'tion. Therapeutic treatment by beating with rods or by strokes of electrodes.

Fus'tin. Yellow dye, $C_{58}H_{46}O_{23}$, from Venetian sumac.

G.

Ga. Chemical symbol of gallium.

Gaboon bark. A poisonous bark of unknown origin.

Gad'berry's mixture. Mixture of quinin sulphate, iron sulphate, nitric acid, and potassic nitrate.

Gad'inin. A poisonous ptomain, $C_7H_{17}N.O_2$, from fish, etc.

Gad'uin (gad'u-in). A basic principle from cod-liver oil.

Ga'dus mor'rhua. The cod, a fish which affords cod-liver oil.

Gaertner's duct (gärt'nerz). See *Gärtner's duct.*

Gaf'sa button. A form of oriental sore or boil.

Gag. Surgical device for holding the mouth open.

Gait (gāt). The manner of progression in walking. **Ataxic g.,** the foot is raised high, and the sole strikes the ground at once and very suddenly. **Cerebellar g.,** a staggering walk indicative of cerebellar disease. **Cow-g.,** a swaying walk due to knock-knee. **Equine g.,** a walk accomplished mainly by flexing the hip-joint, seen in peroneal paralysis. **Frog-g.,** hopping progression resulting from infantile paralysis. **Spastic g.,** walk in which the legs are held together and move in a stiff manner, the toes seeming to drag and catch. **Steppage g.,** one in which the toe is strongly lifted and the heel reaches the ground first.

Galac'tagogue (gal-ak'tag-og). Increasing the flow of milk.

Galacte'mia. Presence of milk in the blood.

Galactidro'sis. The sweating of a milky fluid.
Galac'tin (ga-lak'tin). A basic principle found in milk.
Galac'toblast. A colostrum corpuscle in the gland acini.
Galac'tocele (gal-ak'to-sēl). 1. Milk-containing tumor of the mammary gland. 2. Hydrocele filled with milky fluid.
Galactom'eter. Same as *Lactometer*.
Galactop'athy. The application of a milk-poultice.
Galactoph'agous. Feeding or subsisting upon milk.
Galactoph'igous (gal-ak-tof'ig-us). Arresting the flow of milk.
Galactoph'lysis. Eruption of vesicles with milky contents.
Galactophori'tis. Inflammation of the milk-ducts.
Galactoph'orous (gal-ak-tof'or-us). Conveying the milk.
Galactoph'thisis. Phthisis due to overlactation.
Galactopla'nia (gal-ak-top-la'ne-ah). Secretion of milk in some abnormal part.
Galactopoiet'ic. Concerned in the production of milk.
Galactorrhe'a. Excessive flow of milk.
Galac'toscope (gal-ak'to-skōp). Same as *Lactoscope*.
Galac'tose (ga-lak'tos). A sugar prepared from milk-sugar.
Galactos'tasis (gal-ak-tos'tas-is). 1. Cessation of milk-secretion. 2. Abnormal collection of milk.
Galactother'apy. Treatment of a suckling child by dosing the mother.
Galactu'ria (gal-ak-tu're-ah). See *Chyluria*.
Galan'gal (gal-an'gal). Ginger-like root of *Alpinia officinarum*.
Gal'banum. Gum-resin of *Ferula galbaniflua*.
Galbis'min. A proprietary iodoform-substitute.
Ga'lea aponeurot'ica. The aponeurosis which connects parts of the occipitofrontal muscle.
Galen'ical pharmacy. The old pharmacy which dealt with crude drugs only.
Ga'len's veins. See *Venæ Galeni*.
Gall (gawl). The bile; also, nut-gall; galla. **G.-bladder,** the reservoir for bile, below the liver. **G.-ducts.** See *Bile-ducts*. **G.-stone,** calculus in, or from, the gall-bladder.
Gal'la. Nut-gall; astringent excrescence found on oak-trees.
Gallactophe'none (gal-ak-to-fē'nōn). Yellow powder, used in skin-diseases like pyrogallol.
Gal'lal. Aluminum gallate: used in astringent douches.
Gal'lanol. A powder, $C_{13}H_{11}O_4+2H_2O$, containing anilin and gallic acid: used in skin-diseases.
Gal'late (gal'āt). Any salt of gallic acid.
Gal'lic acid (gal'ik). See *Acid*.
Gal'licin (gal'is-in). Methyl gallate, $C_6H_2(OH)_3COOCH_3$, useful in conjunctivitis.
Gal'lium. A rare metal: some of its salts are poisonous.
Gallobro'mol. A gallic-acid and bromin preparation, $C_6Br_2(OH)COOH$, used as a sedative.
Gal'lon. Four quarts; in the United States, 231 cubic inches.
Gal'loping consumption. Phthisis which takes a rapid course.
Gallotan'nic acid. The tannic acid of nut-galls.
Gal'ton's whistle (gawl'tnz). A whistle used in testing hearing.
Galvan'ic battery. Apparatus for generating galvanic current.
Gal'vanism, Galvan'ic electric'ity. Electricity from a chemical battery; uninterrupted electric current.
Galvaniza'tion (gal-van-iz-a'shun). Treatment by galvanism.
Galvanocau'tery. Cautery by a wire heated by galvanic current.
Galvanocontractil'ity. Contractility on galvanic stimulation.
Galvanofaradiza'tion. Application of continuous and interrupted currents together.
Galvanom'eter. Instrument for measuring galvanic electricity.
Galvanopunc'ture. Puncture and galvanism conjoined.

Galvan'oscope (gal-van'o-skop). Instrument which shows the presence of a galvanic current.

Galvanosur'gery. Surgical application of galvanism.

Galvanotherapeu'tics, Galvanother'apy. Treatment by means of direct battery currents.

Galvan'othermy. Heating by a galvanic battery.

Galvanot'onus. Tonic response to galvanism.

Galvanot'ropism. Movements in organs of animals and plants under the influence of the electric current.

Gamboge (gam-bōj', gum-booj'). Purgative gum-resin of *Garcinia Hanburii.*

Gam'ete (gam'ēt). A conjugative cell-element.

Gam'macism. Imperfect utterances of *g* and *k* sounds.

Gangliasthe'nia. Asthenia due to disease of a ganglion.

Gan'gliated (gang'gle-a-ted). Provided with ganglia. **G. cord,** the main trunk of sympathetic nerve-system.

Gan'gliform (gang'glif-orm). Having the form of a ganglion.

Gang'lioblast. An embryonic cell of the spinal ganglia.

Ganglio'ma (gang-gle-o'mah). Tumor of the lymphatic ganglia.

Gan'glion (gang'gle-on). 1. Any mass of gray nervous substance which serves as a center of nervous influence. 2. A form of cystic tumor on an aponeurosis or a tendon. **Andersch's g.** Same as *Petrous g.* **Arnold's g., Auricular g., Otic g.,** situated below foramen ovale, sends nerves to the tympanic muscles and tensor palati. **Basal ganglia,** the thalami, corpora striata, corpora quadrigemina, tuber cinereum, and geniculate bodies. **Bidder's ganglia,** two ganglia of the auricular septum of a frog's heart. **Bochdalek's g.,** swelling at junction of anterior and middle dental nerves. **Cardiac g., superior,** a ganglion of the superficial cardiac plexus under aortic arch. **Carotid g.,** a ganglion in the lower part of the cavernous sinus. **Carotid g., inferior,** a ganglion of the lower part of the carotid canal. **Carotid g., superior,** one in the upper part of carotid canal. **Casserian g.** Same as *Gasserian g.* **Cephalic ganglia,** the ciliary, otic, sphenopalatine and submaxillary ganglia, all mainly of the trisplanchnic system. **Cervical g., inferior,** between transverse process of lowest cervical vertebra and the neck of the first rib. **Cervical g., Middle,** or **Thyroid g.,** adjacent to fifth cervical vertebra. **Cervical g., superior,** opposite to the second and third cervical vertebra. **Cervical g. of uterus,** near the cervix uteri. **Ciliary g.,** in the posterior part of the orbit. **Cloquet's g.,** swelling of nasopalatine nerve in anterior palatine canal. **Coccygeal g.,** on anterior surface of tip of coccyx. **Ehrenritter's g.** See *Jugular g.* **Gasserian g.,** on larger root of fifth cranial nerve. **Geniculate g.,** on facial nerve in aqueduct of Fallopius. **Hepatic g.,** around the hepatic artery. **G. im'par.** Same as *Coccygeal g.* **Inferior vagal g.,** near the jugular foramen. **Inframaxillary g., anterior.** on inferior maxillary nerve near incisor teeth. **Inframaxillary g., posterior,** near last molar teeth. **Jugular g., Ehrenritter's,** (1) in the upper part of the jugular foramen. **Jugular g.,** (2) in the jugular foramen. **Lenticular g.** Same as *Ciliary g.* **Lingual g.,** on an anterior branch from the superior cervical ganglion. **Ludwig's g.,** at right auricle of heart. **Lumbar ganglia,** 4 or 5 pairs on either side behind abdominal aorta. **Lymphatic g.,** any lymphatic gland. **Meckel's g., Sphenopalatine g.,** in the sphenomaxillary fossa. **Mesenteric g., inferior,** on the inferior mesenteric artery. **Mesenteric g., lateral,** in the superior mesenteric plexus. **Mesenteric g., superior,** in the superior mesenteric plexus. **Nasal g.** Same as *Meckel's g.* **Ophthalmic g., Orbital g.** Same as

Ciliary g. **Otic g.** Same as *Arnold's g.* **Petrous g.**, on glossopharyngeal nerve at lower border of petrous bone. **Pharyngeal g.**, on an anterior branch from the cavernous plexus. **Phrenic g.**, beneath diaphragm at junction of right phrenic nerve and phrenic plexus. **Prostatic g., G. of Müller**, on the prostate gland; connected with prostatic plexus. **Pterygopalatine g.** Same as *Meckel's g.* **Remak's g.**, in the heart near the precava. **Renal g.**, around the renal artery. **Ribes's g.**, the alleged upper ending of the sympathetic nervous system. **Sacral ganglia**, 4 or 5 pairs on ventral face of the sacrum. **Scarpa's g.**, at junction of facial and vestibular branch of auditory nerve. **Schacher's g.** Same as *Ciliary g.* **Semilunar g.**, (1) **Solar g.**, right and left; two ganglia near the suprarenal capsules. **Semilunar g.**, (2) a small ganglion of the fifth nerve. **Sphenopalatine g.** Same as *Meckel's g.* **Spinal ganglia**, on posterior root of each spinal nerve. **Spiral g.**, between plates of the spiral lamina, sending filaments to the organ of Corti. **Splanchnic g.** Same as *Semilunar g.* (1). **Submaxillary g.**, above the submaxillary gland. **Suprarenal g.**, at the junction of the great splanchnic nerves. **Thoracic ganglia**, 12 pairs between transverse processes of vertebræ and head of ribs. **Thyroid g., inferior.** See *Cervical g., middle.* **Thyroid g., superior.** See *Cervical g., superior.* **Tympanic g.**, on the tympanic branch of the glossopharyngeal. **Valentin's g.**, at junction of the posterior and middle dental nerves. **Vestibular g.**, in the aqueduct of Fallopius. **Ventricular g.** Same as *Bidder's g.* **Walter's g.** Same as *G. impar.* **Wrisberg's g.** Same as *Cardiac g.*

Gan'glioneure (gang'gle-o-nūr). Any cell of a nervous ganglion.

Ganglion'ic (gang-gle-on'ik). Pertaining to a ganglion.

Ganglioni'tis (gang-gle-on-i'tis). Inflammation of a ganglion.

Gangrene (gang'grēn). Mortification or non-molecular death of a part. **Diabetic g.**, moist gangrene in some cases of diabetes. **Dry g.**, a hard, shrivelled, and relatively dry form from deficient blood-supply. **Embolic g.** follows cutting off of blood-supply by an embolism. **Hospital g.**, contagious and fatal form in crowded hospital, attacking wounds. **Moist g.**, a form with free offensive watery discharge. **Nosocomial g.** Same as *Hospital g.* **Primary g.**, that which does not follow a local inflammation. **Pulpy g.** Same as *Hospital g.* **Secondary g.**, a form which follows a local inflammation. **Senile g.**, a form that attacks the extremities of the aged. **Symmetric g.**, gangrene of corresponding parts on either side due to vasomotor disturbances. **White g.**, gangrene from local anemia following complete lymphatic obstruction.

Gan'grenous. Affected with gangrene.

Gar'denin. A compound, $C_{23}H_{30}O_{10}$, from resin of *Gardenia lucida*.

Gar'garism (gar'gar-izm). A gargle; a throat wash.

Gar'gle (gar'gl). A throat wash.

Gar'rot. A variety of tourniquet.

Gärtner's duct (gārt'nerz). Persistent relic of the Wolffian duct.

Gas. An elastic aëriform fluid.

Gas'eous (gaz'e-us). Of the nature of a gas.

Gasomet'ric analysis. Analysis by measuring the gas evolved.

Gasse'rian arteries. Arteries which supply the Gasserian ganglion. See *Ganglion*.

Gasterasthe'nia. Gastric ability.

Gasterhysterot'omy. Cesarean section.

Gastral'gia (gas-tral'je-ah). Pain in the stomach.

Gastrecta'sia, Gastrec'tasis. Dilatation of the stomach.

Gastrec'tomy. Excision of part of stomach.

Gas'tric. Pertaining to the stomach.

Gas'tricism (gas'tris-izm). Dyspepsia; indigestion; gastric disorder.

Gastri'tis. Inflammation of the stomach. **Atrophic g.,** chronic gastritis with atrophy of mucous membrane and glands. **Hypertrophic g.,** gastritis with infiltration and enlargement of the glands. **Phlegmonous g.,** a variety with abscesses in the stomach-walls. **Polypous g.,** hypertrophic g. with polypus-like projections within the viscus. **Pseudomembranous g.,** a variety in which false membrane occurs in patches within the stomach.

Gastro-anastomo'sis. Formation of communication between two pouches of stomach in hour-glass contraction.

Gastrobro'sis. Perforation of the stomach.

Gas'trocele (gas'tro-sēl). Hernia of the stomach.

Gastrocne'mius (gas-trok-ne'me-us). See *Muscles, Table of.*

Gastrocol'ic omentum. Same as *Epiploōn.*

Gastrocoli'tis. Inflammation of the stomach and colon.

Gastrocolos'tomy. Creation of an artificial passage from the stomach to the colon.

Gastrocolot'omy. Incision of stomach and colon.

Gastrocolpot'omy. Incision into the vagina through abdomen.

Gastrodi'aphane (gas-tro-di'af-ān). Electric light for use in gastrodiaphany.

Gastrodiaphanos'copy, Gastrodiaph'any. View of the interior of the stomach through its walls rendered translucent by the gastrodiaphane.

Gastrodid'ymus. A double monster with one abdominal cavity.

Gastroduodeni'tis. Inflammation of stomach and duodenum.

Gastroduodenos'tomy. Creation of an artificial opening between the stomach and duodenum.

Gastrodyn'ia (gas-tro-din'e-ah). Pain in the stomach.

Gastro-elytrot'omy. Same as *Gastrocolpotomy.*

Gastro-enter'ic. Pertaining to stomach and intestines.

Gastro-enteri'tis. Inflammation of stomach and intestines.

Gastro-enteros'tomy. Formation of an artificial passage from stomach to intestine.

Gastro-enterot'omy. Incision of stomach and intestine.

Gastro-epiplo'ic. Pertaining to the stomach and epiploōn.

Gastrogastros'tomy. Same as *Gastro-anastomosis.*

Gas'trograph. Apparatus for registering motions of stomach.

Gastrohelco'sis. Ulceration of the stomach.

Gastrohepat'ic. Pertaining to the stomach and liver.

Gastrohysterec'tomy. Removal of uterus through an abdominal section.

Gastrohysterot'omy. Cesarean section.

Gastro-intes'tinal. Pertaining to stomach and intestine.

Gastrojejunos'tomy. Formation of artificial passage between stomach and jejunum.

Gas'trolith (gas'tro-lith). Calculus or concretion in the stomach.

Gastrolithi'asis. Formation of gastroliths.

Gastrol'ogy (gas-trol'o-je). Treatise on the stomach.

Gastrol'ysis. Operation of loosening stomach from adhesions.

Gastromala'cia (gas-tro-mal-a'she-ah). Softening of the wall of the stomach.

Gastrom'elus. A monster with a leg on the abdomen.

Gastrome'nia. Vicarious menstruation through stomach.

Gastrop'athy (gas-trop'ath-e). Any disease of the stomach.

Gastroperiodyn'ia. Periodic distress in the stomach.

Gastrophren'ic. Pertaining to the stomach and diaphragm.

Gas'troplasty. Plastic operation upon the stomach.

Gastroplica'tion. The reefing and stitching of the stomach-wall.

Gastropto′sis. Abnormal depression of stomach.

Gastropylorec′tomy. Excision of pyloric part of the stomach.

Gastrorrha′gia (gas-tror-ra′je-ah). Hemorrhage from stomach.

Gastror′rhaphy (gas-tror′raf-e). The suturing of the stomach.

Gastrorrhe′a (gas-tror-re′ah). Excessive secretion by stomach.

Gastros′chisis (gas-tros′kis-is). Fissure in wall of abdomen.

Gas′troscope. Instrument used in stomach inspection.

Gastros′copy. Inspection of interior of stomach.

Gastrosplen′ic. Pertaining to stomach and spleen.

Gastrosteno′sis. Contraction of the stomach.

Gastros′tomy. Creation of artificial gastric fistula.

Gastrosuccorrhe′a. Continuous secretion of gastric juice.

Gas′trotome. An instrument used in gastrotomy.

Gastrot′omy (gas-trot′o-me). Incision of abdomen or stomach.

Gastrotubot′omy. Incision of an oviduct through the abdominal wall.

Gastrotympani′tes. Tympanitic distention of the stomach.

Gastrox′ia, Gastroxyn′sis. Periodic hyperacidity of stomach.

Gas′trula (gas-tru-lah). That early embryonic stage which follows the blastula.

Gastrula′tion. Passage of ovum from blastula to gastrula stage.

Gath′ering. Popular name for abscess or swelling.

Gaucher's disease (go-shāz′). Epithelioma of the spleen.

Gaulthe′ria procum′bens. Teaberry or wintergreen: its oil is antiseptic and antirheumatic.

Gaul′therin. A glucosid from the bark of the black birch.

Gauze (gawz). Thin fabric used in surgery; carbasus.

Gavage (gah-vahzh′). Feeding by a stomach-tube.

Gawalow′ski's test (gah-vah-lof′skiz). Test for sugar made by use of ammonium molybdate.

Geiss′ler's test (gīs′lerz). A delicate test for albumin in urine.

Geissosper′min. Poisonous alkaloid, $C_{19}H_{24}N_2O_2 + H_2O$, from *Geissospermum læve*, a tree of tropical America.

Gelan′thum. A glycerin and gelatin vehicle used in skin-diseases.

Gel′atin (jel′at-in). An albuminoid from animal tissues. **G.-culture,** a bacterial preparation with a basis of gelatin. **G.-disk,** a disk of medicated gelatin for eye-treatment. **G.-peptone,** a product of the digestion of gelatin. **G.-sugar.** Same as *Glycocoll*.

Gelatinif′erous (jel-at-in-if′er-us). Producing gelatin.

Gelat′inize (jel-at′in-īz). To convert into a jelly.

Gelatino′sa. Same as *Substantia gelatinosa*.

Gelat′inous (jel-at′in-us). Like jelly or softened gelatin.

Gel′atol (jel′at-ol). Ointment-base consisting of glycerin, gelatin, oil, and water.

Ge′lose (je′lōs). A carbohydrate, $C_6H_{10}O_5$, from agar.

Gelo′sin. Mucilage from a Japanese alga.

Gel′semin (jel′sem-in). A poisonous alkaloid, $C_{22}H_{38}N_2O_4$, from gelsemium.

Gelse′mium. The root of *G. semper′virens*, yellow jessamine: a powerful sedative; poisonous.

Gely's suture. See *Suture*.

Gemel′lus (je-mel′lus). See *Muscles, Table of*.

Gem′inate (jem′in-āt). Paired; in twos.

Gemma′tion (jem-ma′shun). Reproduction by budding.

Gem′mule (jem′ūl). A bud produced by gemmation.

Ge′nal (je′nal). Pertaining to the cheek.

Gen′eral anatomy. Same as *Histology*. **G. paralysis, G. paresis.** See *Paralysis*.

Gen′eralize. To change from a local to a general disease.

Gen'erating plate. That plate in an electric cell which is chemically acted upon.

Genera'tion (jen-er-a'shun). An act of reproduction. **Alternate g.** See *Alternation of generation*. **Asexual g.**, reproduction without the union of sexual elements. **Sexual g.**, reproduction by the union of male and female cells. **Spontaneous g.**, the alleged development of living organisms from lifeless matter; abiogenesis.

Gen'erative (jen'er-a-tiv). Pertaining to reproduction of the species.

Gener'ic (jen-er'ik). Pertaining to a genus; also, distinctive.

Gene'sial, Genes'ic. Pertaining to genesis.

Genesiol'ogy (jen-e-se-ol'o-je). The science of generation.

Gen'esis (jen'es-is). Reproduction; origin.

Genet'ic (jen-et'ik). Pertaining to reproduction.

Gen'etous (jen'et-us). Dating from fetal life.

Ge'nial (je'ne-al). Of, or pertaining to, the chin. **G. tubercles**, four tubercles of lower jaw-bone.

Genic'ulate (jen-ik'u-lāt). Bent like a knee.

Geniohyoglos'sus. See *Muscles, Table of*.

Geniohy'oid (je-ne-o-hi'oid). See *Muscles, Table of*.

Ge'nion (je'ne-on). Apex of lower genial tubercle.

Ge'nioplasty (je'ni-o-plas-te). Plastic surgery of the chin.

Gen'ital (jen'it-al). Pertaining to reproduction.

Genita'lia, Gen'itals. Reproductive organs.

Genitocru'ral. See *Nerves, Table of*.

Genito-u'rinary. Of, or pertaining to, genital and urinary organs.

Gen'tian (jen'shan). Root of *Gentiana lutea*: valuable tonic and stomachic. **G. violet**, a violet stain for use in microscopic work.

Ge'nu (je'nu). The knee; articulation of femur with leg-bones. **G. extror'sum, G. va'rum**, bow-leg; out-knee. **G. intror'sum, G. val'gum**, knock-knee; in-knee. **G. recurva'tum**, backward curvation of the knee-joint.

Gen'uclast (jen'u-klast). An instrument for breaking up knee-joint adhesions.

Genupec'toral posture. Position of a patient on knees and chest.

Genyantri'tis (jen-e-an-tri'tis). Inflammation of the maxillary antrum.

Gen'yplasty (jen'e-plas-te). Plastic surgery of the cheek.

Geograph'ical tongue. Presence on the tongue of denudations bordered by thickened epithelium.

Geoph'agism, Geoph'agy (je-of'aj-izm, je-of'aj-e). Habit of eating clay.

Ge'osote (je'o-sōt). Guaiacol valerianate.

Gera'nium. Rhizome or root of *G. maculatum*: a good astringent.

Ger'dy's fibers (zhăr'dēz). The external web or network which connects clefts on palmar surfaces of fingers.

Ger'lach's network (ger'laks). Fibrillous structures in gray substance of the cord.

Gerlier's disease (zhăr-le-āz'). See *Disease*.

Germ (jerm). 1. A microbe or bacillus. 2. A spore; also, the primitive embryo. **G.-cell**, the primitive stage of a spermatozoon or ovum. **G.-disease**, disease caused by microbes. **G. epithelium, G.-ridge**, epithelial ridge on embryonic mesonephros; from it arise the sexual elements. **G.-plasm**, protoplasm of a germ; also, same as *Id*. **G.-theory**. 1. Doctrine that all organisms are developed from the cell. 2. Theory that infectious diseases are of microbic origin.

Ger'man measles. Same as *Rötheln*.

Germicid'al (jer-mis-i'dal). Destructive to disease-germs.
Ger'micide (jer'mis-īd). An agent that destroys microbes.
Ger'minal (jer'min-al). Pertaining to a germ.
Germina'tion. Sprouting of a seed or plant embryo.
Ger'minative. Same as *Germinal.*
Ger'mol (jer'mol). A proprietary bactericide.
Geromor'phism (jer-o-mor'fizm). Premature old age.
Geron'tin. A leucomain, $C_5H_{14}N_2$, from the nuclei of cells of dog's liver.
Gerontox'on. The arcus senilis.
Gesta'tion (jes-ta'shun). Pregnancy; gravidity.
Ghost corpuscle. Same as *Phantom corpuscle.*
Gi'ant-cell. A large multinuclear cell.
Gi'antism (ji'an-tizm). Same as *Gigantism.*
Gianuz'zi's crescents (jan-noot'sēz). Crescentic cell-masses on the basement membrane of the acini of the mucous glands.
Gibbos'ity (gib-bos'it-e). The condition of being humped.
Gib'bous (gib'bus). Humped; protuberant.
Gid'diness. Same as *Vertigo.*
Gigan'tism. Abnormal overgrowth of the body or of a part.
Gigan'toblast. A very large red corpuscle.
Gimbernat's ligament (zhahm-bār-nahz'). See *Ligament.*
Gin (jin). Alcoholic liquor distilled from malt and juniper berries.
Gin-drinkers' liver. A cirrhotic liver; cirrhosis of liver from alcoholism.
Gin'ger (jin'jer). The rhizoma of *Zingiber officinale*, a carminative and stimulant.
Gin'gerol (jin'jer-ol). The oil of ginger.
Gin'gili oil (jin'jil-le). Same as *Sesame oil.*
Gingi'va (jin-ji'vah). The gum; fleshy structure which covers the alveolar border of the jaw.
Gin'gival (jin'jiv-al). Pertaining to the gums.
Gingivi'tis (jin-jiv-i'tis). Inflammation of the gums.
Ginglymo-arthro'dial. Partly ginglymoid and partly arthrodial.
Gin'glymoid. Hinge-like; resembling ginglymus.
Gin'glymus. A hinge-joint like that of wrist or ankle.
Gin'seng (jin'seng). Root of different species of *Aralia*: stimulant and tonic.
Giraldès's organ (zhe-rahl-dez'). A vestige of the Wolffian body at the back of the testicle.
Gir'dle anesthesia. Ring around the body devoid of sensation. **G.-pain,** painful sensation about the body. **G. sensation,** feeling as of a tight belt about the body.
Glabel'la, Glabel'lum. Space between the eyebrows.
Glabrific'ins (glab-rif-is'inz). Antibodies: so-called because they render the bacteria glabrous.
Gla'cial (gla'se-al). Appearing like ice; vitreous.
Gladi'olin. An alkaloid from brain-tissue.
Gladi'olus. The main piece of the sternum.
Glair'in (glar'in). Gelatinous mass of bacteria in water of sulphur-springs.
Glair'y (glar'e). Resembling white of an egg.
Gland. Organ for separating any fluid from the blood. **Absorbent g.,** any lymphatic gland. **Accessory thyroid g.,** a small exclave of the thyroid gland. **Acinous g.,** a gland made up of several acini. **Aggregate g's.,** Peyer's patches. **Agminated g's.,** the glands of Peyer's patches. **Albuminous g's.,** certain glands of the digestive tract secreting a watery fluid. **Axillary g's.,** lymphatic glands situated in the axilla. **G. of Bartholin,** a minute gland on either side of the vagina; vulvovaginal gland. **Bowman's g's.,** glands in the

olfactory region of the nose. **Bronchial g's.**, lymph-glands at the root of a bronchus. **Bruch's g's.**, lymph-follicles in conjunctiva of lower lid. **Brunner's g's.**, glands in the duodenum. **Ceruminous g's.**, glands which secrete cerumen. **Cervical g's.**, lymph-glands of the neck. **Coccygeal g.**, a vascular body near tip of coccyx. **Compound g.**, a gland made up of various pouches or acini. **Conglobate g.**, a lymphatic gland. **Cowper's g's.**, two glands near bulb of corpus spongiosum. **Ductless g.**, a gland-like organ having no true duct. **Duodenal g's.** See *Brunner's g's.* **Duverney's g's.** See *Bartholin's g's.* **Haversian g's.**, folds on synovial surfaces regarded as secretors of synovial fluid. **Hematopoietic g's.**, glands which take a part in the making of the blood, such as spleen, thyroid, and lymphatic glands. **Intestinal g's., solitary**, isolated lymph-glands distributed in intestinal mucous membrane. **Lacrimal g.**, the gland whose function it is to secrete the tears. **Lieberkuhn's g's.** See *Crypts.* **Littré's g's.**, racemose glands in spongy portion of urethra. **Luschka's g.** See *Coccygeal g.* **Lymphatic g's.**, ductless organs in the course of lymphatic vessels. **Mammary g.**, the mamma; the milk-secreting organ. **Meibomian g's.**, sebaceous follicles between the cartilage and conjunctiva of eyelids. **Moll's g's.**, small glands of the eyelid. **Montgomery's g's.**, sebaceous glands in the mammary areola. **Morgagni's g's.** Same as *Littré's g's.* **Muciparous g's.**, **Mucous g's.**, glands which secrete mucus. **Pacchionian g's.** See *Pacchionian bodies.* **Parotid g.**, the large salivary gland in front of the ear. **Peyer's g's.**, lymphatic glands, chiefly in the ileum, partly solitary and partly in patches. **Pineal g.** See *Pineal body.* **Pituitary g.** See *Pituitary body.* **Prostate g.** See *Prostate.* **Pyloric g's.**, the pepsin-secreting glands of the stomach situated near the pylorus. **Racemose g.** Same as *Acinous g's.* **Rivini's g.** See *Sublingual g.* **Salivary g.**, any gland that secretes saliva, as the parotid, submaxillary, or sublingual. **Serous g's.** Same as *Albuminous g's.* **Sublingual g.**, a salivary gland on either side under the tongue. **Submaxillary g.**, a salivary gland on either side under the tongue. **Sudoriparous g's.**, **Sweat g's.**, glands of the skin which excrete sweat. **Thymus g.** See *Thymus.* **Thyroid g.** See *Thyroid body.* **Tubular g's.** Same as *Follicle.* **Tubular g., compound**, one made up of a number of tubules with only one duct. **Urethral g's.** See *Littré's g's.* **Vaginal g.**, any gland of vaginal mucous membrane. **Vulvovaginal g's.** See *Bartholin's g's.*

Glan'ders. Contagious horse-disease, communicable to man.

Glandilem'ma. Capsule or outer envelop of a gland.

Glan'dula (glan'du-lah). A small gland.

Glan'dular. Pertaining to a gland.

Glan'dule (glan'dūl). A small gland.

Glan'dulin. A therapeutic preparation of gland-tissue.

Glans. L. for *Gland.* **G. clito'ridis**, distal end of clitoris. **G. pe'nis**, head of penis.

Glase'rian artery. Branch of internal maxillary: goes to tympanum. **G. fissure.** See *Fissure.*

Glas'sy. Hyaline; vitreous; like glass.

Glau'ber's salt (glaw'berz). Sodium sulphate; a purgative.

Glauco'ma. Excessive pressure within the eye, causing hardness of the eye and blindness.

Glaucom'atous. Of the nature of glaucoma.

Gleet. Chronic gonorrheal urethritis.

Glenard's disease (gla-nahrz'). Same as *Enteroptosis.*

Glenohu'meral ligaments. See *Ligaments.*

Gle'noid. Resembling a pit or socket. **G. cavity.** See *Cavity.*
Gli'a cells (gli'ah). See *Deiters's cells.*
Gli'adin. Tough proteid from wheat gluten.
Gliococ'cus. Micrococcus forming gelatinous matter.
Glio'ma. Malignant sarcoma of a structure like neuroglia.
Gliomato'sis. Over-development of neuroglia in spinal canal.
Gliomyo'ma. Glioma blended with myxoma.
Glioneuro'ma. Glioma with neuromatous elements.
Gliosarco'ma. Glioma combined with sarcoma.
Glisso'nian cirrhosis. Perihepatitis.
Glis'son's capsule. See *Capsule.*
Glo'bin. A proteid from hemoglobin.
Glob'ular (glob'u-lar). Like a globe or globule; spherical.
Glob'ule (glob'ūl). A small spherical mass.
Globulici'dal. Destroying the blood-corpuscles.
Glob'ulin (glob'u-lin). A proteid from the lens; any proteid of the group of which it is the type.
Globulinu'ria. Presence of a globulin or globulins in the urine.
Glob'ulose (glob'u-lōs). A product of the digestion of globulins.
Glo'bus (glo'bus). L. for sphere or ball. **G. hyster'icus,** subjective sensation of choking; lump in the throat. **G. ma'jor,** the head of the epididymis. **G. mi'nor,** distal end of epididymis. **G. pal'lidus,** pale interior of the lenticular nucleus.
Glom'erate. Crowded together in a ball.
Glomer'ular. Formed into a glomerulus.
Glomeruli'tis. Inflammation of glomeruli of kidney.
Glomerulonephri'tis. Same as *Glomerulitis.*
Glomer'ulus, Glom'erule. Any cluster of vascular tufts in Malpighian body of kidney.
Glono'in (glo-no'in). Same as *Nitroglycerin.*
Glos'sal. Of, or pertaining to, the tongue.
Glossal'gia (glos-sal'je-ah). Pain in the tongue.
Glossec'tomy (glos-ek'to-me). Surgical removal of the tongue.
Glossi'tis (glos-i'tis). Inflammation of the tongue.
Glos'socele (glos'o-sēl). Swelling and protrusion of the tongue.
Glosso-epiglottid'ean. Pertaining to the tongue and epiglottis.
Glos'sograph. Apparatus for registering tongue-movements in speech.
Glossohy'al. Pertaining to tongue and hyoid bone.
Glossol'ogy (glos-sol'o-je). 1. Sum of knowledge regarding the tongue. 2. Treatise on nomenclature.
Glossol'ysis (glos-ol'is-is). Paralysis of tongue.
Glossop'athy (glos-sop'ath-e). Diseased state of the tongue.
Glossopharyn'geal. Pertaining to tongue and pharynx. See also *Nerves, Table of.*
Glossophyt'ia (glos-so-fit'e-ah). Dark and foul tongue from the presence of microphytes.
Glos'soplasty (glos'o-plas-te). Plastic surgery of the tongue.
Glossople'gia (glos-so-ple'je-ah). Paralysis of tongue.
Glos'sospasm (glos'so-spazm). Spasm of tongue muscles.
Glossot'omy. Incision or excision of the tongue.
Gloss'y skin. Shining smoothness of skin from nerve-lesion.
Glot'tis. Aperture or chink between the vocal cords.
Glov'er's suture (gluv'erz). A form of continuous surgical suture.
Glucohe'mia. Presence of sugar in the blood.
Glu'cose (glu'kōs). Grape-sugar, $C_6H_{12}O_6$, from honey, fruit, etc.: commercially prepared from maize; found in the animal body.
Glu'cosid (glu'ko-sid). Any vegetable principle decomposable into glucose and another principle.
Glu'cosin. Any one of a group of bases derived from glucose by action of ammonia.
Glucosu'ria. Sugar in the urine in an abnormally high proportion.

Glue-like tumor. Glioma; also, colloma.
Glu'ge's corpuscles. See *Corpuscle.*
Glutæ'us (gloo-te'us). See *Muscles, Table of.*
Glutam'ic acid. Derivative, $C_5H_9NO_4$, from proteid decomposition.
Glutam'in. A principle, $C_5H_{10}N_2O_3$, from juices of many plants.
Glutar'ic acid. Pyrotartaric acid, $C_5H_8O_4$; it exists in decomposing pus.
Glu'teal. Pertaining to the buttocks.
Glu'ten (glu'ten). Glue-like principle of various grains.
Glu'tin. The viscid constituent of wheat-gluten.
Glu'tinous (glu'tin-us). Adhesive; sticky.
Gluti'tis. Inflammation of glutei muscles.
Glu'toform. A gelatin and formaldehyd compound.
Glu'tol. Commercial name of formalin-gelatin, used for antiseptic wound-dressing.
Glycæ'mia (gli-se'me-ah). Presence of glucose or sugar in the blood.
Glyc'erid (glis'er-id). Glycerin compounded with an acid.
Glyc'erin (glis'er-in). Syrupy liquid, $C_3H_8O_3$, from oils and fats. **G.-jelly**, compound of glycerin and gelatin.
Gly'cerite (glis'er-it). Medicated preparation of glycerin.
Glycerophos'phate. A combination of a base with glycerin and phosphoric acid.
Gly'ceryl (glis'er-il). The radical, C_3H_5, of glycerin.
Gly'cin, Glyco'sin (gli'sin, gli-ko'sin). Same as *Glycocoll.*
Gly'cocoll (gli'ko-kol). Gelatin sugar; also, any substance of its group.
Glycocoll'ic acid. See *Acid.*
Gly'cogen (gli'ko-jen). A carbohydrate, $C_6H_{10}O_5$, from liver and other tissues.
Glycogen'esis (gli-ko-jen'es-is). Production of sugar or glycogen.
Glycohe'mia (gli-ko-he'me-ah). Presence of sugar in the blood.
Gly'col (gli'kol). Any diatomic alcohol.
Glycolyt'ic ferment. A sugar-digesting ferment.
Gly'conin. Preparation of glycerin with yolk of eggs.
Glycorrhe'a. Any sugary discharge from the body.
Glycosol'vol (gli-ko-sol'vol). Same as *Antidiabeticum.*
Glycosu'ria (gli-ko-su're-ah). Same as *Glucosuria.*
Glycosu'ric acid. Acid sometimes found in urine.
Gly'cozone (gli'ko-zōn). A proprietary ozone and hydrogen peroxid preparation.
Glycuron'ic acid. See *Acid.*
Glycyrrhi'za (glis-ir-ri'zah). Same as *Liquorice.*
Glycyrrhi'zin. A principle, $C_{24}H_{36}O_9$, from liquorice.
Glyp'tic formula (glip'tik). A formula intended to represent actual arrangement of atoms.
Gm. Abbreviation for gram.
Gna'thic index (na'thik). See *Index.*
Gna'thion (na'the-on). Lowest point of median line of lower jaw.
Gnathi'tis (na-thi'tis). Inflammation of the jaw.
Gnathoceph'alus. Headless monster with jaws.
Gna'thoplasty (na'tho-plas-te). Plastic surgery of jaws or cheek.
Go'a powder. Powder from wood of *Andira araroba:* it affords chrysarobin.
Goat-leap pulse. Same as *Caprizant pulse.*
Gob'let-cells. Mucous epithelial cells of goblet-shape.
Gog'gle-eye. Abnormally protruding eye.
Gog'gles. Spectacles with wire screens for the eye.
Goi'ter, Goi'tre (goi'ter). Great enlargement of thyroid gland. See also *Exophthalmic goiter.*
Gold. Heavy yellow metal: several of its salts are medicinal.

Gold-beaters' skin. Prepared cecum of the ox: used in surgery.
Gol'den seal. See *Hydrastis.*
Gold-thread. Same as *Coptis.*
Goll's column or **tract** (golz). See *Column.*
Gomphi'asis. Looseness of the teeth.
Gompho'sis. Articulation in which a spike of bone fits into a bony socket.
Gon'ad (gon'ad). A reproductive gland.
Gonag'ra (gon-ag'rah). Gouty seizure of the knee.
Gonarthri'tis. Inflammation of the knee-joint.
Gonarthroc'ace (gon-ar-throk'as-e). White swelling of the knee.
Gonarthrot'omy. Incision into the knee-joint.
Gon'ecyst, Gonecys'tis. A seminal vesicle.
Gonecysti'tis. Inflammation of a gonecyst.
Gonei'tis (go-ne-i'tis). Inflammation of the knee.
Gonepoie'sis. The secretion of the semen.
Goniom'eter. An instrument for measuring angles.
Go'nion (go'ne-on). Tip of angle of lower jaw.
Gonococ'cus. The coccus of gonorrhea, a product of *Micrococcus gonorrhœæ*, a schizomycete.
Gonohe'mia (go-no-he'me-ah). General gonorrheal infection.
Gonopep'sin. A proprietary gonorrheal remedy.
Gonorrhe'a. Contagious catarrhal inflammation of the genital mucous membrane.
Gonorrhe'al. Pertaining to gonorrhea. **G. arthritis, G. rheumatism.** See *Arthritis.*
Gon'yocele (gon'i-o-sēl). Synovitis, or tuberculous arthritis, of the knee.
Goose-flesh. Same as *Cutis anserina.*
Gor'get (gor'jet). Wide-grooved lithotomy director.
Gossyp'ium (gos-sip'e-um). 1. Cotton. 2. Cotton-root bark.
Gouge (gowj). An instrument for cutting bone.
Gou'lard's cerate (goo'larz). Cerate of subacetate of lead. **G. extract,** solution of subacetate of lead.
Gout (gowt). Painful constitutional disease with joint inflammation and chalky deposits. **Latent g., Masked g.,** lithemia without the typical features of gout. **Misplaced g., Retrocedent g.,** gout in which the arthritic symptoms have disappeared and are followed by severe constitutional disturbances. **Poor man's g.,** gout ascribed to hard work, exposure, ill-feeding, and excess in the use of malt liquors.
Gout'y. Of the nature of, or affected by, gout. **G. diathesis,** predisposition to gout.
Gow'ers's tract (gow'erz-iz). Ascending anterior lateral tract of the spinal cord.
Gr. Abbreviation for grain.
Graaf'ian vesicles or **follicles** (grah'fe-an). Spherical ovarian bodies each containing an ovum.
Gra'cile (gras'il). Slender; delicate. **G. fasciculus, G. funiculus.** See *Fasciculus gracilis.* **G. nucleus.** Same as *Nucleus gracilis.*
Gra'cilis (gras'il-is). See *Muscles, Table of.*
Grada'tim. Gradually.
Grad'uate (grad'u-āt). 1. A measuring vessel marked by a series of lines. 2. Person who has received a college degree.
Grad'uated. Marked by a succession of lines. **G. tenotomy,** incomplete division of the tendon of an eye-muscle.
Graft. A slip of skin or other tissue for transplantation.
Grain. 1. Seed of a cereal plant. 2. Twentieth part of a scruple; or 0.065 of a gram.
Gram. Metric weight, equal to 15.434 grains.

Gram's solution. One part iodin, 2 of potassium iodid, 300 parts water; used as a stain.
Granato'nin. Same as *Pseudopelletierin.*
Grana'tum. Same as *Pomegranate.*
Gran'cher's disease. See *Splenopneumonia.*
Gran'dry's corpuscles. Tactile corpuscles in birds.
Gran'ular. Made up of, or marked by, granules or grains.
Granula'tion. Formation in wounds of rounded flesh masses; also, a mass so formed.
Gran'ule. 1. A small rounded body. 2. A medicinal pellet. **G. layer.** 1. One of the layers of the retina. 2. Layer next to cortical layer of cerebellum.
Granulo'ma. A tumor of granulation tissue.
Gran'ulose. The more soluble portion of starch.
Gra'num. L. for *Grain.*
Grape cure. Treatment by eating grapes. **G.-sugar.** See *Glucose.*
Graph'ite (graf'īt). A form of carbon.
Graphol'ogy (graf-ol'o-je). The study of handwriting in diagnosis of nerve-disease.
Graph'ospasm. Writers' cramp; spasm from overuse of hand.
Grattage (grah-tahzh'). Removal of granulations by friction with a stiff brush.
Grave. Serious; severe. **G.-wax.** Same as *Adipocere.*
Grave'do. Coryza, or nasal catarrh.
Grav'el. Minor concretions in kidney or bladder.
Graves's disease (grāvz). Exophthalmic goiter.
Grav'id (grav'id). Pregnant; with child.
Grav'idin. A substance from urine of pregnant women; kyestein.
Gravimet'ric. Performed by weight and measure.
Gravita'tion. Force tending to draw all bodies together.
Grav'ity. Weight; tendency toward the center of the earth.
Gray atrophy, or degeneration. See *Atrophy.*
Green-blindness. Lack of perception of green tints. **G. sickness.** See *Chlorosis.* **G. softening,** abscess of brain with greenish pus. **G. vitriol,** ferrous sulphate; copperas.
Green'stick fracture. See *Fracture.*
Gref'fotome. An instrument for cutting grafts of skin, nerve substance, etc.
Gregari'na. A genus of protozoans: parasitic in invertebrates.
Greg'ory's powder. Compound powder of rhubarb with magnesia and ginger.
Griffe des orteils (grēf-da-zor-ta'e). Same as *Claw-foot.*
Grif'fith's mixture. Compound iron mixture.
Grinde'lia robus'ta. A plant: antispasmodic and used in bronchitis and asthma.
Grind'ers (grind'erz). The molar teeth.
Grind'ers' disease. A lung-disease in tool-grinders, due to dust inhalation.
Grip, Grippe. Same as *Influenza.*
Grippotox'in (grip-po-tox'in). The toxin of influenza.
Gro'cer's itch. Eczema of the hands, peculiar to grocers.
Groin. Lower lateral part of the abdominal wall.
Gross anatomy. Macroscopic anatomy of the tissues. **G. appearances,** appearance of a tissue as seen without the microscope.
Ground'-bundle. Either portion of the anterolateral tract of spinal cord.
Grow'ing-pains. Neuralgic or rheumatic pains of young persons.
Gru'el. A decoction of any cereal grain.
Gru'mous (gru'mus). Lumpy or clotted.
Gru'tum (gru'tum). See *Milium.*

Gry'ochrome. A nerve-cell the stainable portion of which consists of minute granules.

Gtt. Abbreviation of *Gutta*, a drop.

Guachama'ca (gwah-chah-mah'kah). A South American plant, *Malouclia nitida;* poisonous.

Gua'co (gwah'ko). The South American plant *Mikania guaco:* teniacidal and febrifugal.

Guai'ac (gwi'yak). Resin from *Guiacum officinale:* alterative, stimulant.

Guaiac'etin (gwi-as'et-in). A derivative of guaiacol used in treating phthisis.

Guai'acol (gwi'ak-ol). Oil-like substance, $C_7H_8O_2$: used in phthisis.

Guai'acum wood (gwi'ak-um). Wood of *G. officinale:* diaphoretic stimulant.

Gua'nin (gwah'nin). Leucomain from guano and other sources.

Gua'no (gwah'no). Dung of sea-fowl; useful in skin-diseases.

Guara'na (gwah-rah'nah). Paste from seeds of *Paullinia cupana;* nerve-stimulant.

Guard-cells. See *Cell.*

Gubernac'ulum tes'tis. Fetal cord between epididymis and bottom of scrotum.

Gub'ler's line (goob'lerz). Line which connects points of origin of fifth nerve. **G.'s paralysis.** Same as *Crossed hemiplegia.* **G.'s tumor,** a swelling on back of wrist in lead-poisoning.

Gud'den's com'missure (gud'denz). Upper and inner fibers of optic tract. Same as *Arcuate commissure.*

Guil'lotine (gil'lo-tēn). Instrument for cutting of the tonsil, etc.

Guin'ea worm (gin'ne). A tropical worm, *Filaria medinensis,* burrowing in the human body.

Gull'et (gul'let). The esophagus; also the pharynx.

Gum. 1. Mucilaginous excretion of various plants. 2. See *Gingiva.* **G. arabic.** See *Acacia.* **Bassora g.,** gum resembling gum arabic from Persia. **British g.,** dextrin. **G. res'in,** concrete vegetable juices, often medicinal. **G. tragacanth.** Same as *Tragacanth.* **G.-boil.** Same as *Parulis.*

Gum'ma. A soft gummy tumor in tertiary syphilis.

Gum'matous (gum'at-us). Of the nature of gumma.

Gum'mi. L. for the *gum of plants.*

Gum'my (gum'e). Resembling gum or gumma.

Gums. See *Gingiva.*

Gun-cotton. See *Pyroxylin.*

Gun-stock deformity. Deformity in which the forearm forms an angle owing to fracture of either condyle of the humerus.

Gur'jun balsam (goor'jun). Oleoresin from *Dipterocarpus lævis,* a tree of Asia: used in gonorrhea and leprosy.

Gus'tatory (gus'tat-o-re). Pertaining to taste.

Gut. The bowel or intestine.

Gut'ta. L. for *Drop.* **G. per'cha,** concrete juice of *Isonandra gutta,* a tree of the East Indies. **G. rosa'cea.** Same as *Acne rosacea.* **G. sere'na,** amaurosis.

Gutta'tim. Drop by drop.

Gut'tur. L. for *Throat.*

Gut'tural (gut'er-al). Pertaining to the throat.

Gutturotet'any. Spasm of the throat with resultant stammer.

Guy'on's sign (ghe-ongz'). Ballottement of floating kidney.

Gymnas'tics (jim-nas'tix). Systematic muscular exercise.

Gymne'mic acid (jim-ne'mik). A principle from *Gymnema palustre,* a shrub of South Asia: it temporarily suspends the sense of taste.

Gym'nocyte (jim'no-sit). A cell with no cell-wall.

Gynan'drism (jin-an'drizm). Hermaphroditism.

Gynatre'sia (jin-at-re'zhe-ah). Imperforate condition of vagina.

Gynecolog'ic, Gynecolog'ical. Pertaining to gynecology.
Gynecol'ogist. Person skilled in gynecology.
Gynecol'ogy (jin-e-kol'o-je). Sum of knowledge of women's diseases.
Gynecomas'tia. Large size of male mammary glands.
Gynepho'bia (jin-e-fo'be-ah). Dread of, or aversion to, society of women.
Gynocar'dia. See *Chaulmugra*.
Gynoplas'tics (jin-o-plas'tix). Plastic surgery of female genitalia.
Gyp'sum (jip'sum). Plaster of Paris; calcium sulphate.
Gyra'tion (ji-ra'shun). Revolving in a circle.
Gyre (jir). Same as *Gyrus*.
Gy'ri (ji'ri). The pl. of *gyrus*.
Gy'romele (ji'ro-mēl). Flexible catheter tipped with sponge.
Gyro'sa (ji-ro'sah). Gastric vertigo in which everything seems to turn round.
Gy'rospasm (ji'ro-spazm). Rotatory spasm of the head.
Gy'rus (ji'rus), pl. *gy'ri*. A convolution of the brain. **G. fornica'tus,** the gyre which makes an arch above the corpus callosum.

H.

H. Symbol of *Hydrogen*.
Habe'na (ha-be'nah). The peduncle of the pineal gland.
Haben'ula. Any frenum (a series of structures in the cochlea are especially known as habenulæ).
Hab'it. 1. A fixed or constant practice established by frequent repetition. 2. Predisposition; bodily temperament. **H.-chorea, H.-spasm,** spasmodic movements which are frequent and seem to be involuntary.
Hab'itat. Natural abode or home of an animal or plant species.
Habit'ual abortion. See under *Abortion*.
Habroma'nia. Insanity with excessive gaiety.
Hachement (ahsh-maw'). See *Hacking*.
Hack'ing. Chopping stroke in massage. **H. cough,** a short, frequent, and feeble cough.
Hæ-. For words thus beginning see *He-*.
Hair. The filamentous outgrowth found mainly upon the scalp. **H.-bulb,** the bulbous expansion at lower end of a hair-root. **H.-cell,** an epithelial cell with hair-like processes or cilia. **H.-follicle,** a depression in the skin which contains a hair-root. **H.-papilla,** a point of corium projecting into a hair-bulb.
Hairy heart. A heart covered with a shaggy exudation. **H. tongue,** one whose papillæ have a hair-like look.
Halistere'sis. Deficiency of mineral salts in a part, as bone.
Hal'itus. An exhalation; an expired breath.
Hal'ler's acid elixir. Sulphuric acid mixture. **H.'s circles,** arterial and venous circles within the eye.
Hall's disease (hawlz). Spurious hydrocephalus.
Hallucina'tion. A sense-perception not founded on an objective reality.
Hal'lus, Hal'lux. The great toe. **H. val'gus,** displacement of the hallux toward the other toes. **H. va'rus,** displacement of hallux away from the other toes.
Ha'lo glaucomato'sus. A whitish ring around the optic disk in glaucoma.
Ha'logen (ha'lo-jen). Any element capable of forming haloid salts; such as chlorin, iodin, bromin, and fluorin.
Ha'lo-symptom. Seeing of colored rings around lights; a symptom of incipient glaucoma.

Ha'loid salt. Any binary compound formed on the type of common salt.
Hal'stern's disease. Epidemic or endemic syphilis.
Ham. 1. The popliteal region. 2. The hip and buttock.
Hamame'lis virginia'na. The witch-hazel: astringent, sedative, and tonic.
Ham'mer-toe. The claw-like bending of the toe.
Ham'string. Either one of the tendons which laterally bound the popliteal space. **Inner h.,** tendons of gracilis, sartorius, and two other muscles. **Outer h.,** tendon of biceps flexor femoris.
Ham'ular. Shaped like a hook.
Ham'ulus. Any hook-shaped process.
Hand-elec'trode. An electrode to be held in the hand.
Hang'ing-drop culture. A bacterial culture made by inoculating a drop of bouillon under a cover-glass.
Hang'-nail. The splitting of epidermis at the side of a finger-nail.
Hanot's disease. Hypertrophic cirrhosis of liver with icterus.
Haphalge'sia (haf-al-je'ze-ah). Pain on touching objects.
Haphepho'bia (haf-ef-o'be-ah). Morbid fear of touching or being touched.
Hap'loscope (hap'lo-skōp). A form of stereoscope.
Hard chancre. True syphilitic chancre.
Hare'lip. Congenitally cleft lip. **H. suture.** Same as *Twisted suture.*
Har'lequin fetus. Child born with ichthyosis.
Harmo'nia, Har'mony. Form of suture in which the articulating surfaces are nearly smooth.
Har'rison's groove. Groove on the thorax caused by the contraction of the diaphragm.
Harts'horn. 1. Horn of the stag. 2. Popular name of ammonia.
Hä'ser's for'mula (ha'serz). Same as *Trapp's formula.*
Hashish', Hasheesh'. Stalks and leaves of *Cannabis indica.*
Has'ner's valve. Membranous fold at the nasal orifice of the nasolacrimal duct.
Has'sal's corpuscles. Nucleated cells in the thymus.
Hat'ter's disease. Mercurial poisoning or lung-disease in hatters.
Haunch-bone. The ilium.
Haus'tus. L. for *Draft.* **H. ni'ger,** black draught; compound infusion of senna.
Haut-mal (ō-mahl). Epileptic attack in its full development.
Haver'sian canals. Anastomosing canals in bony tissue. **H. canaliculi,** system of minute passages connected with a h. canal. **H. glands,** synovial folds within the joints.
Hawk. To clear the throat of mucus.
Hay fever, H. asthma. Acute annually recurrent conjunctivitis with nasal catarrh.
Hay'garth's deformities or **nodosities.** Knobs on joints in arthritis deformans.
Ha'zelin (ha'zel-in). Proprietary extract of witch-hazel.
H. D. Abbreviation for hearing distance.
Head. That part of the organism which contains the brain and the organs of special sense. **H.-drop,** malarial disease of Japan, with drooping of head. **H.-fold,** fold of blastoderm at cephalic end of young embryo. **H.-gut.** Same as *Foregut.* **H. kidney.** Same as *Pronephros.* **H.-lock,** hooking together of chins in twin labor. **H.-louse.** Same as *Pediculus capitis.*
Head'ache (hed'āk). Pain in the head; cephalalgia.
Hea'ling (he'ling). The process of cure; restoration of wounded parts. **H. by first intention,** union which leaves no scar. **H. by second intention,** union by adhesion of granulating

surfaces. **H. by third intention,** union by filling of wound with granulations.

Health (helth). Normal condition of body and mind.

Health'y pus. Same as *Laudable pus.* **H. ulcer,** ulcer that has a tendency to heal.

Hear'ing distance. Utmost distance at which a given sound can be heard.

Heart (hart). Muscular viscus which maintains the circulation of the blood. **H.-clot,** blood-clot within the heart. **Fibroid h.,** heart affected with fibroid degeneration.

Heart'burn. Burning sensation in the esophagus; cardialgia.

Heat (hēt). A form of kinetic energy communicable from one body to another, and appreciable by the thermal sense. **Atomic h.,** the specific heat of an atom of any element. **H.-centers,** centers in brain which regulate heat-production and heat-elimination. **Latent h.,** heat which a body may absorb without changing its temperature. **Molecular h.,** the product of the molecular weight of a substance multiplied by its specific heat. **Prickly h.** See *Lichen tropicus.* **Specific h.,** amount of heat needed to raise the unit volume of any substance through one degree centigrade. **H.-stroke,** insolation; sunstroke or thermic fever. **H.-unit.** Same as *Calory.*

Hebephre'nia. Mental disturbance at the period of puberty.

Heb'erden's asthma. Same as *Angina pectoris.* **H.'s nodes,** nodosities at sides of distal phalanges of fingers.

Heb'etude (heb'et-ūd). Mental dulness.

Hec'tic fever. See *Fever.* **H. flush,** flush of face in wasting diseases.

Hec'togram, Hec'toliter, Hec'tometer. One hundred grams, liters, or meters.

Hedeo'ma pulegioi'des. American pennyroyal: emmenagogue and stimulant.

Hedge'hog crys'tals. Spiny growth of uric acid.

Hed'rocele (hed'ro-sēl). Anal hernia; anal prolapse.

Heel'bone. Same as *Calcaneum.*

Heid'enhain's demilunes (hī'den-hīnz). Same as *Giannuzzi's crescents.* **H.'s rods,** rod-like epithelial striations in tubules of kidney.

Heis'ter's valves (hīs'terz). Folds within the neck and duct of gall-bladder.

Hel'coid (hel'koid). Like an ulcer.

Helcol'ogy (hel-kol'o-je). The science of ulcers.

Hel'coplasty (hel'ko-plas-te). Plastic surgery of ulcers.

Hel'enin (hel'en-in). A principle, C_6H_8O, from elecampane; also, a proprietary derivative from the same: antiseptic.

Hel'icine (hel'is-in). Spiral. **H. arteries,** spiral arteries of the penis.

Hel'icoid (hel'ik-oid). Coiled; spiral.

Helico'sis. The formation of an ulcer.

Helicotre'ma. A foramen between the scala tympani and scala vestibuli.

Heliopho'bia. Morbid fear of sunlight.

Heliother'apy (he-le-o-ther'ap-e). The sun-cure.

He'lium (he'le-um). A gaseous element from the atmosphere.

He'lix (he'lix). The margin of the external ear.

Hel'lebore. Root of *Helleborus niger;* cathartic and emmenagogue.

Heller's test. A test for albumin and blood in urine.

Helm'holtz's ligament. Part of anterior ligament of malleus. **H.'s line.** See *Line.*

Hel'minth. An intestinal worm or worm-like parasite.

Helminth'agogue (hel-minth'ag-og). Same as *Vermifuge.*

Helminthi'asis, Helmin'thism. Morbid state due to infestation with worms.

Helmin'thic. Anthelmintic; vermifugal.

Helminthol'ogy. Sum of knowledge of endoparasitic worms.

Hemabarom'eter. Instrument for ascertaining specific gravity of blood.

Hem'achrome. The red coloring-matter of blood.

Hemachro'sis. Abnormal red coloration of blood.

Hemacy'anin (hem-as-i'an-in). Same as *Hematocyanin.*

Hemacytom'eter. Device used in counting blood-corpuscles.

He'mad (he'mad). Toward the ventral or hemal side.

Hemadromom'eter. See *Hæmodromeler.*

Hemadynam'eter. Instrument for measurement of blood-pressure.

Hemafa'cient. An agent producing blood.

Hem'agogue (hem'a-gog). Promoting the flow of blood.

He'mal (he'mal). Pertaining to blood or blood-vessels. **H. arch,** arch made up of bodies of vertebræ, ribs, and sternum. **H. spine,** sternum and linea alba together.

Hemalbu'min. Albuminate of iron; used as a remedy.

Hemangio-endothelio'ma. A new growth of the endothelium of the capillary vessels.

Hemangio'ma. True angioma.

Hemangiosarco'ma. Same as *Angiosarcoma.*

Hemaphe'in (hem-af-e'in). Brown coloring-matter of blood.

Hemapoie'sis (hem-ap-oi-e'sis). The formation of blood.

Hemapoiet'ic. Same as *Hematopoietic.*

Hemapoph'ysis (hem-ap-of'is-is). A costal cartilage.

Hemarthro'sis. Presence of blood in a joint-cavity.

Hematachom'eter (hem-at-ak-om'e-ter). Instrument for measuring speed of blood-currents.

Hematem'esis (hem-at-em'es-is). The vomiting of blood.

Hematenceph'alon. Effusion of blood in the brain.

Hemather'mous. Warm-blooded; having warm blood.

Hemat'ic (he-mat'ik). Pertaining to the blood.

Hematidro'sis. The excretion of bloody sweat.

Hematom'eter. Device for counting blood-corpuscles.

Hema'tin. A principle from hemoglobin.

Hematin'ic (hem-at-in'ik). Same as *Hematic.*

Hematinom'eter. Instrument used in measuring the hemoglobin of the blood.

Hematinu'ria. Coloration of urine by hematin.

Hemato'bium. Any organism that lives in the blood.

Hem'atoblast. Cell which develops into a red blood-corpuscle.

Hemat'ocele (he-mat'o-sēl). Effusion of blood into a cavity, as the tunica vaginalis testis.

Hematoceph'alus. Fetus born with head distended with blood.

Hematochylu'ria. Discharge of blood and chyle with the urine.

Hematocol'pus. Accumulation of blood in vagina.

Hem'atocrite. Centrifuge for separating corpuscles from blood.

Hematocry'al (hem-at-o-kri'al). Having cold blood.

Hematocrys'tallin (hem-at-o-kris'tal-in). Same as *Hemoglobin.*

Hematocy'anin. Blue coloring-matter of octopus blood.

Hem'atocyst (hem'at-o-sist). Effusion of blood in the bladder or in a cyst.

Hem'atocyte (hem'at-o-sit). Any blood-corpuscle.

Hematocytom'eter. Same as *Hematimeter.*

Hemat'ogen (hem-at'o-jen). A preparation of egg-albumen.

Hematogen'esis (hem-at-o-jen'es-is). The formation of blood.

Hematogen'ic, Hemato'genous (hem-at-od'jen-us). 1. Produced in the blood. 2. Producing blood.

Hematoglob'ulin. Same as *Hemoglobulin.*
Hematohidro'sis. Same as *Hemohidrosis.*
Hem'atoid (hem'at-oid). Like blood; bloody.
Hematoid'in. A reddish principle from blood-clots.
Hematokol'pos. See *Hematocolpus.*
Hem'atokrit (hem'at-o-krit). See *Hematocrite.*
Hematol'ogy. Sum of what is known regarding the blood.
Hematol'ysis. Disintegration and degeneration of the blood.
Hematolyt'ic. Pertaining to hematolysis.
Hemato'ma. Tumor containing effused blood. **H. au'ris,** blood-tumor in the perichondrium of the ear.
Hematomediasti'num. Effusion of blood in the mediastinum.
Hematom'eter. A hemometer; also, hemadynamometer.
Hematome'tra. Accumulation of blood in the uterus.
Hematomphal'ocele. Umbilical hernia containing blood.
Hematomye'lia. Blood effusion in spinal cord.
Hematomyeli'tis. Acute myelitis with bloody effusion.
Hematopericar'dium. Blood effusion in pericardium.
Hematoph'agous (hem-a-tof'ag-us). Subsisting on blood.
Hematophil'ia (hem-at-of-il'e-ah). Same as *Hemophilia.*
Hem'atophyte (hem'at-o-fit). Vegetable parasite in blood.
Hematoplas'tic. Concerned in the elaboration of blood.
Hematopoie'sis. Formation of blood or blood-corpuscles.
Hematopoiet'ic. Making, or regenerating, the blood.
Hematopor'phyrin. Hematin without its iron.
Hematoporphyrinu'ria. Presence of hematoporphyrin in urine: due to unwise use of sulphonal.
Hematopo'sia (hem-a-to-po'ze-ah). Blood-drinking.
Hemator'rhachis, Hemor'rhachis (hem-a-tor'ra-kis, hem-or'ra-kis). Hemorrhage into the spinal membranes.
Hematorrhe'a (hem-at-o-re'ah). Free or copious hemorrhage.
Hematosal'pinx. Collection of blood in oviduct.
Hematos'cheocele. Hematoma of the scrotum.
Hem'atoscope (hem'at-os-kōp). Device used in examining thin layers of blood.
Hematos'copy (hem-at-os'ko-pe). The inspection of blood.
Hematosep'sis (hem-at-o-sep'sis). Same as *Septicemia.*
Hemato'sin (hem-at-o'sin). Same as *Hematin.*
Hemato'sis. The formation or aeration of the blood.
Hematospec'troscope. Spectroscope for examining the blood.
Hematospectros'copy. Use of the hematospectroscope.
Hematosper'mia. Presence of blood in the semen.
Hematother'mal. Having warm blood; hemathermous.
Hematotho'rax. Same as *Hemothorax.*
Hematotox'ic. Pertaining to blood-poisoning.
Hematotym'panum. Hemorrhagic exudation in the drum-cavity.
Hematox'ylin (hem-at-ox'il-in). A stain from logwood.
Hematox'ylon campechia'num. Logwood; a tree and its astringent wood.
Hematozo'on (hem-at-o-zo'on). Animal that lives in the blood.
Hematu'ria (hem-at-u're-ah). Discharge of bloody urine.
Hemau'tograph. Tracing made by an arterial blood-jet.
Hemautog'raphy. Formation of a hemautograph.
Hemeralo'pia. 1. Same as *Day-blindness.* 2. Same as *Nyctalopia.*
Hemiachromatop'sia. Color-blindness in one half, or in corresponding halves, of visual field.
Hemialbu'min (hem-e-al-bu'min). The same as *Antialbumin.*
Hemialbu'mose. A digestion product of certain proteids: normally found in bone-marrow.
Hemialbumosu'ria. Discharge of hemialbumose in urine.

Hemianalge'sia. Analgesia on one side of the body.
Hemianesthe'sia. Anesthesia of either lateral half of body.
Hemiano'pia, Hemianop'sia. Blindness for one half the field of vision in one or both eyes.
Hemiarthro'sis (hem-e-ar-thro'sis). A spurious synchondrosis.
Hemiatax'ia. Ataxia on one side of the body.
Hemiatheto'sis. Athetosis of one side of the body.
Hemiat'rophy. Atrophy of one side of the body.
Hem'ic. Pertaining to or generated in blood.
Hemicepha'lia. Congenital absence of one lateral half of the skull.
Hemiceph'alus. A monster with one cerebral hemisphere.
Hemichore'a (hem-e-ko-re'ah). Chorea which affects but one side.
Hemicra'nia. 1. Headache on one side of the head. 2. Absence of anterior bones of the skull.
Hemidiaphore'sis. Sweating of one side of body.
Hemidro'sis. Same as *Hematidrosis.*
Hemidysesthe'sia. Disorder of sensation affecting one half the head.
Hemienceph'alus. Fetus without the sense-organs of the brain.
Hemiep'ilepsy. Epilepsy of one side of the body.
Hemiglossi'tis. Inflammation of one half of the tongue.
Hemihyperesthe'sia. Abnormal sensitiveness of one side.
Hemihyper'trophy. Overgrowth of one half or side.
Hemim'elus (hem-im'el-us). Fetus with defective limbs.
He'min (he'min). A crystalline salt of hematin.
Hemineurasthe'nia. Neurasthenia exhibited in one side only.
Hemio'pia (hem-e-o'pe-ah). Same as *Hemianopia.*
Hemiop'ic (hem-e-op'ik). Affecting one eye.
Hemip'agus (hem-ip'ag-us). Twin birth joined at the thorax.
Hemiparanesthe'sia. Anesthesia of lower half of one side.
Hemiparaple'gia (hem-e-par-ap-le'je-ah). Paralysis of the lower half of one side.
Hemipar'esis. Paresis affecting one side.
Hemipep'tone. One of the forms of peptone obtained from pepsin digestion.
Hemiple'gia (hem-e-ple'je-ah). Paralysis of one side of the body. **Alternate h.,** that which affects one side of face and opposite of body. **Cerebral h.,** that which is due to brain lesion. **Facial h.,** paralysis of one side of face. **Hephestic h.** See *Hephestic.* **Spastic h.,** h. with spasms and atrophy: usually infantile. **Spinal h.,** h. due to lesion of spinal cord.
Hemipro'tein (hem-e-pro'te-in). Same as *Antialbumid.*
Hemisec'tion. Section of one half; also, bisection.
Hem'ispasm (hem'e-spazm). Spasm affecting only one side.
Hem'isphere (hem'is-fēr). Either lateral half of cerebrum or cerebellum.
Hemisys'tole. Systole of only one side of the heart.
Hemiter'ic. Congenitally deformed, but not monstrous.
Hem'lock. 1. Conium. 2. A fir-tree of the genus *Tsuga.*
Hemocce'lom, Hæmocœ'lom. Part of celom whence the heart is developed.
Hemochromato'sis. Staining with coloring principles of blood.
Hemochro'mogen. A derivative from hemoglobin.
Hemochromom'eter. An instrument for making color-tests of the quality of the blood.
Hemocrys'tallin (hem-o-kris'tal-in). Same as *Hemoglobin.*
Hemocy'anin. Same as *Hematocyanin.*
Hem'ocyte (hem'o-sīt). A blood-corpuscle or blood-cell.
Hemocytol'ysis (hem-o-si-tol'is-is). Disintegration of the blood-corpuscles.

Hemocytom'eter (hem-o-si-tom'et-er). Same as *Hematimeter*.

Hemocytotryp'sis. Disintegration of blood-corpuscles by reason of pressure.

Hemodromom'eter. Instrument for measuring speed of the blood-current.

Hemodynamom'eter. Same as *Hemadynamometer*.

Hemofer'rum (hem-o-fer'um). Oxyhemoglobin.

Hemofus'cin (hem-o-fus'in). Brown coloring-matter of blood.

Hemogal'lol. Medicinal preparation containing hemoglobin.

Hemogen'esis (hem-o-jen'es-is). Formation of blood.

Hemogen'ic. Pertaining to the production of blood.

Hemoglo'bin. Coloring-matter of red blood-corpuscles.

Hemoglobine'mia. Abnormal presence of hemoglobin in the plasma of the blood.

Hemoglobinom'eter. Instrument for measuring the hemoglobin in the blood.

Hemoglobinu'ria. Presence of hemoglobin in the urine. **Epidemic h.**, hemoglobinuria of young infants, with cyanosis, jaundice, etc. **Intermittent,** or **Paroxysmal, h.**, a form with recurrent paroxysms. **Toxic h.**, that which is consequent upon the ingestion of various poisons.

Hemoko'nise. Small refractive bodies in the blood, said to be fragments of blood-corpuscles.

He'mol. Medicinal preparation of hemoglobin.

Hem'olymph. 1. Blood and lymph. 2. Nutrient fluid or blood of certain invertebrates.

Hemol'ysis (hem-ol'is-is). Same as *Hematolysis*.

Hemolyt'ic (hem-o-lit'ik). Breaking down the blood-corpuscles.

Hemomediasti'num. Same as *Hematomediastinum*.

Hemom'eter. Instrument used in inspecting the blood.

Hemome'tra (hem-o-me'trah). Same as *Hematometra*.

Hemopericar'dium. Same as *Hematopericardium*.

Hemoperitone'um. Blood in the peritoneal cavity.

Hemophag'ocyte (hem-o-fag'os-it). A white blood-corpuscle.

Hemophil'ia (hem-o-fil'e-ah). Strong tendency to bleeding.

Hemophthal'mia, Hemophthal'mus. Extravasation of blood inside the eye.

Hemopneumotho'rax. Same as *Hematopneumothorax*.

Hemopoie'sis. Same as *Hematopoiesis*.

Hemop'tysis (hem-op'tis-is). Spitting of blood.

Hem'orrhage (hem'or-ej). Escape of blood from the veins. **Accidental h.**, caused by premature detachment of placenta. **Capillary h.**, oozing from minute vessels. **Concealed h.**, hemorrhage without escape from the body. **Consecutive h.**, that which does not directly follow an injury. **Critical h.**, that which occurs at a crisis. **Petechial h.**, subcutaneous h. occurring in minute spots. **Post-partum h.**, that which follows soon after labor. **Primary h.**, that which soon follows an accident. **Secondary h.**, that which follows an accident after a considerable lapse of time. **Unavoidable h.** follows the detachment of a placenta previa. **Vicarious h.**, flow of blood from a part in consequence of the suppression of a discharge from another part.

Hemorrhag'ic (hem-or-aj'ik). Pertaining to hemorrhage.

Hemorrhe'a (hem-or-e'ah). Copious hemorrhage.

Hemor'rhoid. A pile or vascular tumor of the rectal mucous membrane.

Hemorrhoi'dal. Pertaining to hemorrhoids.

Hemosid'erin. Preparation containing iron from the blood.

Hemospa'sia (hem-os-pa'zhe-ah). Withdrawal of blood.

Hemos'tasis (hem-os'tas-is). 1. The arrest of hemorrhage. 2. Stoppage of the blood-current.

Hemostat′ic (hem-os-tat′ik). Checking the escape of blood.

Hemotachom′eter. Instrument for measuring speed of the blood-current.

Hemotho′rax. Collection of blood in the thoracic cavity.

Hemp. See *Cannabis; also Apocynum.*

Hen′bane. Same as *Hyoscyamus.*

Hen′le's layer. Outermost layer of inner root-sheath of hair-follicle. **H.'s loop,** the U-shaped loop of the uriniferous tubule of kidney. **H.'s membrane,** fenestrated membrane of an artery. **H.'s sheath,** sheath which envelops an isolated nerve-fiber outside of the neurilemma. **H.'s sphincter,** muscular fibers around the prostatic urethra.

He′noch's purpura. Purpura with intestinal disturbances.

Hen′sen's disk. H.'s line. Line which passes transversely through sarcous elements. **H.'s prop-cells,** cylindric cells outside the outer hair-cells in organ of Corti.

He′par (he′par). L. for *Liver.* **H. sulphu′ris,** potassium sulphid with sulphur.

Hepatal′gia (hep-at-al′je-ah). Pain in the liver.

Hepatec′tomy. Excision of part of liver.

Hepat′ic (hep-at′ik). Pertaining to liver. **H. duct.** See *Duct.* **H. lobes,** the five lobes of the liver. **H. veins,** three veins from the liver to postcava. **H. zones,** the arterial, venous, and portal areas of the liver.

Hepaticos′tomy. Creation of artificial fistula into hepatic duct.

Hep′atin (hep′at-in). Glycogen.

Hepati′tis (hep-at-i′tis). Inflammation of the liver.

Hepatiza′tion. Change of tissue into a liver-like substance.

Hepato-. Prefix denoting some relation to the liver.

Hep′atocele (hep′at-o-sēl). Hernia of the liver.

Hepatocirrho′sis (hep-at-o-sir-o′sis). Cirrhosis of liver.

Hepatocys′tic. Pertaining to liver and gall-bladder.

Hepatodyn′ia (hep-at-o-din′e-ah). Pain in the liver; hepatalgia.

Hepatogen′ic, Hepatog′enous. Produced in the liver.

Hep′atolith (hep′at-o-lith). A bile-stone.

Hepatolithi′asis. Formation of calculi in liver or gall-cyst.

Hepatomala′cia (hep-at-o-mal-a′se-ah). Softening of the liver.

Hepatop′athy (hep-at-op′ath-e). Any disease of liver.

Hep′atopexy. Fixation of displaced liver to abdominal wall.

Hep′atophage (hep′at-o-fāj). Giant-cell reputed to destroy liver-cells.

Hepator′rhaphy (hep-at-or′af-e). The suturing of the liver.

Hepatorrhe′a. A morbid flow from the liver.

Hepatorrhex′is. Rupture of the liver.

Hepatot′omy (hep-at-ot′o-me). Surgical incision of liver.

Hephes′tic hemiplegia, H. spasm. A hemiplegia and spasm of blacksmiths.

Hep′tad. Any element having a valency of seven.

Hep′tane. A hydrocarbon, C_7H_{16}, from pine and petroleum.

Her′apathite. Iodosulphate of quinin.

Herb. A plant with a stem not woody.

Herbiv′orous. Living on grasses and herbs.

Hered′itary. Derived from ancestry, or by inheritance. **H. ataxia.** See *Friedreich's disease.*

Hered′ity. Inheritance of qualities from ancestry.

Her′ing's the′ory. Doctrine that color-perceptions are dependent on a visual substance in the retina which is variously modified by anabolism for black, green, or blue, and by catabolism for white, red, and yellow.

Hermaph′rodism. Double, or doubtful, sex. **Complex h.,** when internal and external organs of both sexes are present. **Dimidiate h., Lateral h.,** when the organs of one side are male and of the other female. **Spurious h.**, doubtful sex. **Transverse h.**, when the outward organs appear to be of one sex, and the internal ones are of the other. **True h.**, double sex. **Unilateral h.**, when one side has an ovary or testis, and the other has both an ovary and a testis.

Hermaph'rodite. A person having, or appearing to have, both male and female characters.

Hermaphrod'itism. Same as *Hermaphrodism.*

Hermet'ical (her-met'ik-al). Impervious to air.

Her'nia (her'ne-ah). Protrusion of a loop or knuckle of an organ or tissue through an abnormal opening. **Abdominal h.**, protrusion of some internal structure through the abdominal wall. **H. of bladder**, protrusion of a part of the bladder through any normal or other opening. **H. cer'ebri**, protrusion of brain-substance through the skull. **Cloquet's h.**, a variety of femoral h. **Complete h.**, one in which the sac and its contents have passed through the orifice. **Concealed h.**, hernia not perceptible on palpation. **Congenital h.**, presence at birth of a knuckle of the bowel in the scrotum. **Crural h.** Same as *Femoral h.* **Cystic h.** Same as *Cystocele.* **Diaphragmatic h.**, hernia through the diaphragm. **Diverticular h.**, protrusion of a congenital diverticulum of the gut. **Encysted h.**, scrotal hernia enveloped by the tunica vaginalis. **Femoral h.**, hernia into the femoral canal. **Funicular h.**, h. of the umbilical or spermatic cord. **Holthouse h.**, **Inguinocrural h.**, that which is both inguinal and femoral. **Incarcerated h.**, h. so occluded as to completely obstruct the bowels. **Incomplete h.**, one which has not passed quite through the orifice. **Infantile h.**, oblique inguinal h. behind funicular process of peritoneum. **Inguinal h.**, one into the inguinal canal. **Irreducible h.**, one that cannot be restored by taxis. **Ischiatic h.**, hernia through sacrosciatic foramen. **Labial h.**, protrusion into labium majus. **Lumbar h.**, hernia in the loin. **Mesocolic h.**, hernia into a pouch of the mesocolon. **Nuckian h.**, protrusion into canal of Nuck. **Obturator h.**, protrusion through obturator foramen. **Omental h.**, hernia containing omentum. **Properitoneal h.**, hernia through peritoneum and within the abdominal wall. **Reducible h.**, one that may be returned by manipulation. **Retroperitoneal h.**, hernia of intestine into the duodeno-jejunal fossa. **Richter's h.**, one in which only a part of the caliber of the gut is protruded. **Scrotal h.**, inguinal h. which has passed into the scrotum. **Strangulated h.**, one which is tightly constricted, and has become, or is likely to become, sphacelated. **Umbilical h.**, protrusion at navel. **Vaginal h.**, hernia in the vagina. **Ventral h.**, hernia through abdominal wall.

Hernia'tion (her-ne-a'shun). Formation of hernia.

Hernio-enterot'omy. Herniotomy with enterotomy.

Her'niopuncture. Surgical puncture of a hernia.

Herniot'omy (her-ne-ot'om-e). Same as *Kelotomy.* -

Hero'ic. Severe; rash.

Her'pes (her'pēz). Skin-disease marked by clusters of small vesicles. **H. circina'tus.** Same as *Tinea circinata.* **H. febri'lis**, so-called fever-sores. **H. gestatio'nis**, a herpes peculiar to pregnant women. **H. i'ris**, a form seen in rings on the hands and feet. **H. preputia'lis** occurs on the genitalia. **H. zos'ter**, painful disease known as shingles.

Herpet'ic. Pertaining to herpes. **H. neuralgia**, painful neurosis associated with herpes zoster.

Herpet'iform. Resembling herpes.

Her'petism. Predisposition to chronic skin-disease.

Hess'elbach's hernia. Femoral hernia with a pouch through the cribriform fascia. **H.'s triangle**, the triangular space bounded by Poupart's ligament, rectus muscle, and epigastric artery.

Heteradel'phia. Twin monstrosity in which one fetus is more developed than the other.

Heteradel'phus. Twin monster affected with heteradelphia.

Heterade'nia. Any abnormality of gland-tissue.

Heteraden'ic. Pertaining to heteradenia.

Heteradeno'ma. Any hyaline cylindroma.

Hetera'lius. An extreme example of heteradelphia.

Heterœ'cious (het-er-e'shus). Living upon one host in one stage, or generation, and on another in the next.

Heteroal'bumose. Hemialbumose insoluble in water.

Heteroau'toplasty. Plastic transfer of tissue from one part of the body to another.

Heteroceph'alus. A monster with two unequal heads.

Heterochron'ic. Irregular; occurring at abnormal times.

Heterod'ymus. Monster with a second head on abdomen.

Heteroge'neous (het-er-o-je'ne-us). Of dissimilar nature.

Heterogen'esis. 1. Alternation of generation. 2. Asexual generation.

Heterogenet'ic. 1. Pertaining to heterogenesis. 2. Not arising in the organism.

Hetero-infec'tion. Infection by virus from outside the organism.

Hetero-inocula'tion. Inoculation from any organism.

Heterol'ogous. Made up of tissue not normal to the part.

Heteromor'phous. Of abnormal shape or structure.

Heteron'omous. 1. Not independent. 2. Abnormal.

Heteron'ymous. Reversed; opposite in position.

Heterop'agus. Fetus to which another rudimentary fetus is attached by the abdomen.

Heterop'athy. Abnormal or morbid sensibility to stimuli.

Heteropha'sia. The wrong use of terms.

Heterophe'mia. The saying of one thing for another.

Heterophoral'gia. Heterophoria with pain.

Heteropho'ria. Absence of parallelism between visual lines.

Heterophthal'mos. Condition in which irides differ in color.

Heteropla'sia. Replacement of normal by abnormal tissues.

Heteroplastic (het-er-o-plas'tik). Pertaining to heteroplasia.

Het'eroplasty. Plastic surgery in which tissue is removed from a sound person.

Heterotax'ia. Abnormal position of viscera.

Heterot'opy. Displacement or misplacement of parts.

Heterotro'pia (het-er-o-tro'pe-ah). Same as *Strabismus.*

Heteroxan'thin. A leukomain from urine; methyl-xanthin.

Heub'ner's disease (hoib'nerz). Syphilitic endocarditis.

Hexaba'sic. Having six atoms replaceable by a base.

Hex'ad (hek'sad). A sexvalent element.

Hexamethylenetetram'in. Same as *Urotropin.*

Hexatom'ic (hek-sat-om'ik). Containing six replaceable atoms.

Hexylam'in. Poisonous base, $C_6H_{15}N$, from yeast and cod-liver oil.

Hey's ligament. Part of falciform ligament of fascia lata.

Hg. Symbol of *mercury.*

Hia'tus (hi-a'tus). A fissure or gap. **H. Fallo'pii,** opening for Vidian nerve in petrous bone.

Hiberna'tion. The dormant state in which certain animals pass the winter.

Hic'cup, Hic'cough. Sharp inspiratory sound with spasm of glottis and diaphragm; singultus.

Hide'-bound. Affected with scleroderma.

Hidropoie'sis. The process of the formation of sweat.

Hidropoiet'ic. Concerned in, or relating to, hidropoiesis.

Hidrosadeni'tis. Inflammation of the sweat-glands.
Hi'era pi'era. The powder of aloes and canella.
High lithotomy. Suprapubic lithotomy.
High'more's antrum. See under *Antrum.* **H.'s body.** Same as *Mediastinum testis.*
Hil'ton's muscle. The compressor sacculi laryngis. **H.'s sac.** Same as *Sacculus laryngeus.*
Hi'lum. A depression at the entrance and exit of vessels, nerves, and duct into a gland.
Hind'-brain. See *Epencephalon.* **H.-gut,** embryonic structure whence the colon is formed. **H.-kidney,** the metanephros.
Hinge'-joint. Same as *Ginglymus.*
Hip. The region on either side of the pelvis. **H.-joint,** articulation of the innominate bone and femur. **H.-joint disease.** Same as *Coxalgia.*
Hippocam'pal convolution. See *Convolution.* **H. fissure,** fissure above the temporal lobe on mesial surface of cerebrum.
Hippocam'pus ma'jor. A curved structure on floor of the middle horn of the lateral ventricle. **H. mi'nor,** a white elevation on floor of posterior cornu of lateral ventricle.
Hippocrat'ic face. See *Facies Hippocratica.* **H. sound,** splashing succussion sound.
Hippomel'anin. Black pigment from tumors or marrow of melanotic horses.
Hippu'ria (hip-pu're-ah). Excess of hippuric acid in urine.
Hippu'ric acid. See *Acid.*
Hip'pus (hip'us). Tremor of the iris.
Hir'sute (her'sût). Shaggy; hairy.
Hirsu'ties (hur-su'she-ēz) Excessive hairiness.
Hiru'do (hi-ru'do). L. for *Leech.*
His'tioid. Same as *Histoid.*
Histochem'istry. Chemistry of organized or living tissues.
Histodial'ysis. Disintegration or breaking down of tissue.
Histogen'esis (his-to-jen'es-is). Formation of tissues.
Histogenet'ic (his-to-jen-et'ik). Pertaining to histogenesis.
Histohem'atin. Any one of a group of red tissue-pigments.
His'toid (his'toid). Developed from but one tissue.
Histol'ogy (his-tol'o-je). The science of the minute structure and composition of tissues. **Normal h.,** science of healthy tissues. **Pathological h.,** science of diseased tissues.
Histol'ysis (his-tol'is-is). Dissolution or breaking down of tissues.
His'ton. An albumose from cell-nuclei.
Histon'omy. Statement of the laws of tissue-development.
Histophysiol'ogy. Physiology of the minute elements of tissues.
Histother'apy. Treatment by administration of animal tissues.
His'totome (his'to-tōm). A cutting instrument in microtomy.
Histot'omy (his-tot'om-e). Dissection of tissues; microtomy.
His'tozyme (his'to-zim). Any enzyme which causes a fermentation in a tissue.
Histrion'ic spasm. See *Tic, convulsive.*
Hives (hivz). 1. Urticaria. 2. Croup or laryngitis.
Hl. Symbol for *latent hypermetropia.*
Hm. Symbol for *manifest hypermetropia.*
Hoang nan (ho-ang nahn). Chinese remedy for leprosy and syphilis; bark of *Strychnos Malaccensis.*
Hoarse'ness. Harshness or roughness of voice.
Hob-nail liver. Liver marked with nail-like masses, due to cirrhosis or passive congestion.
Hoch'singer's sign. Indicanuria as a sign of tuberculosis.
Hodg'kin's disease. Pseudoleukemia.
Hoff'man's anodyne. The compound spirit of ether.
Hog-cholera. Contagious febrile disease of swine.

Hol'den's line. See *Line.*

Hol'low-back. Same as *Lordosis.*

Holm'gren's worsteds. Skeins of worsted yarn for testing color-blindness.

Holoblas'tic ova. Ova of which all the yolk undergoes segmentation.

Holoca'in. A derivative of phenetidin: used as a local anesthetic.

Holorrachis'chisis. Fissure of the entire spinal cord.

Holos'chisis (ho-los'kis-is). Same as *Amitosis.*

Holt'house's hernia. Inguinocrural hernia. See *Hernia.*

Hol'zin. A solution of formaldehyd in methyl alcohol.

Hol'zinol. Holzin combined with menthol: used as a germicide and disinfectant.

Homat'ropin (ho-mat'ro-pin). Mydriatic alkaloid from opium.

Homeomor'phous (ho-me-o-mor'fus). Of like form and structure.

Homeop'athy. System which professes to cure by infinitesimal doses of medicines which are capable of producing symptoms like those of the disease treated.

Homeopla'sia. Formation of new tissue like that adjacent to it.

Home'-sickness. Intense longing for home; nostalgia.

Homocen'tric rays. A conic pencil of light-rays.

Homocer'ebrin. Principle obtainable from brain-substance.

Homoge'neous (ho-mo-je'ne-us). Of uniform quality.

Homogen'esis, Homog'eny. Reproduction of the same process in each generation.

Homogentes'ic acid. An acid from urine; of bacterial origin.

Homol'ogous (ho-mol'og-us). Of similar structure or place.

Hom'ologue (hom'ol-og). Any homologous organ or part.

Homol'ogy (ho-mol'o-je). Quality of being homologous.

Homon'omous (ho-mon'om-us). Under the same law.

Homon'ymous (ho-mon'im-us). Of corresponding name or place. **H. diplopia.** See *Diplopia.*

Homosexual'ity. Sexual perversion toward those of same sex.

Homother'mal. Of uniform temperature.

Homoton'ic (ho-mo-ton'ik). Of uniform course or tension.

Ho'motype (ho'mo-tip). A part having reversed symmetry with its fellow.

Hondu'ras bark. Same as *Cascara amarga.*

Hon'ey-comb ringworm. Same as *Favus.*

Honora'rium (hon-or-a're-um). Physician's professional fee.

Hook. Curved instrument for traction or holding.

Hoop'ing-cough. Same as *Whooping-cough.*

Hop. See *Humulus.*

Horde'olum. Sty; inflammation of sebaceous glands of eyelid.

Hor'deum. See *Barley.*

Hore'hound. The plant *Marrubium vulgare:* sudorific, bechic, and tonic.

Hor'mion. Median anterior point of spheno-occipital bones.

Hor'ner's muscle. See *Tensor tarsi* in *Muscles, Table of.*

Hor'ny epithelium. Trachomatous conjunctivitis. **H. layer.** Same as *Stratum corneum.*

Horop'ter. Sum of all points seen in binocular vision with the eyes fixed.

Horripila'tion. Cutis anserina, or goose-flesh.

Horse-pox. A disease of the horse, a modified small-pox.

Horse-rad'ish. A plant, *Cochlearia armoracia:* root stimulant and antiscorbutic.

Horse-shoe fistula. A semicircular fistulous tract about the anus. **H. kidney,** union of the kidneys by the lower ends.

Hos'pital. Institution for treatment of the sick.

Hos'pitalism. Morbid state due to impure air in hospital.

Host. Any animal or plant which supports a parasite.

Hot drops. Tincture of capsicum and myrrh. **H. eye,** temporary congestion of the eye, seen in gouty patients.

Hot′tentot apron. Velamen vulvæ; hypertrophy of nymphæ or labia minora. **H. deformity.** See *Steatopygia.*

Hot′tentotism. Exaggerated form of stuttering.

Hour′-glass contraction. Contraction of the uterus which assumes an hour-glass shape.

House-maid's knee. Inflammation of the bursa of knee-cap.

House-surgeon. Resident surgeon of a hospital.

Hous′ton's muscle (hew′stunz). The compressor venæ dorsalis. **H.'s valves,** folds of mucous membrane in rectum.

How′ship's lacunæ. Depressions in bone beneath periosteum.

Ht. Symbol for *total hypermetropia.*

Huguier's canal (u-gwe-āz′). See *Canal.* **H.'s glands,** two minor vaginal glands.

Hu′manized virus. Vaccine virus for human subject.

Hu′meral (hu′mer-al). Of, or pertaining to, the humerus.

Humerora′dial. Pertaining to humerus and radius.

Hu′merus (hu′mer-us). The bone between shoulder and elbow.

Hu′mid gangrene. See under *Gangrene.*

Humid′ity (hu-mid′it-e). Degree of moisture in the air.

Hu′mor (yu′mor). Any fluid or semifluid of the body.

Hu′moral pathology, Humor′alism. Obsolete doctrine that all diseases arise from some change of the humors.

Hu′mulus. Strobiles of *Humulus lupulus,* or hops; stimulant and sedative.

Hu′mus (hu′mus). Dark mould of decayed vegetable tissue.

Hun′ger-cure. Treatment of disease by severe fasting.

Hunte′rian chancer. True, hard, or syphilitic chancer.

Hun′ter's canal. See *Canal.*

Hunya′di Ja′nos (hun-yah′de yah′nosh). An aperient mineral water.

Huschke's canal (hoosh′kēz). See *Canal.*

Hut′chinson teeth. Notched and narrow-edged teeth indicative of inherited syphilis.

Hux′ham's tincture. Compound tincture of cinchona bark.

Hux′ley's layer. A layer of the root-sheath of a hair-follicle within Henle's layer.

Hy′alin (hi′al-in). A principle obtainable from the products of amyloid degeneration.

Hy′aline. Glassy; pellucid. See *Degeneration.*

Hyalinu′ria. Discharge of hyalin in the urine.

Hyali′tis. Inflammation of hyaloid membrane.

Hy′aloid (hi′al-oid). Pellucid; like glass. **H. artery,** fetal branch of central artery of retina. **H. fossa.** See *Fossa.*

Hyaloidi′tis (hi-al-oi-di′tis). See *Hyalitis.*

Hy′aloplasm (hi′al-o-plazm). Fluid part of cell-protoplasm.

Hy′brid. Animal or plant bred or grafted from two species.

Hydan′toin. A basic substance, $C_3H_4N_2O_2$, from allantoin.

Hydat′id, Hydat′id cyst. A cyst formed by the larva of *Tænia.* **H. of Morgagni,** cyst-like remains of Müllerian duct attached to oviduct or testicle.

Hydatid′iform. Resembling a hydatid in form.

Hydrace′tin. Poisonous antipyretic, $C_6H_5N_2O_2(C_2H_3O)$, from coal-tar.

Hydra′cid. Any hydrogen acid containing no oxygen.

Hydradeni′tis. Inflammation of a lymph-gland.

Hydraëroperitone′um. Collection of water and pus in the peritoneal cavity.

Hy′dragogue (hi′drag-og). Causing watery purgation.

Hydram′nion. Dropsy of the amnion; excess of amniotic fluid.

Hydrargyra'lia. Mercurial medicinal preparations.
Hydrargy'ria, Hydrar'gyrism. Same as *Mercurialism.*
Hydrar'gyrum. L. for *Mercury.*
Hydrarthro'sis, Hydrar'thus. Dropsical effusion into a joint.
Hydras'tin. Medicinal alkaloid; also a precipitate from *Hydrastis canadensis.*
Hydras'tis canaden'sis. Golden seal; a plant with aperient, diuretic, and tonic properties.
Hy'drate (hi'drāt). 1. Compound of hydroxyl with a radical. 2. A salt or other compound which contains water.
Hy'drated (hi'dra-ted). Combined with water.
Hydrau'lics (hi-draw'lix). Science of liquids in motion.
Hy'drazin (hi'dra-zin). A gaseous diamin, H_4N_2; also, any member of a group of its substitution derivatives.
Hydre'mia (hi-dre'me-ah). Excess of water in the blood.
Hydrencephal'ocele. Protrusion of brain-tissue enclosing part of a ventricle.
Hydrenceph'alus (hi-dren-sef'al-us). Same as *Hydrocephalus.*
Hy'drid. Compound of hydrogen with an element or radical.
Hydriod'ic acid. See *Acid.*
Hydro'a. Skin-disease with vesicular patches.
Hydrobiliru'bin. One of the bile-pigments.
Hydrobro'mate. Any salt of hydrobromic acid.
Hydrobro'mic acid. See *Acid.*
Hydrocar'bon. Any compound of hydrogen and carbon.
Hy'drocele (hi'dro-sēl). Collection of fluid about testicle. **H. mulie'bris,** watery dilatation of canal of Nuck.
Hydrocephal'ic. Of, or pertaining to, hydrocephalus.
Hydroceph'alocele. Same as *Hydrencephalocele.*
Hydroceph'aloid. Resembling hydrocephalus. **H. disease,** state simulating hydrocephalus, but with depressed fontanels following diarrhea.
Hydroceph'alus. Fluid effusion within the cranium.
Hydrochlo'rate. Any salt of hydrochloric acid.
Hydrochlo'ric acid. See *Acid.*
Hydrocholecys'tis. Dropsical inflation of gall-bladder.
Hydrocir'socele (hi-dro sir'so-sēl). Hydrocele combined with varicocele.
Hydrocol'lidin. A dangerous ptomain from putrefying flesh.
Hydroco'nion (hi-dro-ko'ne-on). An atomizer or vaporizer.
Hydrocyan'ic acid (hi-dro-si-an'ik). See *Acid.*
Hy'drocyst (hi'dro-sist). Cyst with watery contents.
Hydrocysto'ma. Disease characterized by small hydrocysts.
Hydro-elec'tric bath. Bath in which electricity is administered through water.
Hydro-electriza'tion. Treatment by hydro-electric bath.
Hydrofluor'ic acid. See *Acid.*
Hy'drogen (hi'dro-jen). Light inflammable gaseous element; symbol H. **H. acid.** Same as *Hydracid.* **H. disulphid,** ill-smelling gas, H_2S. **H. monoxid,** water. **H. peroxid,** disinfectant and cleansing liquid, H_2O_2.
Hydrohymeni'tis. Inflammation of a serous membrane.
Hydro'lein (hi-dro'le-in). Cod-liver oil emulsified with borax and pancreatin.
Hydrol'ogy (hi-drol'o-je). The study of water and its uses.
Hy'drolymph. The thin blood of certain animals.
Hydrol'ysis. Decomposition due to absorption of water.
Hydrolyt'ic. Pertaining to hydrolysis.
Hy'dromel (hi'dro-mel). Water sweetened with honey.
Hydromeningi'tis. 1. Meningitis with serous effusion. 2. Descemetitis.

Hydromenin'gocele. Encephalocele; also, spina bifida with protrusion of spinal meninges.
Hydrom'eter. Instrument for finding specific gravities of fluids.
Hydrome'tra. Collection of watery fluid in the uterus.
Hydrom'phalus (hi-drom'fal-us). Watery tumor at navel.
Hydromye'lia, Hydromyel'ocele. Formation of spaces filled with water in spinal cord of children.
Hydronaph'tol. A disinfectant preparation of naphtol.
Hydronephro'sis. Collection of urine in pelvis of kidney.
Hydro-oligocythe'mia. Anemia with excess of serum.
Hydropath'ic. Of, or pertaining to, hydropathy.
Hydrop'athy (hi-drop'ath-e). Water cure; hydrotherapy.
Hydropericar'dium. Dropsy of pericardium.
Hydroperitone'um. Ascites; abdominal dropsy.
Hydroph'ilous (hi-drof'il-us). Absorbing water; bibulous.
Hydropho'bia (hi-dro-fo'be-ah). Same as *Rabies.*
Hydrophobopho'bia. Morbid dread of hydrophobia.
Hydrophthal'mia, Hydrophthal'mus. Distention of eyeball from watery infusion.
Hydrophysome'tra. Presence of gas and water in uterus.
Hydrop'ic (hi-drop'ik). Affected with dropsy.
Hydropneumato'sis. Collection of fluid and gas.
Hydropneumopericar'dium. Gas and fluid in pericardium.
Hydropneumotho'rax. Same as *Pneumohydrothorax.*
Hy'drops (hi'drops). L. for *Dropsy.*
Hydroqui'none. An antipyretic, $C_6H_6O_2$, from quinone.
Hydrorhe'ostat. A rheostat in which water affords resistance.
Hydror'rhachis. Collection of fluid in vertebral canal.
Hydrorrhachi'tis. Hydrorrhachis with inflammation.
Hydrorrhe'a (hi-dror-re'ah). A watery discharge. **H. gravida'rum.** watery discharge from the gravid uterus.
Hydrosal'pinx. Dropsy of an oviduct.
Hydrosar'cocele. Hydrocele and sarcocele together.
Hydro'sis (hi-dro'sis). Incorrect spelling of *Hidrosis.*
Hydrosphyg'mograph. Sphygmograph with water for an index.
Hydrostat'ic test. Floating of lungs on water as a test of live-birth.
Hydrostat'ics. Science of equilibrium of fluids.
Hydrosulphu'ric acid. See *Acid.*
Hydrosyringomye'lia. Distention of central canal of spinal cord, with formation of cavities and degeneration.
Hydrotherapeu'tics, Hydrother'apy. Treatment of disease by means of water.
Hydrothionammone'mia. Ammonium sulphid in the blood.
Hydrothione'mia. Hydrogen sulphid in the blood.
Hydrothionu'ria. Hydrogen sulphid in the urine.
Hydrotho'rax (hi-dro-tho'rax). Effused fluid in pleural cavity.
Hydro'tis (hi-dro'tis). Dropsy of the ear.
Hydrot'omy. Dissection of parts by injections of water.
Hydrotym'panum. Dropsy of the tympanic cavity.
Hydrova'rium (hi-dro-va're-um). Ovarian dropsy.
Hydrox'id. Any compound of hydroxyl with another radical.
Hydrox'yl (hi-drox'il). The univalent radical HO.
Hydroxylam'in hydrochlorid. A preparation useful in skin-diseases.
Hy'drozone (hi'dro-zōn). Water charged with hydrogen peroxid.
Hydru'ria (hi-dru're-ah). Same as *Diabetes insipidus.*
Hygiene (hi-jeen'). Science of health and its preservation.
Hygien'ic (hi-je-en'ik). Pertaining to hygiene or to health.
Hy'grin (hi'grin). A mydriatic base from coca leaves.
Hygro'ma (hi-gro'mah). A sac, cyst, or bursa filled with fluid.
Hygrom'eter. Instrument for measuring moisture of atmosphere.

Hygrom'etry. Measurement of moisture in atmosphere.
Hygroscop'ic (hi-gro-skop'ik). Readily absorbing moisture.
Hygrosto'mia (hi-gro-sto'me-ah). Salivation; ptyalism.
Hy'men. Membranous fold which partly closes vaginal orifice.
Hymeni'tis (hi-men-i'tis). Inflammation of the hymen.
Hymenol'ogy (hi-men-ol'o-je). Science of the membranes.
Hymen'otome. Instrument for cutting membranes.
Hyobasioglos'sus. Basal part of hyoglossal muscle.
Hyocholal'ic acid. An acid from swine's bile.
Hyo-epiglottid'ean. Pertaining to hyoid bone and epiglottis.
Hyoglos'sal. Pertaining to the hyoid and tongue.
Hyoglos'sus. See *Muscles, Table of.*
Hy'oid. 1. Shaped like Greek letter υ. 2. Hyoid bone. **H. arch,** second visceral or branchial arch. **H. bone,** bone at base of tongue.
Hyopharyng'eus. See *Constrictor, Middle,* in *Muscles, Table of.*
Hyos'cin (hi-os'in). A nerve-depressant and mydriatic alkaloid from hyoscyamus.
Hyoscy'amin. Alkaloid like atropin, from hyoscyamus.
Hyoscy'amus ni'ger. Henbane, a poisonous plant: narcotic, sedative, and mydriatic.
Hypacou'sia, Hypacu'sia, Hypacu'sis. Defect of hearing.
Hypalbumino'sis. Deficiency of albumins in blood.
Hypalge'sia, Hypal'gia. Diminished sensibility to pain.
Hypax'ial (hip-ax'e-al). Situated ventrad to bodily axis.
Hypera'cid (hi-per-as'id). Abnormally or excessively acid.
Hyperacid'ity (hi-per-as-id'it-e). Excessive degree of acidity.
Hyperacu'sis. Abnormally acute sense of hearing.
Hyperalbumino'sis. Excess of albuminoids in the blood.
Hyperal'gia (hi-per-al'je-ah). Abnormal sensitiveness to pain.
Hyperbrachycephal'ic. Excessively brachycephalic.
Hypercathar'sis. Excessive purgation.
Hypercemento'sis. Excessive growth of tooth cement.
Hyperchlorhyd'ria. Excess of hydrochloric acid in the gastric juice.
Hyperchromato'sis. Excess of pigment in any part.
Hypercine'sia (hi-per-sin-e'zhe-ah). Preternatural mobility.
Hypercryalge'sia (hi-per-kri-al-je'zhe-ah). Excessive sensitiveness to cold.
Hypercye'sis. Same as *Superfetation.*
Hyperdicrot'ic. Markedly dicrotic.
Hyperdisten'tion (hi-per-dis-ten'shun). Excessive distention.
Hyperdiure'sis. Excessive secretion of urine.
Hyperdyna'mia. Excess of muscular action.
Hyperem'esis (hi-per-em'is-is). Excessive vomiting.
Hypere'mia (hi-per-e'me-ah). Excess of blood in any part of the body.
Hyperenceph'alus. Monster fetus with brain exposed.
Hyperephidro'sis. Too profuse sweating.
Hyperesopho'ria. Extreme upward and inward strabismus.
Hyperesthe'sia. Excessive sensitiveness of the skin.
Hyperesthet'ic. Pertaining to, or affected with, hyperesthesia.
Hyperexopho'ria. Extreme upward and outward strabismus.
Hyperexten'sion. Extreme or excessive extension.
Hypergen'esis (hi-per-jen'es-is). Excessive development.
Hypergeusthe'sia, Hypergeu'sia. Abnormal acuteness of sense of taste.
Hyperglobu'lia. Excess in number of red blood-corpuscles.
Hyperglyce'mia (hi-per-gli-se'me-ah). Excess of glucose in the blood.
Hyperhidro'sis (hi-per-id-ro'sis). Excessive sweating.

Hyperinose'mia, Hyperino'sis. Excess of fibrin in the blood.

Hyperinvolu'tion. Too complete involution, as of the womb.

Hyperkerato'sis. 1. Hypertrophy of cornea. 2. Keratoglobus. 3. Hypertrophy of the stratum corneum.

Hyperkine'sia, Hyperkine'sis. Abnormal mobility.

Hyperleukocyto'sis. Excess in number of leukocytes.

Hypermas'tia. Excessive size of mammary gland.

Hypermature (hi-per-mat-ūr'). Past the stage of maturity.

Hyper'metrope (hi-per'met-rōp). A far-sighted person.

Hypermetro'pia. Far-sightedness; hyperopia.

Hypermyot'rophy. Excessive development of muscular tissue.

Hypernor'mal. In excess of what is normal.

Hyperonych'ia (hi-per-o-nik'e-ah). Hypertrophy of the nails.

Hy'perope (hi'per-ōp). Same as *Hypermetrope.*

Hypero'pia. Far-sightedness; focussing of parallel rays behind the retina. **Absolute h.,** that which can be partially corrected by accommodation. **Axial h.** is due to shortness of the antero-posterior axis of the eye. **Facultative h.** can be entirely corrected by accommodation. **Latent h.,** that part of the total h. which is not corrected by accommodation. **Manifest h.,** that which may be corrected by accommodation aided by convex lenses. **Relative h.,** that in which vision is distinct only when excessive convergence is made. **Total h.,** manifest and latent h. combined.

Hyperorex'ia. Excessive appetite; bulimia.

Hyperos'mia, Hyperosphre'sis. Morbid sensitiveness to odors.

Hyperosto'sis. Excessive growth of bony tissue.

Hyperpep'sia. Dyspepsia with excess of chlorids in gastric juice.

Hyperpho'ria. Elevation of one visual axis above the other.

Hyperpla'sia. Abnormal multiplication of tissue-elements.

Hyperplas'tic (hi-per-plas'tik). Pertaining to hyperplasia.

Hyperpne'a (hi-perp-ne'ah). Exaggerated breathing movements.

Hyperprax'ia. Abnormal activity; restlessness.

Hyperpselaphe'sia (hi-perp-sel-af-e'zhe-ah). Morbid tactile sensitiveness.

Hyperpyret'ic (hi-per-pi-ret'ik). Affected by hyperpyrexia.

Hyperpyrex'ia. Excessively high fever.

Hyperres'onance. Exaggerated resonance.

Hypersecre'tion (hi-per-sek-re'shun). Too copious secretion.

Hypersthe'nia. Exalted strength or tonicity.

Hyperthermalge'sia (hi-per-ther-mal-je'zhe-ah). Abnormal sensitiveness to heat.

Hyperthyroida'tion. Over-action of thyroid gland, as in exophthalmic goiter.

Hyperto'nia. Excessive tonicity, strength, or tension.

Hypertrichi'asis, Hypertricho'sis. Excessive hairiness.

Hypertroph'ic (hi-per-trof'ik). Characterized by hypertrophy.

Hyper'trophy (hi-per'trof-e). Morbid enlargement of an organ or part. **Compensatory h.,** that which results from increased functional activity due to some physical defect. **Concentric h.,** increased thickness of the walls of an organ with no enlargement, but with diminished capacity. **Excentric h.,** hypertrophy with dilatation of cavity. **False h.,** increase in one constituent substance only. **Numeric h.,** that due to increased number of structural elements. **Physiologic h.** Same as *Compensatory h.* **Simple h.** is due to increased size of structural elements. **True h.** is due to increase of all component tissues.

Hypertro'pia. Elevation of one of the visual axes.

Hyphe'mia (hi-fe'me-ah). 1. Hemorrhage within the eye. 2. Same as *Oligemia*.

Hyphidro'sis (hif-id-ro'sis). Too scanty perspiration.

Hypino'sis (hip-in-o'sis). Lack of fibrin in the blood.

Hyp'nal (hip'nal). Hypnotic preparation of antipyrin and chloral.

Hypnogenet'ic. Causing or producing sleep. **H. spots**, superficial areas, stimulation of which brings on sleep.

Hyp'nolepsy (hip'no-lep-se). Abnormal sleepiness.

Hypnol'ogy (hip-nol'o-je). Scientific view of sleep or of hypnotism.

Hyp'none (hip'nōn). Same as *Acetophenone*.

Hypno'sis. The condition of abnormal sleep.

Hypnot'ic. 1. Causing, or resembling, sleep. 2. Agent that induces sleep.

Hyp'notism. Artificially induced state resembling sleep.

Hyp'notize (hip'not-iz). To put into a condition of hypnotism.

Hypo-acid'ity (hi-po-as-id'it-e). Lack or need of an acid.

Hy'poblast (hi'po-blast). The innermost layer of the primitive embryo; the endoderm.

Hypoblas'tic (hi-po-blas'tik). Pertaining to the hypoblast.

Hypochlorhyd'ria. Lack of hydrochloric acid in gastric juice.

Hypochon'driac. 1. Situated under the lowest ribs. 2. A person affected with hypochondriasis. **H. region.** Same as *Hypochondrium*.

Hypochondri'acal. Affected with hypochondriasis.

Hypochondri'asis. Morbid anxiety about the health.

Hypochon'drium. The upper lateral region on either side next below the thorax.

Hypochro'mia, Hypochro'sis. Deficiency of color.

Hypocyto'sis (hi-po-si-to'sis). Deficiency of blood-corpuscles.

Hypodermat'ic, Hypoder'mic (hi-po-der-mat'ik, hi-po-der'-mik). Applied beneath, or situated under, the skin.

Hypodermat'omy (hi-po-der-mat'o-me). Subcutaneous incision.

Hypodermoc'lysis. Injection of fluids into subcutaneous tissues.

Hypogas'tric. Of, or pertaining to, hypogastrium. **H. artery**, umbilical artery of fetus. **H. plexus**, plexus of sympathetic nerve for pelvic viscera. **H. region.** Same as *Hypogastrium*.

Hypogas'trium. The lower middle abdominal region.

Hypogeu'sia (hi-po-jew'ze-ah). Deficient sense of taste.

Hypoglobu'lia. Same as *Hypocytosis*.

Hypoglos'sal. Situated under the tongue.

Hypoglot'tis. Same as *Ranula*.

Hypog'nathus. Monster fetus with a head on lower jaw.

Hypohidro'sis (hi-po-hid-ro'sis). Same as *Hyphidrosis*.

Hypoleukocyto'sis. Deficiency of leukocytes in blood.

Hypoma'nia (hi-po-ma'ne-ah). Mania of a mild type.

Hypomelancho'lia. Melancholia with slight mental disorder.

Hyponi'trous acid. Acid, HNO, forming hyponitrites.

Hypopep'sia. Indigestion from lack of function in stomach.

Hypophos'phite. Any salt of hypophosphorous acid.

Hypophos'phorous acid. See *Acid*.

Hypoph'ysis cer'ebri. Same as *Pituitary body*.

Hypopla'sia. Incomplete or defective structure.

Hypopselaphe'sia (hi-pop-sel-af-e'ze-ah). Dulness of tactile sense.

Hypo'pyon (hi-po'pe-on). Pus in anterior chamber of eye.

Hyposar'ca. Same as *Anasarca*.

Hypos'mia (hi-poz'me-ah). Imperfect sense of smell.

Hypospa'dias (hi-po-spa'de-as). 1. Congenital opening of urethra on under side of penis. 2. Opening of the urethra into the vagina.

Hypos'tasis (hi-pos'tas-is). 1. Deposit or sediment. 2. Formation of a deposit; especially a settling of blood from feeble blood-current.

Hypostat'ic. Of, or pertaining to, hypostasis.
Hyposthe'nia. Enfeebled state; defect of strength.
Hyposul'phurous acid. See *Acid.*
Hypoth'enar. Ridge on palm along bases of fingers and ulnar margin.
Hypother'mal. Moderately warm; deficient in heat.
Hy'pothermy (hi'po-ther-me). Abnormally low temperature.
Hypoto'nia, Hypot'onus, Hypot'ony. Diminished tension, especially intra-ocular tension.
Hypotoxic'ity. Diminished or mitigated toxic quality.
Hypoxan'thin. A leucomain from plant and animal tissue.
Hypsiceph'alus, Hypsoceph'alus. A head having a breadth-height index exceeding 75.
Hysteral'gia (his-ter-al'je-ah). Pain in the uterus.
Hysterec'tomy (his-ter-ek'to-me). Surgical removal of uterus.
Hyste'ria. Disease, mainly of women, characterized by lack of control over emotions and acts. **H. ma'jor.** Same as *Hystero-epilepsy.* **H. mi'nor,** hysteria with mild convulsions, in which consciousness is not lost.
Hyster'ical. Pertaining to, or affected with, hysteria.
Hystericoneural'gic. Resembling neuralgia, but of hysterical origin.
Hysteri'tis (his-ter-i'tis). Inflammation of womb.
Hysterocat'alepsy. Hysteria with cataleptic symptoms.
Hysteroclei'sis. Surgical closure of os uteri.
Hystero-ep'ilepsy. Severe type of hysteria with epileptiform convulsions.
Hysterogastror'rhaphy. Suture of uterus to gastric wall.
Hysterogen'ic. Causing hysterical phenomena or symptoms.
Hys'teroid (his'ter-oid). Like or akin to hysteria.
Hys'terolith (his'ter-o-lith). A uterine calculus.
Hysterol'ogy (his-ter-ol'o-je). The study of the uterus.
Hysterom'eter. Instrument for measuring the womb.
Hysterom'etry. Measurement of uterus, or its length.
Hysteromyo'ma. Myoma of the uterus.
Hysteromyomec'tomy. Excision of uterine myoma.
Hysteroneuro'sis. Nervous disease due to uterine lesion.
Hysterop'athy (his-ter-op'ath-e). Any uterine disease.
Hysteropex'ia. Fixation of uterus to abdominal wall.
Hys'terophore (his'ter-o-fōr). A pessary for uterine support.
Hysteropsycho'sis. Mental disease from disease of uterus.
Hysteropto'sis (his-ter-op-to'sis). Prolapse of the womb.
Hysteror'rhaphy. 1. The stitching of a lacerated uterus. 2. Same as *Hysteropexia.*
Hysterorrhex'is. Rupture of the womb.
Hyster'oscope. Instrument for examining womb.
Hyster'otome. Instrument for incising cervix uteri.
Hysterot'omy (his-ter-ot'o-me). Incision of uterus.
Hysterotrachelor'rhaphy. Plastic surgery of cervix uteri.
Hysterotrachelot'omy. Incision of neck of uterus.
Hysterotraumat'ic. Due to traumatic hysteria.
Hysterotrau'matism. Hysteric symptoms following traumatism.
Hysterotris'mus. Spasm of the uterus.
Hystrici'asis, Hys'tricism. 1. Morbid erection of hairs. 2. Ichthyosis hystrix.

I.

I. Symbol of *iodin*.
Iamatol'ogy (i-am-at-ol'o-je). Science of remedies.
Iatralip'tic method. Frictional application of remedies.
Iatralip'tics. Treatment by inunction and friction.
Iat'ric (i-at'rik). Pertaining to medicine or to a physician.
Iatrochem'istry. Obsolete opinion that chemistry is the basis of all therapeutics.
I'atrol (i'at-rol). Oxyindolmethylanilid; an antiseptic agent.
Iatrol'ogy (i-at-rol'o-je). Science of medicine.
Iatrophys'ics (i-at-ro-fiz'iks). Obsolete treatment of all diseases by physical or mechanical means.
Iatrotech'nics. Practical application of therapeutical principles.
Ic'ajin (ik'aj-in). Poisonous alkaloid from African drug.
Ice-bag, I.-cap, I.-compress. A poultice or bag of pounded ice to reduce the temperature.
Ice'land moss (is'land). See *Cetraria*. **I. spar,** transparent calcium carbonate, used in making Nicol prisms.
I'chor (i'kor). Watery fluid discharged from wounds or sores.
Ichore'mia (i-kor-e'me-ah). Contamination of the blood by septic or toxic material.
I'chorous (i'kor-us). Watery and acrid pus.
Ichorrhe'mia (i-kor-re'me-ah). See *Ichoremia*.
Ich'thidin, Ich'thin, Ich'thulin. Three substances from eggs of fishes.
Ichthyocol'la. Isinglass; gelatin from fish-bladders.
Ich'thyoid (ik'the-oid). Fish-like; shaped-like a fish.
Ich'thyol (ik'the-ol). A thick brownish liquid from a kind of asphalt; useful in skin-diseases.
Ichthyo'sis (ik-the-o'sis). Disease characterized by dryness, roughness, and scaliness of the skin. **I. follicula'ris,** form in which sebum and epithelium are heaped around orifices of hair-follicles. **I. hys'trix,** a variety with dry warty knobs. **I. seba'cea.** See *Seborrhea*. **I. sim'plex.** See *Xeroderma*.
Ichthyot'ic. Pertaining to, or affected with, ichthyosis.
Ichthyotox'icum. A poisonous principle obtainable from fish.
Ichthys'mus. Disease caused by eating rancid or poisonous fish.
I'cing-liver. Liver covered with a white coating like icing.
Icterepati'tis. Hepatitis and jaundice.
Icter'ic (ik-ter'ik). Pertaining to, or affected with, jaundice.
Icteri'tious (ik-ter-ish'us). Of the color of jaundice.
Ic'teroid (ik'ter-oid). Like or resembling jaundice.
Ic'terus. L. for *Jaundice*. **I. febri'lis.** See *Weil's disease*. **I. gra'vis,** acute yellow atrophy of liver. **I. neonato'rum,** jaundice of new-born children.
Ic'tus. A stroke, blow, or sudden attack.
Id. A chromosphere considered as a component of the idants.
I'dant. A chromosome regarded as a factor in heredity.
Ide'al paraplegia. See *Paraplegia*.
Idea'tion (i-de-a'shun). Clear mental presentation of an object.
Iden'tical points. The corresponding points in the retinas of the two eyes.
Ideomo'tion. Muscular action induced by a dominant idea.
Ideomo'tor. Transforming mental energy into motion.
Ideophren'ic insanity. See *Insanity*.
Id'iocy (id'e-o-se). Complete imbecility.
Idioglos'sia. Production of meaningless vocal sounds.
Idiomus'cular contraction. Motion produced by non-nervous stimulus: it is peculiar to degenerated muscles.
Ideoneuro'sis. Any neurosis arising from the nerves themselves.

Idiopath'ic (id-e-o-path'ik). Self-originated; neither sympathetic nor traumatic.

Idiop'athy (id-e-op'ath-e). A peculiar morbid state.

Id'ioplasm. Physical basis of inheritance in a germ or ovum; germ-plasm.

Id'iosome. An ultimate element of living matter.

Idiosyn'crasy. A habit or peculiarity of body or mind characteristic of any individual.

Id'iot (id'e-ot). A person without understanding.

Idor'gan. A potential organ or organism not possessed of personality.

Idro'sis (id-ro'sis). Same as *Hidrosis*.

Igasu'ric acid. An acid derived from nux vomica.

Igasu'rin. Compound of strychnin and brucin from nux vomica.

Igna'tia (ig-na'she-ah). The bean-like seed of *Strychnos ignatia*: used like nux vomica.

Igniextirpa'tion. Excision of an organ by cautery.

Ig'nipuncture. Therapeutic puncture with hot needles.

Ig'nis (ig'nis). L. for *Fire*. **I. sa'cer.** Same as *Herpes zoster*.

Igni'tion (ig-nish'un). The act of burning or of taking fire.

Il'eac passion. Same as *Ileus*.

Ileadel'phus. Monster fetus, double below the pelvis.

Ileec'tomy (il-e-ek'to-me). Surgical removal of the ileum.

Ilei'tis (il-e-i'tis). Inflammation of the ileum.

Ileoce'cal (il-e-o-se'kal). Pertaining to the ileum and cecum.

Ileocol'ic (il-e-o-kol'ik). Pertaining to the ileum and colon. **I. valve.** Same as *Ileocecal valve*.

Ileocoli'tis. Inflammation of ileum and colon.

Ileocolos'tomy. Formation of passage between ileum and colon.

Ileocolot'omy. Surgical incision of the ileum and colon.

Ileo-ileos'tomy. Formation of passage between two parts of the ileum.

Ileoproctot'omy. Formation of passage between ileum and rectum.

Ileorectos'tomy. Same as *Ileoproctostomy*.

Ileos'tomy. Formation of a surgical opening into the rectum.

Il'eum (il'e-um). The distal portion of the small intestine ending in the cecum.

Il'eus. Severe colic due to intestinal obstruction.

Il'iac. Pertaining to the ilium.

Ili'acus (il-i'ak-us). **I. muscle.** See *Muscles, Table of*.

Iliadel'phus (il-e-ad-el'fus). Same as *Ileadelphus*.

Iliocolot'omy. Surgical incision of the colon in the iliac region.

Iliocos'tal muscle. See *Sacrolumbalis*, in *Muscles, Table of*.

Iliofem'oral. Pertaining to the ilium and femur.

Iliohypogas'tric nerve. See *Nerves, Table of*.

Ilio-in'guinal. Pertaining to the iliac and inguinal regions.

Iliopso'as (il-e-o-so'as). The iliacus and psoas magnus muscles taken together.

Iliotib'ial band. Part of fascia lata which forms a sheath for the tensor fasciæ femoris.

Il'ium. 1. The flank. 2. Flat upper part of innominate bone.

Illaquea'tion. Cure of ingrowing eyelash by drawing with a loop.

Illic'ium ve'rum (il-lish'e-um). Asiatic tree affording star-anise and oil of anise.

Illumina'tion (il-lu-min-a'shun). The lighting up of a part, organ, or object for inspection. **Axial i.**, light transmitted or reflected along the axis of a microscope. **Direct i.**, light thrown upon the object from in front. **Focal i.**, when light is thrown upon the focus of a lens or mirror. **Oblique i.**, illumination from one side.

Illu'sion (il-lu'zhun). A false or misinterpreted sensory image.

Illu'sional. Pertaining to, or characterized by, illusions.

Im'age (im'ej). A picture or conception with more or less likeness to an objective reality. **Aerial i.,** image seen as in the air by the ophthalmoscope. **After i.,** retinal impression continued after the image proper has ceased to be visible. **Direct i., Erect i.,** picture from rays not yet focussed. **False i.,** image formed by the deviating eye in strabismus. **Inverted i.,** one which is upside down. **Real i.,** one formed where the emanating rays are collected. **Virtual i.** Same as *Direct i.*

Imbecil'ity. Feebleness of mind; extreme dementia.

Imbed'. To enclose in a fixing substance before section-cutting.

Imbibi'tion (im-bib-ish'un). The absorption of liquids.

Im'bricated. Overlapping like tiles or shingles.

Im'id. A monobasic acid ammonia in which two hydrogen atoms are replaced by an acid radical.

Immature (im-mat-ūr'). Unripe; not fully developed.

Imme'diate. Direct: with nothing intervening. **I. agglutination,** union by first intention. **I. auscultation.** See *Auscultation.* **I. cause,** a cause which directly originates a disease. **I. contagion,** contagion by direct personal contact. **I. union,** union by first intention.

Immed'icable (im-ed'ik-a-bl). Incurable.

Immer'sion. 1. The plunging of a body into a liquid. 2. The use of the microscope with the object and object-glass both covered with a liquid.

Immis'cible. Incapable of being mixed.

Immobiliza'tion. The rendering of a part incapable of being moved.

Immune (im-mûn'). Protected against any particular disease, as by inoculation.

Immu'nity (im-mu'nit-e). The condition of being immune. **Actual i.,** that conferred by recovery from a contagious disease. **Congenital i., Natural i.,** that which is possessed by a person from birth. **Passive i.,** that resulting from inoculation with an antitoxin or an attenuated virus.

Immuniza'tion. The process of rendering a subject immune.

Immunotox'in. Any antitoxin.

Impac'ted. Driven firmly in; closely lodged.

Impac'tion. Firm lodgement; condition of being wedged firmly.

Impal'udism. Malarial cachexia; marsh-poisoning.

Im'par. Not even; unequal; unpaired.

Imper'forate. Not open; abnormally closed.

Imperfora'tion. Abnormal closure or atresia.

Imper'meable. Not permitting a passage, as for fluids.

Imper'vious. Not affording a passage; impenetrable.

Impetig'enous (im-pe-tij'en-us). Pertaining to, or of the nature of, impetigo.

Impeti'go (im-pe-ti'go). A skin-disease characterized by isolated pustules. **I. contagio'sa,** a contagious form of impetigo. **I. herpetifor'mis,** severe disease affecting pregnant women, characterized by pustules in groups. **I. syphilit'ica,** a pustular eruption in syphilis.

Implanta'tion. 1. Transfer of sound teeth. 2. Skin-grafting. 3. The introduction of a solid medicine into the tissue. **Hypodermatic i.,** the putting of a medicine under the skin. **Parenchymatous i.,** the placing of a medicine in the substance of a tumor. **Teratic i.,** the partial blending of an imperfect fetus with one nearly perfect.

Impon'derable. Not capable of being weighed.

Im'potence, Im'potency. Want of power; chiefly of reproductive power.

Impregna'tion. 1. Fertilization of the ovum. 2. Saturation.

Impres'sio col'ica, I. duodena'lis, I. gas'trica, I. rena'lis. Impressions on the liver, made respectively by the colon, duodenum, stomach, and kidney.

Impres'sion (im-presh'un). 1. An indentation or dent. 2. An effect on the mind or senses produced by external objects.

Inac'tose (in-ak'tōs). A variety of optically inactive sugar.

Inad'equacy. Inability to perform allotted function.

Inalimen'tal (in-al-im-en'tal). Not nutritious.

Inan'imate. Lifeless; lacking in animation.

Inani'tion (in-an-ish'un). Lack of food; starvation.

Inap'petence (in-ap'pe-tenz). Lack of appetite or desire.

Inartic'ulate. Not uttered like articulate speech.

In artic'ulo mor'tis. At the very moment of death.

Inassim'ilable. Not susceptible of being utilized as nutriment.

Incandes'cent. Glowing with heat and light.

Incar'cerated. Closely confined; constricted.

Incarcera'tion. Abnormal retention or constriction.

In'ca's bone. The interparietal bone.

In'cident nerve. An afferent or centripetal nerve.

Incinera'tion (in-sin-er-a'shun). The act of burning to ashes.

Incip'ient (in-sip'e-ent). Commencing or beginning.

Incised wound (in-sizd'). A wound made by cutting.

Inci'sion (in-sizh'un). 1. A cut or wound. 2. The act of cutting.

Inci'sive (in-si'siv). 1. Having the power or quality of cutting; sharp. 2. Pertaining to the incisor teeth. **I. bone,** the anterior or medial part of the upper jaw-bone.

Inci'sor (in-si'zor). Any one of the four front teeth of either jaw.

Incisu'ra. A cut; an incision or notch. **I. cerebel'li,** the notch which separates the hemispheres of the cerebellum.

Incis'ures of Schmidt and Lantermann. Oblique slashes or lines on the sheath of the medullated nerve-fibers.

Inclinom'eter. Instrument for determining ocular diameter.

Inclu'sion. Enclosure within something else.

Incoer'cible (in-ko-er'sib-l). Uncontrollable.

Incohe'rent (in-ko-he'rent). Not coherent; incongruous.

Incombus'tible. Not susceptible of being burnt.

Incompat'ible. Mutually repellent, as medicines; not to be conjoined in the same preparation.

Incom'petence. Inadequacy or insufficiency. **I. of the valves,** a defect of heart-valves which causes their imperfect closure.

Incompres'sible. Not susceptible of being compressed.

Incon'tinence. Inability to restrain natural discharges.

Inco-ordina'tion. Lack of normal adjustment of muscular motions; failure to work harmoniously.

Incorpora'tion. Thorough mixing of a substance with another.

In'crement. Increase or augmentative growth.

Incrusta'tion. The formation of a crust; a crust or scab.

Incuba'tion. The period between the implanting of an infectious disease and its manifestation.

In'cubator. Apparatus for rearing prematurely-born infants.

In'cubus (in'ku-bus). 1. Nightmare. 2. A heavy mental burden.

In'cudal. Of, or pertaining to, the incus.

Incudostape'dial. Of, or pertaining to, the incus and stapes.

Incu'rable. Not susceptible of being cured.

In'cus. The anvil-shaped ossicle of the middle ear.

Indaga'tion. Careful search, inquiry, or examination.

Indenta'tion. A pit, dent, or depression.

In'dex. 1. The first or forefinger. 2. The numerical ratio of measurement of any part in comparison with a fixed standard. **Alveolar i.,** degree of prominence of jaws. **Cephalic i.,**

number found by multiplying cranial breadth by 100 and dividing by cranial length. **Cerebral i.,** ratio of greatest transverse to greatest anteroposterior diameter of cranial cavity. **Gnathic i.,** number expressing amount of projection of jaw. **Length-breadth i.** Same as *Cephalic i.* **Length-height i.,** the height of the skull expressed as a percentage of its length. **I.-movement,** a compulsory movement in which an animal turns round and round. **Pelvic i.,** ratio of conjugate and transverse diameters of pelvis. **Refractive i.,** the co-efficient of refraction. **Thoracic i.,** the ratio of the anteroposterior diameter of the thorax to the transverse diameter.

In'dian hemp. See *Cannabis* and *Apocynum.* **I. rubber,** caoutchouc; gum elastic. **I. tobacco.** See *Lobelia.*

In'dican. 1. Yellow glucosid, $C_{26}H_{3}$, from indigo plants. 2. A principle, $C_8H_7NSO_4$, from sweat and urine.

Indicanu'ria. Excess of amount of indican in the urine.

Indica'tion. Anything which shows what ought to be done.

Indif'ferent. Having no preponderating affinity; neutral.

Indig'enous (in-dij'en-us). Native to a place or country.

Indiges'tible (in-dij-es'tib-l). Not susceptible of digestion.

Indiges'tion. Dyspepsia; failure of digestive function.

Indigita'tion. Same as *Intussusception* or *Invagination.*

In'digo. Blue coloring matter from indigo plant (*Isatis, Indigofera,* etc.). **I. blue,** indigotin, $C_{16}H_{10}N_2O_2$, the main constituent of indigo. **I. carmin,** sodium and potassium sulphindigotate: used as a histologic stain.

Indig'ogen (in-dig'o-jen). A crystalline principle from indigo.

Indigo'tin. See *Indigo blue.*

Indigu'ria. The presence of indigo in the urine.

Indirect cell-division. See *Karyokinesis.*

Indisposi'tion. The condition of being ill; slight disease.

In'dol. A crystalline body, $C_8H_7N_1$, from indigo and feces.

In'dolent. With but little pain; sluggish.

Induced (in-dūst'). Produced or brought on by induction. **I. abortion.** See *Abortion.*

Induc'tion (in-duk'shun). 1. The process or act of inducing, or causing to occur. 2. The generation of electrical phenomena in a body by the influence of an electrified body near it.

Induc'togram (in-duk'to-gram). Same as *Skiagraph.*

Inducto'rium. An apparatus for generating induced electric currents.

In'durate, In'durated. Hardened; abnormally hard.

Indura'tion. Quality of being hard; process of hardening; and abnormally hard. **Black i.,** hardening and pigmentation of lung, as in anthracosis. **Brown i.,** deposit of altered blood-pigment in pneumonia. **Gray i.,** induration of lung-tissue in or after pneumonia, without pigmentation. **Red i.,** interstitial pneumonia in which the lung is red and congested.

In'durative. Pertaining to, or marked by, induration.

Ine'briant, An intoxicating agent.

Inebria'tion, Inebri'ety. A condition of drunkenness.

Inelas'tic. Lacking elasticity.

Iner'tia (in-er'she-ah). Inactivity. **I. u'teri,** atony of uterus in labor.

In extre'mis. At the point, or in the article, of death.

In'fant. A babe; a young child.

Infan'ticide (in-fan'tis-id). The murder of an infant.

In'fantile. Pertaining to an infant or to infancy.

In'farct. A mass of extravasated matter, especially in a vessel.

Infarc'tion. 1. The engorgement or stoppage of a canal. 2. An infarct.

Infec'tion. The communication of disease from one person to another, whether by effluvia or by contact, mediate or immediate; also, the implantation of disease from without.

Infec'tious. Liable to be communicated by infection.

Infecund'ity. Sterility or barrenness.

Infibula'tion. The fastening of the foreskin or labia majora with stitches or clasps to prevent copulation.

Infil'trate. Material deposited by infiltration.

Infiltra'tion. The deposit or diffusion of a morbid solid or fluid in any tissue. **I.-anesthesia.** See *Anesthesia.* **Calcareous i.,** deposit of lime and earthy salts in the tissues. **Cellular i.,** infiltration of tissues with round cells. **Fatty i.,** the deposit of fat in the tissues; presence of oil- or fat-globules in cells. **Glycogenic i.,** deposit of glycogen in cells. **Pigmentary i.,** deposits of pigment in tissues. **Purulent i.,** presence of dispersed pus-cells in a tissue. **Serous i.,** abnormal presence of serum in a tissue. **Urinous i.,** the extravasation of urine into a tissue. **Waxy i.,** deposition of amyloid substance.

In'finite distance. In optics any distance of over twenty feet, rays of light from which are practically parallel.

Infir'mary. A hospital, dispensary, or sanitarium.

Inflamma'tion. A morbid condition characterized by redness, pain, heat, and swelling. **Acute i.,** that in which the processes are active. **Adhesive i.,** that which promotes the union of cut surfaces. **Catarrhal i.,** one which affects principally a mucous surface and which is marked by discharge of muco-pus and epithelial debris. **Chronic i.,** inflammation of slow progress, marked by formation of new connective tissue. **Interstitial i.** affects primarily the materials between the essential structural elements. **Parenchymatous i.** affects chiefly the essential structural elements. **Reactive i.,** that which occurs around a foreign body or a focus of degeneration. **Specific i.,** one which is due to a special micro-organism. **Suppurative i.,** one which is characterized by the formation of pus. **Toxic i.,** one which is due to a poison, as to a ptomain or bacterial product. **Traumatic i.,** that which follows a wound or injury.

Inflam'matory. Pertaining to, or marked by, inflammation.

Infla'tion (in-fla'shun). Distention with air, gas, or fluid.

Inflec'tion (in-flek'shun). The act of bending inward or state of being bent inward.

Influen'za. An epidemic disease marked by depression, heaviness over the eyes, and distressing fever.

Influen'zal (in-flu-en'zal). Pertaining to influenza.

Influen'zin. A proprietary influenza cure.

Infra-axil'lary. Situated below the axilla.

Infraclavic'ular region. The region between the clavicle and the third rib.

Infracos'tal (in-fra-kos'tal). Situated below a rib.

Infrahy'oid. Below the hyoid bone.

Inframam'mary region. Space in chest below sixth rib.

Inframar'ginal convolution. See *Convolution.*

Inframax'illary. Situated below the jaw.

Infra-or'bital. Situated beneath the orbit.

Infrascap'ular. Situated beneath the shoulder-blade.

Infraspina'tus. See *Muscles, Table of.*

Infraspi'nous. Situated beneath the spine of the scapula.

Infraster'nal. Situated beneath the sternum.

Infratroch'lear. Situated beneath the trochlea.

Infric'tion. The rubbing of medicaments upon the skin.

Infundib'ular, Infundib'uliform. Shaped like a funnel. **I. fascia, I. process,** a process of the transversalis fascia ensheathing the cremaster muscle.

Infundib'ulum (in-fun-dib'u-lum). A funnel-shaped passage;

a, a canal from the pituitary body to the third ventricle; *b*, any one of the divisions of the pelvis of a kidney; *c*, a passage between the nasal meatus and the ethmoidal cells; *d*, the cavity of the fimbriæ of an oviduct; *e*, any one of the ultimate expansions of a bronchiole; *f*, a cavity at the upper end of the cochlear canal; *g*, the conus arteriosus.

Infu'sible. Not susceptible of being fused.

Infu'sion (in-fu'zhun). The steeping of a substance in water for obtaining its soluble principles; also the solution so obtained.

Infusodecoc'tion. A mixture of the infusion and the decoction of a substance.

Infuso'ria (pl.) (in-fu-zo're-ah). Microscopic protozoan animals, often found in infusions.

Infu'sum (in-fu'zum). L. for *Infusion*.

Inges'ta (in-jes'tah). Food and drink taken into the body.

Inges'tion (in-jes'chun). The act of taking food or drink.

Inges'tol (in-jes'tol). A proprietary dyspepsia cure.

In'gluvin (in'glu-vin). A ferment prepared from chickens' gizzards; used like pepsin.

Ingras'sias's apophysis. The lesser wing of the sphenoid.

Ingraves'cent. Gradually increasing in strength.

In'growing nail. The condition of a toe-nail when edge is overlapped by the flesh.

In'guen (in'gwen). L. for *Groin*.

In'guinal (ing'gwin-al). Pertaining to the groin.

Inhala'tion. The throwing of air or other vapor into the lungs.

Inha'ler. Instrument for administering a medicated vapor.

Inhe'rent. Implanted by nature; intrinsic; innate. **I. cauterization,** that which is deep and thorough.

Inhibi'tion (in-hib-ish'un). Arrest or restraint of a process affected by nervous influences.

Inhib'itory. Restraining or arresting any process.

Inhib'itrope. Persons in whom certain stimuli cause partial inhibition of function.

In'iac, In'ial (in'e-ak, in'e-al). Pertaining to the inion.

Inienceph'alus (in-e-en-sef'al-us). Fetus with a fissured occiput.

Inion (in'e-on). The external occipital protuberance.

Ini'tial (in-ish'al). Beginning or commencing.

Ini'tis (in-i'tis). Inflammation of muscular substance.

Injec'ted. Filled by injection; congested.

Injec'tion. The act of throwing a liquid into a part (as rectum or blood-vessel); also the substance thus thrown in; an enema.

In'let of the pel'vis. The upper limit of the pelvic cavity.

Innerva'tion. Distribution of the nerves.

In'nocent (in'o-sent). Not malignant; benign.

Innom'inate. Nameless or unnamed. **I. bone,** hip-bone; ischium, ilium, and pubes together.

Innox'ious (in-nok'shus). Not hurtful; not injurious.

I'noblast (i'no-blast). Connective-tissue cell in the formative stage.

Inoculabil'ity. Susceptibility of transmission by inoculation.

Inoc'ulable. 1. Transmissible by inoculation. 2. Not immune against a transmissible disease.

Inocula'tion. Insertion of virus into a wound or abrasion in the skin in order to communicate disease.

Ino-epithelio'ma. Epithelioma with fibrous elements.

I'nogen (i'no-jen). The supposed contractile substance of muscle.

Inohymeni'tis. Inflammation of any fibrous membrane.

Inoleiomyo'ma. Myoma containing unstriated muscle-fibers.

Ino'ma (in-o'mah). Same as *Fibroma*.

Inopex'ia. The tendency to spontaneous coagulation of the blood.

Inorgan'ic. 1. Having no organs. 2. Not of organic origin. **I.**

acid, any acid which contains no carbon. **I. compound**, any substance which is not of organic origin.

Inos'culating. Communicating directly; anastomosing.

Inoscula'tion. Anastomosis of the blood-vessels.

In'osite (in'o-sīt). Muscle-sugar, $C_6H_{12}O_6$, from muscle, urine, viscera, and plants.

Inosit'ic acid. An acid from muscle-tissue.

Inositu'ria. Occurrence of inosite in the urine.

Inosteato'ma. Fatty tumor combined with fibroma.

Inosu'ria (i-no'su're-ah). Same as *Inosituria.*

In'quest. Inquiry before a coroner as to manner of death.

Insaliva'tion. Saturation of food with saliva in mastication.

Insalu'brious. Unhealthy; injurious to health.

Insane (in-sān'). Affected with insanity: not of sound mind.

Insan'itary. Not in good sanitary condition.

Insan'ity. Disorder of the mental faculties; lunacy. **Acquired i.**, one arising after a long period of mental soundness. **Affective i.** Same as *Emotional i.* **Circular i., Cyclic i.**, insanity recurring in cycles, melancholia following mania, and being often followed by a lucid interval. **Climacteric i.**, that associated with the menopause. **Communicated i.**, that which is transmitted from one person to another. **Confusional i.**, acute temporary insanity following severe disease or nervous shock. **Doubting i.**, insanity characterized by morbid doubt, suspicion, and indecision. **Emotional i.**, that which is characterized by emotional depression or exaltation. **Epidemic i.**, a form which sometimes affects many persons in a community. **Hereditary i.**, that which is inherited from a parent or grandparent. **Homicidal i.**, insanity marked by a desire to take human life. **Ideational i.**, insanity with perverted ideation. **Ideophrenic i.**, insanity with perverted ideation. **Impulsive i.**, insane tendency to acts of violence. **Menstrual i.**, that which recurs at the menstrual period. **Moral i.**, that which is marked by impairment of the moral sense. **Perceptional i.**, a form marked by hallucination and illusions. **Periodic i.**, that which recurs at regular intervals.

Inscrip'tio tendin'ea. Tendinous cord traversing a muscle and giving attachment to its fibers.

Inscrip'tion. That part of a prescription which contains the names and amounts of ingredients.

In'sect powder. Powdered flowers of *Pyrethrum*, for destroying insects.

Insec'ticide (in-sek'tis-īd). A substance used for killing insects.

Insemina'tion. The fertilization of the ovum.

Insen'sible. 1. Devoid of sensibility or of consciousness. 2. Not perceptible to the senses.

Inser'tion (in-ser'shun). The place of attachment of a muscle to the bone which it moves.

Insid'ious (in-sid'e-us). Stealthy; treacherous.

In si'tu. In its natural or normal place.

Insola'tion. Sunstroke or thermic fever.

Insol'uble (in-sol'u-bl). Not susceptible of being dissolved.

Insom'nia (in-som'ne-ah). Inability to sleep; wakefulness.

Inspec'tion (in-spek'shun). Examination by the eye.

Insper'sion (in-sper'shun). A sprinkling with powder.

Inspira'tion. The act of drawing air into the lungs.

In'spiratory. Pertaining to or subserving inspiration.

In'spissated (in'spis-a-ted). Thickened; made less fluid.

In'step. The dorsal part of the arch of the foot.

Instilla'tion. Act of dropping a liquid into a cavity, as the eye.

Institutes of medicine. The fundamental principles of medical science; especially physiology and pathology.

In'strument. Any mechanical appliance, tool, or apparatus.

Instrumen'tal. Pertaining to, or performed by, an instrument. **I. labor,** parturition facilitated by instruments.

Instrumenta'tion. The use and care of instruments.

Insuffic'iency (in-suf-ish'en-se). Same as *Inadequacy*.

Insuffla'tion. The blowing of a powder, vapor, or gas into a cavity.

Insuffla'tor. An instrument for blowing a powder into a cavity.

In'sula (in'syu-lah). The island of Reil.

In'sular (in'syu-lar). Of, or pertaining to, the insula.

Insula'tion. The prevention of the escape of electricity from a body by means of non-conductors.

Integ'ument. The natural covering of the body; the skin.

Integumen'tary. Pertaining to, or composed of, skin.

In'tellect. The mind, thinking faculty, or understanding.

Intem'perance. Excess in the use of food or drink.

Inten'sity (in-ten'sit-e). A high degree of activity and power.

Inten'sive (in-ten'siv). Increasing in force or intensity.

Inten'tion. The agglutination of the edges of a wound in healing. See *Healing*.

Interang'ular segment. The part of a nerve between any two consecutive nodes of Ranvier.

Interartic'ular. Situated between articulating surfaces.

Interauric'ular. Situated between the auricles.

In'terbrain. Same as *Thalamencephalon*.

Interca'dence. The occurrence of occasional extra beats between any two pulse-beats.

Inter'calary (in-ter'kal-a-re). Inserted between; interposed.

Intercarot'ic ganglion. An enlargement connected with the carotid plexus at the bifurcation of the common carotid.

Intercel'lular. Situated between the cells.

Intercen'tral. Situated between, or connecting, nerve-centers.

Interchon'dral (in-ter-kon'dral). Situated between cartilages.

Intercil'ium (in-ter-sil'e-um). The space between the eyebrows.

Interclavic'ular. Situated between the clavicles.

Intercolum'nar fascia. A membrane situated between the pillars of the abdominal ring and enclosing the spermatic cord.

Intercon'dylar, Intercon'dylous. Between two condyles.

Intercos'tal. Situated between ribs.

Intercosta'les (in-ter-kos-ta'lēz). See *Muscles, Table of*.

Intercostohumera'lis. A branch of the second intercostal nerve going to the skin of the arm.

Intercur'rent. Breaking into and modifying the course of a disease.

Interden'tal. Situated or placed between the teeth.

Interdig'ital. Between any two fingers or toes.

Interdigita'tion. 1. An interlocking of parts by finger-like processes. 2. One of a set of finger-like processes.

Interfib'rillary. Occurring between fibrils.

Interfi'lar. Situated between the fibrils of a reticulum.

Interganglion'ic. Situated between ganglions.

Interglob'ular spaces. The irregular spaces within the dentin.

Interlob'ular emphysema. That which is characterized by the presence of air between the lobules of the lung.

Intermax'illary. Situated between the jaws, or maxilla. **I. bone.** Same as *Incisive bone*.

Intermediolat'eral tract of spinal cord. A tract which is lateral and between the dorsal and ventral horns.

Intermenin'geal. Situated between the meninges.

Intermis'sion. Period between two paroxysms or recurrences; temporary cessation.

Intermit'tent. Having periods of cessation of activity.

Intermus'cular. Situated between muscles.

Intern'(in-tern'). See *Interne.*

Inter'nal capsule. See *Capsule.* **I. ear,** labyrinth of ear.

Interne'(in-tern'). A resident physician or surgeon of a hospital.

In'ternode. Any interannular segment of a nerve-fiber.

Internun'cial fibers. Fibers which connect nerve-cells.

Inter'nus. 1. Internal. 2. The rectus internus muscles of the eye.

Interol'ivary. Situated between the olivary bodies.

Interor'bital. Situated between the orbits.

Interos'seous (in-ter-os'se-us). Situated between bones.

Interos'seus. See *Muscles, Table of.*

Interpari'etal. Situated between parietal bones. **I. suture.** Same as *Sagittal suture.*

Interpedun'cular space. The space bounded by the crura cerebri and optic tracts.

Interpu'bic. Situated between the pubic bones.

Interrup'ter. An automatic device for breaking an electric current.

Interscap'ular. Situated between the scapulæ.

Interspina'lis (in-ter-spi-na'lis). See *Muscles, Table of.*

Interstit'ial (in-ter-stish'al). Pertaining to, or situated in, interstices.

Intertrag'icus (in-ter-traj'ik-us). See *Muscles, Table of.*

Intertransversa'lis. See *Muscles, Table of.*

Intertri'go (in-ter-tri'go). Erythema due to chafing of the skin.

Intertrochanter'ic lines. Two ridges around the base of the neck of the femur.

Intertu'bular (in-ter-tu'bu-lar). Situated between tubules.

Interventric'ular. Situated between the ventricles.

Interver'tebral. Situated between vertebræ.

Intes'tin. A proprietary intestinal antiseptic.

Intes'tinal. Pertaining to the intestines.

Intes'tine. Membranous tube extending from the stomach to the anus. The first, longer and narrower portion is the *small*, the other is the *large* intestine.

In'tima. The innermost coat of a blood-vessel.

Intimi'tis. Inflammation of an intima.

Intol'erance. Inability to endure or withstand.

Intra-abdom'inal. Situated within abdomen.

Intra-arte'rial. Situated within an artery or the arteries.

Intra-artic'ular (in-trah-ar-tik'u-lar). Situated within a joint.

Intracap'sular (in-trah-kap'su-lar). Situated within a capsule.

Intracartilag'inous. Situated or formed within a cartilage.

Intracel'lular (in-trah-sel'u-lar). Situated within a cell or cells.

Intracra'nial. Situated within the cranium.

In'trad (in'trad). Inwardly.

Intrafi'lar mass. Same as *Paramitome.*

Intraligamen'tous. Situated within a ligament.

Intralob'ular. Situated within a lobule.

Intramu'ral. Situated within the walls of an organ.

Intramus'cular. Situated within the muscular substance.

Intra-oc'ular. Situated within the eye.

Intrapari'etal. Situated in the substance of a wall.

Intraperitone'al. Occurring within the peritoneal sac.

Intrathorac'ic (in-trah-tho-ras'ik). Situated within the thorax.

Intra-u'terine. Situated or occurring in the uterus.

Intravasa'tion. Entrance of abnormal material into vessels.

Intrave'nous (in-trah-ve'nus). Situated within the veins.

Intraventric'ular. Situated within a ventricle.

Intrin'sic muscle. Any muscle attached wholly to one organ and its accessories.

Intro'itus. The entrance to a cavity or space.

Intromis'sion. The insertion of one part or thing into another.

Introsuscep'tion. Same as *Intussusception.*
Introver'sion (in-tro-ver'shun). A turning inside out.
Intuba'tion. The insertion of a tube, as into the larynx.
Intumes'cence. A normal or abnormal swelling.
Intumes'cent (in-tu-mes'ent). Swelling or becoming swollen.
Intumescen'tia ganglifor'mis. See *Ganglion, geniculate.*
Intussuscep'tion. The invagination or indigitation of a portion of the intestine into an adjacent portion.
Intussuscep'tum. A portion of intestine which has been pushed into another part.
Intussuscip'iens. That portion of intestine which contains the intussusceptum.
In'ula (in'yu-lah). A genus of plants. See *Elecampane.*
In'ulin. A starch, $C_6H_{10}O_5$, from inula.
In'ulol (in'yu-lol). Same as *Alantol.*
Inunc'tion. The rubbing of the skin with an ointment.
Invag'inated. Thrust inward in the manner of a pouch.
Invagina'tion (in-vad-jin-a'shun). The telescoping of an organ in the manner of a pouch.
In'valid. 1. Not well and strong. 2. A person not in good health.
Inva'sion (in-va'zhun). The attack or onset of a disease.
Invermina'tion. Diseased state induced by worms.
Inver'sion (in-ver'shun). A turning upside down.
Inver'tin. Ferment obtainable from the intestine and from yeast.
In'vert-sugar. 1. Levulose. 2. A mixture of levulose and dextrose.
Invet'erate. Confirmed and chronic; difficult to cure.
In vit'ro. Occurring in a glass, as in a test-tube.
In'volucre, Involu'crum. A covering or sheath, as of a sequestrum.
Invol'untary. Performed independently of the will.
Involu'tion. 1. A rolling or turning inward. 2. Reduction in size. 3. Retrograde change.
I'odal. A hypnotic somewhat like chloral, C_2I_3HO.
Iodantife'brin. A crystalline antipyretic, $C_6H_4INH(C_2H_3O)$.
Iodantipy'rin. Same as *Iodopyrin.*
I'odat (i'od-āt). Any salt of iodic acid.
Iod'ic acid (i-od'ik). See *Acid.*
I'odid (i'od-id). Any binary compound of iodin.
I'odin (i'od-in). A halogen element with peculiar odor and taste: irritant and absorbent: symbol I.
I'odism (i'od-izm). Ill health due to injudicious use of the iodids.
I'odized (i'od-izd). Charged with, or under the influence of, iodin.
Iodoamy'lum. Insoluble iodized starch: a surgical antiseptic.
Iodocaf'fein. White crystalline compound; used in heart-diseases.
Iodoca'sein. A yellow antiseptic powder.
Io'docin. A proprietary antiseptic substance.
Iodocre'sol. Antiseptic compound: used like cresol.
Iododer'ma. Iodin acne.
Iodoeu'genol. An antiseptic preparation of iodin and eugenol.
Iod'oform (i-od'o-form). A crystalline substance, CHI_3, with pungent odor: anesthetic and antiseptic.
Iodofor'min. Antiseptic containing iodoform and urotropin.
Iodofor'mism. Poisoning by iodoform.
Iodog'enin. Charcoal treated with iodin: used in fumigation.
I'odol (i'o-dol). A brownish powder, $C_4O_4NH_4$: used like iodoform.
Iodophena'cetin, Iodophe'nin. An antiseptic powder.
Iodophenochlo'ral. Parasiticide mixture of tincture of iodin, carbolic acid, chloral hydrate.
Iodophe'nol. A carbolic-acid solution of iodin.
Iodopy'rin. An antiseptic compound, $C_{11}H_{11}IN_2O$.

Iodother'apy. Use of iodin and iodids as remedies.
Iodothy'mol. Same as *Aristol.*
Iodothy'rin. Active principle of the thyroid gland.
Iod'ozone. An antiseptic preparation containing iodin and ozone.
Io'dum (i-o'dum). L. for *Iodin.*
I'on (i'on). An element set free by electrolysis.
I'onone (i'o-nōn). Odoriferous derivative of orris-root.
Io'tacism (i-o'tah-sizm). Defective utterance of the *i* sound.
Ip'ecac, Ipecac'uan. Same as *Ipecacuanha.*
Ipecacuan'ha. The root of *Cephaelis ipecacuanha:* diaphoretic, emetic, and expectorant.
Ir. Abbreviation for *Internal resistance.*
Ir'idal. Of, or pertaining to, the iris.
Iridec'tome. A cutting instrument used in iridectomy.
Iridec'tomize. To excise a part of the iris.
Iridec'tomy. Excision of a slip of iris for artificial pupil.
Iridenclei'sis (ir-id-en-kli'sis). Strangulation of a slip of the iris in a corneal incision.
Iridere'mia (ir-id-er-e'me-ah). Absence of the iris.
Irid'esis. Formation of artificial iris.
Irid'ic (i-rid'ik). Pertaining to the iris.
Irid'ocele (i-rid'os-ēl). Hernial protrusion of a slip of the iris.
Iridochoroidi'tis. Inflammation of the iris and choroid.
Iridocolobo'ma. Fissure of the iris.
Iridocycli'tis. Inflammation of the iris and ciliary organs.
Iridod'esis. Formation of artificial pupil by ligating the iris.
Iridodial'ysis. 1. Same as *Corediatysis.* 2. Separation or loosening the iris form its attachments.
Iridodon'esis (i-rid-o-don'es-is). Same as *Hippus.*
Iridople'gia (i-rid-o-ple'je-ah). Paralysis of the pupil. **Accommodative i.,** failure of iris to contract or accommodate effort.
Iridorrhex'is. 1. Rupture of iris. 2. A tearing away of iris.
Iridosclerot'omy. Puncture of the sclerotic and of the edge of the iris.
Irido'sis (i-rid-o'sis). Same as *Iridodesis.*
Iridot'omy. Formation of artificial pupil by cutting.
I'ris. 1. Pigmented membrane behind the cornea, perforated by the pupil. 2. Genus of plants with cathartic rhizome.
I'rish moss. Same as *Chondrus.*
Irit'ic (i-rit'ik). Pertaining to the iris.
Iri'tis (i-ri'tis). Inflammation of the iris.
Irit'omy (i-rit'om-e). Same as *Iridotomy.*
I'ron. A metallic element, symbol Fe: much used in medicine.
Irra'diating. Spreading out, or diverging, as from the center.
Irredu'cible (ir-red-u'sib-l). That which cannot be reduced.
Irres'pirable. Not to be breathed with safety.
Irriga'tion. Washing by a stream of water or other lotion.
Irritabil'ity. Quality of being irritable. **Faradic i.,** condition in which a faradic current will produce a muscular response. **Galvanic i.,** state wherein a galvanic current will cause a muscular response. **Muscular i.,** the normal contractile quality of muscle. **Nervous i.,** the ability of a nerve to transmit impulses.
Ir'ritable. 1. Capable of reacting to a stimulus. 2. Abnormally sensitive to stimuli.
Ir'ritant. 1. Causing irritation. 2. Agent causing irritation.
Irrita'tion. 1. The act of stimulating. 2. A state of over-excitation and undue sensitiveness.
Ir'ritative. Pertaining to irritation; causing irritation.
Isambert's disease (e-zaw-bārz'). Miliary laryngeal tuberculosis.
Ische'mia (is-ke'me-ah). Deficiency of blood-supply of a part.
Ischi'ac, Ischiad'ic (is'ke-ak, is-ke-ad'ik). Same as *Ischiatic.*
Is'chial, Ischiat'ic. Pertaining to the ischium.

Ischidro'sis (is-kid-ro'sis). Suppression of secretion of sweat.
Ischiobul'bar. Pertaining to ischium and bulb of urethra.
Ischiocaverno'sus. See *Erector penis*, in *Muscles, Table of.*
Is'chiocele (is'ke-o-sēl). Hernia at the sacrosciatic notch.
Ischiococcyg'eus. 1. The coccygeus muscle. 2. Posterior part of the levator ani.
Ischiofem'oral. Pertaining to the ischium and femur.
Ischiome'nia. Suppression of the menstrual flow.
Ischioneural'gia (is-ke-o-nu-ral'je-ah). Same as *Sciatica.*
Ischiop'agus. A monster with two heads and bodies and united at hips.
Ischiopu'bic. Pertaining to the ischium and pubes.
Ischiopubiot'omy. Obstetric division of the ischiopubic and horizontal branches of the os pubis.
Ischiorec'tal. Of, or pertaining to, the ischium and rectum.
Is'chium (is'ke-um). The lower hind part of the innominate bone.
Ischuret'ic (is-ku-ret'ik). Pertaining to ischuria.
Ischu'ria (is-ku're-ah). Retention or suppression of the urine.
I'singlass (I'sin-glas). Same as *Ichthyocolla.*
Is'land of Reil. Isolated part of the cerebral cortex in the fissure of Sylvius.
Iso-amylam'in. A ptomain from stale yeast.
Iso-am'ylene (i-so-am'il-ēn). Same as *Pental.*
Isochromat'ic. Of the same color throughout.
Isoch'ronous (i-sok'ro-nus). Performed in equal times.
Isoco'ria (i-so-ko're-ah). Equality of pupils in the two eyes.
Isodiamet'ric. Having a uniform diameter.
Isodynam'ic foods (i-so-di-nam'ik). Foods which generate equal amounts of force in heat units.
Iso-elec'tric (i-so-e-lek'trik). Uniformly electric throughout.
I'solate. To separate from other persons, materials, or objects.
Isola'tion. Separation of persons having infectious disease.
I'somer (i'so-mer). Any isomeric substance.
Isomer'ic. Made up of the same elements in the same proportions, yet unlike.
Isom'erism (i-som'er-izm). Quality of being isomeric.
Isomet'ric. 1. Of equal dimensions. 2. Not isotonic. **I. muscle,** a muscle whose tension is altered on stimulation, its length being unchanged.
Isomor'phism. The quality of being isomorphous.
Isomor'phous (i-so-mor'fus). Having the same form.
Isonaph'tol. An antiseptic derived from naphtalene.
Isonitro'so-antipy'rin. A diuretic and antipyretic compound, $C_{11}H_{11}N_3O_2$.
Isop'athy. Treatment by administering the virus which causes the disease.
Isopep'sin (i-so-pep'sin). Pepsin changed by heat.
Isop'ters (i-sop'terz). Curves in the field of vision, denoting equality of visual acuity.
Isother'mal. Having or indicating the same temperature.
Isoton'ic muscle. Muscle which contracts on stimulation, its tension remaining unchanged.
Isotrop'ic (i-so-trop'ik). Having a single and uniform refraction.
Is'sue (is'u). A suppurating sore, made and kept open by inserting an irritant substance. **I. pea,** a pellet of orris-root or other material used in making and maintaining an issue.
Is'tarin (is'tar-in). A substance obtainable from brain-tissue.
Isthmi'tis (ist-mi'tis). Inflammation of isthmus of fauces.
Isthmus (ist'mus). A narrow strip of tissue or a narrow passage connecting two larger parts. **I. of Eustachian tube,** the narrowest part of the Eustachian tube. **I. fau'cium,** the pas-

sage between the mouth and fauces. **I. of thyroid,** the band or strip of tissue joining the lobes of the thyroid.

Ital'ian leprosy. Same as *Pellagra.* **I. rhinoplasty,** the Taliacotian operation.

Itch. A skin-disease attended with itching; scabies. See *Bakers'*, *Barbers'*, *Grocers'*, etc.

Itch'ing. Pruritus; a teasing irritation of the skin.

I'ter. A way or tubular passage. **I. ad infundib'ulum,** the passage from the third ventricle to the infundibulum. **I. a ter'tio ad quar'tum ventric'ulum.** Same as *Aqueduct of Sylvius.* **I. den'tium,** the passage through which a permanent tooth makes its appearance.

I'trol. Citrate of silver; used in gonorrhea.

I'vain (I'va-in). A yellow material, $C_{24}H_{42}O_5$, from *Achillea moschata.*

I'vory. 1. See *Dentin.* 2. Bone-like material from the tusks of elephants. **I. black.** Same as *Animal charcoal.*

Ixo'des. A genus of ticks parasitic on man and animals.

Ixomyeli'tis. Inflammation of the lumbar part of the cord.

I'zal. A proprietary disinfectant from coke-ovens.

J.

J. Symbol for Joule's equivalent.

Jaboran'di. The shrub *Pilocarpus selloanus,* of South America: sialagogue and sudorific.

Jab'orin. Alkaloid from jaborandi, $C_{11}H_{16}N_2O_2$.

Jacaran'da. Leaves of South American tree: used in syphilis.

Jaccoud's sign (zhah-kooz'). Prominence of aorta in suprasternal notch in leukemia and pseudoleukemia.

Jackso'nian epilepsy. See *Epilepsy.*

Ja'cob's membrane. Same as *Basilar layer.* **J.'s ulcer.** Same as *Rodent ulcer.*

Ja'cobson's cartilage. Hyaline cartilage which supports J.'s organ. **J.'s nerve,** the tympanic branch of the glossopharyngeal. **J.'s organ,** sac in nasal septum, in man rudimentary except in the fetus. **J.'s sulcus,** trench in middle ear which contains branches of tympanic plexus.

Jactita'tion. Tossing to-and-fro in acute sickness.

Jadelot's lines, furrows, or **traits** (zhahd-lōz'). Lines of the face in young children, regarded as indicative of disease.

Jail fever. Same as *Typhus.*

Jaksch's disease (yahkshs). Infantile pseudoleukemia.

Ja'lap, Jala'pa. The root of *Exogonium purga,* of Mexico: actively cathartic.

Jal'apin (jal'ap-in). Cathartic glucosid from *Ipomœa orizabensis.*

Jamai'ca dogwood. The plant *Piscidia erythrina:* sedative.

James's powder. An official antimonial powder.

James'town weed. Same as *Stramonium.*

Jan'iceps (jan'is-eps). Monster fetus with two faces.

Japacon'itin. Poisonous base from Japanese aconite.

Jarjavay's muscle (zhar-zhah-vāz'). The depressor urethræ.

Jas'min, yellow. See *Gelsemium.*

Jat'ropha cur'cas. A tropical tree, affords a purging oil. **J. man'ihot.** See *Cassava.*

Jaun'dice. Yellowness of skin and eyes from bile-pigments. **Catarrhal j.,** that caused by catarrhal inflammation of bile-ducts. **Hematogenous j.,** that which is due to destruction of blood-corpuscles. **Hepatogenous j.,** a form caused by obstruction of the bile-ducts. **Malignant j.** Same as *Icterus gravis.* **J. of the new-born.** See *Icterus neonatorum.*

Jaw, Jaw-bone. See *Maxilla*. **J.-clonus, J.-jerk,** a tendon-reflex obtained by depressing the lower Jaw.

Jec'orin. Proprietary substitute for cod-liver oil.

Je'cur. L. for *Liver*.

Je'junal. Pertaining to the jejunum.

Jejuni'tis. Inflammation of the jejunum.

Jejunocolos'tomy. Formation of artificial opening between jejunum and colon.

Jejuno-ilei'tis. Inflammation of the jejunum and ileum.

Jejuno-ileos'tomy. Formation of artificial opening between jejunum and ileum.

Jejunos'tomy. Surgical creation of opening into jejunum through abdominal wall.

Jeju'num. Second portion of small intestine, between the duodenum and the ileum.

Jenne'rian. Relating to Edward Jenner, who invented vaccination.

Jequir'ity. Seeds of *Abrus precatorius*: used in treating trachoma.

Jerk'ing respiration. See *Respiration*.

Jer'vin. Alkaloid, $C_{26}H_{37}NO_3$, from *Veratrum album* and *V. viride*.

Jes'samine. See *Gelsemium*.

Jes'uit's bark. Same as *Cinchona*.

Jig'ger. Same as *Chigre*.

Jim'son weed. Same as *Stramonium*.

Jobert's suture (zho-bârz'). See *Suture*.

Jo'dum (yo'doom). Ger. for *Iodin*.

Joff'roy's symptom. Absence of facial contraction when patient suddenly turns his eyes upward: seen in exophthalmic goiter.

Joint-disease. Same as *Charcot's arthropathy*.

Joule (jool). Work expended by a current of one ampere flowing for one second against a resistance of one ohm.

Joule's equivalent (joolz). Work expended in raising one gram of water through 1° C.

Ju'gal. Pertaining to the cheek bone. **J. bone.** Same as *Malar bone*. **J. process.** Same as *Zygomatic process*.

Ju'glans cine'rea. The butternut tree: bark mildly aperient.

Ju'gular. Pertaining to the neck. **J. foramen.** See *Foramen*. **J. fossa,** part of j. foramen for passage of j. vein. **J. ganglion.** (1) node of root of vagus, and (2) on glossopharyngeal nerve; both in j. foramen. **J. process,** (1) point of temporal, and (2) of occipital bone at j. foramen. **J. veins,** great veins in the neck conveying most of the blood from the head.

Jugula'tion. Rapid arrest of disease by therapeutic measures.

Ju'gum pe'nis. Forceps for compressing the penis.

Juice (jūs). Fluid from animal or plant tissue. **J.-canals,** spaces in connective tissue forming the origins of lymphatic vessels. **Gastric J.,** the clear liquid secreted by the stomach. **Intestinal J.,** transparent liquid secreted by the follicles of Lieberkühn. **Pancreatic J.,** thick, transparent fluid secreted by pancreas.

Ju'jube. Fruit of *Zizyphus vulgaris*: pectoral.

Ju'lep. Sweetened alcoholic drink or cordial.

Jump'er. Neurotic individual affected with palmus.

Jump'ing disease. Enfeebled will, with jumping movements.

Jun'gle fever. Severe form of tropical remittent.

Ju'niper. A tree, *Juniperus communis*: oil of fruit is a stimulant diuretic.

Junk. Form of cushion used in dressing fractures.

Junk'et. Curds and whey flavored and used as food.

Junod's boot (zhu-nōz'). A case for foot and leg fitted to an air-pump: used in relieving congestions of the head or viscera.

Jurispru'dence (ju-ris-pru'dens). See *Medical Jurisprudence.*
Ju'ry-mast. Upright bar used in supporting head in cases of Pott's disease.
Jus'culum (jus'ku-lum). Soup or broth.
Jus'to ma'jor. Larger than is normal or usual. **J. mi'nor,** smaller than is normal or usual.
Jute (jût). Fiber of *Corchorus olitorius:* used in surgical dressings.
Ju'vantia (ju'van-she-ah). Adjuvant and palliative medicines.
Juxta-artic'ular. Near a joint; in the region of a joint.
Juxtaposi'tion. Adjacent situation; apposition.

K.

K. The symbol of *Potassium.*
Ka. Abbreviation of *Kathode* (cathode).
Kaif (kif) [Arab.]. Dreamy tranquillity from use of drugs.
Kai'rin. An antipyretic alkaloid, $C_{10}H_{13}ON.ACl + H_2O$, from quinolin.
Kai'rolin. Antipyretic medicine, $C_{10}H_{15}N$, from kairin.
Kak'ke. Same as *Beriberi.*
Kakos'mia (kak-os'me-ah). Foul or disagreeable smell.
Kakot'rophy (kak-ot'rof-e). Same as *Cacotrophy.*
Ka'li (kal'le). Ger. for *Potash.*
Kalim'eter (kal-im'et-er). Same as *Alkalimeter.*
Ka'lium (ka'le-um). Same as *Potassium.*
Kam'ala. Hairs and capsular glands of *Mallotus philippinensis:* purgative and anthelmintic.
Kam'alin. Alkaloid from kamala.
Kan'dahar sore. A form of oriental sore.
Kangaroo' ligature. Ligature from tail-tendons of kangaroo.
Ka'olin. Fine clay used in skin-disease and in pharmacy.
Kapo'si's disease (kah-po'sēs). Same as *Xeroderma pigmentosum.*
Kar'yochrome. Nerve-cell with an easily staining nucleus.
Karyokine'sis, Karyol'ysis. Indirect nuclear division.
Kar'yolymph. The nuclear sap.
Kar'yomite. Same as *Chromosome.*
Karyomi'tome (kar-e-om'it-ōm). Nuclear chromatin network.
Karyomito'sis (kar-e-o-mit-o'sis). Same as *Karyokinesis.*
Kar'yon (kar'e-on). The nucleus of a cell.
Kar'yophage. An intracellular sporozoon.
Kar'yoplasm. Nucleoplasm; nuclear substance.
Karyothe'ca. The nuclear membrane of a cell.
Kat-, Kata-. For words thus beginning, see *Cat-, Cata-.*
Ka'va-Ka'va (kah'vah-kah'vah). Root and resin of *Piper methysticum:* used for cystitis, gout, and wasting diseases.
Keep'er. The armature of a magnet.
Ke'fir, Ke'phyr (ke'fer). A preparation of fermented milk.
Kel'ectome. Device used in removing samples of tumor-tissue.
Ke'lene, Ke'lin. Same as *Chelene.*
Ke'lis (ke'lis). Same as *Keloid;* also *Morphea.*
Ke'loid, Ke'los. Multiple formation of skin-tumors.
Keloso'mus (ke-lo-so'mus). Same as *Celosomus.*
Kelot'omy. Relief of hernial strangulation by cutting.
Kenopho'bia. Morbid dread of large open spaces.
Keph'alin (kef'al-in). Same as *Cephalin.*
Ke'phyr. Same as *Kefir.*
Ker'asin (ker'as-in). Same as *Cerasin.*
Keratal'gia (ker-at-al'je-ah). Pain in the cornea.
Kerateeta'sia. Protrusion of the cornea.
Ker'atin. Substance which forms the base of horny tissues.

Kerat'inous (ker-at'in-us). Composed of keratin.

Kerati'tis. Inflammation of the cornea. **K. bullo'sa,** presence of large or small blebs upon the cornea. **Interstitial k.,** when the entire cornea becomes hazy. **Neuroparalytic k.,** that which follows disease of the trifacial nerve. **Phlyctenular k.,** a variety marked by formation of pustules or papules on the cornea. **Punctate k.** Same as *Descemetitis*. **Purulent k.,** that in which pus is formed. **Sclerosing k.,** k. with scleritis. **Trachomatous k.** Same as *Pannus*. **Traumatic k.,** that which results from a wound of the cornea.

Ker'atocele (ker'at-o-sēl). Corneal protrusion of Descemet's membrane.

Keratoco'nus (ker-at-o-ko'nus). Cone-shaped corneal deformity.

Keratog'enous (ker-at-oj'en-us). Producing a horny tissue.

Keratoglo'bus. Globular corneal enlargement.

Keratohelco'sis (ker-at-o-hel-ko'sis). Ulceration of the cornea.

Kerato-iri'tis. Inflammation of the cornea and iris.

Keratol'ysis (ker-at-ol'is-is). Peeling off of the skin.

Kerato'ma (ker-at-o'mah). Any growth of horny tissue.

Keratomala'cia (ker-at-o-ma-la'she-ah). Softening of cornea.

Ker'atome (ker'at-ōm). A knife for incising the cornea.

Keratom'eter. An instrument for measuring the curves of the cornea.

Keratom'etry. Measurement of corneal curves.

Keratomyco'sis. Fungous disease of the cornea.

Keratonyx'is (ker-at-o-nik'sis). Puncture of the cornea.

Ker'atoplasty. Plastic surgery of the cornea.

Ker'atoscope. Instrument for examining cornea.

Keratos'copy. 1. Inspection of the cornea. 2. Skiascopy.

Kerato'sis. Formation of horny growth or tissue. **K. pila'ris,** formation of a hard elevation around each hair-follicle. **K. seni'lis,** a harsh, dry state of skin in old age.

Kerat'otome (ke-rat'o-tōm). See *Keratome*.

Keraunoneuro'sis. Nerve disorder from lightning-stroke.

Keraunopho'bia. Morbid dread of lightning.

Kerec'tomy (ke-rek'to-me). Removal of a part of the cornea.

Ke'rion (ke're-on). A pustular disease of the scalp.

Kerk'ring's valves. Same as *Valvulæ conniventes*.

Ker'mes. An insect found on leaves of various oaks: used as a dye-stuff. **K. mineral,** antimony oxysulphid.

Ke'tone. Any compound of the radical CO with two alcohol radicals.

Key and Retzius's foram'ina. Two passages from cisterna magna to the fourth ventricle.

Kibe (kīb). Same as *Chilblain*.

Kid'ney (kid'ne). Either one of two glandular bodies in the lumbar region which secrete the urine. **Amyloid k.,** one which is the seat of amyloid degeneration. **Fatty k.,** one which is affected with fatty degeneration. **Floating k.,** one which is loosened and displaced. **Gouty k., Granular k.,** one affected with chronic interstial inflammation. **Horse-shoe k.,** union of the ends of the two kidneys. **Large white k.,** one affected with chronic interstitial nephritis. **Pigback k.,** congestion of kidney in chronic alcoholism. **Red contracted k.** See *Gouty k.* **Small white k.,** atrophied and degenerated state following chronic interstitial nephritis. **Surgical k.,** suppurative pyelonephritis after operation on a urinary organ. **Wandering k.,** Same as *Floating k.* **Waxy k.** Same as *Amyloid k.*

Kies'tein (ki-es'te-in). Same as *Kyestein*.

Kil'ian's pelvis. Pelvis affected with osteomalacia.

Kil'ogram, Kiloli'ter, Kil'ometer. One thousand grams, liters, or meters.

Kinemat'ics. Science of motion, including bodily movements.
Kinesal'gia (kin-e-sal'je-ah). Pain on muscular exertion.
Kinesiat'rics (kin-es-e-at'rix). Same as *Kinesitherapy.*
Kinesim'eter, Kinesiom'eter. Instrument for the quantitative measurement of motions.
Kinesioneuro'sis. Disordered movements from nervous disease.
Kinesip'athy (kin-e-sip'ath-e). Same as *Kinesitherapy.*
Kinesither'apy. Treatment of disease by movements; Lingism.
Kinesod'ic. Pertaining to the conveyance of motor impulses.
Kinesthe'sia, Kinesthe'sis. The sense by which muscular movements are perceived.
Kinesthesiom'eter. Device for testing the muscular sense.
Kinesthet'ic. Pertaining to kinesthesia.
Kinet'ic energy. See under *Energy.*
King's evil. Scrofula. **K.'s yellow.** See *Orpiment.*
Ki'no. Dried juice of *Pterocarpium marsupium* and of other trees: astringent.
Kinom'eter. Device for measuring womb-displacements.
Ki'none (ki'nōn). Same as *Quinone.*
Ki'noplasm. The substance giving origin to the spindle-fiber of cytoplasm.
Kiono, etc. See under *Ciono.*
Ki'otome. Instrument for amputation of uvula.
Kiot'omy. Removal of the uvula or part of it.
Kis'singen water (kis'sing-en). Saline, laxative, and tonic water from Bavaria.
Kitasa'to's bacillus. Bacillus of bubonic plague.
Klebs-Lœffler bacillus. The bacillus of diphtheria.
Kleptoma'nia. Insane propensity to steal.
Kleptopho'bia. Insane dread of becoming a thief.
Klump'ke's paralysis (kloomp'kiz). See *Paralysis.*
Knee. Joint between femur and tibia. **K.-cap, K.-pan.** Same as *Patella.* **K.-jerk,** upward twitch of foot on striking the patellar ligament, the leg being flexed.
Kneip'pism. Cure by walking barefooted in the morning dew.
Knife-rest crystals. Peculiar indented crystals of triple phosphate in the urine; coffin-lid crystals.
Knit'ting. The repair of a fractured bone.
Knock-knee. Condition in which the knees are bent inward.
K. O. C. Abbreviation of *Cathodal opening contraction.*
Koch's lymph. Same as *Tuberculin.*
Kohl'rausch's fold (kōhl'rowsh's). Fold of mucous membrane extending from right side into rectum; called also the third sphincter.
Ko'la (ko'lah). Seeds of *Sterculia acuminata:* cardiac and nerve-stimulant.
Ko'lanin. One of the active principles of kola.
Kolp-. For words beginning thus, see *Colp-.*
Kolpi'tis. See *Colpitis.*
Kolpot'omy. See *Colpotomy.*
Kolysep'tic (ko-lis-ep'tik). Hindering septic processes.
Koos'so. See *Kousso.*
Kopf-tet'anus. Tetanus from head wounds.
Kopio'pia (ko-pe-o'pe-ah). Same as *Copiopia.*
Koro'nion. Point at apex of coronoid process of inferior maxilla.
Koros'copy (ko-ros'ko-pe). Same as *Skiascopy.*
Ko'sin. Same as *Brayerin.*
Kosotox'in. A poisonous active principle from kousso flowers.
Kou'miss (koo'mis). Fermented drink prepared from milk.
Kous'so (koos'so). Flowers of *Hagenia Abyssinica:* good against tapeworm.

Krame'ria. Genus of South American plants; rhatany: root of *K. triandra*, is astringent.

Kraure'sis vul'væ. Shrivelling and dryness of vulva.

Krau'se's bulbs or **corpuscles** (krow'sez). See *Corpuscles*. **K.'s line,** line passing through white bands of a muscular fibril. **K.'s membrane,** membrane believed to separate disks of sarcous muscular material.

Kre'atin (kre'at-in). Same as *Creatin*.

Kreat'inin (kre-at'in-in). Same as *Creatinin*.

Kres'apol. Antiseptic solution of cresol in potassium soap.

Kres'in. Same as *Cresin*.

Kre'sol (kre'sol). Same as *Cresol*.

Kris'haber's disease (kris'hah-berz). See *Disease*.

Krön'lein's hernia (kren'linz). See *Hernia*.

Kryp'ton. A gaseous element found in the atmosphere.

Kubisga'ri. Endemic paralytic vertigo of Japan.

Ku'miss, Ku'myss (koo'mis). Same as *Koumiss*.

Kuss'maul's coma (koos'mawlz). See *Coma*.

Kyes'tein (ki-es'te-in). An albuminoid which floats on the urine of pregnant women.

Kyllo'sis (kil-o'sis). Club-foot.

Ky'mograph (ki'mo-graf). Instrument for registering undulations, arterial or other.

Ky'moscope. Device used in observing the blood-current.

Kynoceph'alus. A monster with head like a dog's.

Kynuren'ic acid. Same as *Cynurenic acid*.

Kyphoscolio'sis. Kyphosis blended with scoliosis.

Kypho'sis (ki-fo'sis). Hump-back or hunch-back.

Kyphot'ic (ki-fot'ik). Pertaining to, or affected with, kyphosis.

Kysthi'tis (kis-thi'tis). Same as *Vaginitis* or *Colpitis*.

L.

L. Abbreviation for *left*, *lithium*, and *light-sense*.

Lab, Lab-ferment. The ferment of rennet, causing the coagulation of milk. **L.-zymogen,** proenzyme in stomach, which is transformed into lab-ferment by the acids of the gastric juice.

Labarraque's solution (lah-bah-rahks'). Solution of chlorinated soda.

Lab'be's vein. Posterior anastomosing vein of cerebral cortex.

La'bia. Pl. of *labium*, lip.

La'bial. Pertaining to a lip, or labium.

La'bialism. Defective speech with use of labial sounds.

Labidom'eter. Forceps for measuring fetal head in the pelvis.

La'bile (la'bil). Gliding; not fixed to one point.

Labiochore'a. A choreic affection of the lips, with stammering.

Labioglossopharyn'geal. Pertaining to lips, tongue, and pharynx.

La'bioplasty (la'be-o-plas-te). Same as *Cheiloplasty*.

Labiotenac'ulum. Instrument for holding the lip.

La'bium. A lip or lip-shaped organ. **L. cer'ebri,** margin of the cerebral hemisphere which overlaps the callosum. **L. ma'jus,** pl. *labia majora*, the hairy fold of the skin on either side of the slit of the vulva. **L. mi'nor,** pl. *labia minora*, fold of mucous membrane within the labia majora. **L. tympan'icum,** the lower border of the sulcus spiralis. **L. vestibula're,** the upper part of sulcus spiralis.

La'bor. Child-birth; bringing forth of a child. **Artificial l.,** that which is facilitated or induced by mechanical or other extraneous means. **Dry l.,** that in which the liquor amnii escapes too soon. **Induced l.,** that which is artificially brought on. **Instrumental l.,** one which is facilitated by the use of instruments. **Missed l.**, retention of the dead fetus *in utero* after the cessation of the time of normal gestation. **Postponed l.**, that which takes place later than the normal limit. **Precipitate l.**, that in which delivery is accomplished with undue celerity. **Premature l.**, that which takes places too soon. **Protracted l.**, labor protracted beyond the ordinary limit. **Spontaneous l.**, that which requires no artificial aid.

Lab'oratory. A place for experimental work.

Lab'yrinth. The internal ear, made up of the vestibule, cochlea, and canals. **Bony l.** Same as *Osseous l.* **Cortical l.**, a network of tubules and blood-vessels in the cortex of the kidney. **Ludwig's l's.**, spaces between Bertin's columns and the cortical arches. **Membranous l.**, space within the osseous labyrinth. **Osseous l.**, bony part of internal ear.

Labyrin'thine. Pertaining to the labyrinth.

Labyrinthi'tis. Inflammation of the labyrinth.

Lac. L. for *Milk.*

Lac'erated (las'er-a-ted). Torn; of the nature of a rent.

Lacera'tion (las-er-a'shun). A wound produced by tearing.

Lacer'tus fibro'sus. Aponeurotic band from the tendon of the biceps to the fascia of the forearm.

Lac'rimal (lak'rim-al). Pertaining to tears. **L. bone**, bone of inner angle of orbit.

Lacrima'tion. The secretion and discharge of tears.

Lacrimot'omy. Incision of lacrimal duct or sac.

Lac'tagogue (lak'tag-og). Same as *Galactagogue.*

Lactalbu'min. A proteid found in milk.

Lac'tate (lak'tāt). Any salt of lactic acid.

Lacta'tion. 1. Secretion of milk. 2. The suckling of a child. 3. Period of secretion of milk.

Lac'teal. 1. Pertaining to milk. 2. Any one of the intestinal lymphatics which take up chyle.

Lac'tein (lak'te-in). Same as *Lactolin.*

Lactes'cence (lak-tes'ens). Resemblance to milk.

Lac'tic acid. See *Acid.* **L.-a. fermentation.** See *Fermentation.*

Lactif'erous, Lactig'erous. Producing or conveying milk.

Lac'tifuge (lak'tif-ūj). Lessening the secretion of milk.

Lac'tin (lak'tin). Sugar of milk or lactose.

Lac'tinated. Containing sugar of milk.

Lactiv'orous (lak-tiv'or-us). Subsisting upon milk.

Lac'tocele (lak'to-sēl). Same as *Galactocele.*

Lac'tochrome (lak'to-krōm). An alkaloid of milk, $C_6H_{18}NO_6$.

Lactoglob'ulin. Same as *Lactalbumin.*

Lac'tol. Naphthyl lactate: an antiseptic preparation.

Lac'tolin (lak'to-lin). Condensed milk.

Lactom'eter. Instrument for measuring specific gravity of milk.

Lac'tone. An aromatic liquid from lactic acid.

Lactopep'sin. A proprietary dyspepsia remedy.

Lactophe'nin. An antipyretic and hypnotic compound.

Lactophos'phate. A salt of lactic and phosphoric acids.

Lactopro'teid (lak-to-pro'te-id). Any proteid from milk.

Lacto'scope. Device showing proportion of cream in milk.

Lac'tose. Milk-sugar; a sugar derived from milk.

Lactosu'ria (lak-to-su're-ah). Presence of milk-sugar in urine.

Lactuca'rium. Sedative drug from juice of *Lactuca.*

Lactu'ca viro'sa. A species of lettuce which affords lactucarium.

Lactuce'rin. Waxy principle from lactucarium.

Lacu'na. A small pit, hollow, or depression. **L. cer'ebri**, the cerebral infundibulum. **Howship's l.**, any depression of bone under the periosteum. **Intervillous l.**, any one of the blood-spaces of the placenta in which the fetal villi are found. **L. mag'na,** largest of the orifices of the glands of Littre. **L. pharyn'gis,** depression at the pharyngeal end of Eustachian tube.

Lacu'nar. Having, pertaining to, or resembling lacunæ.

Lacu'nula. A small or minute lacuna.

La'cus lacrima'lis. The triangular space at the inner canthus between the two eyelids.

Lad'anum. A resin from species of *Cistus.*

Lady Web'ster pills. Dinner pills of aloes and mastic.

Læ-. For words thus beginning, see *Le-.*

Lafayette's mixture (lah-fah-yets'). Preparation of copaiba, cubebs, spirit of nitrous ether, and liquor potassæ.

Lage'na (laj-e'nah). Part of upper extremity of scala media.

Lagophthal'mus. Inability to shut the eyes.

La Grippe. Same as *Influenza.*

La'ky blood. Blood, the serum of which is charged with hemoglobin from broken-down red corpuscles.

Lalla'tion, Lal'ling. Babbling, semi-infantile speech.

Laloneu'rosis. Speech-disorder of nervous or central origin.

Lalop'athy (lal-op'ath-e). Any speech-disorder.

Lalopho'bia. Dislike of speaking, often with extreme stuttering.

Lamb'da. Point of union of lambdoid and sagittal sutures.

Lamb'dacism. Inability to utter the *l* sound.

Lamb'doid, Lambdoid'al. Shaped like the Greek letter Λ. **L. suture,** suture between the parietal and occipital bones.

Lamel'la, pl. *lamel'læ.* 1. A thin scale or plate. 2. A medicated disk. **Concentric lamellæ,** bony plates around the Haversian canal. **Intermediate l.,** any one of the plates between the concentric layers of a bone. **Triangular l.,** a layer joining the choroid plexuses of the third ventricle. **Vitreous l.** Same as *Bruch's membrane.*

Lamel'lar. Pertaining to, or composed of, lamellæ.

Lam'in. Hemostatic alkaloid from flowers of *Lamium album.*

Lam'ina (lam'in-ah). A thin layer or plate. **Bowman's l.** See *Bowman's membrane.* **L. cine'rea,** layer of gray matter between the callosum and optic chiasma. **L. cribro'sa.** 1. The fascia which covers the saphenous opening. 2. Either one of the perforated spaces in the brain. 3. Part of sclera perforated for passage of optic nerve. **L. fus'ca,** the pigmentary layer of the sclera. **L. pro'pria,** the middle or fibrous layer of the tympanic membrane. **L. reticula'ris,** the perforated hyaline membrane which covers the organ of Corti. **L. spira'lis,** partition which divides the cochlea into the two scalæ. **Vitreous l.** Same as *Bruch's membrane.*

Lamina'ria digita'ta. A seaweed, used in making tents and bougies.

Lam'inated. Made up of laminæ or layers.

Lamina'tion. 1. Laminar structure, or arrangement. 2. The slicing of the fetal head in embryotomy.

Laminec'tomy, Lamnec'tomy. Excision of posterior arch of a vertebra.

Lamini'tis. Inflammation of the laminæ of a horse's foot.

Lamp'black. Powdered carbon from combustion of oils, etc.

Lan'ain (lan'a-in). Purified wool-fat.

Lan'cet. Small pointed two-edged surgical knife. **Gum l.,** knife for incising the gums. **Spring l.,** one, the blade of which is held by a spring. **Thumb l.,** one with a wide two-edged blade.

Lan'cinating. Tearing, darting, or sharply cutting.

Lanci'si's nerves (lahn-che'sēz). Same as *Striæ longitudinales.*

Landou'zy-Deje'rine atrophy (lahn-doo'zē-dezh'rēn). See *Atrophy.*

Landry's paralysis (lahn-drēz'). Acute ascending paralysis.
Land'-scurvy. Same as *Purpura hæmorrhagica.*
Lang'han's layer. The deep, cellular layer of chorionic villi.
Lannai'ol. An iodocresol; used as a substitute for iodoform.
Lan'olin. Rectified wool-fat; used externally.
Lan'termann's incisures (lan'ter-mahnz). See *Incisures.*
Lan'tonin. Alkaloid from a Brazilian tree: used like quinin.
Lanu'go. The fine hair on the body of the fetus.
Laparocholecystot'omy. Laparotomy with incision of the gall-bladder.
Laparocolos'tomy. Colostomy by an abdominal incision.
Laparocolot'omy. Laparotomy combined with colotomy.
Laparocystec'tomy. Laparotomy and removal of a cyst.
Laparocystot'omy. Laparotomy and removal of cyst-contents.
Laparo-elytrot'omy. Laparotomy and vaginal incision for removing fetus.
Laparo-enterot'omy. Laparotomy with incision into intestine.
Laparogastrot'omy. Laparotomy with incision into stomach.
Laparohysterec'tomy. Laparotomy with excision of uterus.
Laparohystero-oöphorec'tomy. Laparotomy with removal of uterus and ovaries.
Laparohysterot'omy. Laparotomy with incision of uterus.
Laparo-ileot'omy. Laparotomy with incision of ileum.
Laparokelyphot'omy. Same as *Laparocystotomy.*
Laparomyomec'tomy, Laparomyot'omy. Laparotomy with removal of myoma.
Laparonephrec'tomy. Laparotomy with removal of kidney.
Laparosalpingec'tomy. Laparotomy with excision of an oviduct.
Laparos'copy. Instrumental abdominal exploration.
Laparosplenec'tomy. Laparotomy with excision of a spleen.
Laparot'omy. Surgical incision through abdominal wall.
La'pis (la'pis). L. for *Stone.*
Lap'pa. The burdock *Arctium lappa:* diuretic and tonic.
Lard. The fat of the swine; adeps.
Larda'cein. A proteid found in amyloid degenerations.
Larda'ceous (lar-da'shus). Resembling lard; amyloid.
Lark'spur. The plant *Delphinium consolida:* diuretic and antasthmatic.
Larrey's amputation (lah-rāz'). Double-flap amputation at shoulder-joint or hip-joint. **L.'s spaces,** spaces between parts of diaphragm attached to sternum and those which are attached to ribs.
Laryn'geal (lar-in'je-al). Pertaining to the larynx.
Laryngec'tomy (lar-in-jek'tom-e). Excision of the larynx.
Laryngis'mus strid'ulus. Sudden laryngeal spasm in children, with crowing inspiration.
Laryngi'tis (lar-in-ji'tis). Inflammation of the larynx.
Laryn'gocele. Protrusion of mucous membrane across cricothyroid space.
Laryngocente'sis. Surgical puncture of the larynx.
Laryn'gofissure. Surgical splitting of thyroid cartilage.
Laryn'gograph. Device for recording laryngeal movements.
Laryngog'raphy. A description of the larynx.
Laryngol'ogy. Sum of what is known regarding the larynx.
Laryngoparal'ysis. Paralysis of the larynx.
Laryngop'athy. Any disorder of the larynx.
Laryngophan'tom. An artificial model of the larynx.
Laryngopharyn'geal. Pertaining to the larynx and pharynx.
Laryngophar'ynx. The lower portion of the pharynx.
Laryngoph'ony. Sound heard in auscultating the pharynx.
Laryn'goplasty. Plastic surgery of larynx.

Laryngople'gia (lar-in-go-ple'je-ah). Paralysis of the larynx.
Laryn'goscope. Apparatus for inspecting the larynx.
Laryngos'copy (lar-in-gos'ko-pe). Inspection of the larynx.
Laryn'gospasm (lar-in'go-spasm). See *Laryngismus stridulus.*
Laryngosteno'sis. Narrowing or stricture of larynx.
Laryngostrob'oscope. Apparatus for observing the vibrations of vocal cords and other intralaryngeal phenomena.
Laryngot'omy. The act of incising the larynx.
Laryngotrachei'tis. Inflammation of the larynx and trachea.
Laryngotracheot'omy. Incision of the larynx and trachea.
Lar'ynx (lar'inx). Air-passage and vocal organ between the tongue and trachea.
La'ta, Latah. Form of palmus or jumping-disease, endemic in Java.
La'tent (la'tent). Concealed; not manifest. **L. heat,** heat which is absorbed by bodies which are not thereby rendered warmer. **L. period,** period after application of a stimulus and before its result is manifest.
Lat'erad. Toward a side or lateral aspect.
Lat'eral. Pertaining to a side. **L. sinuses.** See *Sinus.*
Lateriti'ous (lat-er-ish'us). Like brick-dust.
Lateroflex'ion (lat-er-o-flex'shun). Flexion to either side.
Lateropul'sion. Involuntary tendency to go to one side.
Laterover'sion (lat-er-o-ver'shun). Abnormal inclination to one side.
Lath'yrism (lath'ir-izm). Poisoning by chick pea; lupinosis.
Latis'simus col'li. See *Platysma myoides,* in *Muscles, Table of.* **L. dor'si.** See *Muscles, Table of.*
Laud'able pus. Pus of a kind thought to indicate an improving condition.
Laud'anin. An alkaloid from opium, $C_{20}H_{25}NO_4$.
Lau'danum (law'dan-um). Tincture of opium.
Laugh'ing gas. Nitrogen monoxid, N_2O_2; anesthetic.
Laurocer'asus. Same as *Cherry laurel.*
Lavage (la'vaj, lah-vahj'). A washing out or irrigation.
Lavan'dula. Lavender; a plant with a carminative oil.
Laveran's bodies (lahv-rahnz'). See *Plasmodium malariæ.*
Law. A uniform or constant fact or principle. **Avogadro's l.,** equal volumes of gases with the same pressure and temperature contain an equal number of molecules. **Behring's l.,** blood and serum of an immunized person when transferred to another subject will render the latter immune. **Bell's l.,** anterior roots of spinal nerves are motor, and posterior sensory. **Berthollet's l.,** if two salts in solution by double decomposition can produce a salt less soluble than either, such a salt will be produced. **Boyle's l.,** at any stated temperature a given mass of gas varies in volume inversely as the pressure. **Charles's l.,** equal increments of temperature add equal amounts to the product of the volume and pressure of a given mass of any gas. **Colles's l.,** a child who is affected with congenital syphilis, its mother showing no signs of the disease, will not infect its mother. **Dalton's l.,** though the volume of a gas absorbed by a liquid remains constant, the weight of the absorbed gas rises and falls in proportion to the pressure. **Fechner's l.,** if a stimulus is increased, the sensation increases as the logarithm of the stimulus. **Gay-Lussac's l.** Same as *Charles's l.* **Graham's l.,** the rate of diffusion of a gas through porous membranes is in inverse ratio to the square root of their density. **Henry's l.** See *Dalton's l.* **Hilton's l.,** a nerve-trunk which supplies any given joint, also supplies the muscles which move the joint and the skin over the insertion of such muscles. **Listing's l.,** when the eyeball is moved from a resting position, the rotational angle in the second position is the

same as if the eye were turned about a fixed axis perpendicular to the first and second positions of the visual line. **Mariotte's l.** Same as *Boyle's l.* **Ohm's l.**, strength of an electric current varies directly as the electromotive force and inversely as the resistance. **Profeta's l.**, a non-syphilitic child born of syphilitic parents is immune. **Ritter-Valli l.**, the primary increase and secondary loss of irritability in a nerve, produced by a section which separates it from the nerve-center, travel in a peripheral direction. **L. of sines**, the sine of the angle of incidence is equal to the sine of the angle of reflection multiplied by a constant quantity. **Weber's l.**, the variation of stimulus which causes the smallest appreciable change in sensation maintains an approximately fixed ratio to the whole stimulus.

Lax. Slack; not tense.

Lax'ative. Mildly aperient; also, an aperient medicine.

Lax'ator tym'pani. See *Muscles, Table of.*

Lay'er. A stratum of nearly uniform thickness. **Bacillar l.**, the rod and cone layer of the retina. **Ganglionic l.**, a stratum of angular cells in the cerebral cortex. **Horny l.**, the outer layer of the skin; stratum corneum. **Osteogenetic l.**, the innermost layer of the periosteum. See also *Stratum.*

Lazaret'to. A quarantine station; also, a pest-house.

Lb., Lib. Abbreviation for *Libra*, a pound.

Lead. A soft gray-blue metal with poisonous salts. **L., black**, See *Graphite.* **L. colic**, colic resulting from lead-poisoning. **L. encephalopathy**, brain-disease caused by lead-poisoning. **L.-pipe contraction**, cataleptic condition in which the limbs remain in any position in which they may be placed.

Le'ber's disease (la'berz). Hereditary atrophy of the optic nerve.

Lec'ithin (les'ith-in). Fatty principle, $C_{44}H_{90}NPO_9$, found in animal tissues; also, any principle of the group to which normal lecithin belongs.

Lec'tual. Pertaining to a bed or couch.

Leech. An aquatic platyhelmian *Hirudo medicinalis:* used for drawing blood.

Lees. The dregs or sediment of wine.

Left-lateral position. See *Sims's position.*

Leg. The lower extremity, especially the part between knee and ankle. **Badger l.**, inequality in the length of the legs. **Baker's l.**, knock-knee or genu valgum. **Bandy-l.** Same as *Bow-l.* **Barbadoes l.**, elephantiasis. **Black l.**, symptomatic anthrax. **Bow-l.**, out-knee or genu varum. **Milk-l.**, phlegmasia dolens. **Scissor-l.**, deformity with crossing of the legs.

Legit'imacy. Condition of having been born in wedlock.

Leg'umin. A principle from plants like casein.

Leiomyo'ma. Myoma of the non-striated muscle-fibers.

Leiphe'mia (li-fe'me-ah). Thinness of the blood.

Lei'ter's coil (li'terz). Coiled metallic tube used in warming or cooling a part.

Lembert's suture (lem'bertz). See *Suture.*

Lemnis'cus. White band on outer surface of peduncles of cerebellum.

Lemoparal'ysis. Esophageal paralysis.

Length-breadth index. See *Index.*

Len'itive. 1. Demulcent; soothing. 2. A soothing medicine.

Lens. A lentil-shaped glass for refracting light. **Achromatic l.**, a lens corrected for chromatic aberration. **Apochromatic l.**, one corrected for chromatic and spheric aberration. **Biconcave l., Concavoconcave l.**, a lens concave on both faces. **Biconvex l.**, one with two convex faces. **Bifocal l.**, one with two foci. **Converging l., Convex l.**, one which focuses light. **Convexoconcave l.**, one which has one convex and one concave face. **Crystalline l.**, eye-lens, the transparent lenticular organ behind the pupil. **Cylindric l.**, one which has one surface plane and another concave or convex. **Decentered l.**, one in which the visual line does not pass through the center. **Dispersing l., Concave l.**, one which disperses light. **Orthoscopic l.**, a form of lens which gives a very flat and undistorted field of vision. **Periscopic l.**, a concavoconvex, or convexoconcave lens. **Spheric l.**, one which has a surface which is the segment of a sphere.

Lentico'nus. Exaggerated curvation of the eye-lens.

Lentic'ular. Having the form of a lens. **L. arteries**, arteries which supply l. nucleus.

Lenticulostri'ate. Pertaining to lenticular nucleus and corpus striatum.

Lenti'go (len-ti'go). L. for *Freckle.*

Leonti'asis. Form of leprosy with lion-like expression about face.

Le'per. A person who is affected with leprosy.

Lepido'sis (lep-id-o'sis). Any scaly eruption.

Lep'ocyte. A nucleated cell having a cell-wall.

Le'pra. Same as *Leprosy;* also, *Psoriasis.* **L. anesthet'ica**, leprosy with anesthetic spots. **L. maculo'sa**, in which the skin is marked with spots of pigmentation. **L. mu'tilans**, the final stage of true leprosy, with mutilation of extremities.

Lep'rosy. A chronic transmissible disease with anesthesia, maculæ, and frequent loss of digits.

Lep'rous. Pertaining to, or affected with, leprosy.

Leptan'dra. Root of *Veronica virginica:* purgative and cholagogue.

Leptoceph'alus (lep-to-sef'al-us). Fetus with very small head.

Leptomeningi'tis. Inflammation of the arachnopia.

Lep'torrhine (lep'to-rin). Having a very slender nose.

Lep'tothrix. Genus of schizomycetes from tartar of teeth.

Lep'tus autumna'lis. The harvest-bug; a mite infesting the skin.

Le'sion. Any hurt, wound, or local degeneration. **Local l.**, one in the nervous system which gives origin to distinctive local symptoms. **Indiscriminate l.**, lesion affecting distinct parts. **Initial syphilitic l.**, true or hard chancre. **Irritative l.**, a lesion which excites the functions of the part where it is situated. **Peripheral l.**, a lesion of nerve-endings. **Structural l.**, one that produces an obvious change in a tissue. **Systematic l.**, one limited to a system or set of organs with a common function. **Toxic l.**, one due to a poison.

Le'thal (le'thal). Deadly; fatal.

Leth'argy. Stupor or coma; also, hypnotic trance.

Le'thin (le'thin). Proprietary narcotic.

Let'ter-blindness. State due to central lesion in which the sight of letters conveys no impression to the mind.

Let'tuce (let'is). See *Lactuca.*

Leucce'mia, Leucæ'mia. Same as *Leukemia.*

Leu'cin (lu'sin). Crystalline substance, $C_6H_{13}NO_2$, found in the body.

Leuci'tis (lu-si'tis). Same as *Scleritis.*

Leuco-. For words beginning thus, see those beginning *Leuko-.*

Leucocythe'mia. Same as *Leukemia.*

Leukas'mus. Same as *Leukoderma.*

Leuke'mia, Leukæ'mia (lu-ke'me-ah). Fatal disease, with marked increase in number of blood leukocytes. **Lymphatic l.**, that associated with disease of lymphatic organs. **Myelogenic l.**, that due to disease of bone-marrow. **Splenic l.**, that associated with splenic enlargement.

Leukem'ic. Pertaining to, or affected with, leukemia.

Leu'kin. A crystalline material found in various organs.

Leu'koblast (lu'ko-blast). An immature leukocyte.

Leu'kocyte (lu'ko-sit). Any coloring ameboid mass, like a white blood-corpuscle. **Beta l.,** leukocyte which does not disintegrate during coagulation of blood.

Leukocythe'mia. Same as *Leukemia.*

Leukocytogen'esis. The formation of leukocytes.

Leukocytol'ysis. Breaking down or destruction of leukocytes.

Leukocyto'ma. Tumor-like mass of leukocytes.

Leukocytom'eter. Instrument for counting leukocytes.

Leukocytopla'nia. Wandering of leukocytes; passage of leukocytes through a membrane.

Leukocyto'sis. Increase in number of blood leukocytes.

Leukocytu'ria. Discharge of leukocytes in the urine.

Leukoder'ma. Abnormal whiteness: albinism in patches.

Leukokerato'sis (lu-ko-ker-at-o'sis). Same as *Leukoplakia.*

Leu'kol, Leu'kolin. Same as *Quinolin.*

Leukol'ysis (lu-kol'is-is). Same as *Leukocytolysis.*

Leuko'ma. White corneal opacity.

Leukoma'in. Any one of a group of alkaloids normally present in organic tissues.

Leukomaine'mia. Excess of leukomains in blood.

Leukom'atous. Pertaining to, or of the nature of, leukoma.

Leukomyeli'tis. Inflammation of white substance of myelon.

Leukonecro'sis. Gangrene, with formation of white slough.

Leukonu'clein. Nuclein from digested leukocytes.

Leukopathi'a, Leukop'athy. Same as *Leukoderma.*

Leukope'nia. Deficiency in number of leukocytes.

Leukophlegma'sia. A variety of white non-dropsical edema.

Leukopla'cia, Leukoplak'ia, Leukopla'sia. Formation of white patches, as mucous membrane of cheeks and tongue.

Leukoplas'tid. Any one of the white granules of plant-cells whence the starch-forming elements are formed.

Leukop'sin. A visual white derived from rhodopsin by bleaching on exposure to light.

Leukorrhe'a. Whitish discharge from vagina.

Leukosar'coma. Any uncolored or colorless sarcoma.

Leva'tor. Any lifting or raising muscle. See *Muscles, Table of.*

Leviga'tion. The grinding of moist substances.

Levogy'rous (le-vo-ji'rus). Rotating polarized light-rays to the left.

Levoro'tatory (le-vo-ro'ta-to-ri). Same as *Levogyrous.*

Levulo'san. A carbohydrate, $C_6H_{12}O_5$, from fruit-sugar.

Lev'ulose. A sugar, $C_6H_{12}O_6$, from fruits, honey, and the intestines.

Levulosu'ria. Presence of levulose in urine.

Lew'inin. Locally anesthetic resin from kava.

Ley'den jar (li'dn). Device for accumulation of static electricity.

Li. Symbol for *Lithium.*

Libid'inous. Lustful; salacious.

Li'bra. L. for *Pound* and for *Balance.*

Li'chen. 1. Any one of a group of plants believed to be composed of symbiotic algæ and fungi. 2. Papular skin-disease of many kinds. **L. acumina'tus,** a grave form, with papulosquamous eruption. **L. ag'rius,** a severe form of eczema. **L. dissemina'tus,** a form with irregularly placed eruption. **L. pila'ris,** a form which especially affects the hair-follicles. **L. pla'nus,** an inflammatory skin-disease with wide flat papules, often in circumscribed patches. **L. ru'ber,** a papulosquamous disease with grave constitutional symptoms and sometimes fatal wasting:

named from the red color of the eruption. **L. scrofulo'sus,** a form which is peculiar to persons of a strumous habit. **L. trop'-icus,** prickly heat; a form with a red itching eruption.

Li'chenoid (li'ken-oid). Resembling the disease called lichen.

Licorice (lik'or-is). The plant *Glycyrrhiza glabra:* root and extract sweet and demulcent.

Lie'ben's test (le'benz). A test for acetone by ammonia and iodin.

Lie'berkühn's crypts or **glands** (le'ber-kunz). The tubular intestinal glands.

Lie'big's extract. A form of beef-extract.

Li'en (li'en). L. for *Spleen.*

Lien'adin. Proprietary remedy made from the spleen.

Li'enal. Of, or pertaining to, the spleen.

Lieni'tis (li-en-i'tis). Same as *Splenitis.*

Lienomala'cia. Softening of the spleen.

Lienomyelo'genous (li-en-o-mi-el-o'jen-us). Originating in the spleen and bone-marrow.

Lienter'ic (li-en-ter'ik). Pertaining to, or affected with, lientery.

Li'entery (li'en-ter-e). Diarrhea with passage of undigested food.

Lig'ament. A tough band connecting bones or supporting viscera. **Accessory l.,** one which strengthens or supplements another. **Adipose l.,** the mucous ligament of the knee. **Alar l's.,** the two folds of synovial membrane on either side of the adipose ligament. **Annular l.,** any ring-shaped ligament, as of the wrist or ankle. **Arcuate l's.,** the arched ligaments which connect the diaphragm with the lowest ribs and the first lumbar vertebra. **Atlo-axoid l.** connects the atlas and axis. **Auricular l's.,** the three ligaments which unite the external ear to the side of the head. **Barkow's l.,** anterior and posterior l's. of elbow-joint. **Berard's l.,** suspensory l. of pericardium. **Bertin's l.,** iliofemoral ligament. **Bigelow's l.,** the iliofemoral ligament. **Broad l.** 1. The peritoneal fold which supports the uterus on either side. 2. The suspensory ligament of the liver. **Burns's l.,** the falciform process of the fascia lata. **Camper's l.,** the deep perineal fascia. **Capsular l.,** the tough fibrous framework which surrounds every joint. **Carcassonne's l.,** triangular ligament of urethra. **Central l.** Same as *Filum terminale.* **Check l's.,** Same as *Odontoid l's.* **Ciliary l.,** l. joining iris to corneosclera. **Conoid l.,** inner part of coracoclavicular ligament. **Coraco-clavicular l.** extends from the clavicle to the coracoid process. **Coronary l.,** a peritoneal fold, extends from posterior border of liver to diaphragm. **Costocolic l.** attaches the spleen to the diaphragm. **Costocoracoid l.** joins the first rib to the coracoid process. **Cotyloid l.,** a ring at the margin of the acetabulum. **Crucial l's.,** two ligaments of the knee. **Cruciform l.,** the transverse ligament of the atlanto-axoid joint. **Crural l.** Same as *Poupart's l.* **Deltoid l.,** the internal lateral ligament of the ankle-joint. **Falciform l.,** the broad ligament of the liver. **Flood's l.** See *Glenohumeral l.* **Gimbernat's l.,** triangular expanse of the aponeurosis of the external oblique muscle, anteriorly joined to Poupart's l., and going to the iliopectineal line. **Glenohumeral l's.,** three ligaments strengthening capsule of shoulder. **Glenoid l.** 1. A ring of fibrocartilage connected with the rim of the glenoid fossa. 2. The anterior l's of the metacarpo-phalangeal joints. **Hey's l's.,** a falciform expansion of the fascia lata. **Iliofemoral l.,** an important ligament of the hip-joint, from the ilium to the lesser trochanter. **Iliotrochanteric l.,** portion of capsular l. of hip-joint. **Interclavicular l.** joins the two clavicles to each other and the sternum. **Lateral l.,** a peritoneal fold, one on either side of the liver, joining it to the diaphragm. **Odontoid l's.,** one on either side of the odontoid process, which connect the atlas to the skull. **Poupart's l.,**

lower border of aponeurosis of external oblique muscle between anterior spine of ilium and the spine of the pubis. **Pterygomaxillary l.** connects the apex of internal pterygoid plate and the posterior end of the internal oblique line of lower jaw. **Pubic l's.**, three ligaments (anterior, posterior, and superior) of the symphysis pubis. **Rhomboid l.** connects cartilage of the first rib to under surface of clavicle. **Round l.** 1. See *Ligamentum teres*. 2. A fibrous cord which represents the umbilical vein from the navel to anterior border of liver. 3. One of the ligaments of the radio-ulnar articulation. 4. Either of two cords from cornua of uterus to the mons Veneris. **Sacrosciatic l's.**, two ligaments (great, or posterior, and lesser, or anterior) from the sacrum to the ischium. **Stylohyoid l.**, a fibrous cord from the styloid process to the lesser cornu of the hyoid. **Stylomaxillary l.** extends from the styloid process to ramus of the lower jaw. **Suspensory l.** See *Zinn's zonule*. **Transverse l.**, name of various ligaments, as of atlas, knee, hip, and scapula. **Trapezoid l.**, forward and outward part of coracoclavicular ligament. **Triangular l.**, name of various ligaments, as of urethra, tympanic bones, uterus, and the vertebræ. **Vesico-umbilical l.** Same as *Urachus*. **Vesico-uterine l.**, from front of uterus to the bladder. **Winslow's l.**, posterior ligament of the knee. **Zinn's l.** See *Zinn's zonule*.

Ligamen'tous. Pertaining to, or of the nature of, a ligament.

Ligamen'tum. L. for *Ligament*. **L. arcua'tum**, an arched ligament of the lumbar region. **L. denticula'tum**, serrated lengthwise band on either side within the spinal dura. **L. muco'sum**, synovial fold in knee-joint. **L. nu'chæ**, tough band at the nape of neck, uniting the two trapezius muscles. **L. patel'læ**, the ligament which connects the patella and tibia. **L. spira'le**, the ligamentous part of the basilar membrane of the cochlea. **L. te'res.** Same as *Round ligament*. See *Ligament*.

Liga'tion. The application of a ligature.

Lig'ature. Thread or wire for tying a part. **Double l.**, ligation of an artery at two places and division between them. **Elastic l.**, caoutchouc band used to strangulate hemorrhoids and pedunculated growths. **Erichsen's l.**, a double thread of white and black for ligating nævi. **Intermittent l.**, a tourniquet applied to interrupt the blood-current, but occasionally relaxed to renew the circulation. **Kangaroo l.**, tendons of kangaroo's tail used as a ligature. **Lateral l.**, a ligature so applied as to check, but not to interrupt, the blood-current. **L.-forceps**, a forceps for holding delicate parts. **Provisional l.**, one applied at the beginning of an operation, but removed before its close.

Light (lit). Ethereal vibration which gives origin to the visual sense. **Axial l.**, **Central l.**, light whose rays are parallel to each other and to optic axis. **Diffused l.**, that which has been scattered by reflection and refraction. **Oblique l.**, light falling obliquely on a surface. **Polarized l.**, light of which the vibrations are made over one plane or in circles or ellipses. **Reflected l.**, light turned back from an illuminated surface. **Refracted l.**, light whose rays have bent out of their original course by passing through a transparent medium. **L.-sense**, faculty by which varying degrees of light or brightness may be perceived. **Transmitted l.**, light which passes or has passed through an object.

Light'ning pains. Cutting pains of locomotor ataxia.

Lignosul'phin. A disinfectant product of manufacture of sulphicellulose.

Lig'num (lig'num). L. for *Wood*.

Lig'ula. A strip of white substance near the lateral border of the fourth ventricle.

Limatu'ra fer'ri. Iron filings.

Limb. An arm or leg; an extremity.

Lim'bic. Marginal; pertaining to a limbus.

Lim'bus. A rim or border. **L. lam'inæ spira'lis.** Same as *Crista spiralis*. **L. lu'teus.** Same as *Macula lutea*.

Lime. 1. Calcium oxid; also calcium hydrate. 2. The acid fruit of *Citrus acidi:* refrigerant and antiscorbutic.

Li'men na'si. The boundary line between the bony and cartilaginous portions of the nasal cavity.

Lim'inal. Barely perceptible; pertaining to a threshold.

Lim'itans (lim'it-anz). Same as *Membrana limitans*.

Limo'sis (lim-o'sis). Extreme hunger.

Limotherapy. Treatment by fasting; starvation cure.

Linc'ture, Linc'tus. An electuary; a medicine to be taken by licking.

Line. A stripe, streak, or narrow mark. **Abdominal l's.,** lines on abdomen, indicating the boundaries of muscles. **Alveobasilar l.,** from nasion to alveolar point. **Alveolonasal l.,** from alveolar to nasal point. **Auriculobregmatic l.,** from auricular point to bregma. **Axillary l's.** (anterior and posterior), from axilla downward. **Base l.,** from infra-orbital ridge to external auditory meatus and to middle line of occiput. **Basiobregmatic l.,** from basion to bregma. **Baudelocque's l.,** external conjugate diameter of pelvis. **Biauricular l.,** from one auditory meatus over vertex to the other. **Blue l.,** characteristic line on gums showing chronic lead-poisoning. **Bryant's l.,** a test-line for detecting shortening of the femur. **Burton's l.** Same as *Gingival l.* **Camper's l.,** from external auditory meatus to a point just below the nasal spine. **Clapton's l.,** green line on gums in copper-poisoning. **Corrigan's l.,** purplish line on gums in copper-poisoning. **Costo-articular l.,** from sternoclavicular joint to point of eleventh rib. **Costoclavicular l., Parasternal l.,** line midway from nipple-line and border of sternum. **Curved l's. of ilium** (superior, middle, and inferior), three prominent lines of the ilium. **Curved l's. of occipital bones** (superior and inferior), two lines on either half of outer surface of occipital bones. **Douglas's l.,** curved lower edge of inner layer of aponeurosis of internal oblique muscle. **Ellis's l.,** curved line at upper border of a pleuritic effusion. **Embryonic l.,** primitive trace in center of germinal area. **Facial l.,** straight line touching the glabella and a point at lower border of face. **Fraunhofer's l's.** See *Fraunhofer's lines*. **Genal l.,** one of Jadelot's lines, from malar surface to nasal line. **Gingival l.,** a reddish streak on edge of the gum. **Gubler's l.,** line connecting apparent origin of roots of fifth nerve. **Haller's l.,** the linea splendens. **Helmholtz's l.,** line perpendicular to plane of axis of rotation of eyes. **Hilton's l.,** white line which shows the point of junction of the skin of perineum with the anal mucosa. **Holden's l.,** sulcus below the inguinal fold, crossing the capsule of hip. **Iliopectineal l.,** ridge on ilium and pubes, showing the brim of true pelvis. **Incremental l's.,** lines supposed to indicate laminar structure of dentin. **Intertrochanteric l's.** (anterior and posterior), traces on anterior and posterior surfaces of femur between the trochanters. **Jadelot's l's.** See *Jadelot's l's.* **Mammary l.,** line from one nipple to the other. **Mammillary l.,** vertical line through center of nipple. **Mylohyoidean l.,** a ridge on inner surface of lower jaw. **Nasobasilar l.,** line through basion and nasal point. **Nélaton's l.,** from anterior superior process of ilium to most prominent part of tuberosity of ischium. **Nuchal l's.** (inferior, median, and superior), lines on outer surface of occiput. **Oblique l's.,** name of many lines, as of fibula, radius, thyroid cartilage, tibia, etc. **Ogston's l.**, line from tubercle of femur to the intercondylar notch. **Parasternal l.** Same as *Costoclavicular l.* **Pectineal l.**, portion of iliopectineal line on the pubic bone. **Primitive l.** Same as *Primitive streak.* **Profile l.** Same as *Camper's l.* **Quadrate l.**, line on posterior surface of femur. **Respiratory l.**, line which connects bases of up-strokes in a sphygmogram. **Roser's l.** Same as *Nélaton's l.* **Salter's l.** Same as *Incremental l.* **Scapular l.**, vertical downward line from lower angle of scapula. **Semicircular l.** See *Douglas's l.* **L. of sight**, straight line from center of pupil to object viewed. **Sternal l.**, median line of sternum. **Sternomastoid l.**, line from heads of sternomastoid to the mastoid process. **Supra-orbital l.**, line across forehead just above root of external angular process of frontal bone. **Sylvian l.**, line upon the head indicating direction of fissure of Sylvius. **Thompson's l.**, red line on gums in pulmonary tuberculosis. **Trapezoid l.**, mark of attachment of trapezoid ligament to the clavicle. **Virchow's l.**, line from root of nose to lambda. **Visual l.**, line from object seen through nodal point of eye to macula lutea. **Zöllner's l's.**, a set of lines of peculiar arrangement for purposes of an ocular test.

Lin'ea (lin'e-ah), pl. *lin'eæ.* L. for *Line.* **L. al'ba**, tendinous mesial line down the front of the belly. **L. albican'tes**, white abdominal lines seen after pregnancy. **L. as'pera**, a rough longitudinal line on the back of the femur. **L. quadra'ti**, a line on the femur which marks the insertion of the quadratus femoris. **L. semiluna'res**, a pair of curved lines, one on either side of the linea alba. **L. splen'dens**, fibrous band down the anterior surface of the pia mater of the spinal cord.

Lin'ear. Pertaining to, or resembling, a line.

Ling's cure, L.'s system, Ling'ism. Kinesitherapy; movement cure.

Ling'ua (ling'gwah). L. for *Tongue.* **L. geograph'ica.** Same as *Geographical tongue.*

Lin'gual. Of, or pertaining to, the tongue. **L. bone.** Same as *Hyoid bone.* **L. delirium**, delirious utterance of meaningless words.

Lingua'lis (ling-gua'lis). See *Muscles, Table of.*

Lin'gula. An anterior lobule of the cerebellum. **L. of sphenoid**, ridge between the body and greater wing of the sphenoid. **L. Wrisber'gi**, fibers joining the motor and sensory roots of the trifacial nerve.

Lin'iment, Linimen'tum. An oily liquid preparation to be rubbed upon the skin.

Li'nin. Substance of the achromatic nuclear reticulum of the cell.

Lini'tis. Inflammation of gastric cellular tissue.

Lin'seed. Seeds of flax, *Linum usitatissimum:* demulcent and emollient. **L. oil**, fixed drying oil from the same.

Lint. Absorbent dressing made by picking apart woven linen; also, a specially finished woven fabric for surgical dressing.

Lin'tine. Cotton lint from which fats and oils are removed.

Li'num. L. for *Flax*, and for *Linseed.*

Lipacide'mia. Presence of any fatty acid in the blood.

Lipacidu'ria. Presence of any fatty acid in the urine.

Lip'anin. Olive oil mixed with oleic acid; used like cod-liver oil.

Lipar'ocele. Fatty scrotal tumor; also hernia containing fatty material.

Lipe'mia. Presence of fat or oil in the blood.

Lip'ochrin. Pigment from retinal fat-globules.

Lip'ochrome. Any one of a special group of animal fat-pigments.

Lipofibro'ma. Lipoma with fibrous elements.

Lipo'ma (li-po'mah). A fatty tumor.
Lipomato'sis. Excessive proportion of fat in the tissues.
Lipomyxo'ma. Lipoma with myxomatous elements.
Lipothym'ia. A swooning; faintness.
Lip'plug. Development of a bony lip in osteo-arthritis.
Lip'pitude. Marginal blepharitis; blear eye.
Lipu'ria (lip-u're-ah). Presence of fat or oil in the urine.
Liquefa'cient. Changing into a liquid; liquefying.
Liquefac'tion. Change into a liquid form.
Liquidam'bar. Genus of trees affording storax, etc.
Li'quor (li'kwor). A liquid. **L. am'nii,** fluid contained in the amnion. **L. Cotun'nii.** Same as *Perilymph.* **L. pu'ris,** the more liquid or sanious portion of pus. **L. san'guinis,** the plasma, or serum, of the blood. **L. Scar'pæ.** Same as *Endolymph.*
Liq'uorice (lik'or-is). See *Licorice.*
Lis'franc's amputation. A form of amputation at joints. **L.'s tubercle,** tubercle for the scalenus anticus on the first rib.
Lisp'ing. Substitution of *th* sound for *s* and *z.*
Lis'sauer's zone (lis'sowrz). The area of white matter at tip of posterior cornu of gray matter of spinal cord.
Lis'terine. A proprietary antiseptic compound.
Lis'terism. The principles and practice of antiseptic and aseptic surgery.
Lis'tol. Antiseptic combination of thyroid gland and iodin.
Li'ter (le'ter). One thousand cubic centimeters; or 1.056 quarts wine measure.
Lit'eral agraphia. See under *Agraphia.*
Lith'agogue (lith'ag-og). Expelling calculi.
Lith'arge (lith'arj). Lead protoxid.
Lith'ate (lith'āt). Same as *Urate.*
Lithec'tasy. Removal of calculus by perineal incision.
Lithe'mia. Excess of uric acid and water in the blood.
Lith'ia (lith'e-ah). Lithium oxid, Li_2O.
Lithi'asis. Formation of calculi and concretions.
Lithi'atry. The medical treatment of calculus.
Lith'ic acid. Same as *Uric acid.* **L.-a. diathesis,** tendency to lithemia, or gout.
Lith'ium. A white metal, Li: its salts are medicinal.
Lithocenо'sis (lith-o-sen-o'sis). Same as *Lithotrity.*
Lith'oclast (lith'o-klast). Same as *Lithotrite.*
Lith'oclasty. Same as *Lithotrity.*
Lith'oclysmy. Injection of solvents into urinary bladder.
Lithodial'ysis. Same as *Litholysis,* or as *Lithotrity.*
Lithol'apaxy. The crushing of a stone in the bladder and washing out of fragments.
Litho'lein. An oily product from petroleum: used in dermatology.
Lithol'ogy. The sum of what is known about calculi.
Lithol'ysis. The dissolving of calculi.
Lithontrip'tic. Effecting solution of stone in bladder.
Lithope'dium. A stony or petrified fetus.
Lith'ophone. Device for detecting stone in the bladder by means of sound.
Lith'oscope. Instrument for examining calculus in bladder.
Lith'otome (lith'o-tōm). A knife for lithotomy.
Lithot'omy. Removal of stone by cutting into the bladder. **Bilateral l.** is done through a transverse incision in front of rectum. **Lateral l.,** one where the cut is before the rectum and to the left of the raphe. **L.-position,** position with the patient on his back, the thighs and legs flexed, and the knees held widely apart. **Marian l., Median l.,** one made on the raphe before the anus. **Mediolateral l.,** a combination of the lateral and

median operations. **Rectal l.**, one performed by an incision through the rectum. **Suprapubic l.**, one done with a cut above the pubes. **Vaginal l.**, one performed by an incision through vaginal wall.

Lithotre'sis. The drilling or boring of holes in a calculus.

Lith'otripsy. The crushing of a calculus in the bladder.

Lithotrip'tic. An agent dissolving vesical calculus.

Lith'otrite. Instrument for crushing calculi.

Lithot'rity (lith-ot'rit-e). Same as *Lithotripsy.*

Lith'ous. Pertaining to a calculus or stone.

Lithure'sis. Passage of gravel in the urine.

Lithu'ria. Excess of uric acid or urates in the blood.

Lit'mus. A blue stain from lichens, turned red by acids. **L.-paper,** paper stained with litmus.

Li'tre (le'ter). Fr. for *Liter.*

Litten's diaphragm phenomenon. Movable horizontal depression on lower sides of thorax, seen in respiration.

Lit'ter. A couch for transporting the sick or wounded.

Lit'tle's disease. Spasmodic paraplegia of infants.

Littré's colotomy. Colotomy in the groin. **L.'s glands,** muciparous glands in spongy portion of urethra. **L.'s hernia.** Same as *Diverticular hernia.*

Live'do. A discolored patch on the skin.

Liv'er. A glandular viscus which secretes bile. **Albuminoid l.**, **Amyloid l.**, one which is a seat of albuminoid or amyloid degeneration. **Beaver-tail l.**, one with a peculiarly deformed left lobe. **Biliary cirrhotic l.**, one wherein the bile-ducts are clogged and distended, and the substance of the organ inflamed. **Cirrhotic l.**, one which is the seat of a chronic inflammation with overgrown connective tissue and distended bile-ducts. **Degraded l.**, liver divided into an unusual number of lobes. **Fatty l.**, one affected with fatty degeneration and infiltration. **Gin-drinker's l.** Same as *Hobnail l.* **Hobnail l.**, liver whose surface is marked with nail-like points from atrophic cirrhosis. **L.-fluke.** See *Distoma* and *Bilharzia.* **L.-spot.** See *Chloasma* and *Morphea.* **L.-wort.** See *Hepatica.* **Nutmeg l.**, a liver presenting a mottled appearance when cut. **Tight-lace l.**, one which is deformed by use of tight corsets. **Wandering l.**, a displaced liver. **Waxy l.** See *Amyloid l.*

Livid'ity. Li'vor. Discoloration, as from a bruise or congestion.

Lixivia'tion. Leeching of ashes to obtain lye.

Lixiv'ium (lik-siv'e-um). L. for *Lye.*

Lo'bar. Of, or pertaining to, a lobe.

Lo'bate. Provided with lobes.

Lobe. Part of an organ or viscus demarkated by fissures or divisions. **Caudate l.**, the tail-like process of the liver. **Slender l.**, the fourth of the five lobes on under surface of cerebellar hemisphere.

Lobe'lia infla'ta. A North American herb: emetic, expectorant, and depressant.

Lo'belin. A poisonous alkaloid from lobelia; also, a resinoid from the same.

Lob'ular. Pertaining to a lobule or to lobules.

Lob'ulated. Made up of lobules.

Lob'ule (lob'ūl). Any small lobe. **Fusiform l.**, the inferior temporo-occipital convolution. **Paracentral l.**, the superior connecting convolution of the ascending frontal and ascending parietal convolutions.

Lobulette (lob-u-let'). A minute lobule or acinus.

Lo'bus. L. for *Lobe.* **L. cauda'tus.** Same as *Caudate lobe.*

Lo'cal. Pertaining to one place or spot. **L. asphyxia.** Same as *Raynaud's disease.*

Localiza'tion. The discovery of the locality of a disease or process. **Cerebral l.,** localization of various faculties in particular parts of the brain.

Lo'calized. Not general; restricted to a limited region.

Lo'chia (lo'ke-ah). Vaginal discharge which follows childbirth. **L. al'ba,** whitish discharge, normal after about six days. **L. cruen'ta, L. ru'bra,** sanguineous flow of first week. **L. sero'sa,** a serous or ichorous discharge.

Lochiome'tra. The retention or non-discharge of the lochia.

Lochiorrhe'a. Abnormally free lochial discharge.

Lochios'chesis. Retention of the lochia.

Lochometri'tis (lo-ko-met-ri'tis). Puerperal metritis.

Lock'jaw. See *Tetanus* and *Trismus.*

Lo'co. Various plants of the United States, poisonous to cattle, horses, and sheep.

Lo'coism. Disease of live-stock ascribed to poisoning by loco.

Locomo'tion. Movement from one place to another.

Locomo'tor. Of, or pertaining to, locomotion. **L. ataxia.** See *Ataxia.*

Loc'ular (lok'u-lar). Containing loculi.

Lo'cus. L. for *Place.* **L. cine'reus, L. cœru'leus, L. ferrugin'eus,** pigmented eminence in the fourth ventricle. **L. mino'ris resisten'tiæ,** spot of lessened resistance. **L. ni'ger,** dark spot in the section of crus cerebri. **L. perfora'tus,** anterior and posterior perforated spaces at base of brain through which blood-vessels pass. **L. ru'ber,** the red nucleus.

Lœmol'ogy (le-mol'o-je). Science of contagious disease.

Löffl'eria (lef-le're-ah). Disease in which the diphtheria-bacillus is present without the ordinary symptoms of diphtheria.

Löffler's bacillus (lef'lerz). The microbe of diphtheria.

Logoneuro'sis. Any neurosis with speech disorder.

Logop'athy. Any disorder of speech of central origin.

Logople'gia (log-o-ple'je-ah). 1. Any paralysis of speech-organs. 2. Inability to speak, while words are remembered.

Logorrhe'a. Excessive or abnormal volubility.

Log'wood. Same as *Hematoxylon.*

Loi'mic (loi'mik). Pertaining to the plague.

Loimol'ogy. Scientific study of the plague.

Loin. Part of back between thorax and pelvis.

Lom'bardy leprosy. Same as *Pellagra.*

Lon'don paste. Mixture of caustic soda and lime.

Longev'ity (lon-jev'it-e). Long life.

Longis'simus dor'si. See *Muscles, Table of.*

Longsight'edness. See *Hypermetropia.*

Lon'gus col'li. See *Muscles, Table of.*

Loop of Henle. Same as *Henle's loop.*

Lordo'ma, Lordo'sis. Curvation of spinal column with forward convexity.

Lordoscolio'sis. Lordosis complicated with scoliosis.

Lore'ta's operation. Gastrotomy and dilatation of pylorus.

Lore'tin (lo-re'tin). A proprietary antiseptic powder.

Los'ophan. Cresol iodid, $C_6HI_3(CH_3)OH$, used in skin-diseases.

Los'torfer's corpuscles. See *Corpuscles.*

Lo'tion (lo'shun). A liquid preparation for bathing a part.

Louse. See *Pediculus.*

Lou'siness. Infestation with lice.

Low'er's tubercle. A tubercle in the right auricle of the heart, between the openings of the venæ cavæ.

Löwe's ring (la'vez). See *Ring.*

Lox'a bark. Pale Peruvian bark; cinchona pallida.

Loxar'thron. Oblique deformity of a joint without luxation.

Loz'enge (loz'enj). A form of medicated troche.

Lu'cid interval. The period between paroxysms of insanity.
Lud'wig's angina. See *Angina Ludwigii.*
Lu'es. Plague; more frequently syphilis.
Luet'ic. Pertaining to, or affected with, syphilis.
Lu'gol's caustic. One part each of iodin and potassium iodid with two parts of water. **L.'s solution,** the official compound solution of iodin.
Lumba'go (lum-ba'go). Neuralgia of the loins.
Lum'bar (lum'bar). Pertaining to the loins. **L. puncture.** See *Quincke's puncture.*
Lumbocolos'tomy. Colostomy by incision in the loin.
Lumbocolot'omy. An incision into the colon through the loin.
Lumbocos'tal. Pertaining to the loins and ribs.
Lumbrica'lis. See *Muscles, Table of.*
Lum'bricoid (lum'brik-oid). Resembling the earthworm.
Lumbri'cus. 1. The earthworm. 2. Same as *Ascaris.*
Lu'men. Transverse section of a tube.
Luminiferous ether. The medium whose vibrations constitute light.
Lump'y-jaw. Same as *Actinomycosis.*
Lu'nacy. Insanity; mental disorder.
Lu'nar caustic. Silver nitrate, A_gNO_3.
Lung. Either one of the pair of thoracic organs which serve for the aeration of the blood. **L. fever.** Same as *Pneumonia.*
Lu'nula. The whitish crescent at root of nail.
Lu'piform. 1. Resembling lupus. 2. Resembling a wen.
Lu'pinin. A poisonous alkaloid; also a glucosid from lupines.
Lupino'sis. Poisoning by lupines, or chickpea; lathyrism.
Lu'pulin. Yellow resinous powder from hops: sedative and stomachic.
Lu'pulus. Hops. See *Humulus.*
Lu'pus. Tuberculosis of the skin. **Disseminated follicular l.,** lupus of the face with large and small papules. **Erythematous l., Cazenave's l.,** non-tubercular disease like lupus. **L. ex'edens. L. vulga'ris,** true or typical tuberculous lupus. **L. hypertroph'icus, L. veg'etans,** a kind marked by formation of vegetations. **L. maculo'sus,** a variety characterized by maculæ. **L. non-ex'edens,** a variety with no ulceration. **L. serpigino'sus,** a variety which spreads by serpiginous growth. **L. tu'midus,** a variety with edematous infiltration. **L. verruco'sus,** a kind with warty growths.
Luschka's bursa (loosh'kaz). Same as *Bursa pharyngea.* **L.'s gland.** Same as *Coccygeal gland.* **L.'s tonsil.** See *Tonsil.*
Lu'sus natu'ræ. A freak of nature; a teratism.
Lute. Paste for covering joints of vessels.
Lu'tein. Pigment from egg-yolk and corpus luteum.
Luxa'tion. Same as *Dislocation.*
Lux'us consumption. The eating or digestion of food in excess of the real needs of the body. **L. heart,** dilatation with hypertrophy of left ventricle.
Lycan'thropy. Delusion in which patient believes himself a wolf.
Lyce'tol. Preparation of piperazin: used for lithemia and gout.
Lycopo'dium. Sporules of *L. clavatum:* used mainly in pharmacy; also, a homeopathic remedy from the same.
Lye. An alkaline percolate from wood-ashes; lixivium.
Ly'ing-in. The puerperal state; childbed.
Lymph. The fluid taken up and discharged by the lymphatics; also, any clear watery liquid resembling the typical lymph. **Animal l.,** vaccine lymph from an animal. **L.-cell, L.-corpuscle,** a leukocyte from lymph. **L.-channels, L.-sinuses,** open irregular spaces in and about lymphoid structures. **Humanized l.,** vaccine virus from the human subject. **Inflam-**

matory l., lymph produced by inflammation, as in wounds. **Koch's l.** See *Tuberculin*. **Plastic l.**, that from which embryonic tissue is formed. **L.-scrotum**, dilatation of scrotal lymphatics: seen in filariasis. **L.-spaces**, open spaces in connective or other tissue filled with lymph; especially those of the brain and meninges.

Lymphadenec'tasis. Dilatation of a lymphatic gland.

Lymphadeni'tis. Inflammation of lymphatic glands.

Lymphadeno'ma. Same as *Lymphoma*.

Lymphangiec'tasis. Dilatation of a lymphatic.

Lymphangiog'raphy. Description of lymphatic organs.

Lymphangio'ma. Tumor made up of lymphatic vessels.

Lymphangi'tis. Inflammation of a lymphatic vessel.

Lymphat'ic. 1. Pertaining to lymph. 2. A lymphatic vessel. **L. system**, the lymphatic glands, vessels, spaces, sinuses, and lacteals collectively. **L. vessels**, vessels that convey lymph.

Lym'phatism. Lymphatic temperament; slowness or sluggish habit.

Lymphati'tis. Same as *Lymphangitis*.

Lymphede'ma. Edema from clogging of efferent lymphatic.

Lymphe'mia (lim-fe'me-ah). Presence of lymphocytes in blood.

Lymphiza'tion. The production of lymph.

Lym'phocyte (lim'pho-sit). A leukocyte of the lymph.

Lymphocythe'mia. Excess of lymph-corpuscles in the blood.

Lymphocyto'sis. Same as *Lymphocythemia*.

Lymphoder'mia. Any disease of the skin lymphatics.

Lymphog'enous (lim-foj'en-us). Lymph-producing.

Lym'phoid. Resembling lymph; also, adenoid.

Lympho'ma. Any tumor of lymphoid tissue.

Lymphorrha'gia, Lymphorrhe'a. Flow of lymph from cut or ruptured lymph-vessels.

Lymphosarco'ma. Sarcoma of any lymph-organ.

Lym'photome. Instrument for excising adenoid growths on tonsils.

Lymphot'omy. The anatomy of lymphatics.

Lymphot'rophy. Attractive energy of cancer-cell for lymph.

Lypema'nia. Melancholia; insanity with despondency.

Lypothym'ia. Morbid despondency; melancholia.

Ly'ra. A triangular striated depression on lower side of fornix.

Lys'atin (lys'at-in). A basic principle derivable from casein.

Lys'idin. A diamin, $C_6H_{13}N_3O_2$, solvent for calculi and tophi.

Ly'sin. Any bacterial product which destroys alexins.

Ly'sis. Gradual abatement of a disease.

Ly'sol. An antiseptic preparation of tarry oils.

Lys'sa (lis'ah). Hydrophobia, or rabies.

Lys'sin. The specific hydrophobia virus.

Lyte'rian. Indicative of the approach of lysis.

M.

M. Abbreviation for *mille*, thousand; *misce*, mix; *minim*, *myopia*, *molar*, and *meter*.

μ. Symbol for *micron*, or *micromillimeter*.

MM. Abbreviation for *millimeter*.

MMM. Abbreviation for *micromillimeter*.

Maca'co worm. Larva of South American fly, which burrows under the skin.

Macal'lin. Alkaloid from bark of a tree of Yucatan: used like quinin.

McBur'ney's point. Superficial point marking most frequent position of appendix vermiformis.

Macdowel's frenum. Fibers which strengthen the intermuscular septum of the arm.

Mace (mās). A spice; the aril which envelops nutmeg.

Ma'cene (ma'sēn). Essential oil, $C_{20}H_{16}$, from nutmeg-flowers.

Macera'tion (mas-er-a'shun). The softening of a solid by soaking.

Ma'cies (ma'she-ēz). L. for *Wasting*.

Macrobio'sis (mak-ro-bi-o'sis). Long life; longevity.

Macroceph'alous. Having an abnormally large head.

Macroceph'aly (mak-ro-sef'al-e). Excessive size of head.

Macrochei'lia (mak-ro-ki'le-ah). Excessive size of lip.

Macrochi'ria. Oversize of the hands.

Macrococ'cus. A coccus of the largest recognized type.

Mac'rocyte (mak'ro-sit). A red blood-corpuscle of largest type.

Macrocythe'mia. Abnormal size of red blood-corpuscles.

Macrodactyl'ia. Abnormal largeness of fingers.

Mac'rodont (mak'ro-dont). Possessing large teeth.

Macroesthe'sia. Sensation as if things were larger than they really are.

Macroglos'sia (mak-ro-glos'se-ah). Hypertrophy of the tongue.

Macromas'tia, Macroma'zia. Oversize of the breasts.

Macrom'elus. Fetus with abnormally large limbs.

Mac'romere (mak'ro-mēr). A large blastomere.

Macronu'cleus. The larger of two paired nuclei.

Mac'rophage, Macroph'agus. A large cytophagous leukocyte.

Macropho'tograph. An enlarged photograph.

Macrop'sia. State in which objects appear larger than they are.

Macrosce'lia (mak-ro-se'le-ah). Excessive size of the legs.

Macroscop'ic. Seen by the unaided eye.

Macrosomа'tia, Macroso'mia. Great bodily size.

Macrosto'mia. Abnormally large size of mouth.

Mac'ula, pl. *mac'ulæ.* A stain or spot. **M. acus'tica,** terminations of acoustic nerve in utricle and saccule. **M. cor'neæ,** a corneal opacity. **M. cribro'sa,** area on wall of vestibule perforated for passage of filaments of the auditory nerve. **M. lu'tea,** the point of clearest vision at the center of retina. **M. sola'ris,** a freckle.

Mac'ular (mak'u-lar). Characterized by maculæ.

Mac'ulate (mak'u-lāt). Spotted or blotched.

Macula'tion. The condition of being spotted.

Mad. Insane; crazy.

Madaro'sis (mad-ar-o'sis). Loss of eyelashes or eyebrows.

Mad'der. The root of *Rubia tinctorum;* a red dye.

Madu'ra foot, M. disease. Same as *Mycetoma.*

Magen'die's foramen (mah-zhon-dēz'). See *Foramen.* **M.'s solution,** 3 per cent. aqueous solution of morphin sulphate.

Magen'ta (ma-jen'tah). Fuchsin or other salt of rosanilin.

Mag'istery (mad'jis-ter-e). A precipitate; any subtle or masterly preparation.

Mag'ma. Any pulpy mass or residue.

Magne'sia. Magnesium oxid, MgO: aperient and antacid.

Magne'sium (mag-ne'se-um). A white metal. **M. carbonate, M. citrate, M. sulphate,** medicinal salts of the same.

Mag'net. Electro-, soft iron rendered temporarily magnetic by an electric current in a helix around the iron. **Horse-shoe m.,** a magnet having the shape of a horse-shoe. **M. operation,** removal of iron particles by the magnet. **Permanent m.,** one with permanent magnetic qualities. **Temporary m.,** a substance which is magnetic during the passage of an electric current or when a fixed magnet is near it.

Mag'neto-electric'ity. Electric current induced by a magnet.

Magnetother'apy. Treatment of diseases by magnets.
Magnifica'tion. Apparent increase of size under microscope.
Mai'denhead. 1. The hymen. 2. Virginity.
Ma'idism (ma'id-izm). Pellagra; poisoning by damaged maize.
Main en griffe (man-on-grif'). Same as *Claw-hand*
Main succulente (man suk-ku-lant'). Edema of the hands.
Maize (māz). Indian corn; *Zea mays.* See *Zea.*
Make. Closure and completion of an electric circuit.
Makro-. See under *Macro-.*
Mal (mahl). Illness; disease. **M. de mer** (mahl-de-mār'), seasickness. **M. de los Pintos,** contagious psoriasis in Mexico.
Ma'la. 1. The cheek. 2. Malar bone.
Mal'abar itch. Skin-disease of India.
Mala'cia (ma-la'she-ah). Morbid softening of a part.
Mal'acin. A crystalline antipyretic and analgesic; salicyl-phenetidin.
Malaco'ma, Malaco'sis. Same as *Malacia.*
Malacos'teon. Softening of the bones; osteomalacia.
Malacot'omy. Incision of the abdominal wall.
Mal'ady (mal'ad-e). Any disease or illness.
Malaise (mal-āz'). Any uneasiness or indisposition.
Mal'akin. A salicylic derivative; used as antipyretic, antirheumatic, and antineuralgic.
Ma'lar (ma'lar). Pertaining to the cheek. **M. bone,** the cheek-bone; mala.
Mala'ria (mal-a're-ah). A febrile disease due to poisonous emanations from damp ground; or, more correctly, the emanations themselves.
Mala'rial. Pertaining to malaria.
Mal'arin. A proprietary antipyretic and antineuralgic.
Malassimila'tion. Defective or faulty assimilation.
Ma'late (ma'lāt). Any salt of malic acid.
Malaxa'tion. A kneading; kneading movement in massage.
Male (māl). One of the sex that begets young; masculine. **M. fern.** Same as *Aspidium.*
Malforma'tion. A defective formation.
Malgaigne's hooks (mal-gānz'). Adjustable double hooks for treating fractured patella.
Malias'mus. Glanders, or farcy.
Ma'lic acid. See *Acid.*
Malig'nancy. Tendency to react and to progress in virulence.
Malig'nant. Virulent, and tending to go from bad to worse.
Malin'gerer (ma-lin'jer-er). One who feigns illness.
Mallea'tion. Sharp and swift muscular twitching of hands.
Mal'lein (mal'le-in). Pathogenic lymph from cultures of glanders-bacillus.
Malleo-in'cudal. Of, or pertaining to, malleus and incus.
Malle'olar (mal-le'o-lar). Pertaining to malleolus.
Malle'olus, inner. Lower point of tibia. **M., outer,** lower end of fibula.
Mal'let-finger. Permanent flexion of a distal phalanx. **M.-toe.** Same as *Hammer-toe.*
Mal'leus. 1. Mallet-shaped ossicle of middle-ear. 2. Glanders, or farcy.
Malnutri'tion. Imperfect assimilation and nutrition.
Malpig'hian bodies. Bodies at beginning of uriniferous tubules of kidney. **M. capsule,** a pouch-like envelop of a M. body. **M. tuft,** the interior capillary part of a M. body.
Malposi'tion (mal-po-zish'un). Abnormal placement.
Malprac'tice (mal-prak'tis). Wrong or injurious treatment.
Malpresenta'tion. Faulty fetal presentation.
Malt (mawlt). Grain which has been sprouted and dried. **M.**

liquor, any fermented beverage prepared from malt, as ale, beer, porter. **M.-sugar.** Same as *Maltose.*

Mal'ta fever (mawl'tah). Same as *Mediterranean fever.*

Mal'ted milk. A proprietary food-preparation.

Mal'tine. A proprietary food-preparation of malt.

Maltodex'trin. A dextrin convertible into maltose.

Mal'tol. A constituent, $C_6H_6O_3$, of malt-caromel.

Mal'tose. Malt-sugar, a glucose from malt or digested starch.

Ma'lum. L. for *Disease.* **M. per'forans pe'dis,** perforating ulcer of the foot.

Mam'ma. The mammary gland; the breast.

Mam'mary. Pertaining to the mammary gland.

Mammil'la (mam-il'ah). See *Nipple.*

Mam'millary (mam'il-a-re). Like a nipple.

Mam'millated. Having nipple-like projections.

Mammil'liplasty. Plastic surgery of the nipple.

Mammi'tis (mam-i'tis). Inflammation of the mamma.

Mam'mose. Having unusually large mammæ.

Mammot'omy. Surgical incision of a mamma.

Man'aca. A South American plant, *Franciscea uniflora:* diuretic and cathartic.

Man'dible (man'dib-l). The lower jaw-bone.

Mandib'ular. Pertaining to the lower jaw-bone.

Mandrag'ora officina'lis. True mandrake; a narcotic and purgative plant.

Mandrag'orin. A poisonous alkaloid, $C_{17}H_{23}NO_3$, from mandragora.

Man'drake. See *Mandragora* and *Podophyllum.*

Man'drin. A metal guide for a flexible catheter.

Manduca'tion. The chewing of food.

Man'ganese (man'gan-ēs). A whitish metal; symbol Mn. **M. dioxid,** black oxid of manganese, MNO_2. **M. sulphate,** a purgative and cholagogue, $MnSO_4$.

Mange (mānj). Skin-disease of domestic animals, due to mites.

Ma'nia (ma'ne-ah). Violent insanity with wild excitement. **Alcoholic m.,** insanity from misuse of alcoholic stimulants. **M. a potu,** delirium tremens. **Bell's m.,** acute periencephalitis. **Dancing m.** See *Choromania.* **Epileptic m.,** maniacal attack in an epileptic. **Puerperal m.,** insanity which sometimes follows childbirth. **Religious m.,** mania with abnormal or perverted religious impulses. **Transitory m.,** severe frenzied mania, the attacks of which are of short duration.

Ma'niac. One affected with mania.

Mani'acal. Affected with mania.

Man'icure. 1. Process of caring for and embellishing the hand. 2. One who professionally cares for the hands and nails.

Man'ihot. See *Cassava* and *Jatropha.*

Man'ikin (man'ik-in). A model to illustrate anatomy.

Manipula'tion. Skilful or dextrous treatment by the hands.

Manip'ulus. L. for *Handful.*

Man'na (man'nah). Sweet concrete aperient exudation from *Fraxinus ornus.*

Man'nite. Manna sugar, $C_6H_{14}O_6$: used like manna.

Man'nitose. A carbohydrate, $C_6H_{12}O_6$, derived from mannite.

Manom'eter. Instrument for ascertaining the pressure of liquids.

Man'ual. Pertaining to, or performed by, the hands.

Manu'brium. 1. The uppermost piece of the sternum. 2. The inferior part of the malleus.

Man'us. L. for *Hand.*

Manustupra'tion. Masturbation; self-pollution.

Maran'ta. Same as *Arrow-root.*

Maran'tic. Pertaining to, or of the nature of, marasmus.

Maraschi'no (mah-rahs-ke'no). A liqueur containing cherries.
Maras'mic. Pertaining to, or affected with, marasmus.
Maras'mus. Progressive wasting, especially in young infants.
Marc (mark). The refuse after the pressing of grapes or olives.
Margar'ic acid. A mixture of stearic and palmitic acids.
Mar'garin. A mixture of stearin and palmitin.
Mar'ginal (mar'jin-al). Pertaining to a margin.
Margin'oplasty. Surgical renewal of a margin or border.
Mar'go (mar'go). L. for *Border.*
Marie's disease (mah-rēz'). Same as *Acromegaly.*
Mariotte's law mah-re-ots'). Same as *Boyle's law.* **M.'s spot.** Same as *Blind spot.*
Maritonu'cleus. Nucleus of the ovum after the sperm-cell has entered it.
Mar'kasol (mar'kas-ol). Bismuth borophenate.
Marmor'ekin. Antistreptococcin.
Mar'row (mar'o). Soft material which fills most of the cavities and cancelli of bones. **Spinal m.,** the spinal cord.
Marru'bium. Same as *Horehound.*
Mar'shall's fold. Same as *Vestigial fold.* **M.'s vein,** a vein of the left side of the heart.
Marsh fever. Malarial or paludal fever. **M. gas.** Same as *Methane.*
Marsh'mallow. Same as *Althæa.*
Marsh's test. A test for the presence of arsenic.
Marsupializa'tion. Operative formation of a pouch in abdominal cavity in treatment of cysts or other tumors.
Marsu'pia patella'ria. The alar ligaments of the knee.
Mar'tial (mar'shal). Containing iron; ferruginous.
Mar'tin's bandage. India-rubber bandage for varicose veins, etc. **M.'s depilatory,** calcium sulphydrate. **M.'s hemostatic,** agaric or punk charged with ferric chlorid.
Mas'culine. Pertaining to the male sex; male.
Mask. Appliance for shading, protecting, or medicating the face.
Masked. Hidden; not obvious.
Mas'ochism (mas'ok-izm). Sexual perversion with enjoyment of being cruelly treated.
Mas'ochist (mas'o-kist). A person given to masochism.
Mass. A body made up of coherent particles.
Mas'sa. L. for *Mass:* chiefly a plastic mass to be made into pills.
Massage (mahs-sahzh'). Systematic therapeutical friction, stroking, and kneading the body.
Mas'sering ball. A ball rolled on surface of body for massage.
Mass'eter. See *Muscles, Table of.*
Masseur (mas-er'). A man who performs massage.
Masseuse (mas-es'). A woman who performs massage.
Mas'sicot (mas'se-kot). Yellow lead monoxid, PbO.
Mas'sive pneumonia. See *Pneumonia.*
Massother'apy. Treatment of disease by massage.
Mastal'gia (mas-tal'je-ah). Pain in mammary gland.
Mast-cells. See *Cells.*
Mas'tic. Resin of *Pistacia lentiscus:* stimulant and stomachic.
Mastica'tion (mas-tik-a'shun). The act of chewing.
Mas'ticatory. 1. Pertaining to mastication. 2. A substance to be chewed but not swallowed.
Masti'tis. Inflammation of the mammary gland.
Mastodyn'ia (mas-to-din'e-ah). Pain in the mamma.
Mas'toid. Nipple-shaped. **M. antrum.** Same as *Antrum mastoideum.* **M. bone,** the m. process of the temporal bone. **M. cells.** The same as *M. sinuses.* **M. disease.** Same as *Mastoiditis.* **M. operation,** drainage from without of m. cells in mastoiditis.

Mastoideocente'sis. Paracentesis of the mastoid cells.
Mastoidi'tis. Inflammation of the mastoid antrum and cells.
Mastome'nia. Vicarious menstruation from the breast.
Masto-occip'ital. Pertaining to the mastoid process and occipital bone.
Masturba'tion. Self-pollution; causation of orgasm by hand.
Ma'té. Dried leaves of *Ilex Paraguayensis*: used like tea.
Mate'ria med'ica. Branch of medical study which deals with drugs, their sources, preparations, and uses.
Mate'ries mor'bi. The substance, virus, or principle which causes a disease.
Mater'nal. Pertaining to the mother.
Mati'co (mah-ti'ko). A shrub of tropical America, *Piper augustifolium*: leaves stimulant and astringent.
Matrica'ria chamomil'la. German chamomile: mild tonic and febrifuge.
Matricula'tion. Enrollment as a student in a college.
Ma'trix. 1. Womb, or uterus. 2. Groundwork in which cells, etc., are embedded.
Mat'toid (mat'oid). A paranoiac, or crank.
Mat'tress suture. See *Suture.*
Matura'tion. 1. Stage or process of becoming mature. 2. The formation of pus.
Mature (ma-tūr'). Ripe; fully developed.
Matu'tinal (mat-u'tin-al). Pertaining to the morning.
Matzoon (mat-zoon'). A drink prepared from fermented milk.
Maxil'la. A jaw-bone; especially the upper (superior m.). **Inferior m.,** the lower jaw-bone, or mandible.
Max'illary. Pertaining to a jaw or jaw-bone. **M. bone.** See *Maxilla.* **M. fissure,** fissure on superior maxilla for m. process of the palatal bone.
Max'imal. Greatest possible, allowable, or appreciable; the reverse of *minimal* and of *liminal.*
Max'imum. 1. Greatest possible or actual effect or quantity. 2. The acme of a disease or process.
Max'well's ring. A variety of visual ring, smaller and fainter than Löwe's ring.
May-apple. Same as *Podophyllum pellatum.*
Me'able. Susceptible of being passed through.
Mead'ow saf'fron. See *Colchicum.*
Mea'sles (me'zlz). 1. A contagious eruptive fever with coryza and catarrhal symptoms. 2. Cysticercal disease of domestic animals.
Mea'tal (me-a'tal). Of, or pertaining to, a meatus.
Meatom'eter, Device used in measuring a meatus.
Meatot'omy (me-at-ot'om-e). The cutting of urinary meatus.
Mea'tus (me-a'tus). L. for *Passage.* **M. audito'rius,** the passage of the ear in two parts (internal and external). **M. of the nose,** either of the three passages of the nasal cavity. **M. urina'rius,** the orificial part of the urethra (chiefly used of the male).
Mec'ca bal'sam. See under *Balsam.*
Mechan'ical antidote (me-kan'ik-al). See *Antidote.*
Mechan'ics (me-kan'ix). The science of force and matter.
Meckelec'tomy. Surgical removal of Meckel's ganglion.
Meckel's cartilage. Ventral segment of the first visceral arch of embryo. **M.'s diverticulum,** an occasional cecal appendage of the ileum: a relic of the vitelline duct. **M.'s ganglion,** the sphenopalatine ganglion. **M.'s space,** recess in dura which lodges the Gasserian ganglion.
Mecom'eter. An insrument for measuring an infant.
Meconar'ceïn. An alkaloidal mixture from opium; narcotic.

Mec'onate (mek'o-nāt). Any salt of meconic acid.

Mecon'ic acid (me-kon'ik). See *Acid*.

Mec'onin. A neutral substance, $C_{10}H_{10}O_4$, in opium.

Mec'onism. Opium-poisoning; the opium habit.

Meco'nium. Fecal matter discharged by new-born children.

Me'dia. The middle tunic of a blood- or lymph-vessel.

Me'dial (me'de-al). Pertaining to the middle.

Me'dian. Situated in the middle; mesial. **M. artery,** a branch of the interosseous. **M. nerve.** See *Nerves, Table of.*

Medias'tinal. Of, or pertaining to, the mediastinum.

Mediastini'tis. Inflammation of mediastinum.

Mediastinopericardi'tis. Inflammation of mediastinum and pericardium.

Mediasti'num. The median septum between the lateral cavities of the thorax. **M. tes'tis,** partial septum of the testicle.

Me'diate. Indirect; accomplished by means of a medium.

Med'ic. Any plant of the genus *Medicago*, including lucerne, nonesuch, shamrock, etc.

Med'ical. Pertaining to medicine. **M. jurisprudence,** the application of the principles of medicine to questions of law and justice.

Medic'ament (me-dik'am-ent). A medicinal agent.

Med'icated. Imbued with a medicinal substance.

Medica'tion (med-ik-a'shun). Administration of remedies.

Medic'inal (med-is'in-al). Having healing qualities.

Med'icine. 1. A drug or remedy. 2. The art of healing disease. **Clinic m.,** study of m. at the bedside. **Forensic m., Legal m.,** medical jurisprudence. **Galenical m.,** obsolete practice on the principles of Galen. **Patent m.,** a medicine whose manufacture is protected by letters patent. **Preventive m.,** that which aims at preventing disease. **Proprietary m.,** a remedy whose formula is private property. **Spagyric m.,** the obsolete school of Paracelsus. **State m.,** that which deals with the public health, sanitation, etc.

Medicine'rea (med-e-se-ne're-ah). Internal gray matter of brain.

Medicochirur'gical. Pertaining to medicine and surgery.

Medicole'gal. Pertaining to medical jurisprudence.

Med'icus (med'ik-us). L. for *Physician.*

Medi'na worm (me-de'nah). Same as *Guinea worm.*

Mediolat'eral lithotomy. See *Lithotomy.*

Mediopon'tine. Pertaining to the center of the pons.

Mediotar'sal. Pertaining to the center of the tarsus.

Mediterra'nean fever. See *Fever.*

Me'dium, pl. *me'dia.* Conditions and environment of the body. See also under *Culture.*

Medul'la. L. for *Marrow.* **M. neph'rica.** the pyramids of the kidneys collectively. **M. oblonga'ta,** the organ of brain directly continuous with spinal cord. **M. os'sium,** bone-marrow. **M. spina'lis,** spinal cord, or myelon.

Medul'lary. Pertaining to the marrow or to any medulla.

Med'ullated nerve-fiber. Any one of the white fibers of a nerve.

Medullispi'nal. Pertaining to the spinal cord.

Medulli'tis. Same as *Osteomyelitis;* also, *Myelitis.*

Medulliza'tion. Abnormal enlargement of marrow-spaces in cancellous bone.

Megabacte'rium. A large bacterium.

Megacephal'ic (meg-as-ef-al'ik). Having an abnormally big head.

Megacoc'cus. A coccus of large size. See *Macrococcus.*

Meg'aloblast (meg'al-o-blast). Same as *Macrocyte.*

Megalocephal'ic. Having a large skull.

Megalocor'nea. Bulging of the cornea.
Meg'alocyte (meg'al-o-sīt). See *Megaloblast.*
Megalodac'tylous. Having very large fingers.
Megalogas'tria. Abnormal size of the stomach.
Megaloglos'sia (meg-al-o-glos'e-ah). Same as *Macroglossia.*
Megaloma'nia (meg-al-o-ma'ne-ah). Delirium of grandeur.
Megalop'sia (meg-al-op'se-ah). Same as *Macropsia.*
Meg'aloscope. A magnifying speculum; a large magnifying lens.
Meg'aseme (meg'as-ēm). Having an orbital index exceeding 89.
Megas'toma intestina'le. A pathogenic protozoan of the intestine.
Megophthal'mus (meg-of-thal'mus). Same as *Buphthalmus.*
Me'grim (me'grim). Same as *Migraine.*
Meibo'mian glands (mi-bo'me-an). See *Gland.*
Meiocar'dia (mi-o-kar'de-ah). Contraction of the heart; systole.
Meio'sis (mi-o'sis). Same as *Miosis.*
Meiot'ic (mi-ot'ik). Same as *Miotic.*
Meiss'ner's corpuscles (mis'nerz). The tactile corpuscles. **M.'s ganglion, M.'s plexus,** plexus of nerve-fibers in submucous intestinal tissue.
Mel. L. for *Honey.*
Melæ'na (mel-e'nah). Blackening of feces from blood-pigments.
Melanede'ma (mel-an-e-de'mah). Same as *Anthracosis.*
Melane'mia. Presence of black pigmentary masses in blood.
Melancho'lia. Insanity with depression of spirits or gloomy forebodings. **M. agita'ta,** m. with strong motor excitement. **M. atton'ita. M. stuporo'sa,** motionless and silent melancholy. **M. sim'plex,** mild form, with neither delusions nor great excitement.
Melanephidro'sis. Discharge of black sweat.
Mel'anin. A dark pigment from choroid, hair, and other dark tissues; also, from melanotic tumors.
Mel'anism (mel'an-izm). Excessive pigmentation; blackening of the integuments.
Melanocarcino'ma. A pigmented cancer.
Mel'anocyte. A dark-colored leukocyte.
Melanoder'ma. Black discoloration of the skin.
Mel'anoid. Pertaining to, or resembling, melanosis.
Melano'ma. Melanotic or discolored tumor.
Melanop'athy. Excess of skin-pigmentation.
Melanorrha'gia, Melanorrhe'a. Passage of feces darkened with blood-pigments.
Melanosarco'ma. Sarcoma with pigmentary elements.
Melanoschir'rhus. Same as *Melanocarcinoma.*
Melano'sis. Condition characterized by pigmentary deposits.
Melanot'ic. Characterized by dark pigmentation.
Melanu'ria. The discharge of darkly-stained urine.
Melas'ma (me-laz'mah). Dark pigmentation of the skin. **M. Addiso'nii.** Same as *Addison's disease.*
Mele'na (mel-e'nah). Darkening of feces by blood-pigments.
Melez'itose. A sugar from Briançon manna, $C_{18}H_{32}O_{16}$.
Melicc'ra, Melice'res. 1. A cyst filled with honey-like substance. 2. Viscid syrupy sweating.
Melis'sa officina'lis. Lemon-balm, an aromatic and carminative herb.
Melitag'ra (mel-it-ag'rah). Eczema with honey-comb crusts.
Melite'mia. Excessive amount of sugar in the blood.
Mel'itose. A sugar from Australian manna, $C_{12}H_{22}O_{11}$.
Melitu'ria (mel-it-u're-ah). Same as *Diabetes mellitus.*
Mel'lite (mel'īt). Any preparation of medicated honey.
Meloma'nia. Insane fondness for music.
Melom'elus. Monstrous fetus with supernumerary limbs.

Mel'on-seed bodies. Small bodies in joints and tendon-sheaths.

Mel'oplasty (mel'op-las-te). Plastic surgery of a cheek.

Melt'ing-point. The temperature at which a solid melts.

Membra'na. L. for *Membrane.* **M. adventit'ia.** See *Adventitia.* **M. basila'ris.** Same as *Basilar membrane.* **M. choriocapilla'ris,** innermost vascular layer of the choroid. **M. decid'ua.** Same as *Decidua.* **M. eb'oris,** investing membrane of the tooth-pulp, made up of relics of the odontoblasts. **M. flac'cida.** Same as *Shrapnell's membrane.* **M. granulo'sa,** cell-layer which limits the Graafian vesicle. **M. nic'titans.** See *Nictitating membrane.* **M. pituito'sa.** See *Schneiderian membrane.* **M. pro'pria.** Same as *Basement membrane.* **M. Reissne'rii.** See *Reissner's membrane.* **M. tecto'ria.** Same as *Corti's membrane.* **M. tym'pani,** drum of the membranous ear. **M. vi'brans, M. ten'sa,** the tenser portion of the drum-membrane of the ear.

Membrane. A thin layer of tissue which covers a surface or divides an organ. **Animal m.,** a thin diaphragm of membrane, as of bladder, used as a dialyzer. **Basement m.,** delicate layer underlying epithelium. **M.-bone,** a bone ossified within, or developed from, a membrane. **Bruch's m.,** inner layer of choroid coat. **Corti's m.,** membrane over Corti's organ. **Costocoracoid m.,** fascia between pectoralis minor and subclavius muscles. **Cricothyroid m.,** membrane which connects the thyroid and cricoid cartilages. **Croupous m.,** false membrane of true croup. **Debove's m.,** delicate layer between the epithelium and tunica propria of broncial, tracheal, and intestinal mucous membrane. **Descemet's m.,** posterior lining membrane of the cornea. **Diphtheritic m.,** the peculiar false membrane characteristic of diphtheria. **Drum m.** See *Membrana tympani.* **Elastic m.,** a membrane made up largely of elastic fibers. **False m.,** membranous exudate, like that of diphtheria. **Fenestrated m.,** the elastic inner membrane of the arterial intima. **Fetal m's.,** chorion, amnion, and allantois. **Germinal m.,** the blastoderm. **Huxley's m.,** cellular membrane of root-sheath and proximal end of a hair. **Hyaline m.** 1, Membrane between outer root-sheath and inner fibrous layer of hair-follicle. 2. Basement membrane. **Jacob's m.,** the rod-and-cone layer of the retina. **Krause's m.,** membrane supposed to separate disks of sarcous matter in muscle. **Meconic m.,** a layer within the fetal rectum. **Medullary m.** Same as *Endosteum.* **Mucous m.,** membrane covered with epithelium lining canals and cavities which communicate with external air. **Nasmyth's m.,** membrane covering enamel of an unworn tooth. **Nictitating m.,** the so-called third eyelid of various animals. **Obturator m.,** the tough membrane which closes the obturator foramen. **Periodontal m.,** membrane which covers the cement of a tooth. **Pupillary m.,** delicate membrane which closes the fetal pupil. **Pyogenic m.,** old name for prophylactic membrane. **Pyophylactic m.,** fibrous membrane lining a pus-cavity, and tending to prevent reabsorption of injurious materials. **Ruyschian m.** Same as *Entochoroidea.* **Schneiderian m.,** mucous membrane which lines the nose. **Serous m.,** the lining membrane of any one of the great splanchnic or lymph-cavities. **Shrapnell's m.,** the thin upper part of the membrana tympani. **Synovial m.,** the membrane which lines joint-cavities and tendon-sheaths. **Tenon's m.** See *Tenon's capsule.* **Thyrohyoid m.,** membrane which connects thyroid cartilage and hyoid bone. **Tympanic m.** Same as *Membrana tympani.*

Membranocartilag'inous. Pertaining to, or developed in, membrane and cartilage.

Mem'branous. Of, or pertaining to, membrane.
Mem'brum viri'le. The penis.
Menidro'sis. Bloody sweat replacing the menstrual discharge.
Ménière's disease (men-e-ârz'). See *Disease*.
Menin'geal (me-nin'je-al). Of, or pertaining to, the meninges.
Menin'ges (me-nin'jēz), pl. of *meninx*. The membranes of the brain and cord; the dura, pia, and arachnoid.
Menin'gism. Hysteric simulation of meningitis.
Meningit'ic. Of, or pertaining to, meningitis. **M. streak,** streak on skin when the nail is drawn over it in meningitis.
Meningi'tis (men-in-ji'tis). Inflammation of the meninges. **Cerebral m.,** inflammation of the membranes of the brain, acute or chronic. See *Leptomeningitis*, *Pachymeningitis*. **Cerebrospinal m.,** epidemic inflammation of meninges of the brain and spinal cord. **Otitic m.,** that which may complicate an attack of otitis. **Septicemic m.,** that which is due to septic blood-poisoning. **Spinal m.,** that which affects the membranes of spinal cord. **Tubercular m.** Same as *Acute hydrocephalus*.
Meningitopho'bia. Condition simulating meningitis, due to dread of that disease.
Menin'gocele (me-nin'go-sēl). Hernial protrusion of meninges.
Meningocerebri'tis. Inflammation of brain and meninges.
Meningococ'cus. A micro-organism causing meningitis.
Meningo-encephal'ocele. Protrusion of brain and meninges.
Meningomyeli'tis. Inflammation of spinal cord and its membranes.
Meningomyel'ocele. Protrusion of spinal cord and membranes.
Meningorhachid'ian. Pertaining to spinal cord and meninges.
Meningo'sis. Union or attachment of bones by membrane.
Meningu'ria. Presence of shreds in urine.
Me'ninx (me'ninx), pl. *meninges*. A membrane, especially one of the brain or spinal cord.
Menis'cus. 1. A crescentic interarticular fibrocartilage. 2. A concavo-convex (positive m.) or convexo-concave (negative m.) lens.
Menisper'mum. The root of *Menispermum canadense*, or moonseed: it is tonic.
Menocee'lis (men-o-se'lis). Spotting of skin from stoppage of the menses.
Men'opause. Period when menstruation ceases; change of life.
Menopla'nia. Metastasis or aberration of menses.
Menorrha'gia, Menorrhe'a. Immoderate flow of menses.
Menosep'sis. Septic poisoning from retained menses.
Menos'tasis (men-os'tas-is). Suppression of the menses.
Men'ses (men'sēz). The monthly courses of women.
Mens'trual. Pertaining to the menses.
Menstrua'tion. The monthly sanguineous discharge peculiar to women. **Climacteric m.,** time of first menstruation. **Vicarious m.,** menstrual flow from some part or organ other than the vagina.
Men'struum (men'stru-um). A solvent medium.
Mensura'tion. The act or process of measuring.
Mentag'ra (men-tag'rah). Same as *Sycosis*.
Mentagrophy'ton. The fungus *Microsporon mentagrophytes* causing sycosis.
Men'tal. 1. Pertaining to the mind. 2. Pertaining to the chin.
Men'tha. L. for *Mint*. **M. piperi'ta,** peppermint. **M. pule'gium,** true pennyroyal. **M. vir'idis,** spearmint.
Men'thene (men'thēn). A hydrocarbon, $C_{10}H_{18}$, from menthol.
Men'thol. A stearoptene from peppermint oil: locally anodyne.
Menthophe'nol. An antiseptic containing menthol and phenol.
Men'tum (men'tum). L. for *Chin*.

Mephit'ic (me-fit'ik). Noxious; foul; of an ill odor.
Meral'gia (me-ral'je-ah). Pain in a thigh.
Mercap'tan. Any alcohol in which oxygen is replaced by sulphur.
Mercier's bar (mer-se-āz'). A bar or fold at neck of bladder.
Mercu'rial (mer-ku're-al). 1. Pertaining to, or containing, mercury. 2. A preparation containing mercury. **M. palsy**, paralysis caused by mercurial poisoning. **M. rash**, rash caused by local application of mercurials.
Mercu'rialism. Chronic poisoning from misuse of mercury.
Mercu'ric chlorid. Corrosive sublimate, $HgCl_2$: poisonous, antiseptic. **M. oxid**, a red or yellow powder, HgO.
Mercuroidolhe'mol. Brown powder, containing hemol, mercury, and iodin: used as alterative and hematinic.
Mer'curous chlorid. Calomel, Hg_2Cl_2; a white cholagogue purgative powder.
Mer'cury. A bivalent liquid metal, symbol Hg.
Meriat'chenje. See *Miryachit.*
Merismope'dia. A genus of bacteria said to be pathogenic.
Mer'ispore. A spore produced by the division of another spore.
Meroblas'tic ovum. One in which only a part of the yolk undergoes segmentation.
Mer'ocele (mer'o-sēl). Femoral hernia.
Merorrhachis'chisis. Fissure of a part of the spinal cord.
Merot'omy (me-rot'o-me). A cutting into segments.
Mer'ycism (mer'is-izm). Rumination; regurgitation of food from stomach and chewing it again.
Mer'ycole. One who ruminates.
Mes'ad. Toward a center or mesial line.
Me'sal (me'sal). See *Mesial.*
Mesame'boid. A cell given off from the epiblast or hypoblast to become a part of the mesoblast or mesoderm.
Mesara'ic (mes-ar-a'ik). Same as *Mesenteric.*
Mesarteri'tis. Inflammation of the middle coat of an artery.
Mesaticephal'ic. With a length-breadth index of 75° to 80°.
Mescal buttons. Tops of *Anhalonium Lewinii* of Mexico: they are poisonous.
Mes'calin. An alkaloid from mescal buttons.
Mesenceph'alon (mes-en-sef'al-on). The corpora quadrigemina and crura cerebri together.
Mesen'chyma (mes-en'kim-ah). Embryonic connective tissue.
Mesenter'ic (mes-en-ter'ik). Pertaining to the mesentery.
Mesenteri'tis. Inflammation of the mesentery.
Mesen'teron. The part of the body-cavity whence alimentary canal, lungs, liver, and pancreas are derived.
Mes'entery (mes'en-ter-e). Fold of peritoneum which attaches the mesentery to the abdominal wall.
Me'siad (me'se-ad). Toward the middle; mesad.
Me'sial (me'se-al). Situated in the middle; median.
Me'sion (me'se-on). The plane which divides the body into right and left symmetrical halves.
Mes'merism (mes'mer-izm). Hypnotism, or animal magnetism.
Mesoappen'dix. The peritoneal fold which connects the appendix to the ileum.
Meso'rium (mes-o-a're-um). Same as *Mesovarium.*
Mes'oblast. The middle layer of the primitive embryo.
Mesobronchi'tis. Inflammation of middle coat of bronchia.
Mesocæ'cum, Mesocæ'cum. Peritoneal fold which gives attachment to the cecum.
Mesocephal'ic. 1. Pertaining to the mesocephalon. 2. Having a head of medium size.
Mesoceph'alon. Same as *Mesencephalon.*
Mesocol'ic hernia. Hernia into a pouch of the mesocolon.

Mesoco'lon. Peritoneal process by which colon is attached.
Mes'ocord. An umbilical cord adherent to the placenta.
Mes'oderm (mes'o-derm). Same as *Mesoblast.*
Mesodmi'tis. Inflammation of the mediastinum.
Mesogas'ter (mes-o-gas'ter). Same as *Midgut.*
Mesogas'tric. Pertaining to mesogastrium or to umbilical region.
Mesogas'trium. The embryonic mesentery of the stomach.
Mesogna'thic. With a gnathic index between 98 and 103.
Mesogna'thion (mes-og-na'the-on). The premaxillary bone.
Mesol'obus (me-sol'o-bus). The corpus callosum.
Mes'on (mes'on). Same as *Mesion.*
Mesoneph'ric. Pertaining to the mesonephron. **M. duct.** Same as *Wolffian duct.*
Mesoneph'ron, Mesoneph'ros. Same as *Wolffian body.*
Mesoneuri'tis. 1. Inflammation of the substance of a nerve. 2. Inflammation of the lymphatics of a nerve.
Mesoph'ryon (mes-of're-on). Central point of the glabellum.
Mesopneu'mon. Fold of pleura which attaches the lung.
Mesor'chium. Peritoneal fold which holds in place the fetal testicle.
Mesorec'tum. The mesentery of the rectum.
Mesoret'ina (mes-o-ret'in-ah). The middle layer of the retina.
Mes'orrhine. With a nasal index between 47 and 51.
Mes'oseme. Within an orbital index between 83 and 90.
Mes'ostate. Any product of metabolism which represents an intermediate stage in the formation of another product.
Mesoster'num. The middle piece or body of the sternum.
Mesothe'lium (mes-o-the'le-um). Part of mesoblast whence the serous cavities and muscles are developed.
Mesoth'enar (mes-oth'en-ar). The adductor pollicis.
Mesova'rium. Peritoneal fold which holds ovary in place.
Metab'asis (met-ab'as-is). Change of disease or of place.
Metabol'ic (met-ab-ol'ik). Pertaining to metabolism.
Metab'olin (met-ab'o-lin). A product of metabolism.
Metab'olism. Change in living organism induced by the action of cells. **Constructive m.** See *Anabolism.* **Destructive m.** See *Catabolism.*
Metab'olite. Any substance derived by metabolism.
Metacar'pal (met-ak-ar'pal). Pertaining to the metacarpus.
Metacar'pus. Part of hand between the wrist and phalanges.
Met'acele (met'as-ēl), **Metacœ'le** (met-ah-se'le). Same as *Fourth ventricle.*
Metachlo'ral. A remedy, C_2Cl_3HO, not unlike chloral hydrate.
Metach'ysis (me-tak'is-is). Transfusion of blood.
Metacine'sis. Separation of daughter-stars from each other.
Metagas'ter. The permanent intestinal canal of the embryo.
Metagas'trula. Gastrula with cleavage differing from the standard type.
Metagen'esis (met-aj-en'es-is). Alternation of generation.
Met'al. Any element marked by luster, malleability, ductility, and conductivity of electricity and heat.
Metalbu'min (met-al-bu'min). A proteid found in ovarian cysts.
Metal'lic. Pertaining to, or composed of, metal. **M. tinkling,** a peculiar ringing auscultatory sound in pneumothorax, and over large lung-cavities.
Met'alloid. 1. Any non-metallic element. 2. Any metal that has not all the characters of a typical metal.
Metallos'copy. Observation of the effects of applying metals to the body.
Metallother'apy. Treatment of disease by applying metals to the integument.
Metamer'ic. Of, or characterized by, metamerism.

Metam'erid (met-am'er-id). A metameric substance.

Metam'erism. Isomerism when the component elements are identical, but the structural arrangement is not the same.

Metamorphop'sia. State of the eye in which objects looked at seem to be distorted.

Metamor'phosis. Change of structure or shape. **Fatty m.** Same as *Fatty degeneration.* **Regressive m., Retrograde m.**, a degeneration; also, a catabolic change. **Viscous m.**, the massing of blood-plaques in thrombosis.

Metaneph'ron, Metaneph'ros. The hindmost segment of the primitive embryonic kidney.

Metaphosphor'ic acid. Glacial phosphoric acid, HPO_3.

Metapla'sia. Change of one kind of tissue into another.

Metaplas'tic. Formed by metaplasia.

Metapneumon'ic. Succeeding or following pneumonia.

Metapoph'ysis. Any tubercle on the superior articular processes of a vertebra.

Metapyret'ic. Performed or occurring after the advent (otherwise, after the decline) of septic fever.

Metas'tasis. Transfer of disease from one organ to another.

Metastat'ic. Pertaining to, or due to, metastasis.

Metaster'num. Same as *Ensiform cartilage.*

Metasyph'ilis. Congenital syphilis with general degeneration, and with no appreciable local lesions.

Metatarsal'gia. Pain in metatarsus.

Metatarsophalan'geal. Pertaining to metatarsus and phalanges.

Metatar'sus. Part of foot between tarsus and toes.

Metath'esis. 1. Artificial transfer of morbid process. 2. Replacement of molecular atoms by other atoms.

Metenceph'alon. 1. Hind-brain; part of embryonic brain whence the pons and part of cerebellum are developed. 2. After-brain; part of embryonic brain whence are developed the oblongata and part of the fourth ventricle.

Me'teorism. Tympanites; gas in the abdomen or intestine.

Me'ter. Measure of length, 39.371 inches. **M.-angle**, angle of visual axes when viewing a point one meter distant.

Methac'etin. An antipyretic and anodyne, $C_7H_{11}NO_2$.

Meth'ane. Marsh gas, CH_4, from decayed organic matter.

Methemoglo'bin. Hemoglobin from decomposing blood.

Methemoglobine'mia. Methemoglobin in the blood.

Methemoglobinu'ria. Methemoglobin in the urine.

Methoma'nia. Insanity from alcoholic drinks.

Metho'zin (meth-o'zin). Same as *Antipyrin.*

Me'thyl. An atom-group, CH_3, from wood-spirit. **M. alcohol,** wood-spirit, CH_3OH; distilled from wood: sedative, narcotic, and poisonous. **M. ether,** colorless anesthetic gas $(CH_3)_2O$. **M. oxid,** gaseous or liquid substance: strongly refrigerant. **M. salicylate,** artificial oil of gaultheria: found also in natural oil of wintergreen. **M. violet,** blue pyoktanin.

Meth'ylal. Same as *Formal.*

Methyl'amin. Gaseous ptomain from decaying fish and from comma-bacillus cultures.

Meth'ylated spirit. Mixture of ethyl and methyl alcohols.

Meth'ylen blue. Blue stain and analgesic. **M. dichlorid,** an anesthetic liquid, CH_2Cl_2.

Methylguan'idin, Methyluram'in. A poisonous ptomain, $C_2H_7N_3$, from spoiled fish, etc.

Metop'agus (me-top'ag-us). Twin fetuses united at forehead.

Meto'pion (me-to'pe-on). Point in median line of forehead, between frontal eminences.

Me'tra (me'trah). The womb, or uterus.

Me'tre (me'ter). Same as *Meter.*
Metrec'topy (me-trek'to-pe). Uterine displacement.
Met'ric system. System of measures and weights having the meter as a basis. See *Weights and Measures, Tables of.*
Metri'tis. Inflammation of the womb.
Met'roclyst. Device for irrigating the womb.
Metrocol'pocele (met-ro-kol'po-sēl). Hernia of uterus into vagina.
Metrocysto'sis. Formation of cysts in the womb.
Metrodyn'ia (met-ro-din'e-ah). Pain in the uterus.
Metrop'athy (met-rop'ath-e). Any uterine disorder.
Metroperitoni'tis. Inflammation of uterus and peritoneum.
Metrophlebi'tis. Inflammation of uterine veins.
Metrorrha'gia (met-ror-ra'je-ah). Uterine hemorrhage.
Metrorrhe'a. Free or abnormal uterine discharge.
Metrortho'sis. Rectification of uterine displacement.
Metrosalpingi'tis. Inflammation of womb and oviducts.
Met'roscope (met'ros-kōp). Instrument for examining the uterus.
Metrostax'is (met-ros-tax'is). Slow loss of blood from uterus.
Met'rotome (met'ro-tōm). Same as *Hysterotome.*
Metrot'omy (met-rot'o-me). Same as *Hysterotomy.*
Metro-ureth'rotome (met-ro-u-reth'ro-tōm). A urethrotome with a device which regulates the amount of cutting.
Meynert's commissure (mi'nerts). Commissure from subthalamic body to floor of third ventricle.
Meze'reon, Meze'reum. Diaphoretic, diuretic, and alterative bark of *Daphne Mezereum.*
Mg. Symbol for *Magnesium.*
Mi'asm, Mias'ma. A noxious effluvium.
Miasmat'ic. Of, or pertaining to, miasm.
Mi'ca pa'nis. L. for *Bread-crumb.*
Micel'la. Same as *Tagma.*
Microenceph'alon. Abnormal smallness of brain; cretinism.
Mi'crobe (mi'krōb). A vegetable micro-organism.
Microbe'mia (mi-kro-be'me-ah). Same as *Microbiohemia.*
Microb'ic (mi-krob'ik). Of, or pertaining to, microbes.
Microbici'dal (mi-krob-is-i'dal). Destroying microbes.
Microb'icide (mi-krob'is-id). An agent that destroys microbes.
Microbici'din. A compound, $C_{10}H_7ONa$, used as external antiseptic, and internally as antipyretic and antiseptic.
Microbiohe'mia. Disease due to microbes in the blood.
Microbiol'ogy (mi-kro-be-ol'o-je). Study of the microbes.
Microbiopho'bia. A morbid dread of microbes.
Mi'crobism (mi'kro-bizm). Disease due to microbes.
Mi'croblast (mi'kro-blast). Same as *Microcyte.*
Microbleph'arism, Microbleph'ary (mi-kro-bleph'ar-e). Abnormal smallness of eyelids.
Microbra'chius. Fetus with preternaturally small arms.
Microcephal'ic, Microceph'alous. Having a small head.
Microceph'alus. Idiot or fetus with very small head.
Microceph'aly (mi-kro-sef'al-e), **Microceph'alism** (mi-kro-sef'al-izm). Abnormal smallness of head.
Microchem'istry (mi-kro-kem'is-tre). Chemical work carried on by the aid of the microscope.
Microc'idin (mi-kros'id-in). Sodium naphtolate; an antiseptic.
Micrococ'cus (mi-kro-kok'kus). A minute bacterial coccus or cell-form; generally regarded as a genus of schizomycetes. **M. a'cidi lac'tici,** a coccus in fresh milk, causing lactic-acid fermentation. **M. ag'ilis,** a species from water, producing a rosy pigment. **M. amylov'orus,** coccus which causes apple and pear blight: produces fermentation in saccharine solutions. **M. aquat'ilis,** coccus found in water. **M. ascofor'mans,** a kind

found in diseased tissues of the horse: causes septicemia. **M. can'dicans,** saprophytic coccus from air, water, etc. **M. capillo'rum,** a kind from the scalp: alters color of the hair. **M. car'neus,** from flowing water: produces a red pigment. **M. chlori'nus,** a coccus which produces a yellowish pigment. **M. cit'reus,** found in water and in osteomyelitis. **M. comula'tus ten'uis,** in nasal mucus. **M. concen'tricus,** in water: not pathogenic. **M. cremoi'des,** in water: named from its creamy pigment. **M. cya'neus,** in the air: forms a blue pigment on potato. **M. dif'fluens,** in air, dust, and feces. **M. endocardi'tidis ruga'tus,** on the valvular vegetations of ulcerative endocarditis. **M. fervido'sus,** in water: not pathogenic. **M. Floc'cii,** from conjunctival sac. **M. fla'vus conjuncti'væ,** from the human conjunctiva: pathogenic in rabbits. **M. fla'vus liquefa'ciens,** from air, water, and the air-passages. **M. fœ'tidus,** ill-smelling form from nasopharynx, and from rotten teeth. **M. fus'cus,** from water. **M. gelatino'sus,** from milk. **M. gingi'væ pyo'genes,** from alveolar abscess: pathogenic. **M. hæmato'des,** from hair of persons with a red sweat: also from sweat of the armpit. **M. liquefa'ciens conjuncti'væ,** from normal human conjunctiva. **M. Lœwenber'gii,** from nose in ozena; pathogenic. **M. of mastitis of cow,** produces mastitis in cows. **M. masto'bius,** from milk of sheep with gangrenous mastitis. **M. nasa'lis,** from nasopharynx: non-pathogenic. **M. nitrif'icans,** from soil: changes various nitrogen compounds to nitrates. **M. of osteomyelitis,** pathogenic form from osteomyelitis. **M. Pasteu'ri,** from saliva. **M. Pflü'geri,** from decaying flesh and potatoes. **M. plumo'sus,** from water. **M. porcello'rum,** from swine with hepatitis. **M. of progressive lymphoma of animals,** found in sputa of pneumonia after measles: dangerously pathogenic. **M. pyo'genes ten'uis,** from large abscesses. **M. radia'tus,** from air and water. **M. restit'uens,** changes peptone into albumin. **M. Rosenbach'ii,** from pus of abscesses. **M. rosetta'ceus,** from water. **M. ro'seus,** from sputum of influenza. **M. saliva'rius sep'ticus,** from sputum of puerperal septicemia. **M. tetra'genus,** from sputum of phthisis and lung-cavities: pathogenic. Other forms referred to this species from smallpox, yellow fever, the stomach-contents, nasal mucus, etc. **M. ure'æ,** produces ammoniacal fermentation in urine. **M. urinal'bus,** from urine in cystitis and pyelonephritis. **M. uri'næ al'bus, M. uri'næ fla'vus, M. uri'næ ma'jor,** three forms from urine of cystitis, etc. **M. versat'ilis,** found in the healthy skin and in the viscera after death from yellow fever. **M. viniper'da,** found in spoiled wine. **M. vir'idis flaves'cens,** from lymph of varicella. **M. visco'sus,** from diseased wine. **M. xanthogen'icus,** from yellow-fever patients.

Microcor'nea (mi-kro-kor'ne-ah). Unusual smallness of cornea.

Microcos'mic salt. Sodium and ammonium phosphate.

Microcou'lomb. The millionth part of a coulomb.

Mi'crocrith. The weight of one atom of hydrogen.

Microcrys'talline. Made up of minute crystals.

Mi'crocyst (mi'kro-sist). A very small cyst.

Mi'crocyte (mi'kro-sit). An undersized red blood-corpuscle.

Microcythe'mia, Microcyto'sis. Condition in which the red blood-corpuscles are undersized.

Microdactyl'ia. Unusual smallness of fingers or toes.

Mi'crodont (mi'kro-dont). Having very small teeth.

Microglos'sia (mi-kro-glos'e-ah). Undersize of the tongue.

Microgna'thia (mi-krog-na'the-ah). Undue smallness of jaws.

Mi'crogram. The one-millionth part of a gram.

Microg'raphy (mi-krog'raf-e). Same as *Microscopy.*

Microgyr'ia (mi-kro-jir'e-ah). Undersize of brain-convolutions.
Microl'ogy. A treatise on microscopy.
Microma'nia (mi-kro-ma'ne-ah). Insane belief that one's body has been reduced in size.
Microm'elus. Fetus with undersized limbs.
Microm'eter. Instrument for measuring microscopical objects.
Microm'etry. Measurement of microscopic objects.
Micromil'limeter. Same as *Micron.*
Micromye'lia (mi-kro-mi-e'le-ah). Abnormal smallness of spinal cord.
Mi'cron (mi'kron). One-millionth part of a meter.
Micro-or'ganism. Any microscopic animal or plant.
Micropathol'ogy. Pathology of diseases caused by micro-organisms.
Mi'crophage, Microph'agus. A phagocyte of small size.
Mi'crophone. Device for rendering feeble sounds audible.
Micropho'noscope. A binaural stethoscope having a membrane in the chest-piece, this accentuates the sound.
Micropho'tograph. 1. Same as *Photomicrograph.* 2. Photograph of microscopic size.
Microphthal'mia. Abnormal smallness of the eyes.
Microphthal'mus. Person with abnormally small eyes.
Mi'crophyte (mi'kro-fit). A microscopic plant.
Microp'sia (mi-krop'se-ah). State in which objects seen appear to be smaller than they really are.
Mic'ropus. A person with abnormally small feet.
Mi'cropyle (mi'kro-pil). Opening through which spermatozoon, in some animals, enters the ovum.
Mi'croscope (mi'kro-skōp). Instrument which magnifies minute objects for visual inspection. **Binocular m.,** microscope to be used with both eyes together. **Compound m.,** one that consists of two or more lenses or lens-systems. **Simple m.,** one which consists of a simple lens or of several lenses acting at once.
Mi'croscopic, Microscop'ical. Pertaining to, or visible only by aid of, the microscope.
Micros'copy. Observation by means of the microscope.
Mi'croseme (mi'kro-sēm). Having the orbital index less than 83.
Microso'mia (mi-kro-so'me-ah). Undersized state of the body.
Microspec'troscope. Spectroscope and microscope combined.
Micros'poron. Genus of fungi producing tinea, sycosis, etc,
Microsto'mia. Undue smallness of the mouth.
Micro'tia (mi-kro'she-ah). Undersize of external ear.
Mi'crotome (mi'kro-tōm). Instrument for making thin slips for microscopic study.
Microt'omy (mi-krot'om-e). The cutting of thin sections.
Mic'rovolt (mik'ro-volt). One-millionth part of a volt.
Mi'crozyme. A microbe which causes fermentation.
Micturi'tion (mik-tu-rish'un). The passage of urine.
Mid'brain. See under *Mesencephalon.*
Mid'gut (mid'gut). Embryonic structure whence the jejunum and ileum are developed.
Mid'riff (mid'rif). The diaphragm.
Mid'wife (mid'wif). A woman who delivers parturient women.
Midwif'ery (mid-wif'er-e). Same as *Obstetrics.*
Migraine (me-grān'). Periodic sick headache, often one-sided.
Mig'ranine. A preparation of antipyrin and caffein.
Migra'tion (mi-gra'shun). Change of place or of seat.
Mi'grosin. Analgesic mixture of menthol and acetic ether.
Mikro-. For words thus beginning, see *Micro-.*
Mik'ulicz's disease. Enlargement of lacrimal and salivary glands, due to replacement of tissue by lymph-cells.

Mil'dew. A parasitic fungus of many species; also a plant-disease caused by it.

Mil'foil. Yarrow. See *Achillea.*

Milia'ria (mil-e-a're-ah). 1. Prickly heat. 2. Miliary fever.

Mil'iary (mil'e-a-re). Like millet-seeds. **M. fever.** See *Fever.*

Mil'ium. A small, white tumor beneath the epidermis.

Milk. The fluid secretion of the mammary gland. **After-m.,** the strippings or last milk taken at any one milking. **Butter-m.,** milk or cream from which the fat has been removed. **Condensed m.,** milk which has been partly evaporated and sweetened with sugar. **M.-crust.** Same as *Crusta lactea.* **M.-cure.** treatment of disease by a milk-diet. **M.-cyst.** a cyst which contains milk; caused by stoppage of a milk-duct. **M.-fever.** See *Fever.* **Fore-m.** 1. The first milk that is taken at any milking. 2. Same as *Colostrum.* **M.-leg.** Same as *Phlegmasia dolens.* **M.-sickness,** poisoning by using contaminated milk. **Skim-m.,** milk after the cream is removed. **M.-spot.** Same as *Strophulus.* **M.-spots,** spots of localized pericarditis. **M.-sugar.** Same as *Lactose.* **M.-teeth,** teeth of the first set. **M.-tumor,** swollen mammary gland with retention of milk.

Milliam'pere. One-thousandth part of an ampere.

Mil'ligram. One-thousandth part of a gram.

Millili'ter. One-thousandth part of a liter.

Mil'limeter. One-thousandth part of a meter.

Mil'lon's reagent. A mixture of mercurous and mercuric nitrates.

Milos'sin. A crystalline substance from the leaves of *Taxus baccata,* or yew-tree.

Mimet'ic, Mim'ic. Marked by simulation of another disease. **M. convulsion,** chronic spasm of facial muscles. **M.-labor,** spurious or false labor.

Min. Abbreviation for *Minim.*

Mind-blindness. Blindness due to brain-lesion. **M.-cure,** pretended cure of disease by mental influence. **M.-deafness,** deafness due to some brain-lesion.

Min'derer's spirit. The solution of ammonium acetate.

Min'eral. A non-organic homogeneous substance. **M. oil.** Same as *Petroleum.* **M. pitch,** a kind of bitumen. **M. water,** water charged with inorganic salts.

Miners' anemia. Same as *Ankylostomiasis.* **Ms'. cachexia, Ms'. elbow,** bursal swelling over olecranon in miners. **Ms'. nystagmus.** See *Nystagmus.* **Ms'. phthisis.** See *Phthisis.*

Min'im. One-sixtieth part of a fluidrachm.

Min'imal dose. The least which will produce a given effect.

Min'imum. Smallest amount or lowest limit.

Min'ium. Lead tetroxid, Pb_3O_4; red lead.

Mi'nor surgery. Bandaging, dressing, catheterization, etc.

Miod'ymus. Fetus with two heads joined at the occiputs.

Mio'pus. Fetal monster with two fused heads, one face being rudimentary.

Mio'sis. Excessive contraction of pupil.

Miot'ic. Causing the pupil to contract.

Miry'achit. A form of palmus with jumping movements and infirm will, endemic in Siberia. See *Palmus* and *Lata.*

Miscar'riage. Abortion; premature expulsion of fetus.

Mis'ce (mis'e). L. for *Mix.*

Missed labor. Cessation of labor-pains and retention of fetus.

Mis'tletoe. A parasitic plant, *Viscum album,* with nervine leaves.

Mistu'ra. L. for *Mixture.*

Mite. A minute insect; an acarus.

Mithrid'atism. Immunity to a poison secured by giving it in increasing doses.

Mit'igated. Rendered more mild or less painful.

Mito'ma, Mi'tome. Thready network of protoplasm.

Mi'tral. Shaped somewhat like a miter. **M. disease,** disease of mitral valve.

Mixed. Affecting various parts at once; showing two or more characteristics.

Mix'ture. A preparation of various ingredients.

Mm. Abbreviation for *Millimeter.*

Mn. Symbol for *Manganese.*

Mnemon'ics. Cultivation of the memory.

Mo'bile spasm. Tonic spasm with irregular movements of the extremities after hemiplegia.

Mobil'ity. Susceptibility of being moved.

Mobiliza'tion. The rendering of a fixed part movable.

Modi'olus (mo-di'ol-us). Central pillar or columella of the cochlea.

Mogigra'phia (mod-je-gra'fe-ah). Writer's cramp.

Mogila'lia (mod-je-la'le-ah). Difficult utterance.

Mogipho'nia. Difficulty in making vocal sounds.

Mogito'cia (mod-je-to'she-ah). Difficult parturition.

Moh'renheim's space (mo'ren-himz). Depression of deltoid muscle and between cephalic artery and vein.

Moist chamber. Form of culture-glass for bacteriological uses. **M. gangrene.** See under *Gangrene.* **M. râle.** See under *Râle.*

Mo'lar. 1. A grinder tooth. 2. Pertaining to a mole or a mass.

Mole. 1. A nævus; also, a brownish spot on the skin. 2. Fleshy mass in the uterus. **Blood-m.,** a mass made up of blood-clots, placenta, and fetal membranes after abortion. **Carneous m., Fleshy m.,** a blood-mole which has assumed a flesh-like appearance; also, a mole formed by a dead ovum in the uterus. **False m.,** mole formed from a polypus or tumor. **Hydatid m.,** a true mole. **Hydatidiform m.,** myxoma formed by cystic generation of villi of chorion. **True m.,** mole from an abortive ovum.

Molec'ular layer. Cortical layer of the cerebral or cerebellar substance. **M. layer, inner,** inner plexiform layer of retina. **M. layer, outer,** outer plexiform layer of retina. **M. lesion,** lesion not visible even by aid of microscope.

Mo'lecule. A very small mass of matter; an aggregation of atoms.

Moli'men (mo-li'men). The monthly effort to establish menstrual flow.

Mol'lin. A soft soap; used as a base for ointments.

Mol'lisin (mol'is-in). Wax and oil preparation; used in ointments.

Molli'ties (mol-lish'e-ēz). Softness; abnormal softening. **M. os'sium.** Same as *Osteomalacia.*

Mollus'cous (mol-lus'kus). Pertaining to molluscum.

Mollus'cum epithelia'le, M. contagio'sum. Disease with rounded skin-tubercles containing a semifluid. **M. fibro'sum, M. sim'plex,** multiple fibroma of the skin.

Molybde'num. A white metallic element; symbol Mo.

Momen'tum. Quantity of motion; product of mass by velocity.

Mo'nad. 1. A single-celled protozoon. 2. A univalent radical or element.

Monar'da puncta'ta. A stimulant and carminative plant; horsemint.

Monartic'ular. Pertaining to one joint.

Monas'ter. The single star-shaped figure in karyokinesis.

Monatheto'sis. Athetosis of one part of the body.

Monatom'ic. Same as *Univalent.*

Moner'ula. Impregnated ovum with as yet no nucleus.

Money-jingle sound. Same as *Cracked-pot sound.*

Monil'iform. Beaded; necklace-shaped.

Monil'ithrix. Infantile disease in which the hair becomes brittle and beaded.
Monks'hood. Same as *Aconite*.
Mono-anesthe'sia. Anesthesia of but one part or organ.
Monoba'sic. Having but one atom of replaceable hydrogen.
Monoblep'sia. Blindness to all colors but one.
Monobra'chius (mon-o-bra'ke-us). Fetus with but one arm.
Monoceph'alus. Monster with two bodies and but one head.
Monochlorphe'nol. Volatile liquid, C_6H_4ClOH, inhaled in lung-disease.
Monochore'a. Chorea affecting but one part.
Monochromat'ic. Having but one color.
Monococ'cus (mon-o-kok'us). A form of coccus consisting of single cells, or of cells neither doubled, grouped, nor in chains.
Monoc'ranus. Monster with one head and double face.
Monoc'ular. Pertaining to or having but one eye.
Monoc'ulus. A bandage for but one eye.
Monogen'esis (mon-o-jen'es-is). Non-sexual reproduction.
Mon'ograph (mon'o-graf). A treatise on but one subject.
Monohy'drated. United with a single molecule of water or of hydroxyl.
Monoloc'ular. Having but one cell or cavity.
Monoma'nia. Insanity on a single subject.
Monom'phalus. Twin fetuses joined at the navel.
Mononu'clear. Having but one nucleus; uninuclear.
Monoparesthe'sia. Paresthesia of a single part or limb.
Monopar'esis. Paresis of a single part.
Monopha'sia. Aphasia with ability to utter but one word or phrase.
Monopho'bia (mon-of-o'be-ah). Morbid dread of solitude.
Monoplasmat'ic. Made up of but one substance.
Mon'oplast. A single constituent cell.
Monople'gia. Paralysis of but a single part.
Mon'ops. A fetus with but a single eye.
Mon'opus. A fetus with but one foot.
Monor'chis. A person having but one testis.
Monoso'mian. Double fetus with only one body.
Mon'ospasm. Spasm of a single part or organ.
Monosymptomat'ic. Having one symptom only.
Monox'id. An oxid with but one oxygen atom.
Monro's foramen. See *Foramen*.
Mons Ven'eris. A rounded prominence in front of the pubes of a woman.
Mon'sel's salt. Basic ferric sulphate (subsulphate or persulphate). **M.'s solution,** a styptic solution of the above.
Mon'ster. Fetus malformed, or with an excess or deficiency of parts.
Monstros'ity. 1. Great congenital deformity. 2. A monster or teratism.
Montgom'ery's glands. Sebaceous glands of mammary areola.
Month'lies, Monthly sickness. The menses.
Montic'ulus cerebel'li. Projecting part of superior vermiform process of cerebellum.
Moon-blind'ness. Amblyopia from sleeping in moonlight.
Mor'al insanity. Insane perversion of the moral sense.
Morand's disease (mor-ōz'). Paresis of the extremities.
Mor'bid. Pertaining to disease; diseased.
Morbid'ity. 1. Condition of being diseased. 2. Proportion of disease to health in a community; sick-rate.
Morbif'ic. Causing or inducing disease.
Morbil'li. L. for *Measles*.
Mor'bus. L. for *Disease*. **M. cadu'cus,** epilepsy. **M. ceru'-**

leus, cyanosis. **M. coxa'rius,** hip-joint disease. **M. mise'-riæ,** any disease due to want and neglect.

Morcella'tion, Morcellement. Act of dividing a tumor or organ and removing it piecemeal.

Mor'dant. A substance used to fix a stain or dye.

Morgagni's caruncle (mor-gahn'yēz). Middle lobe of the prostate gland. **M.'s hydatid.** See under *Hydatid.* **M.'s liquor,** fluid between eye-lens and its capsule. **M.'s sinuses,** three dilatations near commencement of the aorta.

Morgagn'ian cataract (mor-gahn'yan). A fluid cataract with translucent nucleus.

Morgue (morg'). Place where dead bodies are sent for identification.

Mo'ria (mo're-ah). Fatuity or dementia.

Mor'ibund (mor'ib-und). In a dying state.

Mo'rioplasty. Restoration of lost parts by plastic surgery.

Morn'ing sickness. Vomiting and nausea of early pregnancy, occurring chiefly in the morning.

Morphe'a. See *Morphœa.*

Mor'phin. The principal and most active alkaloid of opium.

Mor'phinism, Mor'phism. Morbid state due to misuse of morphin.

Morphinoma'nia, Morphioma'nia. Morbid and habitual crave for morphin.

Mor'phism (mor'fizm). See *Morphinism.*

Morphœ'a. Disease marked by pinkish patches bordered by a purplish areola.

Morphol'ogy (mor-fol'o-je). Science of organic forms and structure.

Morphom'etry. The measurement of forms.

Mor'phon. An individual organism or person.

Morpho'sis. Process of formation; also, a morbid structure.

Morphot'ic. Taking part in, or pertaining to, morphosis.

Mor'rhuin. A ptomain, $C_{19}H_{27}N_3$, from rancid cod-liver oil.

Mor'rhuol. An aromatic, medicinal principle from cod-liver oil.

Mors. L. for *Death.*

Mor'sus diab'oli. Fimbriæ of an oviduct.

Mor'tal. 1. Destined to die. 2. Causing death.

Mortal'ity. Same as *Death-rate.*

Mor'tar. A vessel in which drugs are beaten with a pestle.

Mortifica'tion. Gangrene; a sphacelus; molar death.

Mor'tuary. Pertaining to death.

Mor'ula. The segmented ovum in the mulberry stage.

Mor'ulin. The nucleolus in *Gregarinæ.*

Mor'van's disease. Paresis of the upper or lower extremity with analgesia and trophic lesions.

Mos'chus (mos'kus). L. for *Musk.*

Moth. Same as *Chloasma.*

Moth'er. 1. The female parent. 2. The vinegar-fungus, *Mycoderma aceti.* **M.-liquor,** the liquor which remains after removal of crystals from a solution. **M.-star.** Same as *Monaster.* **M.'s mark.** Same as *Nævus.*

Mo'tile. Having a spontaneous movement.

Motil'ity (mo-til'it-e). The ability to move.

Mo'tor. A muscle, nerve, or center that affects movements; also used adjectively. **M. area,** the ascending frontal and parietal convolutions; Rolandic area. **M. center,** any nerve-center that regulates motions. **M. oc'uli.** See *Nerves, Table of.*

Moto'rial end-plate. See *End-plate.*

Moto'rium. The motor apparatus of the organism.

Moto'rius. Any motor nerve. **M. oc'uli commu'nis.** Same as *Motor oculi.*

Mould (mōld). Any one of a large group of minute parasitic and saprophytic fungi.
Mound'ing. The rising in a lump of a wasting muscle when struck.
Moun'tain fever. 1. A typhoidal fever of mountain regions. 2. See *M. sickness.* **M. sickness,** nausea, vertigo, and headache in climbers of high mountains.
Mount'ing. The preparation of specimens and slides for study.
Mouth. The cavity which contains the tongue and teeth.
Move'ment. An act of moving; motion. **Ameboid m.,** movement of an ameba, or leukocyte, by the protrusion of a pseudopodium. **Angular m.,** movement which increases the angle between two bones. **Associated m.,** movement of parts which act together, as the eyes. **Brownian m.,** dancing motion of minute particles suspended in a liquid. **Ciliary m.,** lashing movement of cilia in some of the tissues. **Circus-m.,** peculiar tumbling movement caused by injuries of the basal ganglia. **Communicated m.,** that produced by a force acting from without. **Fetal m.,** that of a fetus in the womb. **Forced m.,** movement caused by injury to motor centers or conducting paths. **Index m.,** movement of the cephalic part of a body about the fixed caudal part. **Ling m.** Same as *Kinesitherapy.* **Molecular m.** Same as *Brownian m.* **M.-cure.** Same as *Kinesitherapy.* **Rolling m.,** rolling of an animal about its long axis.
Mox'a. Any soft material to be burned upon the skin.
Moxibus'tion. Burning with a moxa.
Moyrapua'ma. Brazilian tree with tonic and aphrodisiac roots.
Muce'din. An amorphous proteid from gluten.
Mu'cic acid. An acid, $C_6H_{10}O_8$, derivable from gums and sugars.
Mucif'erous (mu-sif'er-us). Secreting mucus.
Mu'ciform (mu'sif-orm). Resembling mucus.
Mu'cigen. Substance convertible into mucin and mucus.
Mu'cilage (mu'sil-ej). A slimy paste of gum or dextrin.
Mucilag'inous. Slimy and adhesive.
Mu'cin (mu'sin). The main constituent of mucus.
Mucin'ogen (mu-sin'o-jen). Same as *Mucigen.*
Mu'cinoid (mu'sin-oid). Resembling mucin.
Mucinu'ria. Discharge of mucin in the urine.
Mucip'arous (mu-sip'ar-us). Producing mucin.
Muci'tis. Inflammation of a mucous membrane.
Mu'cocele (mu'ko-sēl). Catarrhal dilatation of lacrimal sac.
Mu'coid (mu'koid). Resembling mucus or jelly.
Mucomem'branous. Composed of mucous membrane.
Mucopu'rulent. Containing mucus and pus.
Mu'copus. Mucus blended with pus.
Mu'cor. A genus of saprophytic mould fungi.
Mu'corin. An albuminous substance from moulds.
Muco'sa. L. for *Mucus;* also mucous membrane.
Mu'cosin. Peculiar mucin of tenacious mucus.
Mucosol'ven. A proprietary diphtheria remedy.
Mu'cous. Pertaining to, or resembling, mucus.
Mucu'na pru'riens. Cowage, a plant with vermifugal spicules.
Mu'cus. The viscid watery secretion of mucous glands.
Mul'berry calculus. See *Calculus.* **M. mark.** Same as *Nævus.* **M. mass.** Same as *Morula.*
Mul'der's test. Indigo-carmin test for glucose.
Mul'lein. Same as *Verbascum.*
Mülle'rian duct, Müller's duct. See *Duct.* **M.'s fluid,** a fluid for hardening microscopic objects. **M.'s muscle.** 1. Circular fibers of ciliary. 2. Inferior and superior palpebral muscles. 3. Muscular layer over the sphenomaxillary fissure. **M.'s ring,**

a ring of muscular fibers at junction of the cervical canal and body of gravid uterus.

Multicap'sular. Having many capsules.

Multicel'lular (mul-tis-el'u-lar). Composed of many cells.

Multicus'pidate. Having numerous cusps.

Mul'tifid (mul'tif-id). Cleft into many parts.

Multigrav'ida. A woman who has often been pregnant.

Multilob'ular (mul-til-ob'u-lar). Having many lobules.

Multiloc'ular. Having many loculi or cells.

Multinu'clear (mul-tin-u'kle-ar). Having many nuclei.

Multip'ara. A woman who has had several children.

Multipar'ity. The condition of being a multipara.

Multip'arous. Having born several children.

Mul'tiple. (For phrases, see the nouns.)

Multipo'lar. Having more than two poles or processes.

Mummifica'tion (mum-if-ik-a'shun). Dry gangrene.

Mumps. Contagious parotiditis.

Mu'ral (mu'ral). Pertaining to a wall.

Murex'id. Ammonium purpurate, $C_8H_8N_6O_6$, a salt from guano: used in testing for uric acid.

Mu'riate. Obsolete synonym for *chlorid.*

Mu'riated (mu're-a-ted). Charged with chlorin.

Muriat'ic acid. Obsolete name of hydrochloric acid.

Mur'mur. A gentle blowing auscultatory sound. **Accidental m.**, one due to some temporary and insignificant circumstance. **Anemic m.**, one due to a watery state of the blood. **Aneurysmal m.**, one due to an aneurysm. **Arterial m.**, one caused by the arterial current. **Blood-m.** Same as *Anemic m.* **Cardiac m.**, any adventitious sound heard over the region of the heart. **Cardiopulmonary m.**, one produced by the impact of the heart against the lung. **Diastolic m.**, one at diastole, from aortic or pulmonary insufficiency. **Direct m.**, murmur produced by obstruction to blood-current. **Duroziez's m.**, double murmur in femoral artery from aortic regurgitation. **Dynamic m.**, one caused by irregular pulsation of the heart. **Endocardial m.**, one produced within the heart-cavities. **Exocardial m.**, a heart-murmur produced outside of the heart's cavities. **Flint's m.**, a peculiar murmur at the apex in aortic regurgitation. **Friction m.**, one due to the rubbing together of two serous surfaces. **Functional m.**, cardiac m. from excited action of heart or from anemia. **Hemic m.**, a sound caused by changes in the amount or quality of blood. **Indirect m.**, one caused by reversal of the direction of blood-current. **Inorganic m.**, murmur not due to valvular lesions. **Mitral m.**, murmur due to diseased mitral valve. **Musical m.**, a cardiac murmur with a musical quality. **Organic m.**, one due to structural change in the heart. **Presystolic m.**, one before systole, from mitral or tricuspid obstruction. **Regurgitant m.**, due to a dilated valvular orifice. **Systolic m.**, one at systole, from aortic, tricuspid, or pulmonary obstruction. **Vesicular m.**, that of normal breathing.

Mur'phy's button. A metallic device used in connecting ends of a divided intestine.

Mur'rain. Any destructive cattle plague.

Mus'cæ volitan'tes. Specks seen as floating before the eyes.

Mus'carin. A deadly alkaloid, $C_5H_{13}NO_2$, from agaric, etc.

Mus'cle. An organ which by contraction produces the movements of an animal organism. [See *Table of the Muscles*, pp. 278-296.] **M.-curve.** Same as *Myogram.* **M.-plasma**, a liquid expressible from muscle-tissue. **M.-plate**, an embryonic muscular segment derived from a protovertebra. **M.-serum**, muscle-plasma deprived of its myosin. **M.-sugar.** Same as *Inosite.*

A TABLE OF THE MUSCLES.

NAME.	ORIGIN.	INSERTION.	INNERVATION.	FUNCTION.
Abduc'tor hallu'cis.	Inner tuberos. of os calcis.	First phalanx of great toe.	Internal plantar.	Abducts great toe.
Abduc'tor lon'gus pol'licis.	Same as *Extensor ossis metacarpi pollicis.*			
Abduc'tor min'imi di'giti.	Pisiform bone.	First phalanx of little finger.	Ulnar.	Abducts little finger.
Abduc'tor min'imi di'giti.	Outer tuberosity of os calcis and plantar fascia.	First phalanx of little toe.	External plantar.	Abducts little toe.
Abduc'tor pol'licis.	Trapezium.	First phalanx of thumb.	Median.	Abducts thumb.
Accelera'tor uri'næ.	Central tendon of perineum and medium raphe.	Bulb, spongy and cavernous part of penis.	Perineal.	Ejects urine.
Adduc'tor bre'vis.	Ramus of pubes.	Upper part of linea aspera of femur.	Obturator.	Adducts and flexes thigh.
Adduc'tor hallu'cis.	Tarsal ends of three middle metatarsals.	Base of first phalanx of great toe.	External plantar.	Adducts great toe.
Adduc'tor lon'gus.	Front of pubes.	Middle of linea aspera of femur.	Obturator.	Adducts and flexes thigh.
Adduc'tor mag'nus.	Rami of pubes and ischium.	Linea aspera of femur.	Obturator and great sciatic.	Adducts thigh and rotates it outward.
Adduc'tor min'imus.	Upper portion of adductor magnus.			
Adduc'tor pol'licis.	Third metacarpal.	First phalanx of thumb.	Ulnar.	Draws thumb to median line.
Ancone'us.	Back of external condyle of humerus.	Olecranon and shaft of ulna.	Musculospiral.	Extends forearm.
Arrecto'res pi'li.	Pars papillaris of skin.	Hair-follicles.	Sympathetic.	Elevate hairs of skin.
Aryte'no-epiglottid'eus infe'rior.	Arytenoid (anteriorly).	Epiglottis.	Recurrent laryngeal.	Compresses saccule of larynx.

Aryte'no-epiglottid'eus superior.	Apex of arytenoid.	Aryteno-epiglottidean folds.	Recurrent laryngeal.	Constricts aperture of larynx.
Arytenoi'deus.	Posterior and outer border of one arytenoid.	Back of other arytenoid.	Superior and recurrent laryngeal.	Closes back part of glottis.
Attol'lens au'rem.	Occipitofrontalis aponeurosis.	Pinna.	Branch cervical plexus.	Elevates pinna.
At'trahens au'rem.	Lateral cranial aponeurosis.	Helix.	Facial.	Advances pinna.
Az'ygos u'vulæ.	Posterior nasal spine of palate bone.	Uvula.	Facial through spheno-palatine ganglion.	Raises uvula.
Bi'ceps (*2 heads*) (hu'meri).	1. Long—Glenoid cavity. 2. Short—Coracoid process.	Tuberosity of radius.	Musculocutaneous.	Flexes and supinates forearm.
Bi'ceps (*2 heads*) (fem'oris).	1. Ischial tuberosity. 2. Linea aspera.	Head of fibula.	Great sciatic.	Flexes and rotates leg outward.
Biven'ter cervi'cis.	Transverse processes, two to four upper dorsal.	Superior curved line of occipital bone.	Portion of complexus.	Retracts and rotates head.
Biven'ter maxil'læ.	Same as *Digastric*.			
Bowman's.	See *Ciliary*.			
Brachia'lis anti'cus.	Lower half of shaft of humerus.	Coronoid process of ulna.	Musculocutaneous, musculospiral.	Flexes forearm.
Brücke's.	See *Ciliary*.			
Buccina'tor.	Alveolar process of maxillary bones and pterygomaxillary ligament.	Orbicularis oris.	Facial.	Compresses cheeks.
Bulbocaverno'sus.	Same as *Accelerator urinæ*.			
Cephalopharyn'geus.	Same as *Constrictor, superior*.			
Ceratoglos'sus.	Portion of hyoglossus attached to great horn of hyoid bone.			

A TABLE OF THE MUSCLES (*continued*).

NAME.	ORIGIN.	INSERTION.	INNERVATION.	FUNCTION.
Cervica′lis ascen′dens.	Angles of five upper ribs.	Transverse processes of fourth, fifth, and sixth cervical.	Branches of cervical.	Keeps neck erect.
Cil′iary.	1. *Longitudinal* part (Brücke's), junction of cornea and sclera. 2. *Circular* part (Müller's), fibers forming a circle.	1. External layers of choroid. 2. Ciliary processes.	Ciliary.	Performs visual accommodation.
Coccy′geus.	Ischial spine.	Coccyx.	Sacral.	Supports coccyx, and closes pelvic outlet.
Complex′us.	Transverse process seventh cervical and three upper dorsal, and articular processes of fourth to sixth cervical.	Occipital bone.	Suboccipital, great occipital, and branches of cervical.	Retracts and rotates head.
Compres′sor na′ris.	Superior maxillary.	Fellow muscle.	Facial.	Dilates nostril.
Compres′sor na′rium mi′nor.	Alar cartilage.	Skin at end of nose.	Facial.	Dilates nostril.
Compres′sor sac′culi laryn′gis.	Aryteno-epiglottideus.		Laryngeal.	Compresses the saccule of the larynx.
Compres′sor ure′thræ.	Ramus of pubes.	Fellow muscle.	Perineal.	Compresses urethra.
Constric′tor (inferior).	Cricoid and thyroid cartilages.	Pharyngeal raphe.	Glossopharyngeal, pharyngeal plexus, and external laryngeal.	Contracts pharyngeal caliber.
Constric′tor (middle).	Cornua of hyoid and stylohyoid ligament.	Pharyngeal raphe.	Glossopharyngeal and pharyngeal plexus.	Contracts pharyngeal caliber.

Constric'tor (superior).	*Internal pterygoid plate*, pterygomax. lig., jaw, and side of tongue.	Pharyngeal raphe.	Glossopharyngeal and pharyngeal plexus.	Contracts pharyngeal caliber.
Coracobrachia'lis.	Coracoid process of scapula.	Inside shaft of humerus.	Musculocutaneous.	Draws arm forward and inward.
Cor'rugator cu'tis a'ni.	Submucous tissue interior of anus.	Subcutaneous tissue on opposite side of anus.	Sympathetic.	Corrugates skin of anus.
Corruga'tor supercil'ii.	Superciliary ridge.	Orbicularis palpebrarum.	Facial.	Draws eyebrow down and in.
Cremas'ter.	Surface of middle of Poupart's ligament.	Pubic boue and fascia propria.	Genital branch of genitocrural.	Raises testicle.
Crico-arytenoi'deus latera'lis.	Side of cricoid.	Angle and external surface of aryteuoid.	Recurrent laryngeal.	Closes glottis.
Crico-arytenoi'deus posti'cus.	Back of cricoid.	Base of arytenoid.	Recurrent laryngeal.	Opens glottis.
Cricothy'roid.	Cricoid cartilage.	Thyroid cartilage (lower inner border).	Superior laryngeal.	Tightens vocal cords.
Crure'us.	See *Vastus internus*.			
Del'toid.	Clavicle, acromion, and spine of scapula.	Shaft of humerus.	Subscapular.	Rotates humerus inward.
Depres'sor a'læ na'si.	Incisive fossa of superior maxillary.	Septum and ala of nose.	Facial.	Contracts uostril.
Depres'sor an'guli o'ris.	External oblique line of inferior maxillary.	Angle of mouth.	Facial.	Depresses angle of mouth.
Depres'sor la'bii inferio'ris.	External oblique line of inferior maxillary.	Lower lip.	Facial.	Depresses lip.
Depres'sor ure'thræ.	Ramus of ischium near deep transversus perinei.	Fibers of constrictor vaginæ.		
Di'aphragm.	Ensiform cartilage, six or seven lower ribs, ligamenta arcuata, bodies of lumbar vertebræ.	Central tendon.	Phrenic.	Respiration and expulsion.

A TABLE OF THE MUSCLES (*continued*).

NAME.	ORIGIN.	INSERTION.	INNERVATION.	FUNCTION.
Digas'tric (anterior belly).	Inner surface inf. maxillary, near symphysis.	Hyoid bone.	Inferior dental.	Elevates hyoid and tongue.
Digas'tric (posterior belly).	Digastric groove of the mastoid process.	Hyoid bone.	Facial.	Elevates hyoid and tongue.
Dila'tor na'ris ante'rior.	Alar cartilage.	Border of ala.	Facial.	Dilates nostril.
Dila'tor na'ris poste'rior.	Nasal notch of the superior maxillary.	Skin at margin of nostril.	Facial.	Dilates nostril.
Dorsal interos'sei, four.	Sides of metacarpal.	Bases of phalanges.	Ulnar.	Abduct fingers from median line.
Dorsal interos'sei.	Sides of metatarsals.	Base of first phalanx of corresponding toe.	External plantar.	Abduct toes.
Erec'tor clito'ridis.	Tuberosity of ischium.	Each side of crus of clitoris.		Erects clitoris.
Erec'tor pe'nis.	Ischial tuberosity, crus penis, and pubic ramus.	Crus penis.	Perineal.	Maintains erection.
Erecto'res pi'li.	Same as *Arrectores pili*.			
Erec'tor spi'næ.	Iliac crest, back of sacrum, lumbar and three lower dorsal spines.	Divides into sacrolumbalis and longissimus dorsi.		
Exten'sor bre'vis digito'rum.	Os calcis, externally.	First phalanx of great toe and tendons of extensor longus.	Anterior tibial.	Extends toes.
Exten'sor car'pi radia'lis bre'vior.	External condyloid ridge of humerus.	Base of third metacarpal.	Posterior interosseous.	Extends wrist.
Exten'sor car'pi radia'lis lon'gior	Lower third of ext. condyloid ridge of humerus.	Base of the second metacarpal.	Musculospiral.	Extends wrist.
Exten'sor car'pi ulna'ris.	Ext. condyle of humerus.	Base of fifth metacarpal.	Posterior interosseous.	Extends wrist.

Exten′sor coc′cygis.	Last bone of sacrum or first of coccyx.	Lower part of coccyx.	Sacral branches.	Extends coccyx.
Exten′sor commu′nis digito′rum.	External condyle of the humerus.	All second and third phalanges.	Posterior interosseous.	Extends fingers.
Exten′sor in′dicis.	Back of the ulna.	Second and third phalanges of index.	Posterior interosseous.	Extends index.
Exten′sor lon′gus digito′rum.	Outer tuberosity of tibia and shaft of fibula.	Second and third phalanges of toes.	Anterior tibial.	Extends toes.
Exten′sor min′imi di′giti.	External condyle of the humerus.	Second and third phalanges of little finger.	Posterior interosseous.	Extends little finger.
Exten′sor os′sis metacar′pi pol′licis.	Back of radius and ulna.	Base of metacarpal of the thumb.	Posterior interosseous.	Extends thumb.
Exten′sor pri′mi interno′dii pol′licis.	Back of the radius.	Base of first phalanx of the thumb.	Posterior interosseous.	Extends thumb.
Exten′sor pro′prius min′imi di′giti.	Lower part of ulna or posterior ligament of wrist-joint.	Base of first phalanx of little finger.		Extends little finger.
Exten′sor pro′prius pol′licis.	Middle of the fibula.	Base of last phalanx of the great toe.	Anterior tibial.	Extends toe.
Exten′sor secun′di interno′dii pol′licis.	Back of the ulna.	Base of last phalanx of the thumb.	Posterior interosseous.	Extends thumb.
Flex′or accesso′rius (*2 heads*).	1. Inner, and, 2. outer surface of os calcis.	Tendon of flexor longus digitorum.	External plantar.	Accessory flexor of toes.
Flex′or bre′vis digito′rum.	Inner tuberosity of os calcis and plantar fascia.	Second phalanges of lesser toes.	Internal plantar.	Flexes lesser toes.
Flex′or bre′vis hallu′cis.	Under surface of cuboid and external cuneiform bones.	First phalanx of great toe.	Internal plantar.	Flexes great toe.
Flex′or bre′vis min′imi di′giti.	Unciform bone.	First phalanx of the little finger.	Ulnar.	Flexes little finger.
Flex′or bre′vis min′imi di′giti.	Base of fifth metatarsal.	Base of first phalanx of the little toe.	External plantar.	Flexes little toe.

A TABLE OF THE MUSCLES (*continued*).

NAME.	ORIGIN.	INSERTION.	INNERVATION.	FUNCTION.
Flex′or bre′vis pol′licis.	Trapezium, trapezoid, os mag., base 3d metacarp.	Base of first phalanx of the thumb.	Median and ulnar.	Flexes thumb.
Flex′or car′pi radia′lis.	Internal condyle.	Metacarpal bone of index.	Median.	Flexes wrist.
Flex′or car′pi ulna′ris (2 *heads*).	1. Internal condyle. 2. Olecranon and ulna.	Fifth metacarpal, annular lig., and pisiform bone.	Ulnar.	Flexes wrist.
Flex′or lon′gus digito′-rum.	Shaft of the tibia.	Last phalanges of toes.	Posterior tibial.	Flexes phalanges and extends toes.
Flex′or lon′gus hallu′cis.	Lower two-thirds of shaft of fibula.	Last phalanx of great toe.	Posterior tibial.	Flexes great toe.
Flex′or lon′gus pol′licis.	Shaft of radius.	Last phalanx of thumb.	Anterior interosseous.	Flexes phalanx.
Flex′or profun′dus digi-to′rum.	Shaft of the ulna.	Last phalanges by four tendons.	Ulnar and anterior interosseous.	Flexes phalanges.
Flex′or subli′mis digito′-rum (*3 heads*).	1. Inner condyle. 2. Coronoid process. 3. Oblique line of radius.	Second phalanges by four tendons.	Median.	Flexes second phalanges.
Gastrocne′mius (*2 heads*).	Condyle of femur.	Os calcis by tendo Achillis.	Internal popliteal.	Extends foot.
Gemel′lus infe′rior.	Tuberosity of ischium.	Great trochanter.	Sacral.	Ext. rotator of thigh.
Gemel′lus supe′rior.	Ischial spine.	Great trochanter.	Sacral.	Ext. rotator of thigh.
Geniohyoglos′sus.	Superior genial tubercle of inferior maxillary.	Hyoid and bottom of tongue.	Hypoglossal.	Retracts and protrudes tongue.
Geniohy′oid.	Inferior genial tubercle of inferior maxillary.	Body of hyoid.	Hypoglossal.	Elevates and advances hyoid.
Glutæ′us max′imus.	Superior curved iliac line and crest, sacrum and coccyx.	Fascia, and femur below great trochanter.	Inferior gluteal and sacral plexus.	Extends, abducts, and rotates thigh outward.
Glutæ′us me′dius.	Ilium between sup. and middle curved lines.	Oblique line of great trochanter.	Superior gluteal.	Rotates, abducts, and advances thigh.

Ilium between middle and int. curved lines.	Great trochanter.	Superior gluteal.	Rotates, abducts, and draws thigh forward.
Rami of pubes and ischium.	Tibia, upper and inner part.	Obturator.	Flexes and abducts leg.
See *Cremaster*.			
Same as *Transversus perinei*.			
Tubercle on helix.	Rim of helix near summit.	Auriculotemporal and posterior auricular.	
Cornua of hyoid.	Side of tongue.	Hypoglossal.	Depresses side of tongue.
Iliac fossa, crest, base of sacrum.	Lesser trochanter.	Anterior crural.	Flexes and rotates femur outward.
Inner surface of ribs.	Inner surface of two or three ribs below.	Intercostal.	Inspiration.
Infraspinous fossa.	Great tuberosity of humerus.	Suprascapular.	Rotates humerus outward.
Outer lip of inferior costal border.	Superior border of ribs above.	Intercostal.	Raise ribs in inspiration.
Inner lip of inferior costal border.	Superior border of ribs below.	Intercostal.	Depress ribs in expiration.
Between spines of contiguous vertebræ.			
Between transverse processes of contiguous vertebræ.			
Spines of six lower dorsal and lumbar and sacral vertebræ, crest of ileum, and three or four lower ribs.	Bicipital groove of humerus.	Subscapular.	Draws arm backward and downward.
Spinous process of sphenoid and tube.	Neck of malleus.	Facial.	Relaxes membrana tympani.
Canine fossa of superior maxillary.	Angle of mouth.	Facial.	Elevates angle of mouth.

A TABLE OF THE MUSCLES (*continued*).

NAME.	ORIGIN.	INSERTION.	INNERVATION.	FUNCTION.
Leva′tor an′guli scap′ulæ.	Transverse processes of four upper cervical vertebræ.	Posterior border of scapula.	Fifth cervical and cervical plexus.	Elevates upper angle of scapula.
Leva′tor a′ni.	Posterior body and ramus of pubes, pelvic fascia, ischial spine.	Rectum, coccyx, and fibrous raphe.	Sacral and perineal.	Supports rectum, vagina, etc.
Leva′tor la′bii inferio′ris.	Incisive fossa of inferior maxillary.	Skin of lower lip.	Facial.	Elevates lower lip.
Leva′tor la′bii superio′ris.	Lower margin of orbit.	Upper lip.	Facial.	Elevates lip.
Leva′tor la′bii superio′ris alæ′que na′si.	Nasal process of superior maxillary.	Alar cartilage and upper lip.	Facial.	Elevates lip, dilates nostril.
Leva′tor men′ti.	Same as *Levator labii inferioris.*			
Leva′tor pala′ti.	Petrous portion of temporal.	Soft palate.	Sphenopalatine ganglia (facial).	Elevates soft palate.
Leva′tor pal′pebræ superio′ris.	Lesser wing of sphenoid.	Upper tarsal cartilage.	Third.	Lifts upper lid.
Levato′res costa′rum, 12.	Transverse processes of last cervical and dorsal vertebræ.	Each one to the rib below it.	Intercostal.	Raise the ribs.
Lingua′lis.	Under surface of tongue.		Chorda tympani.	Elevates center of tongue.
Longis′simus dor′si.	Erector spinæ.	Transverse processes of the lumbar and dorsal vertebræ, 7th to 11th rib.	Branches of lumbar and dorsal.	Erects spine and bends trunk backward.
Lon′gus col′li:				
1. Superior oblique portion.	Transv. processes third to fifth cervical vertebra.	Anterior tubercle of atlas.		

Lon'gus col'li:				
2. Inferior oblique portion.	Bodies of first to third dorsal vertebra.	Transverse processes of fifth and sixth cervical.	Lower cervical.	Flexes cervical vertebræ.
3. Vertical portion.	Bodies of three dorsal and two cervical.	Bodies of second to fourth cervical.		
Lumbrica'les, 4 (of hand).	Tendons of deep flexor.	Tendons of common extensor.	Median and ulnar.	Flex first phalanges.
Lumbrica'les, 4 (of foot).	Teudons of flexor longus.	Second phalanges of lesser toes.	Internal and external plantar.	Accessory flexors.
Masse'ter.	Zygomatic arch.	Angle and ramus of jaw.	Inferior maxillary.	Muscle of mastication, molar teeth.
Multif'idus spi'næ.	Sacrum, iliac spine, artic. proc. lumbar and cervical vertebræ, and transverse proc. of dorsal.	Laminæ and spines of next four vertebræ above.	Posterior spinal branches.	Erects and rotates spinal column.
Mus'culus accesso'rius ad sacrolumba'lem.	Angles of six lower ribs.	Angles of six upper ribs.	Branches of dorsal.	Erects spine and bends trunk backward.
Mylohy'oid.	Mylohyoid ridge of inferior maxillary.	Body of hyoid and raphe.	Inferior dental.	Elevates and advances hyoid. Forms floor of mouth.
Nasolabia'lis.	Nasal septum.	Upper lip.	Facial.	Joins upper lip with septum of nose.
Obli'quus au'ris.	Conch of the ear.	Fossa of antihelix.	Temporal and posterior auricular.	
Obli'quus cap'itis infe'rior.	Spinous process of atlas.	Transverse process of atlas.	Suboccipital and great occipital.	Rotates atlas and cranium.
Obli'quus cap'itis supe'rior.	Transverse process of atlas.	Occipital bone.	Suboccipital and great occipital.	Draws head backward.
Obli'quus exter'nus.	Eight lower ribs.	Middle line, iliac crest, Poupart's ligament.	Intercostal, iliohypogastric, ilio-inguinal.	Compresses viscera and flexes thorax.
Obli'quus infe'rior.	Orbital plate of superior maxillary.	Sclerotic.	Third.	Rotates eyeball up and out.

A TABLE OF THE MUSCLES (*continued*).

NAME.	ORIGIN.	INSERTION.	INNERVATION.	FUNCTION.
Obli′quus inter′nus.	Lumbar fascia, iliac crest, Poupart's ligament.	Four lower ribs, linea alba, pubic crest, pectineal line.	Intercostal, iliohypogastric, ilio-inguinal.	Compresses viscera and flexes thorax.
Obli′quus supe′rior.	Above optic foramen, through pulley.	Sclerotic.	Fourth.	Rotates eyeball down and out.
Ob′turator exter′nus.	Obturator foramen and membrane.	Digital fossa, base of great trochanter.	Obturator.	External rotator of thigh.
Ob′turator inter′nus.	Obturator foramen and membrane.	Great trochanter.	Sacral.	External rotator of thigh.
Occipita′lis.	See *Occipitofrontalis*.			
Occipitofronta′lis.	Superior curved line of occiput and angular process of frontal.	Aponeurosis.	Posterior auricular, small occipital, facial.	Moves scalp. Facial expression.
Omohy′oid.	Upper border of scapula.	Body of hyoid.	Descendens and communicans noni.	Depresses and retracts hyoid.
Oppo′nens min′imi di′giti.	Unciform bone.	Fifth metacarpal.	Ulnar.	Flexes little finger.
Oppo′nens pol′licis.	Trapezium.	Metacarpal of thumb.	Median.	Flexes thumb.
Orbicula′ris o′ris.	Nasal septum and canine fossa of inferior maxillary, by accessory fibers.	Forms lips and sphincter of mouth.	Facial.	Closes mouth.
Orbicula′ris palpebra′rum.	Internal margin of orbit.	Outer margin of orbit.	Facial.	Closes eyelids.
Palatoglos′sus.	Soft palate.	Side and dorsum of tongue.	Sphenopalatine ganglion.	Constricts fauces.
Palatopharyn′geus.	Soft palate.	Thyroid cartilage and pharynx.	Sphenopalatine ganglion.	Closes posterior nares.

Palma'res interos'sei.	Palmar surfaces, second, fourth, and fifth metacarpals.	Bases of first phalanges of corresponding fingers.	Ulnar.	Adductors of fingers.
Palma'ris bre'vis.	Annular ligament and palmar fascia.	Skin of palm of hand.	Ulnar.	Corrugates skin of palm.
Palma'ris lon'gus.	Internal condyle.	Annular ligament and palmar fascia.	Median.	Tightens fascia.
Pectine'us.	Iliopectineal line and pubes.	Femur below lesser trochauter.	Anterior crural, obturator.	Flexes thigh and rotates it outward.
Pectora'lis ma'jor.	Clavicle, sternum, and costal cartilages.	External bicipital ridge of humerus.	Anterior thoracic.	Draws arm down and forward.
Pectora'lis mi'nor.	Third, fourth, and fifth ribs.	Coracoid process.	Anterior thoracic.	Depresses point of shoulder.
Perone'us bre'vis.	Middle third of shaft of fibula, externally.	Base of fifth metatarsal.	Musculocutaneous.	Extends foot.
Perone'us lon'gus.	Head and shaft of fibula.	First metatarsal of great toe.	Musculocutaneous.	Extends and everts foot.
Perone'us ter'tius.	Lower fourth of fibula.	Fifth metatarsal bone.	Anterior tibial.	Flexes tarsus.
Planta'res interos'sei.	Shafts of third, fourth, and fifth metatarsals.	Base of first phalanges of same.	External plantar.	Adducts toes.
Planta'ris.	Outer bifurcation of linea aspera and posterior ligament of knee.	Os calcis by tendo Achillis.	Internal popliteal.	Extends foot.
Platys'ma myoi'des.	Clavicle, acromion, and fascia.	Inferior maxillary, angle of mouth, etc.	Facial and superficial cervical.	Wrinkles skin and depresses mouth.
Poplite'us.	External condyle of femur.	Shaft of tibia above oblique line.	Internal popliteal.	Flexes leg.
Prona'tor quadra'tus.	Lower fourth of ulna.	Lower fourth of shaft of radius.	Anterior interosseous.	Pronates hand.
Prona'tor ra'dii te'res.	Internal condyle and coronoid process.	Outer side of shaft of radius.	Median.	Pronates hand.

A TABLE OF THE MUSCLES (*continued*).

NAME.	ORIGIN.	INSERTION.	INNERVATION.	FUNCTION.
Pso′as mag′nus.	Bodies and trans. processes of last dorsal and all lumbar vertebræ.	Lesser trochanter.	Lumbar.	Flexes and rotates thigh outward, and flexes trunk on pelvis.
Pso′as par′vus.	Bodies of last dorsal and first lumbar vertebræ.	Iliopectineal eminence and iliac fascia.	Lumbar.	Tensor of iliac fascia.
Pter′ygoid (external).	1. Ext. pterygoid plate of sphenoid. 2. Great wing.	Neck of condyle.	Inferior maxillary.	Draws inferior maxillary forward.
Pter′ygoid (internal).	Pterygoid fossa of sphenoid.	Inner surface of angle of jaw.	Inferior maxillary.	Raises and draws inferior maxillary forward.
Pyramida′lis.	Pubes.	Linea alba.	Iliohypogastric.	Tightens linea alba.
Pyramida′lis na′si.	Occipitofrontalis.	Compressor naris.	Facial.	Depresses eyebrow.
Pyrifor′mis.	Front of sacrum, through great sciatic foramen.	Great trochanter.	Sacral.	External rotator of thigh.
Quadra′tus fem′oris.	Tuberosity of ischium.	Quadrate line of femur.	Sacral.	External rotator of thigh.
Quadra′tus lumbo′rum.	Crest of ilium, transverse processes of lower three lumbar vertebræ.	Last rib, transverse processes of last three lumbar vertebræ.	Lumbar.	Flexes thorax laterally.
Quad′riceps exten′sor fem′oris.	Includes the rectus, vastus int. and ext., and crureus muscles. Common tendon contains the patella.			
Rec′tus abdom′inis.	Pubic crest.	Cartilages of fifth to seventh rib.	Intercostal, iliohypogastric, ilio-inguinal.	Compresses viscera and flexes thorax.
Rec′tus cap′itis anti′cus ma′jor.	Transverse processes of third to sixth cervical.	Basilar process.	Cervical plexus.	Flexes head.
Rec′tus cap′itis anti′cus mi′nor.	Transverse process and lateral mass of atlas.	Basilar process.	Cervical plexus.	Flexes head.
Rec′tus cap′itis latera′lis.	Transverse process of atlas.	Jugular process.	Cervical plexus.	Draws head laterally.

Rec'tus cap'itis posti'cus ma'jor.	*Spine of axis.*	*Inferior curved line of occipital bone.*	*Suboccipital and great occipital.*	*Rotates head.*
Rec'tus cap'itis posti'cus mi'nor.	Posterior arch of atlas.	Below inferior curved line of occipital bone.	Suboccipital and great occipital.	Draws head backward.
Rec'tus exter'nus.	Two heads, outer margin of optic foramen.	Sclerotic coat of eyeball.	Sixth.	Rotates eyeball outward.
Rec'tus fem'oris.	Anterior inferior iliac spine, brim acetabulum.	Tuberosity of tibia.	Anterior crural.	Extends leg.
Rec'tus infe'rior.	Lower margin of optic foramen.	Sclerotic coat of eyeball.	Third.	Rotates eyeball downward.
Rec'tus inter'nus.	Inner margin of optic foramen.	Sclerotic coat of eyeball.	Third.	Rotates eyeball inward.
Rec'tus supe'rior.	Upper margin of optic foramen.	Sclerotic coat of eyeball.	Third.	Rotates eyeball upward.
Ret'rahens au'rem.	Mastoid process.	Concha.	Posterior auricular.	Retracts pinna.
Rhombol'deus ma'jor.	Spines of five upper dorsal.	Root of spine of scapula.	Fifth cervical.	Elevates and retracts scapula.
Rhombol'deus mi'nor.	Spines of seventh cervical and first dorsal.	Root of spine of scapula.	Fifth cervical.	Retracts and elevates scapula.
Riso'rius.	Fascia over masseter.	Angle of mouth.	Facial.	Draws out angle.
Rotato'res spi'næ.	Transverse processes of second to twelfth dorsal.	Lamina of next dorsal above.	Dorsal branches.	Rotate spinal column.
Sacrolumba'lis.	Erector spinæ.	Angles of six lower ribs.	Branches of dorsal.	Erects spine and bends trunk backward.
Sarto'rius.	Ant. sup. spine of ilium.	Upper int. shaft of tibia.	Anterior crural.	Flexes and crosses legs.
Scale'nus anti'cus.	Tubercle on first rib.	Transverse processes of third to sixth cervical.	Lower cervical.	Flexes neck laterally.
Scale'nus me'dius.	First rib.	Transverse processes of six lower cervical.	Lower cervical.	Flexes neck laterally.
Scale'nus posti'cus.	Second rib.	Transverse processes of three lower cervical.	Lower cervical.	Bends neck laterally.

A TABLE OF THE MUSCLES (*continued*).

NAME.	ORIGIN.	INSERTION.	INNERVATION.	FUNCTION.
Semimembrano′sus.	Tuberosity of ischium.	Inner tuberosity of tibia.	Great sciatic.	Flexes leg and rotates it inward.
Semispina′lis col′li.	Transverse processes of four upper dorsal and articular processes of four lower cervical.	Spines of second to fifth cervical.	Cervical branches.	Erects spinal column.
Semispina′lis dor′si.	Transverse process of lower dorsal.	Spines of last two cervical and four upper dorsal.	Branches of dorsal.	Erects spinal column.
Semitendino′sus.	Tuberosity of ischium.	Upper and inner surface of tibia.	Great sciatic.	Flexes leg on thigh.
Serra′tus mag′nus.	Eight upper ribs.	Inner margin of posterior border of scapula.	Posterior thoracic.	Elevates ribs in inspiration.
Serra′tus posti′cus infe′rior.	Spines of last two dorsal and first three lumbar.	Four lower ribs.	Posterior branches of dorsal.	Depresses ribs in expiration.
Serra′tus posti′cus supe′rior.	Spines of seventh cervical and two upper dorsal.	Second, third, fourth, and fifth ribs.	Posterior branches of cervical.	Raises ribs in inspiration.
So′leus.	Shaft of fibula, oblique line of tibia.	Os calcis by tendo Achillis.	Internal popliteal.	Extends foot.
Sphinc′ter a′ni, external.	Tip of coccyx.	Tendinous center of perineum.	Hemorrhoidal.	Closes anus.
Sphinc′ter a′ni, internal.	Thickening of circular fibers of intestine above anus.		Hemorrhoidal nerves.	Constricts rectum.
Sphinc′ter vagi′næ.	Central tendon of perineum.	Corpora cavernosa and clitoris.	Homologue of accelerator urinæ in male.	
Spina′lis col′li.	Spines of fifth and sixth cervical.	Into spine of axis, or third and fourth cervical spines.	Cervical branches.	Steadies neck.

Spina'lis dor'si.	Last two dorsal and first two lumbar spines.	Remaining dorsal spines.	Dorsal branches.	Erects spinal column.
Sple'nius cap'itis et col'li.	Half of ligamentum nuchæ and spines of six upper dorsal.	Into occiput and mastoid, also trans. processes of fourth upper cervical.	Posterior branches of cervical.	Retracts head and keeps neck erect.
Stape'dius.	Interior of pyramid.	Neck of stapes.	Facial.	Depresses base of stapes.
Sternocleidomas'toid.	Two heads, sternum and clavicle.	Mastoid process.	Spinal accessory and cervical plexus.	Depresses and rotates head.
Sternohy'oid.	Sternum and clavicle.	Hyoid bone.	Descending and communicating branches of hypoglossal.	Depresses hyoid.
Sternothy'roid.	Sternum and cartilage of first rib.	Side of thyroid cartilage.	Hypoglossal.	Depresses larynx.
Styloglos'sus.	Styloid process.	Side of tongue.	Hypoglossal.	Elevates and retracts tongue.
Stylohy'oid.	Styloid process.	Body of hyoid.	Facial.	Draws hyoid up and back.
Stylopharyn'geus.	Styloid process.	Thyroid cartilage.	Glossopharyngeal and pharyngeal plexus.	Elevates pharynx.
Subancone'us.	Humerus above olecranon fossa.	Posterior ligament of elbow.	Musculospiral.	Tensor of ligament.
Subcla'vius.	Cartilage of first rib.	Under surface of clavicle.	Fifth and sixth cervical.	Draws clavicle downward.
Subcrure'us.	Anterior inferior part of femur.	Synovial sac behind patella.	Anterior crural.	Draws sac up.
Subscap'ularis.	Subscapular fossa.	Lesser tuberosity of humerus.	Subscapular.	Rotates head of humerus inward.
Su'pinator bre'vis.	Ext. condyle of humerus, oblique line of ulna.	Neck of radius and its bicipital tuberosity.	Posterior interosseous.	Supinates hand.
Su'pinator lon'gus.	External condyloid ridge of humerus.	Styloid process of radius.	Musculospiral.	Supinates hand.
Supraspina'les.	Lie on spinous processes in cervical region.			

A TABLE OF THE MUSCLES (*continued*).

NAME.	ORIGIN.	INSERTION.	INNERVATION.	FUNCTION.
Supraspina'tus.	Supraspinous fossa.	Great tuberosity of humerus.	Suprascapular.	Supports shoulder-joint, raises arm.
Tem'poral.	Temporal fossa and fascia.	Coronoid process of inferior maxillary.	Inferior maxillary.	Brings incisor teeth together.
Ten'sor pala'ti.	Scaphoid fossa of sphenoid.	About hamular process into soft palate.	Otic ganglia.	Renders palate tense.
Ten'sor tar'si.	Lacrimal bone.	Tarsal cartilages.	Facial.	Compresses puncta and lacrimal sac.
Ten'sor tym'pani.	Temporal bone, Eustachian tube and canal.	Handle of malleus.	Otic ganglia.	Renders tense membrana tympani.
Ten'sor vagi'næ fem'oris.	Iliac crest and anterior superior spinous process.	Fascia lata.	Superior gluteal.	Tensor of fascia.
Te'res ma'jor.	Inferior angle of scapula.	Internal bicipital ridge of humerus.	Subscapular.	Draws arm down and back.
Te'res mi'nor.	Axillary border of scapula.	Great tuberosity of humerus.	Circumflex.	Rotates humerus outward.
Thyro-arytenoid'eus.	Thyroid and cricothyroid membrane.	Arytenoid, inferior and anterior surface.	Recurrent laryngeal.	Rotates vocal cords.
Thyro-epiglottid'eus.	Inner surface of thyroid.	Epiglottis.	Recurrent laryngeal.	Depresses epiglottis.
Thyrohy'oid.	Side of thyroid cartilage.	Body and greater cornu of hyoid.	Hypoglossal.	Elevates larynx.
Tibia'lis anti'cus.	Outer tuberosity and upper part of shaft of tibia.	Internal cuneiform and first metatarsal.	Anterior tibial.	Flexes tarsus and elevates inner border of foot.
Tibia'lis posti'cus.	Shaft of fibula and tibia.	Tuberosity scaphoid and internal cuneiform.	Posterior tibial.	Extends tarsus and inverts foot.

Tibio-accesso′rius.	See *Flexor accessorius longus digitorum.*			
Trachea′lis.	A layer of unstriped muscular fibers at dorsal part of trachea.		Sympathetic.	
Trachelomas′toid.	Transverse process of third to sixth dorsal, and articular process of three or four lower cervical.	Mastoid process.	Branches of cervical.	Steadies head.
Tra′gicus.	Tragus.	Tragus.	Temporal and posterior auricular.	
Transversa′lis.	Poupart's ligament, iliac crest, six lower ribs, lumbar vertebræ.	Linea alba, pubic crest, pectineal line.	Intercostal, iliohypogastric, ilio-inguinal.	Compresses viscera and flexes thorax.
Transversa′lis col′li.	Transverse processes of third to sixth dorsal.	Transverse processes of five lower cervical.	Cervical branches.	Keeps neck erect.
Transver′sus au′ris.	Convexity of concha.	Convexity over groove of helix.	Temporal and posterior auricular.	Retracts helix.
Transver′sus pe′dis.	Head of fifth metatarsal.	First phalanx of the great toe.	External plantar.	Adducts great toe.
Transver′sus perinæ′i.	Ramus of ischium.	Central tendon.	Perineal.	Tensor of the central tendon.
Trape′zius.	Superior curved line of occipital, spinous processes of last cervical and all dorsal vertebræ.	Clavicle and spine of scapula, and acromion.	Spinal accessory and cervical plexus.	Draws head backward.
Triangula′ris men′ti.	Same as *Depressor anguli oris.*			
Triangula′ris ster′ni.	Ensiform cartilage, costal cartilage of three or four lower ribs and sternum.	Edge of inner surfaces of second, third, fourth, and fifth costal cartilages.	Intercostal.	Expiration.

A TABLE OF THE MUSCLES (*continued*).

NAME.	ORIGIN.	INSERTION.	INNERVATION.	FUNCTION.
Tri′ceps (*3 heads*).	External and internal heads near musculospiral groove, shaft of humerus. Middle or long head, lower edge of glenoid cavity.	Olecranon process of ulna.	Musculospiral.	Extends forearm.
Trochlea′ris.	See *Obliquus superior*.			
Ulna′ris.	Lower fourth of anterior surface of ulnar.	Unciform bone.	Ulnar.	Flexes wrist.
Ulna′ris gra′cilis.	Same as *Palmaris longus*.			
Uvula′ris.	See *Azygos uvulæ*.			
Vas′tus exter′nus.	Anterior edge of great trochanter and linea aspera.	Tuberosity of tibia.	Anterior crural.	Extends leg.
Vas′tus inter′nus and crure′us.	Inner lip of linea aspera.	Tuberosity of tibia.	Anterior crural.	Extends leg.
Vesicopu′bic.	Urachus.	Back of pubic bones.	Sympathetic.	Compresses vesical wall.
Wil′son's.	A part of the compressor urethræ.			
Zygomat′icus ma′jor et mi′nor.	Malar bone.	Angle of mouth.	Facial.	Elevates lip outward.
Zygomato-auricula′ris.	Same as *Attrahens aurem*.			

Mus'cular. Of, or pertaining to, a muscle.

Muscula'ris muco'sæ. A layer of non-striated muscular fibers in a mucous membrane.

Muscula'tion. The muscular system or apparatus.

Mus'culature. The muscles collectively of a part of the body.

Mus'culi papil'lares. Name for some of the columnæ carneæ of the heart-ventricles. **M. pectina'ti,** muscular columns within the heart-auricles.

Mus'culin. Therapeutic extract of muscle-tissue.

Musculocuta'neous. See *Nerves, Table of.*

Musculomem'branous. Pertaining to muscle and membrane.

Musculospi'ral (mus-ku-lo-spi'ral). See *Nerves, Table of.*

Mus'culus (mus'ku-lus). L. for *Muscle.*

Musicoma'nia. Insane fondness for music.

Musicother'apy. Treatment of disease by music.

Mu'sin. A proprietary cathartic from tamarinds.

Musk. Dried secretion of male musk deer: fragrant, restorative, and stimulant.

Mussita'tion. Movement of lips with no utterance of sounds.

Must. Unfermented juice of grapes.

Mu'tacism. Improper pronunciation of sounds of mute letters.

Mute. 1. Unable to speak. 2. One who cannot speak.

Mu'tism. Dumbness; inability to speak.

My. Abbreviation for *Myopia.*

Myal'gia (mi-al'je-ah). Muscular pain.

Myasthe'nia (mi-as-the'ne-ah). Muscular debility.

Myce'lium (mi-se'le-um). The filamentary part of a fungus.

Myceto'ma. Tumor caused by a parasitic plant-growth; Madura foot, or fungus-foot.

Mycoder'ma. Genus of fungi. **M. ace'ti,** mother of vinegar.

Mycodes'moid. A colony of *Micrococcus ascoformans* in horses' lungs.

Mycofibro'ma. Same as *Mycodesmoid.*

Mycohe'mia, Mycohæ'mia. The presence of fungi or microbes in the blood.

Mycolo'gy. The study of fungi.

Mycomyringi'tis. Fungous inflammation of drum-membrane.

Mycophylax'in. Any phylaxin that destroys microbes.

Mycopro'tein. A proteid, $C_{25}H_{42}N_6O_9$, from bacteria of putrefaction.

Myco'sis. Any disease caused by microbes. **M. favo'sa.** Same as *Favus.* **M. fungoi'des,** a very fatal disease, with fungous tumors, cachexia, and much pain.

Mycoso'zin. Any sozin that destroys microbes.

Myda'lein. A poisonous ptomain from putrefied viscera.

Mydatox'in. Deadly ptomain, $C_6H_{13}NO_2$, from decaying flesh.

My'din. A ptomain, $C_9H_{11}NO_2$, from dead bodies: not poisonous.

Mydri'asis (mid-ri'as-is). Great dilatation of the pupil.

Mydriat'ic. 1. Dilating the pupil. 2. A drug that dilates the pupil.

Myd'rin. Mydriatic compound of ephedrin and homatropin.

My'drol. A non-toxic, mydriatic phenol compound.

Myecto'pia. Displacement of a muscle.

Myelal'gia (mi-el-al'je-ah). Pain in the spinal cord.

Myelap'oplexy. Hemorrhage in the spinal cord.

Myelat'rophy (mi-el-at'rof-e). Atrophy of the myelon.

Myelenceph'alon. After-brain; after part of posterior cerebral vesicle of embryo.

My'elin. 1. Same as *Medullary sheath.* 2. Any one of a certain group of principles from nerve-substance.

Myelin'ic. Of, or pertaining to, myelin.

Myeli'tis. Inflammation of spinal cord or of bone-marrow.

Acute m., simple m. due to exposure, disease, or injury. See *Poliomyelitis, Leukomyelitis, Osteomyelitis.* **Ascending m.**, that which moves cephalad along the cord. **Bulbar m.**, that which involves the oblongata. **Cavitary m.** is accompanied by formation of cavities. **Central m.** affects chiefly the gray substance of the cord. **Chronic m.**, a slowly progressing form. **Compression m.**, a form due to pressure on the cord, as of a tumor. **Concussion m.** is caused by spinal concussion. **Cornual m.**, that which chiefly affects the cornua. **Descending m.**, a form which progresses caudad along the cord. **Diffuse m.** involves large and variously placed sections of the cord. **Disseminated m.**, that which has several distinct foci. **Focal m.**, one which affects a small area. **Hemorrhagic m.**, that which is associated with hemorrhage. **Parenchymatous m.** attacks mainly the proper nerve-substance. **Sclerotic m.**, that which is marked by hardening of the cord and overgrowth of interstitial tissue. **Systemic m.**, a variety which affects distinct tracts or systems in the cord. **Transverse m.**, that which extends across the cord. **Traumatic m.**, that which follows direct injury of the cord.

My'elocele, Myelocœ'le. Central canal of myelon.

My'elocele (mi'el-os-ēl). Hernial protrusion of spinal cord.

Myelocys'tocele. Cystic tumor of the myelon.

Myelocystomenin'gocele. Myelocystocele blended with meningocele.

My'elocyte. 1. Any marrow-cell. 2. Any cell of the gray matter of nervous system.

Myelogen'ic, Myelog'enous. Produced in bone-marrow.

My'eloid. Resembling marrow. **M. cell.** Same as *Myeloplax.*

Myelo'ma. 1. Any medullary tumor. 2. Giant-celled sarcoma.

Myelomala'cia. Morbid softening of spinal cord.

Myelomeningi'tis. Inflammation of spinal cord and meninges.

Myelomenin'gocele. Same as *Spina bifida.*

Myelomy'ces. Same as *Encephaloma.*

My'elon (mi'el-on). The spinal cord.

Myelop'athy (mi-el-op'ath-e). Any disease of spinal cord.

My'eloplast. Any leukocyte of the bone-marrow.

My'eloplax. Any multinuclear giant-cell of bone-marrow.

Myelosclero'sis. Sclerosis of the myelon.

Myelo'sis. Formation of a tumor of the medulla.

Myelospon'gium. A network developing into the neuroglia.

Myi'asis (mi-i'as-is). Any disease due to maggots of flies.

Myiodeop'sia. The seeing of muscæ volitantes.

Myi'tis (mi-i'tis). Inflammation of muscle.

Myko-. For words thus beginning, see under *Myco-.*

Mylohy'oid. Pertaining to the hyoid bone and to molar teeth. **M. muscle, M. mylohyoideus.** See *Muscles, Table of.*

Myoal'bumose. A proteid from muscle-juice.

My'oblast. An embryonic cell which becomes a cell of muscle-fiber.

Myocardi'tis. Inflammation of the myocardium.

Myocard'ium. The muscular substance of the heart.

Myocelluli'tis. Myositis conjoined with cellulitis.

My'ochrome (mi'ok-rōm). Same as *Myohematin.*

Myochron'oscope. Device for measuring time required for a motor impulse to become effective.

Myoc'lonus. Same as *Paramyoclonus.*

Myocom'ma. The septum which separates the myotomes.

Myoc'tonin. A poisonous principle from aconite.

My'ocyte (mi'o-sit). A cell of muscular tissue.

Myodesop'sia (mi-o-des-op'se-ah). See *Myiodeopsia.*

Myodynamom'eter. Device for testing power of muscles.

Myodyn'ia. Pains in a muscle; myalgia.
Myo-ede'ma. 1. Same as *Mounding*. 2. Edema of a muscle.
Myofibro'ma. Myoma combined with fibroma.
Myoglob'ulin. A globulin from muscle-juice.
My'ogram (mi'o-gram). The record made by a myograph.
My'ograph. Apparatus for recording effects of muscular contraction.
Myograph'ic tracing. A myogram.
Myog'raphy. 1. The use of a myograph. 2. Description of muscles.
Myohem'atin (mi-o-hem'at-in). Same as *Histohematin*.
My'oid (mi'oid). Resembling, or like, a muscle.
Myoide'ma (mi-oi-de'mah). Same as *Mounding*.
Myolem'ma (mi-o-lem'ah). The sarcolemma.
My'olin. The supposed material of muscular fibrils.
Myolipo'ma. Myoma with fatty elements.
Myol'ogy. Sum of knowledge regarding muscles.
Myo'ma. Any tumor formed of muscular tissue. **M. telangiecto'des,** tumor made up of a coil of blood-vessels in a network of muscular fibers.
Myomala'cia. Morbid softening of a muscle.
Myom'atous. Of, or pertaining to, myoma.
Myomec'tomy. Surgical removal of a myoma.
My'omere (mi'om-ēr). A protovertebra, or embryonic muscular segment.
Myometri'tis. Inflammation of muscular substance of the uterus.
Myome'trium. The muscular substance of the uterus.
Myomohysterec'tomy. Hysterectomy for myoma of uterus.
Myomot'omy (mi-o-mot'o-me). Same as *Myomectomy*.
Myoneural'gia. Neuralgic pain in a muscle.
My'oneure (mi'on-ūr). A nerve-cell which supplies a muscle.
Myoparal'ysis. Paralysis of a muscle.
Myopath'ic (mi-op-ath'ik). Of the nature of a myopathy.
Myop'athy (mi-op'ath-e). Any disease of a muscle.
My'ope (mi'ōp). A near-sighted person; one affected with myopia.
Myopericardi'tis. Myocarditis blended with pericarditis.
My'ophone. A device which renders audible the sound of muscular contraction.
My'opia (mi-o'pe-ah). Near-sightedness; short-sight.
Myop'ic (mi-op'ik). Affected with myopia. **M. crescent,** posterior staphyloma with myopia.
Myorrhex'is (mi-o-rek'sis). Rupture of a muscle.
Myosarco'ma. Myoma blended with sarcoma.
Myo'seism (mi'o-sizm). Jerky, irregular muscular contractions.
My'osin. A proteid from muscle-juice, etc.
Myosin'ogen. A muscle-proteid from which myosin is formed.
Myos'inose (mi-os'in-ōs). An albumose produced by the digestion of myosin.
Myo'sis (mi-o'sis). Same as *Miosis*.
Myosi'tis. Inflammation of a muscle. **Interstitial m.,** inflammation of connective and septal muscular tissue. **M. ossif'icans,** that which is marked by bony deposits. **Parenchymatous m.,** that which affects the essential substance of a muscle. **Specific m., Syphilitic m.,** that which is due to syphilis. **Trichinous m.,** that which is caused by presence of trichina.
My'ospasm (mi'o-spazm). Spasm of a muscle.
My'osuture (mi'o-su-cher). The suturation of a muscle.
Myotat'ic. Performed by stretching a muscle.
Myotenot'omy. Surgical division of muscles and tendons.
Myot'ic (mi-ot'ik). See under *Miotic*.

My'otome (mi'ot-ōm). 1. Instrument for dividing muscles. 2. Same as *Myomere*.
Myot'omy (mi-ot'o-me). The cutting or dissection of muscle.
Myoto'nia (mi-ot-o'ne-ah). Tension or spasm of a muscle. **M. congen'ita.** Same as *Thomsen's disease*.
Myr'cia ac'ris. Shrub producing oil of bay and bay rum.
Myr'icin. 1. A crystalline principle from beeswax. 2. A medicinal precipitate derived from *Myri'ca cerif'era* or wax-myrtle.
Myringi'tis. Inflammation of the membrana tympani.
Myringodec'tomy. Removal of the membrana tympani.
Myringodermati'tis. Inflammation of outer layer of drum-membrane with formation of blebs.
Myringomyco'sis. Disease of membrana tympani caused by growth of fungi.
Myrin'goplasty. Surgical restoration of membrana tympani.
Myrin'gotome. Knife for performing myringotomy.
Myringot'omy. Incision of the membrana tympani.
Myrist'ic acid. Crystalline acid, $C_{14}H_{28}O_2$, from nutmeg butter, spermaceti, etc.
Myris'tica fra'grans. The tree that produces nutmeg.
Myro'sin. A proteid ferment from mustard seed.
Myrrh (mur). A gum-resin from *Commiphora myrrha:* astringent and stimulant.
Myr'rholin. Preparation of castor oil and myrrh.
Myr'tiform. Myrtle-shaped. **M. caruncles.** See *Carunculæ myrtiformes*.
Myr'tol. An antiseptic oil from myrtle; stimulant.
Mysopho'bia. Insane dread of contamination and filth.
My'tacism (mi'tas-izm). Too free use of *m*-sound in speaking.
Mytilotox'in. A poisonous leukomain, $C_6H_{15}NO_2$, from mussels.
Myxede'ma, Myxœde'ma. General swelling, especially of face and hands, from presence of a mucous fluid in subcutaneous tissues.
Myxochondro'ma. Myxoma blended with chondroma.
Myxofibro'ma. Myxoma blended with fibroma.
Myxoidede'ma. Influenza of a severe type.
Myxo-ino'ma. Myxoma blended with inoma.
Myxolipo'ma. Myxoma blended with lipoma.
Myxo'ma (mik-so'mah). A mucous tumor.
Myxomyce'tes. A group of fungoid organisms.
Myxoneuro'ma. Myxoma blended with neuroma.
Myxosarco'ma. Sarcoma blended with mucous tissue.

N.

N. Symbol of *Nitrogen*.
Na. Symbol of *Sodium*.
Nabo'thian follicles, N. glands. Distended mucous glands within the cervix and about the os uteri.
Naegle's pelvis. Distorted pelvis from arrest of development and fusion of sacrum with ilium.
Næ'void, Næ'vus, etc. See *Nevoid, Nevus*, etc.
Nail. Horny dorsal plate on the last phalanx of a finger or toe. **N.-bed,** the surface covered by a nail. **N.-culture,** a form of bacterial culture in which the growing colony becomes nail-shaped. **N.-fold,** a fold of connective tissue which embraces the base and sides of a nail. **Hang-n.,** an agnail; shred of epidermis at side of nail. **Ingrowing n.,** an overlapping of a nail by the flesh. **N.-matrix,** proximal end of n.-bed. **Parrot-beak n.,** curvation of finger-nail like that of a parrot's beak. **Reedy n.,** nail marked by longitudinal furrows. **Turtle-back n.,** a nail greatly distorted.

Na'nism (na'nizm). Dwarfishness; marked undersize.
Nanoceph'alous. Having a very small head.
Nanocor'mia (na-no-kor'me-ah). Dwarfishness of body.
Na'noid (na'noid). Dwarfish; like a dwarf.
Nanom'elus. A fetus with stunted limbs.
Nanoso'mia (na-no-so'me-ah). Dwarfish habit of body.
Na'nous (na'nus). Dwarfed.
Na'nus. 1. A dwarf. 2. Stunted; dwarfish.
Nape. The back or scruff of the neck; nucha.
Napel'lin. Analgesic alkaloid, $C_{26}H_{39}NO_{11}$, from aconite.
Naph'talin (naf'tal-in). Same as *Naphthalene.*
Naph'tha. Crude petroleum; also, a light petroleum distillate.
Naph'thalene (naf'thal-ēn). A hydrocarbon, $C_{10}H_8$, from coal-tar oil; antiseptic.
Naph'thalol (naf'thal-ol). Same as *Betol.*
Naph'thol (naf'thol). Same as *Naphtol.*
Naphthopy'rin. A compound of naphthol and antipyrin.
Naphthosal'ol (naf-tho-sal'ol). Same as *Betol.*
Naph'tol. A crystalline antiseptic medicine from coal-tar, $C_{10}H_7OH$. See also *Alpha-naphtol.*
Nar'cein. A hypnotic alkaloid from opium.
Narcohyp'nia. Numbness felt on waking from sleep.
Nar'colepsy (nar'ko-lep-se). Disease marked by recurrent states of profound sleep.
Nar'cose. 1. Somewhat narcotic. 2. Drowsy.
Narco'sis (nar-ko'sis). Same as *Narcotism.*
Narcot'ic. Producing narcotism or stupor.
Nar'cotin. Antiperiodic and tonic alkaloid, $C_{22}H_{23}NO_7$, from opium.
Nar'cotism. Unconsciousness or stupor produced by a drug.
Nar'cotize. To put under the influence of a narcotic.
Na'ris, ante'rior. A nostril. **N., poste'rior,** either one of the posterior openings of the nasal fossæ.
Na'sal. Pertaining to the nose. **N. bones,** the two bones that form the arch of the nose. **N. fossæ,** cavities beyond nose and nasopharynx. **N. line,** one of Jadelot's furrows.
Nas'cent state. Condition of a substance or element just escaping from a chemical combination.
Na'sion. The middle point of the frontonasal suture.
Nasi'tis. Inflammation of the nose.
Nas'myth's membrane. See under *Membrane.*
Naso-antri'tis. Inflammation of the nose and antrum of Highmore.
Nasolabia'lis (na-zo-la-be-a'lis). See *Muscles, Table of.*
Nasopal'atine. Of, or pertaining to, nose and palate.
Nasopharyn'geal. Pertaining to the nasopharynx.
Nasopharyngi'tis. Inflammation of the nasopharynx.
Nasophar'ynx. Part of pharynx above the soft palate.
Nas'rol (nas'rol). Same as *Symphorol.*
Natal' boil, Natal' sore. An ulcerative disease endemic in South Africa.
Natal'oin. Aloin derived from Natal aloes.
Na'tes (na'tēz). The buttocks; also, anterior pair of corpora quadrigemina.
Na'tive albumin. See *Albumin.*
Na'trium (na'tre-um). Same as *Sodium.*
Na'tron. Native sodium carbonate; also, soda or sodium oxid.
Nat'ural. Neither artificial nor pathological. **N. philosophy,** physics; also, philosophy of nature.
Naupathi'a. Seasickness; nausea navalis.
Nau'sea. Tendency to vomit. **N. nava'lis,** seasickness.
Nau'seant. Inducing nausea; also, an agent so acting.

Nau'seous (naw'shus). Producing nausea or disgust.

Na'vel. The umbilicus. **N. string,** umbilical cord.

Navic'ular. Boat-shaped. **N. bone,** scaphoid bone of the tarsus. **N. fossa.** 1. Cavity behind vaginal aperture. 2. Expansion of urethra in glans penis. 3. Fossa between the helix and antihelix. 4. Depression on internal pterygoid process of sphenoid bone.

Neapol'itan fever. Same as *Mediterranean fever.*

Near-point. Nearest point of clear vision; *absolute,* for either eye alone; *relative,* for both eyes together.

Near-sight. Same as *Myopia.*

Near-sighted. Same as *Myopic.*

Nearthro'sis. A false or artificial joint.

Neb'ula. 1. Slight corneal opacity. 2. Cloudiness in urine.

Neb'ulizer. An atomizer; device for throwing a spray.

Neck. 1. Part between head and thorax. 2. The narrow part near the extremity of an organ or bone. **Anatomic n.,** constriction of the humerus just below its proximal articular surface. **Derbyshire n.** See *Goiter.* **Surgical n.,** constricted part of neck just below the tuberosities. **Wry n.** Same as *Torticollis.*

Necrobio'sis. The progressive atrophy and decay of an organ.

Necrol'ogy. Statistics or records of death.

Necrom'eter. Device for measuring organs of a dead body.

Necroph'agous. Feeding upon carrion.

Necroph'ilism. Insane sexual love for the dead.

Necropneumo'nia. Gangrene of lung.

Nec'ropsy, Necros'copy. Post-mortem examination.

Necro'sis. Molar or non-molecular death of a tissue, especially of a bone. **Balser's fatty n.,** necrosis of pancreas, spleen, and omentum. **Central n.** affects the central portion of an affected bone. **Cheesy n.,** tuberculous necrosis, as of the lung, with formation of a cheesy deposit. **Coagulation-n., Coagulative n.,** variety characterized by formation of fibrous infarcts: often associated with thrombosis. **Colliquative n., Liquefactive n.,** necrosis in an organ marked by the collection of a fluid exudate. **Dry n.,** that in which the dead bone becomes dry. **Fat-n.,** necrosis of fatty tissue in small white areas. **Mercurial n.,** that which is due to mercurial poisoning. **Moist n.,** that in which the dead bone is wet and soft. **N. ustilagin'ea,** dry gangrene from ergot-poisoning. **Phosphorus n.,** in the upper jaw, from exposure to fumes of phosphorus. **Superficial n.** affects the surface of a bone. **Syphilitic n.** is caused by syphilis. **Total n.** affects an entire bone.

Necrot'ic. Pertaining to necrosis.

Necrot'omy. Dissection of a dead body; also, excision of a sequestrum.

Nectan'dra. See *Bebeeru.*

Nee'dle. Sharp instrument for sewing or puncturing. **Aneurysm-n.,** one used in ligating blood-vessels. **Cataract-n.,** one designed for operating upon the cataractous lens. **Discission-n.,** a special form of cataract n. **Exploring n.,** one used in determining the presence of a fluid. **Hagedorn's n.,** a form of flat suture needle. **Hypodermic n.,** needle-pointed tube attached to the barrel of a hypodermic syringe. **N.-holder,** an instrument for drawing or guiding a needle. **N.-knife,** a cutting-edged needle used in operation.

Need'ling. Discission or puncturing with a needle.

Neg'ative electricity. Static electricity like that produced by friction of rosin or sealing-wax. **N. electrode, N. pole.** Same as *Cathode.*

Ne'gro lethargy. Same as *African lethargy.*

Neisse'ria. A genus of schizomycetes made up of biscuit-shaped diplococci. **N. gonorrhœ'æ.** Same as *Gonococcus.*

Nélaton's cath'eter. A soft rubber catheter. **N.'s line,** line from tuberosity of ischium to anterior superior spinous process of ilium. **N.'s probe,** a bullet probe with porcelain tip. See *Probe.*

Nem'atoblast (nem'at-o-blast). Same as *Spermatoblast.*

Nem'atode, or **Nem'atoid.** 1. Like a thread. 2. A thread-like parasitic worm.

Neoarthro'sis (ne-o-ar-thro'sis). Same as *Nearthrosis.*

Neoforma'tion. A new growth; neoplasm.

Neomem'brane (ne-o-mem'brān). A false membrane.

Neona'tal. Of, or pertaining to, the new-born.

Ne'oplasm. Any new and abnormal formation.

Neoplas'tic. Pertaining to, or like, a neoplasm.

Ne'oplasty (ne'op-las-te). Plastic replacement of lost parts.

Nephral'gia (nef-ral'je-ah). Pain in a kidney.

Nephral'gic crises. Paroxysmal pain of kidney-region in tabes.

Nephrat'ony (nef-rat'o-ne). Atony of the kidney.

Nephraux'e. Enlargement of kidney.

Nephrec'tomy (nef-rek'to-me). Removal of a kidney.

Nephrelco'sis. Ulceration of the kidney.

Neph'ric (nef'rik). Pertaining to the kidney.

Nephrid'ium. Embryonic tube whence the kidney is developed.

Neph'rin (nef'rin). Same as *Cystin.*

Neph'rism (nef'rism). Cachexia due to kidney-disease.

Nephrit'ic (nef-rit'ik). Pertaining to nephritis.

Nephri'tis (nef-ri'tis). Inflammation of the kidney. **Acute n.,** suppurative n. of short and severe course. **Albuminous n.,** that in which albuminuria occurs. **Bacterial n.,** that which is caused by micro-organisms. **Capsular n.** affects specially Bowman's capsules. **Catarrhal n.** Same as *Parenchymatous n.* **Cheesy n.,** a chronic suppurative form with caseous deposits. **Chronic n.,** any variety of relatively slow course. **Croupous n.** Same as *Acute n.* **Desquamative n.,** acute catarrhal n. **Diffuse n.,** one which affects both parenchyma and stroma. **Fibrous n.,** that which specially affects the stroma. **Glomerular n.** affects specially the glomeruli. **Glomerulocapsular n.** affects primarily the glomeruli and Bowman's capsules. **Interstitial n.** Same as *Fibrous n.* **Parenchymatous n.** affects specially the parenchyma of kidney. **Saturnine n.,** that due to chronic lead-poisoning. **Scarlatinal n.,** an acute n. due to scarlet fever. **Suppurative n.,** a form accompanied by abscess of kidney. **Tubal,** or **Tubular n.** affects especially the tubules. **Tuberculous n.,** a kind due to the bacillus of tubercle.

Neph'rocele (nef'ro-sēl). Hernia of a kidney.

Nephrogen'ic, Nephrog'enous. Arising in or from a kidney.

Neph'rolith (nef'ro-lith). A renal calculus; gravel in a kidney.

Nephrolithi'asis. Condition marked by presence of renal calculi.

Nephrolithot'omy. Removal of renal calculus by cutting.

Nephrol'ogy (nef-rol'o-je). Scientific study of the kidney.

Neph'ropexy. Surgical fixation of a floating kidney.

Nephropto'sis. Prolapse of a kidney.

Nephropyeli'tis. Nephritis complicated with pyelitis.

Nephropyo'sis (nef-ro-pi-o'sis). Suppuration of a kidney.

Nephror'rhaphy. Same as *Nephropexy.*

Neph'rostome (nef'ros-tōm). The internal orifice of the nephridium.

Nephrot'omy (nef-rot'om-e). Surgical incision of a kidney.

Nephroty'phus (nef-ro-ti'fus). Typhus with renal hemorrhage.

Nephro-ureterec'tomy. Excision of kidney and whole ureter.

Nephroz'ymase. A ferment-like diastase found in urine.

Ner'oli (ner'ol-e). Oil of orange flowers.

A TABLE OF THE NERVES.

Nerve.	Function.	Origin.	Distribution.	Branches.
Abdu'cens (sixth cranial).	Motion.	Fourth ventricle.	External rectus of eye.	None.
Ar'nold's.	See *Auricular.*			
Au'ditory (eighth cranial, portio mollis of seventh).	Hearing.	Fourth ventricle.	Internal ear.	Vestibular, cochlear.
Auric'ular (Arnold's).	Sensation.	Pneumogastric.	External ear.	Filaments.
Auric'ular (posterior).	Motion.	Facial.	Retrahens aurem, occipito-frontalis.	Auricular, occipital.
Auricula'ris mag'nus.	Sensation.	Cervical plexus, second and third cervical.	Parotid gland, face, ear.	Facial, posterior mastoid.
Auriculotem'poral.	Sensation.	Inferior maxillary.	Pinna and temple.	Anterior and posterior temporal.
Buc'cal.	Motion.	Inferior maxillary.	Cheek.	Superior and inferior buccinator and external pterygoid.
Calca'nean, internal.	Sensation.	Posterior tibial.	Fascia and integument of heel and sole.	
Car'diac (cervical and thoracic).	Motion.	Pneumogastric.	Heart.	Branches to cardiac plexuses.
Cer'vical, 8.	Motion and sensation.	Cord.	Trunk and upper extremities.	Anterior and posterior divisions.
Cervical, first (anterior division).	Motion and sensation.	Cord.	Rectus lateralis and two anterior recti.	Branches and communicating to pneumogastric, hypoglossal, sympathetic.
Cervical, first (posterior division).	Motion and sensation.	Cord.	Recti, obliqui, complexus.	Branches, communicating and cutaneous filaments.

Cervical, second (anterior division).	Motion and sensation.	Cord.	Communicating.	Ascending, descending, communicating, and filaments.
Cervical, second (posterior division).	Motion and sensation.	Cord.	Oblique inferior, scalp, ear, complexus, splenius, trachelomastoid.	Internal or occipitalis major, and external.
Cervical, third (anterior division).	Motion and sensation.	Cord.	Communicating.	Ascending, descending, and communicating filaments.
Cervical, third (posterior division).	Motion and sensation.	Cord.	Occiput, etc., splenius, complexus, etc.	Internal, external, and filaments.
Cervical, fourth (anterior division).	Motion and sensation.	Cord.	Shoulder and communicating.	Communicating filaments, muscular, etc.
Cervicals, fifth to eighth (anterior division).	Motion and sensation.	Cord.	Brachial plexus.	Communicating.
Cervicals, fourth to eighth (posterior division).	Motion and sensation.	Cord.	Muscles and skin of neck.	Internal and external branches.
Cervicofa′cial.	Motion.	Facial.	Lower part of face and part of neck.	Buccal, supramaxillary, inframaxillary.
Chor′da tym′pani.	Motion.	Facial.	Tongue, etc.	Filaments.
Cil′iary.	Sensation, motion, nutrition.	Ciliary ganglion.	Eyeball.	
Cir′cumflex.	Motion and sensation.	Brachial plexus.	Teres minor and deltoid.	Upper and lower.
Coccyg′eal.	Motion.	Coccygeal plexus.	Coccygeus and gluteus max.	
Coch′lear.	Hearing.	Auditory.	Cochlea.	
Col′li, superficia′lis.	Sensation.	Cervical plexus.	Platysma muscle and anterolateral parts of neck.	Ascending and descending branches and filaments.
Commu′nicans no′ni.	Motion and sensation.	Second cervical, third cervical.	Descendens noni.	Omohyoid and filaments.
Commu′nicating.	Motion and sensation.	Cervical plexus.	Spinal accessory.	Branches.
Commu′nicating.	Sensation and motion.	First and second cervical.	Pneumogastric, hypoglossal, sympathetic.	Three branches and filaments.

A TABLE OF THE NERVES (*continued*).

NERVE.	FUNCTION.	ORIGIN.	DISTRIBUTION.	BRANCHES.
Cotun′nius.	See *Nasopalatine nerve.*			
Cru′ral, anterior.	Motion and sensation.	Lumbar plexus.	Thigh.	Middle and internal cutaneous, long saphenous, muscular, articular.
Cuta′neous.	Sensation.	Musculospiral.	Skin of arm, radial side of forearm.	One internal, two external.
Cutaneous.	Sensation.	Ulnar.	Wrist and palm.	First and palmar cutaneous.
Cutaneous (dorsal).	Sensation.	Ulnar.	Little and ring fingers.	Filaments and communicating branches.
Cutaneous (external).	Sensation.	Second and third lumbar.	Skin of thigh.	Anterior, posterior.
Cutaneous (internal).	Sensation.	Brachial plexus.	Forearm.	Anterior and posterior branches and filaments.
Cutaneous (lesser internal) ("Wrisberg").	Sensation.	Brachial plexus.	Inner side of arm.	Filaments.
Cutaneous (middle and internal).	Sensation.	Anterior crural.	Thigh and communicating.	Communicating and filaments.
Den′tal (inferior).	Sensation.	Inferior maxillary.	Teeth, muscles, gland.	Mylohyoid, incisor, mental, dental.
Dentals (posterior and anterior).	Sensation.	Superior maxillary.	Teeth.	Filaments.
Depres′sor.	Lowers blood-pressure.	Vagus.	Heart.	
Descen′dens hypoglos′si.	Motion.	Cervical plexus.	Omohyoid, sternohyoid, sternothyroid, thyrohyoid, hyoglossus, and tongue-muscles.	Muscular, lingual.

Descen'dens no'ni.	Same as *Descendens hypoglossi.*			
Digas'tric.	Motion.	Facial.	Posterior belly of digastric.	Filaments.
Dor'sal, 12 (anterior and posterior divisions).	Motion and sensation.	Cord.	Muscles and skin of chest and trunk.	External, internal, cutaneous, etc.
Esoph'ageal.	Motion.	Vagus.	Muscular and mucous coats of esophagus.	Esophageal plexus.
Fa'cial (seventh cranial, portio dura).	Motion.	Fourth ventricle.	Face, ear, palate, tongue.	Petrosals, tympanic, chorda tympani, posterior auricular, digastric, stylohyoid, temporofacial, cervicofacial.
Fron'tal.	Sensation.	Ophthalmic.	Forehead and lids.	Supra-orbital, supratrochlear.
Gas'tric.	Motion.	Pneumogastric.	Stomach.	Filaments.
Genitocru'ral.	Motion and sensation.	Second lumbar.	Cremaster and thigh.	Genital, crural, communicating.
Glossopharyn'geal (ninth cranial).	Sensation and taste.	Fourth ventricle.	Tongue, middle ear, tonsils, pharynx.	Tympanic, carotid, pharyngeal, muscular, tonsillar, lingual.
Glu'teal (superior).	Motion.	Sacral plexus.	Glutæi, tensor vaginæ femoris.	Filaments.
Gus'tatory.	Taste and sensation.	Inferior maxillary.	Tongue and mouth.	Branches and filaments.
Hemorrhoi'dal.	Sensation and motion.	Pudic.	External sphincter ani and integument adjacent.	
Hepat'ic.		Pneumogastric.	Liver.	Hepatic plexus.
Hirsch'feld's.	Motion.	Facial.	Styloglossus and palatoglossus.	
Hypogas'tric.	Sensation.	Iliohypogastric.	Skin around external abdominal ring.	
Hypoglos'sal (twelfth cranial).	Motion.	Fourth ventricle.	Hyoglossus and hyoid muscles.	Descendens noni, muscular, thyrohyoid.

A TABLE OF THE NERVES (*continued*).

NERVE.	FUNCTION.	ORIGIN.	DISTRIBUTION.	BRANCHES.
Iliohypogas′tric.	Motion and sensation.	First lumbar.	Abdominal and gluteal regions.	Iliac, hypogastric, communicating.
Ilio-in′guinal.	Motion and sensation.	First lumbar.	Inguinal region and scrotum.	Muscular, cutaneous, and communicating.
Infra-or′bital.	Sensation.	Superior maxillary.	Nose and lip.	Palpebral, nasal, labial.
Intercos′tal.	Motion and sensation.	Spinal cord.	Muscles and integuments of thorax.	Muscular, anterior, and lateral cutaneous.
Interosseous (anterior).	Motion.	Median.	Deep muscles of forearm.	Branches and filaments.
Interosseous (posterior).	Motion and sensation.	Musculospiral.	Carpus and radial and posterior brachial regions.	Branches and filaments.
Lacri′mal.	Sensation.	Ophthalmic.	Gland and conjunctiva.	Filaments.
Laryn′geal (recurrent or inferior).	Motor.	Pneumogastric.	Larynx.	Branches to all muscles except cricothyroid.
Laryn′geal (superior).	Sensation and motion.	Pneumogastric.	Larynx.	External—cricothyroid muscle and thyroid gland. Internal—mucous membrane, larynx, etc.
Lum′bar, 5.	Motion and sensation.	Cord.	Lumbar and genital tissues, etc.	Anterior and post. divisions, lumbar plexus, etc.
Mandib′ular.	Same as *Maxillary, inferior.*			
Masseter′ic.	Motor.	Inferior maxillary.	Masseter muscle.	Filaments.
Max′illary (inferior).	Sensation, motion, and taste.	Trigeminus.	Muscles of mastication, ear, cheek, tongue, teeth.	Masseteric, auriculotemporal, buccal, gustatory, inferior dental.

Trigeminus.	*Cheek, face, teeth.*	*Orbital, sphenopalatine, dentals, infra-orbital.*
Brachial plexus.	Pronator radii teres, flexors, two lumbricales, fingers, palm, etc.	Muscular, anterior interosseous, palmar cutaneous.
Floor of aqueduct of Sylvius.	Muscles of eye, except rectus ext., obliquus sup., and orbicularis palpebrarum.	Filaments.
First and second cervical.	Muscles.	Rectus capitis lateralis, rectus anterior major and minor.
Cervical plexus.	Sternomastoid, levator anguli scapulæ, scalenus medius, trapezius.	Branches.
Brachial plexus.	Longus colli, scaleni, rhomboidei, subclavius.	Branches.
Musculospiral.	Triceps, anconeus, supinator longus, extensor carpi radialis longus, brachialis anticus.	Internal, posterior, external.
Median.	Superficial muscles of forearm.	Branches and filaments.
Ulnar.	Flexor carpi ulnaris, flexor profundus digitorum.	Two branches.
Great sciatic.	Biceps, semimembranosus, semitendinosus, adductor magnus.	Filaments.
Sacral plexus.	Pyriformis, obturator internus, gemelli, quadratus femoris.	Filaments.
Anterior crural..	Pectineus and muscles of thigh.	Filaments.

A TABLE OF THE NERVES (*continued*).

Nerve.	Function.	Origin.	Distribution.	Branches.
Musculocuta'neous.	Motion and sensation.	Brachial plexus.	Coracobrachial, biceps, brachialis anticus, forearm.	Branches, anterior and posterior.
Musculocuta'neous.	Motion and sensation.	External popliteal.	Muscles of fibular side of leg, skin of dorsum of foot.	Internal, external.
Musculospi'ral.	Motion aud sensation.	Brachial plexus.	Back of arm and forearm, skin of back of haud.	Muscular, cutaneous, radial, posterior interosseous.
Mylohy'oid.	Motion.	Inferior maxillary.	Mylohyoid and digastric muscles.	Filaments.
Na'sal.	Sensation.	Ophthalmic.	Iris, ciliary ganglion, nose.	Ganglionic, ciliary, infratrochlear.
Obtura'tor.	Motion and sensation.	Lumbar plexus.	Obturator externus, adductor, joint and skin.	Anterior and posterior articulating and communicating.
Obtura'tor (accessory).	Motion and sensation.	Lumbar plexus.	Pectineus and hip-joint.	Branches and filaments.
Occipita'lis mi'nor.	Sensation.	Second cervical.	Occipitofrontalis, ear, etc.	Communicating, auricular filaments.
Oculomo'tor.	See *Motor oculi*.			
Œsopha'geal.	See *Esophageal*.			
Olfac'tory (first cranial).	Smell.	Frontal lobe, optic thalamus, island of Reil.	Schneiderian membrane of nose.	Twenty branches.
Ophthal'mic.	Sensation.	Trigeminus.	Forehead, eyes, nose.	Frontal, lacrimal, nasal.
Op'tic (second cranial).	Sight.	Cortical center in occipital lobe.	Retina.	None.
Or'bital.	Sensation.	Superior maxillary.	Temple and cheek.	Temporal and malar.
Pal'atine, anterior or great.	Sensation.	Meckel's ganglion.	Hard palate, gums, nose.	Two inferior nasal.
Pal'mar cuta'neous.	Sensation.	Median.	Thumb and palm.	Outer and inner.

Motion.	Ulnar.	Little finger, dorsal and palmar interosseous, two inner lumbricales, abductor pollicis, etc.	Branches and filaments.
Sensation and motion.	Ulnar.	Palmaris brevis, inner side of hand and little finger.	Filaments and two digital branches.
Motion.	Valve of Vieussens.	Superior oblique of eye.	None.
Motion.	Facial.	Ganglia and plexus.	Great, small, external to Meckel's ganglion, otic ganglion, and meningeal plexus, respectively.
Motion.	Pneumogastric.	Pharynx.	Pharyngeal plexus.
Motion and sensation.	Third, fourth, and fifth cervical.	Diaphragm, pericardium, pleura, etc.	Branches and filaments.
Motion and sensation.	Posterior tibial.	Little toe and deep muscles of foot.	Superficial and deep.
Sensation and motion.	Posterior tibial.	Sole of foot, adductor pollicis, flexor brevis digitorum, toes, etc.	Cutaneous, muscular, articular, digital.
Sensation and motion.	Fourth ventricle.	Ear, pharynx, larynx, heart, lungs, esophagus, etc.	Articular, pharyngeal, superior laryngeal, recurrent laryngeal, cardiac, pulmonary, esophageal, gastric, hepatic.
Sensation and motion.	Great sciatic.	Extensors of skin of foot.	Anterior tibial, musculocutaneous.
Motion and sensation.	Great sciatic.	Knee, gastrocnemius, tibialis, plantaris, soleus, popliteus, skin of foot, etc.	Articular, muscular cutaneous, external saphenous, plantar.
Motion and sensation.	Sacral plexus.	Perineum, anus, genitalia.	Inferior hemorrhoidal, perineal, cutaneous, dorsal of penis.

A TABLE OF THE NERVES (*continued*).

NERVE.	FUNCTION.	ORIGIN.	DISTRIBUTION.	BRANCHES.
Pul′monary (anterior and posterior).		Pneumogastric.	Lungs.	Branches to pulmonary plexuses.
Ra′dial.	Sensation.	Musculocutaneous.	Thumb and three fingers.	External and internal.
Sa′cral, 5.	Motion and sensation.	Cord.	Multifidus spinæ, skin, gluteal region, etc.	Filaments and sacral plexus.
Saph′enous (long or internal).	Sensation.	Anterior crural.	Knee, ankle, etc.	Cutaneous, patellar, communicating filaments.
Sciat′ic (great).	Motor and sensation.	Sacral plexus.	Skin of leg, muscles of back of thigh and muscles of leg and foot.	Articular, muscular, popliteals.
Sciat′ic (small).	Sensation and motion.	Sacral plexus.	Perineum, back of thigh and leg, and gluteus maximus.	Muscular, cutaneous.
Sphenopal′atine.	Sensation.	Superior maxillary.	Meckel's ganglion.	
Spi′nal acces′sory (eleventh cranial).	Motor.	Fourth ventricle.	Sternocleidomastoid, trapezius.	Branches and filaments.
Splanch′nic (great).	Sympathetic.	Thoracic ganglia.	Semilunar ganglion, renal and suprarenal plexus.	Communicating and filaments.
Splanch′nic (lesser).	Sympathetic.	Tenth and eleventh thoracic ganglia, great splanchnic.	Celiac plexus and great splanchnic.	Communicating and filaments.
Splanch′nic (renal).	Sympathetic.	Last thoracic ganglion.	Renal and celiac plexus.	Communicating and filaments.
Stylohy′oid.	Motion.	Facial.	Stylohyoid muscle.	Filaments.
Subscap′ular, 3.	Motion.	Brachial plexus.	Subscapular, teres major, and latissimus dorsi.	Filaments.

Supraclavic'ular (descending).	Sensation.	Third and fourth cervical.	Skin of neck, breast, and shoulder.	Sternal, clavicular, acromial.
Supramandib'ular.	See *Maxillary, superior.*			
Supra-or'bital.	Sensation.	Frontal.	Upper lid, forehead.	Muscular, cutaneous, and pericranial branches.
Suprascap'ular.	Motion and sensation.	Brachial plexus.	Scapular muscles.	Branches and filaments.
Supratroch'lear.	Sensation.	Frontal.	Forehead.	Muscular and skin branches.
Sympathet'ic.	A series of joined ganglia extending along the vertebral column and connected with spinal nerves.			
Temporofa'cial.	Motion.	Facial.	Upper part of face.	Temporal, malar, infra-orbital.
Temporoma'lar.	Same as *Orbital.*			
Thora'cic (post. or long).	Motion.	Brachial plexus.	Serratus magnus.	Filaments.
Thora'cics (ant. and ext.).	Motion.	Brachial plexus.	Pectoralis major and minor.	Branches and filaments.
Tib'ial (anterior).	Motion and sensation.	External popliteal.	Tibialis anticus, extensor longus digitorum, peroneus tertius, etc., joints of foot, skin of great toe, etc.	Muscular, external, internal.
Tib'ial (posterior).	Motion and sensation.	Great sciatic.	Tibialis posterior, flexor longus digitorum, flexor longus pollicis, skin of heel and sole, knee-joint.	Plantars, muscular, cutaneous, articular.
Trigem'inus or trifacial (fifth cranial).	Motion and sensation (taste).	Medulla.	Skin and structures of face, tongue, and teeth.	Ophthalmic, superior and inferior maxillary divisions.
Troch'lear.	See *Patheticus.*			
Tympan'ic.	Motion.	Facial.	Stapedius and laxator tympani muscles.	Filaments.
Ul'nar.	Motion and sensation.	Brachial plexus.	Muscles, etc., shoulder- and wrist-joints, and skin of little finger.	Two articular, muscular, cutaneous, dorsal, superior palmar, deep palmar.
Va'gus.	See *Pneumogastric.*			

Nerve. A cord-like organ which conveys impulses. [See *Table of the Nerves*, pp. 301-313.] **Afferent n.**, any n. which transmits impulses from the periphery intrad. **Calorific n.**, any n. whose stimulation increases heat. **Centrifugal n.**, any n. which carries impulse to the periphery. **Centripetal n.**, any afferent n. **Cranial n.**, any nerve arising from the brain direct. **Depressor n.**, any afferent n. whose stimulation depresses a motor-center. **Efferent n.** Same as *Centrifugal n.* **Esodic n.** Same as *Afferent n.* **Frigorific n.**, any sympathetic n. stimulation of which lowers temperature. **Inhibitory n.**, one whose stimulation inhibits or reduces the activity of an organ. **Mixed n.**, one which is both sensory and motor. **Motor n.**, one which contains wholly or chiefly motor fibers. **N.-cell**, any cell of a nerve, nerve-center, or ganglion. **N.-center**, any group of cells of gray matter having a common function. **N.-corpuscles**, nucleated corpuscles lying between the neurilemma and medullary sheath. **N.-ending**, any terminus of a nerve, especially if peripheral. **N.-fiber**, any one of the fibers which make up a funiculus of n. substance. **N.-grafting**, replacement of a piece of defective nerve by a segment from a sound one. **N.-head**, papilla or optic disk. **N.-plexus.** See *Plexus.* **N.-storm**, sudden outburst of nervous disorder. **N.-stretching**, the stretching of a nerve, chiefly to relieve pain. **N.-tire.** See *Neurasthenia.* **N.-tumor.** See *Neuroma.* **Pressor n.**, any afferent n. whose irritation stimulates a vasomotor center. **Secretory n.**, any efferent n. whose stimulation increases glandular activity. **Sensory n.** Same as *Afferent n.* **Spinal n.**, any nerve which makes its exit from the vertebral column. **Sympathetic n.**, any nerve of the sympathetic system. See *Sympathetic.* **Thermic n.** Same as *Calorific n.* **Trisplanchnic n.**, a general name for the system of sympathetic nerves. **Trophic n.**, one which regulates nutrition. **Vasoconstrictor n.**, one whose stimulation contracts blood-vessels. **Vasodilator n.**, one whose stimulation dilates blood-vessels. **Vasomotor n.**, any nerve concerned in controlling the caliber of vessels.

Ner′vi nervo′rum. Nerve-filaments going to nerves and nerve-sheaths.

Ner′vine (ner′vin). 1. Allaying nervous excitement. 2. A remedy for nervous disorders.

Ner′vous. 1. Pertaining to a nerve or nerves. 2. Unduly excitable. **N. debility.** Same as *Neurasthenia.* **N. system**, the brain, cord, nerves, and ganglia collectively.

Ner′vousness (ner′vus-nes). Morbid or undue excitability.

Ner′vus. L. for *Nerve.*

Ness′ler's reagent. Mercuric chlorid, potassium iodid, and potash dissolved in water: a chemical test.

Nestother′apy. The hunger-cure.

Net′tle-rash. Same as *Urticaria.*

Neu (nu). Same as *Neurilemma.*

Neu′mann's disease (noi′mahnz). Pemphigus characterized by vegetation.

Neu′rad. Toward the neural axis or aspect.

Neuradyna′mia. Same as *Neurasthenia.*

Neurag′mia. The tearing of a nerve-trunk from its ganglion.

Neu′ral. Of, or pertaining to, nerves. **N. groove.** See *Medullary groove.* **N. plate.** See *Medullary plate.* **N. spine**, the spinous process of a vertebra.

Neural′gia (nu-ral′je-ah). Pain in a nerve.

Neural′gic (nu-ral′jik). Of, or pertaining to, neuralgia.

Neural′gin. An antipyretic and anodyne remedy.

Neuramebim′eter. Device used in measuring the reaction-time of nerves.

Neurapoph'ysis. Structure forming either side of the neural arch.

Neurasthe'nia. Depression due to exhausted nerve-energy. **Cerebral n.,** variety characterized by mental and visual disturbances and other head-symptoms. **Gastric n.,** a form marked by functional stomach-complications. **Sexual n.,** a variety associated with disorders of the sexual function.

Neuratro'phia. Impaired nutrition of nervous system.

Neurax'is. An axis-cylinder; also the cerebrospinal axis.

Neurax'on. Any axis-cylinder process.

Neurec'tasis (nu-rek'tas-is). Same as *Nerve-stretching.*

Neurec'tomy (nu-rek'to-me). Excision of part of a nerve.

Neurenter'ic canal. Canal of the embryo from the archenteron to the medullary tube.

Neuri'atry. Treatment of nervous diseases.

Neu'ridin. A ptomain, $C_5H_{14}N_2$, from decaying animal matter.

Neurilem'ma. The sheath of a nerve-fiber; also, the epineurium.

Neurilemmi'tis (nu-ril-em-mi'tis). Inflammation of neurilemma.

Neuril'ity (nu-ril'it-e). Functional attributes of nerve-tissue.

Neu'rin. 1. An albuminous substance from nerve-tissue. 2. A deadly ptomain, $(CH_3)_3C_2H_3NOH$, from decayed nerve-tissue, etc.

Neu'rit, Neu'rite. Any axis-cylinder process from a nerve-cell.

Neurit'ic. Of, or pertaining to, neuritis.

Neuri'tis. Inflammation of a nerve. **Alcoholic n.,** that due to alcoholism. **Ascending n.,** that which progresses centrad, or centripetally. **Axial n.,** inflammation of central part of a nerve. **Degenerative n.** is marked by degeneration of the parenchyma. **Descending n.,** that which progresses centrifugally. **Diabetic n.,** that which follows diabetes. **Diphtheritic n.,** one of the sequels of diphtheria. **Epidemic n.** See *Beriberi.* **Facial n.,** Bell's palsy. **Interstitial n.,** inflammation of the connective tissue of a nerve-trunk. **Leprous n.** is associated with true leprosy. **Lipomatous n.,** that in which the nerve-fibers are destroyed and a fatty connective tissue takes their place. **Lymphatic n.** See *Mesoneuritis.* **Malarial n.,** a form due to malarial poisoning. **N. mi'grans,** a form which ascends one nerve to a center and then descends another nerve. **Multiple n.** affects several nerves at once. See *Polyneuritis, Perineuritis.* **N. nodo'sa** is marked by the formation of nodes on the nerves. **Optic n.,** that of the optic nerve. **Parenchymatous n.** affects primarily the medullary substance and axis-cylinders. **Post-febrile n.** mostly follows an attack of severe exanthematous disease. **Pressure-n.,** that due to compression. **Retrobulbar n.** Same as *Optic n.* **Rheumatic n.,** a form associated with rheumatic symptoms. **Sciatic n.** Same as *Sciatica.* **Segmentary n.** attacks segments of a nerve. **Senile n.** attacks the legs and feet of aged people. **Sympathetic n.** is that which involves an opposite nerve without invading the nerve-center. **Tabetic n.,** that associated with locomotor ataxia. **Toxic n.,** that due to some poison. **Traumatic n.,** that which is cased by an injury.

Neu'roblast (neu'ro-blast). An embryonic or repair-cell from which nervous tissue is formed.

Neu'rocele, Neurocœ'le. Ventricles of brain and central canal of the cord taken together.

Neurochoroidi'tis. Inflammation of the choroid coat and ciliary nerves.

Neu'rocyte (nu'ro-sit). A nerve-cell of any kind.

Neuroden'drite, Neuroden'dron. Process of a nerve-cell combining features of a neuron and a dendron.

Neurodermati'tis. A neurotic skin-inflammation.

Neu'rodin (nu'rod-in). A proprietary antineuralgic remedy.

Neurodyn'ia (nu-rod-in'e-ah). Pain in a nerve or in nerves.
Neuro-epider'mal layer. Same as *Epiblast.*
Neuro-epithe'lium. 1. A specialized epithelium of eye and ear. 2. Epithelium of the epiblast whence the cerebrospinal axis is developed.
Neurofibro'ma. Neuroma with fibromatous elements.
Neurogen'esis, Neurog'eny. Formation of nerves and nervous organs.
Neurog'enous. Arising from some lesion of the nervous system.
Neurog'lia (nu-rog'le-ah). The supporting structure of the nervous system.
Neurog'liar, Neurog'lic. Of, or pertaining to, neuroglia.
Neuroglio'ma. Glioma in which there are nerve-cells. **N. ganglionа're,** glioma in which ganglion-cells are embedded.
Neurog'raphy. Treatise on, or description of, nerves.
Neu'roid (nu'roid). Resembling a nerve.
Neuroker'atin. Substance of which the neuroglia is composed.
Neurol'ogist (nu-rol'o-jist). An expert in neurology.
Neurol'ogy (nu-rol'o-je). Scientific study of the nerves.
Neurol'ysis (nu-rol'is-is). 1. Liberation of a nerve from adhesions. 2. Relief of tension upon a nerve obtained by stretching. 3. Exhaustion of nervous energy.
Neuro'ma. Tumor made up largely of nerve-substance. **Amputation-n.,** n. of a stump after amputation. **Amyelinic n.,** one containing only non-medullated nerve-fibers. **N. cu'tis,** neuroma seated in the skin. **Cystic n.,** a false n. which has become cystic. **False n.,** one which does not contain genuine nerve-fiber. **Ganglionated n., Ganglionic n.** is composed of true nerve-cells. **Myelinic n.** contains medullated nerve-fibers. **Plexiform n.** is marked by multiple nodulous enlargements along the course of the cutaneous nerves. **N. telangiecto'des** contains an excess of blood-vessels.
Neuromala'cia (nu-ro-mal-a'se-ah). Softening of the nerves.
Neurom'atous (nu-rom'at-us). Of the nature of, or pertaining to, neuroma.
Neu'romere (nu'ro-mēr). A segment or section of the cerebrospinal axis.
Neuromime'sis. Hysteric simulation of organic disease.
Neuromus'cular. Pertaining to nerves and muscles.
Neuromyeli'tis. Inflammation of nervous and medullary substance.
Neuromyosi'tis. Neuritis blended with myositis.
Neu'ron. A nerve-cell with all its processes.
Neuroparal'ysis. Paralysis due to disease of a nerve or nerves.
Neuropath'ic. Pertaining to a nervous disorder.
Neuropathol'ogy. Pathology of nerves and nerve-centers.
Neurop'athy (nu-rop'ath-e). Any nervous disorder.
Neuropho'nia. A nervous disorder marked by peculiar outcries.
Neurophysiol'ogy. Physiology of nervous system.
Neu'roplasty. Plastic surgery of a nerve or nerves.
Neuropsycho'sis (nu-rop-si-ko'sis). Nervous disease complicated with mental disorder.
Neuroretini'tis. Inflammation of optic nerve and retina.
Neuror'rhaphy. The stitching together of a cut nerve.
Neurosar'coma. A sarcoma with neuromatous elements.
Neuro'sis (nu-ro'sis). A nervous disease, especially a functional disease.
Neuroskel'eton (nu-ro-skel'et-on). Same as *Endoskeleton.*
Neurostear'ic acid. A fatty acid, $C_{18}H_{36}O_2$, from brain: isomeric with stearic acid.
Neurosthe'nia. Excessive nervous power.
Neu'rosuture (nu'ro-sūt-yur). Same as *Neurorrhaphy.*

Neurota'bes (nu-ro-ta'bes). Tabes due to peripheral neuritis.
Neuroten'sion. Nerve-stretching; neurectasis.
Neurot'ic (nu-rot'ik). Pertaining to, or affected by, neurosis.
Neurotiza'tion. Restoration of a divided nerve.
Neu'rotome (nu'ro-tōm). Needle-like knife for nerve-dissection.
Neurot'omy (nu-rot'om-e). Dissection or cutting of nerves.
Neu'rotripsy (nu'ro-trip-se). The crushing or bruising of a nerve.
Neu'tral. Neither basic nor acid.
Neu'tralize (nu'tral-īz). To deprive of acid or alkaline qualities.
Neu'trophil (nu'tro-fil). Stainable by neutral dyes.
Ne'void. Resembling a nevus. **N. elephantiasis.** Same as *Lymph-scrotum*.
Nevolipo'ma. Venous nevus associated with lipoma.
Ne'vus, Næ'vus. Pigmented spot on the skin. **N. ara'neus.** Same as *Acne rosacea*. **Capillary n.,** one that involves the skin capillaries. **Cutaneous n.,** a skin nevus. **N. lipomato'-des,** one which contains a mass of fat. **N. mater'nus,** congenital angioma, mother's mark, or birthmark. **N. pigmento'-sus,** a pigmented mole. **N. vascula'ris,** an angiomatous n. or birthmark. **Venous n.,** one composed mainly of veins.
New growth. A neoplasm or neoformation.
New'ton's rings. Concentric colored rings reflected from very thin transparent surfaces.
Ni. Symbol of *Nickel*.
Nick'el. A white metal with medicinal salts.
Ni'col prism. Two slabs of Iceland spar for polarizing light.
Nicotian'in. A fragrant principle from tobacco.
Nic'otin (nik'ot-in). Poisonous fluid base, $C_{10}H_{14}N_2$, from tobacco.
Nicotin'ic acid. An acid, $C_6H_5NO_2$, from nicotin, bone oil, etc.
Nic'otinism (nik'ot-in-izm). Poisoning by tobacco or by nicotin.
Nic'oulin. An antitetanic drug, $C_3H_4O_5$.
Nic'tating, Nic'titating. Winking; winking rapidly.
Nicta'tion, Nictita'tion. The act of winking.
Ni'dus (ni'dus). A nest; point of origin or focus of a morbid process. **N. hirun'dinis,** the swallow's nest; a depression in the cerebellum, between the posterior velum and uvula.
Nie'meyer's pill (ne'mi-erz). A pill of quinin, digitalis, and opium.
Night'-blindness. Defect or failure of vision in the night. **N.-soil,** the ordure of a privy. **N.-sweat,** copious sweating in bed at night, as in tuberculosis. **N.-terrors,** a kind of nightmare in children; pavor nocturnus.
Night'mare. Oppressive dreams attended with fright and sense of suffocation.
Nigro'sin. Anilin black, $C_{36}H_{27}N_3$; a microscopic stain.
Ninth nerve. See *Glossopharyngeal* in *Nerves, Table of.*
Niphablep'sia (nif-ah-blep'se-ah). Same as *Snow-blindness.*
Nip'ple. The conical organ which gives outlet to the milk; mammilla or teat. **N.-line,** vertical line through the nipple.
Ni'sus (ni'sus). An effort, tendency, or molimen.
Nit. The egg of a louse.
Ni'ter. Potassium nitrate; saltpeter.
Ni'trate. Any salt of nitric acid.
Ni'trated. Combined with nitric acid or niter.
Ni'tre (ni'ter). Same as *Niter*.
Ni'tric acid (ni'trik). See *Acid.*
Ni'tril. Any combination of nitrogen with a trivalent radical.
Ni'trite (ni'trīt). Any salt of nitrous acid.
Nitrobacte'ria. Bacteria changing ammonia into nitrogen acids.
Nitroben'zol. A poisonous benzol derivative, $C_6H_5NO_2$, used in perfuming soap.
Nitrocel'lulose. Pyroxylin or gun-cotton.

Ni'troform. Trinitrobenzene; an inflammable substance, $CH(NO_2)_3$.

Ni'trogen. A colorless gas found free in the air: symbol N.

Nitrog'enous (ni-trod'je-nus). Containing nitrogen.

Nitrogly'cerin (ni-tro-glis'e-rin). An explosive liquid, $C_3H_5N_3O_9$: a vasodilator.

Nitrohydrochlo'ric acid. See *Acid.*

Nitrosac'charose (ni-tro-sak'ka-rōs). A resinous explosive and a vasodilator like nitroglycerin.

Nitrosal'ol. Yellow crystalline powder used in making salophen.

Ni'trous acid. See *Acid.* **N. oxid,** laughing-gas, N_2O; an anesthetic.

Noctambula'tion. Sleep-walking; somnambulism.

Noctur'nal. Pertaining to the night. **N. emission,** involuntary escape of semen in sleep.

No'dal points. Same as *Cardinal points.*

Nod'ding spasm. Clonic spasm of the sternomastoid muscles; salaam convulsion.

Node. A swelling, knot, or protuberance. **Heberden's n.,** an overgrowth of tubercle of digital phalanges in rheumatoid arthritis. **N. of Ranvier.** See *Ranvier's nodes.* **Parrot's n.,** a syphilitic node on outer table of cranium. **Schmidt's n.,** the medullated interannular segment of a nerve-fiber.

No'dose (no'dōs). Having nodes or projections.

Nodos'ity. 1. A node. 2. The quality of being nodose.

Nod'ular. Marked with, or resembling, nodules.

Nod'ule. 1. A small node or boss. 2. Anterior segment of the inferior vermis of the cerebellum in fourth ventricle.

Noematach'ograph. Device for registering time required in mental operations.

Noematachom'eter. Instrument for measuring the time required in mental operation.

No'li me tan'gere. Rodent ulcer; malignant ulceration.

No'ma (no'mah). Gangrenous sore mouth. **N. puden'di, N. vul'væ,** ulceration of the pudenda of young children.

No'menclature (no'men-kla-chur). System of technical terms; terminology.

No'nan. Recurring every ninth (eighth) day.

Non com'pos men'tis [L.]. Not of sound mind.

Non-conduc'tor. Any substance that does not readily transmit electricity, light, or heat.

Nonip'ara. A woman pregnant for the ninth time.

Non-med'ullated nerve-fiber. Gray nerve-fiber of the sympathetic nerves and ganglia.

Non-met'al. Any element which is not a metal.

No'nus. L. for *ninth;* the hypoglossal nerve.

Non-vi'able. Not capable of living.

No'ri. A Japanese culture-gelatin.

Norm. A fixed or ideal standard.

Nor'ma. A line established to define the aspects of the cranium.

Nor'mal. Agreeing with the regular and established type.

Nor'moblast, Nor'mocyte. A nucleated red blood-corpuscle of the ordinary size.

Norris's corpuscles. Decolorized blood-corpuscles.

Norwe'gian itch. Scabies characterized by pustules and crusts.

Nose. The special organ of the sense of smell. **N.-piece,** device for attaching several objectives to a microscope.

Nose'ma (no-se'mah). Illness or disease.

Nosenceph'alus. A fetus with defective cranium and brain.

Nosochthonog'raphy. Geography of endemic diseases.

Nosog'eny (no-soj'en-e). Same as *Pathogenesis.*

Nosog'raphy (no-sog'raf-e). A description of diseases.

Nosol'ogy (no-sol'o-je). The scientific classification of disease.
Nosoma'nia. Insane belief that one is diseased.
Noson'omy. The classification of diseases.
Nosopar'asite. An organism found in conjunction with a disease which it is able to modify but not to produce.
Nos'ophene (nos'o-fēn). A yellow antiseptic powder.
Nosopho'bia (nos-o-fo'be-ah). Morbid dread of sickness.
Nosopoiet'ic. Causing or producing disease.
Nosotoxico'sis. Poisoning by retained bodily waste.
Nostal'gia. Homesickness or longing for one's native land.
Nostoma'nia. Intense or insane nostalgia.
Nos'trils (nos'trilz). The anterior nares.
Nos'trum. A quack, patent, or secret remedy.
No'tal. Of, or pertaining to, the back; dorsal.
Notal'gia (no-tal'je-ah). Pain in the back.
Notancepha'lia (no-tan-se-fa'le-ah). Absence of back of skull.
Notch. An indentation on the edge of a bone or other organ. **Intervertebral n.,** depression of intervertebral pedicles on upper or lower surface. **Ischiatic n.** See *Sacrosciatic n.* **Jugular n.,** notch forming posterior boundary of jugular foramen. **Nasal n.,** interval between internal angular processes of frontal bone. **Popliteal n.,** depression of posterior surface of head of tibia between two tuberosities. **N. of Rivinus,** defect in osseous tympanic ring filled with Shrapnell's membrane. **Sacrosciatic n.,** one of two notches on posterior border of innominate bone. **Sigmoid n.,** deep impression separating coronoid and condyloid processes. **Suprarenal n.,** depression at top of manubrium. **Suprascapular n.,** notch in superior border of scapula.
Note-blindness. Inability to read musical notes, due to a central lesion.
Notencephal'ocele. Hernial protrusion of brain at the back of the head.
Notenceph'alus. Fetus affected with notencephalocele.
No'tochord (no'to-kord). Rod-shaped body below the primitive groove of the embryo, defining the primitive axis.
Notom'elus. A fetus with accessory limbs attached to the back.
Nox'ious (nox'shus). Hurtful; not wholesome.
Nubec'ula. Slight cloudiness, as of the cornea, or the urine.
Nubil'ity. Marriageableness; fitness to marry: used of the female.
Nu'cha (nu'kah). The nape, back, or scruff of the neck.
Nuck's canal or **diverticulum** (nooks). See *Canal.*
Nu'clear. Of, or pertaining to, a nucleus. **N.-cell,** a nerve-cell made up of a nucleus surrounded by branching protoplasm.
Nu'cleated (nu'kle-a-ted). Having a nucleus or nuclei.
Nucle'ic acid. An acid, $C_{30}H_{62}N_9P_3O_{17}$, derivable from nuclein.
Nu'clein (nu'kle-in). A proteid found in cell-nuclei.
Nuclein'ic acid (nu-kle-in'ik). Same as *Nucleic acid.*
Nucleo-al'bumin. A nuclein from cell-protoplasm.
Nucleohis'ton. A substance from leukocytes, made up of nuclein and histon.
Nucle'olar. Of, or pertaining to, a nucleolus.
Nucle'olus. A nucleus-like body within the nucleus of a cell.
Nucleomi'crosome. Any one of the minute segments of a chromatin fiber.
Nucleop'etal movement. The movement of a male pronucleus toward the female.
Nu'cleoplasm. The achromatin, or unstainable part of a nucleus.
Nucleopro'teid. A nuclein with a relatively large amount of albumin.
Nucleother'apy. Nuclein therapy. See *Therapy.*
Nucleotox'in. A toxin from cell-nuclei; also, any toxin which affects cell-nuclei.

Nu'cleus. 1. A spheroid body within a cell; the core or center of a cell. 2. A mass of gray matter in the central nervous system. **N. abducen'tis**, nucleus of origin of the abducens nerve, a gray mass in the lower part of the pons, near floor of fourth ventricle. **N. ambig'uus**, n. of glossopharyngeal in oblongata. **N. amyg'dalæ**, mass at lateral end of descending horn of lateral ventricle of brain. **N. angula'ris, Bechterew's n.**, group of cells placed dorsad to *Deiters's n.* **Burdach's n.** See *N. funiculi cuneati.* **Caudal n.**, the oculomotor n. **N. cauda'tus**, part of striated n. seen in lateral ventricle. **Cinereous n.**, gray matter of restiform bodies. **Deiters's n.**, in the oblongata, near entry of auditory nerve-roots. **Dentate n.**, gray lamina in central trunk of either hemisphere of cerebellum. **N. embolifor'mis**, small mass near dentate n. and N. fastigii. **N. fasti'gii**, flat mass of gray matter in cerebellum, over roof of fourth ventricle. **Germinal n.**, result of union of male and female pronuclei. **N. gra'cilis**, column of gray substance in the dorsal pyramid of oblongata. **Gray n.**, gray substance of spinal cord. **Hypoglossal n.**, nucleus in the oblongata forming origin of hypoglossal nerve. **Intraventricular n.** Same as *N. caudatus.* **Kölliker's n.**, gray mass around canal of cord. **Laryngeal n.**, n. of origin of nerve-fibers to larynx. **Lenticular n.**, part of corpus striatum external to the third ventricle. **Motor n.**, any collection of cells in central nervous system giving origin to a motor nerve. **Oculomotor n.**, n. of oculomotor nerve under aqueduct of Sylvius. **Olivary n.**, mass of gray matter in oblongata producing a swelling on the surface; olivary body. **Polypous n.**, pulpy mass in center of intervertebral disks. **Pyramidal n.**, inner accessory olivary n. **N. quin'tus**, nucleus of trigeminal nerve. **Red n.**, reddish mass in tegmentum of crus cerebri. **Vesicular n.**, cell-n., the membrane of which stains deeply, while central part is rather pale. **N. vestibula'ris.** Same as *Bechterew's n.* **Vitelline n.**, nucleus produced by fusion of male and female pronuclei in vitellus. **Westphal's n.**, origin of part of trochlear fibers; situated posterior to trochlear n. **White n.**, white part of dentate body.

Nu'el's space. See *Space.*

Nuhn's gland (noonz). Mucous gland on either side of frenum of tongue.

Nullip'ara. A woman who has never born a child.

Nullipar'ity. Condition of being nulliparous.

Nullip'arous (nul-lip'ar-us). Having never born a child.

Numer'ical at'rophy. Atrophy from loss in size and in number of anatomic elements.

Num'miform, Num'mular. Resembling a pile of coins.

Nummula'tion. The assumption of a nummular form.

Nur'ses' contracture. Tetany of nursing women.

Nuta'tion (nu-ta'shun). The act of nodding; to-and-fro movement.

Nut'gall. See *Galla.*

Nut'meg. See *Myristica.* **N. liver**, liver passively congested, often from cardiac disease.

Nu'trient (nu'tre-ent). Nourishing; aiding nutrition.

Nu'triment (nu'trim-ent). Nourishment; nutritious material.

Nu'trin. A nutritive albuminous substance.

Nutri'tion. The process of assimilating food.

Nutri'tious (nu-trish'us). Affording nourishment.

Nu'tritive. Pertaining to, or affording, nutrition.

Nutrito'rium. The apparatus of nutrition.

Nu'trose. A proprietary sodium salt of casein.

Nux vom'ica. Poisonous seed of *Strychnos nux vomica:* it yields strychnin and brucin.

Nyctalo'pia. Night-blindness (less correctly, day-blindness; hemeralopia).
Nyctopho'bia (nik-to-fo'be-ah). Morbid dread of darkness.
Nyctu'ria (nik-tu're-ah). Nocturnal incontinence of urine; habitual urination in bed.
Nym'pha (nim'fah). A labium minus.
Nymphi'tis. Inflammation of a nympha.
Nympho'lepsy. 1. Ecstatic frenzy; morbid exaltation. 2. Surgical removal of the nymphæ.
Nymphoma'nia. Insane sexual desire in a female.
Nymphoma'niac. One who is affected with nymphomania.
Nymphon'cus. Swelling or enlargement of the nymphæ.
Nymphot'omy (nim-fot'om-e). Excision of nymphæ or clitoris.
Nys'sa. Genus of trees. See *Tupelo.*
Nystag'mus. Continuous rolling movement of eyeball. **Cheyne's n.,** a peculiar rhythmical eye-movement. **Lateral n.,** a rolling of the eyes horizontally, or to right and left. **Miners' n.,** a variety of n. peculiar to miners. **Rotatory n.,** rotation of eyes about the visual axis. **Vertical n.,** up-and-down movement of eyes.

O.

O. Symbol of *oxygen;* abbreviation for *oculus,* eye; *octarius,* pint; *opening.*
Oak. See *Quercus.*
Oak'um (o'kum). Prepared fiber from old ropes.
Oa'rium (o-a're-um). Same as *Ovary.*
Ob-. Prefix, signifying *against;* in *front* of, etc.
Obdormi'tion (ob-dor-mish'un). Local numbness from nerve-pressure.
Obduc'tion (ob-duk'shun). A medico-legal autopsy.
Obe'lion. A point on the sagittal suture where it is crossed by line between the parietal foramina.
Obes'ity (o-bes'it-e). Fatness; corpulence.
O'bex. A thickening of ependyma over the calamus scriptorius.
Obfusca'tion. The act of rendering or becoming obscure; a darkening.
Object-blind'ness. Condition in which objects seen make no impression on the mind.
Ob'ject-glass. The lens of a microscope nearest the object.
Objec'tive. 1. Perceptible to the senses. 2. Same as *Object-glass.*
Ob'ligate. Necessary; compulsory. **O. aerobion,** a microbe that cannot live without free oxygen. **O. parasite,** a parasite that is always and necessarily a parasite.
Oblique (ob-leek'). Slanting; inclined.
Obli'quus. See *Muscles, Table of.*
Oblitera'tion. Complete removal, surgical or other.
Oblonga'ta (ob-long-ga'tah). Same as *Medulla oblongata.*
Obses'sion (ob-sesh'un). Demoniacal possession.
Obstet'ric, Obstet'rical. Pertaining to obstetrics.
Obstetric'ian (ob-stet-rish'un). One who practises obstetrics.
Obstet'rics (ob-stet'rix). The art of managing childbirth cases.
Obstipa'tion (ob-stip-a'shun). Intractable constipation.
Obstruc'tion. The act of blocking or clogging; state of being clogged. **Intestinal o.,** any hindrance to the passage of the feces.
Ob'struent. 1. Causing obstruction. 2. An astringent remedy.
Obtund'. To dull or blunt.
Obtun'dent, Obtun'der. A soothing or demulcent agent.
Ob'turator. A disk or plate that closes an opening.

Obtu'sion. A deadening or blunting of sensitiveness.
Occip'ital. Of, or pertaining to, the occiput. **O. lobe,** the posterior portion of the cerebellum, somewhat more extensive than the o. area.
Occipita'lis. The posterior part of the occipitofrontalis.
Occlu'sion. The act of closure, or state of being closed.
Occult'. Obscure or hidden from view.
Occupa'tion neurosis or **disease.** Any affection of nerves due to employment. **O. neuralgia,** pain associated with certain occupation neuroses.
Ocel'lus (o-sel'lus). A simple eye; one of the constituents of a compound eye.
Ochle'sis (ok-le'sis). Disease caused by overcrowding of houses or ships.
Ochron'osus (o-kron'o-sus). A disease marked by yellowness.
Oc'tad. Any octavalent element or radical.
Oc'tan. Recurring on the eighth (seventh) day.
Octa'rius (ok-ta're-us). L. for *Pint.*
Octav'alent. Having the quantivalence of eight.
Octip'ara. A woman pregnant for the eighth time.
Oc'ular. 1. Pertaining to the eye. 2. Same as *Eye-piece.*
Oc'ulist. One who is expert in eye-diseases.
Oculomo'tor. Pertaining to eye-movements. **O. nerve,** the third cranial nerve.
Oculomoto'rius. The oculomotor nerve.
Oculozygomat'ic line. One of Jadelot's lines, said to indicate spinal disease in children.
Oc'ulus (ok'u-lus). L. for *Eye.*
O. D. Abbreviation for *oc'ulus dex'ter,* "right eye."
O'dol. A proprietary salol mouth-wash.
Odontag'ra. Toothache originating from gout.
Odontal'gia. Toothache; pain in a tooth or teeth.
Odonti'asis. Dentition; also, disorder caused by dentition.
Odon'tinoid. A tumor composed of tooth-substance.
Odonti'tis (o-don-ti'tis). Inflammation of a tooth.
Odon'toblast. A connective cell of the kind that forms dentin.
Odontobothri'tis. Inflammation of alveoli of teeth.
Odon'toclast. A cell that helps to absorb the roots of a milk-tooth.
Odontog'eny (o-don-toj'en-e). The development of teeth.
Odontog'raphy (o-don-tog'raf-e). A description of the teeth.
Odon'toid (o-don'toid). Like a tooth.
Odon'tol. A proprietary toothache cure.
Odontol'ogy (o-don-tol'o-je). Scientific study of the teeth.
Odonto'ma (o-don-to'mah). An exostosis on a tooth.
Odontonecro'sis. Necrosis, or massive decay of a tooth.
Odontop'athy (o-don-top'ath-e). Any disease of the teeth.
Odontop'risis. Grinding of the teeth.
Odontortho'sis. The straightening of dental irregularities.
Odonto'sis (o don-to'sis). Dentition; odontogeny.
Odontother'apy. Treatment of diseased teeth.
Odontot'rypy. The boring or drilling of a tooth.
Odorif'erous. Fragrant; emitting an odor.
Odynopha'gia (o-din-o-fa'je-ah). Painful swallowing of food.
Œcoid, Œdema, and other words in **Œ-.** See *Ecoid, Edema,* etc.
Oehl's layer. The stratum lucidum of the epidermis.
Œnantholox'in. Poisonous resin, $C_{17}H_{22}O_5$, from *Œnanthe crocata.*
Offic'ial (of-fish'al). Authorized by pharmacopeias and recognized formularies.
Offic'inal. Regularly kept in stock in druggists' shops.
Ohm (ōm). Electric resistance of a column of mercury one square

millimeter in diameter and 106 centimeters long. **O.'s law.** See *Law.*

Oid'ium al'bicans (o-id'e-um). The fungus that causes thrush.

Oi'koid. Same as *Ecoid.*

Oil. An inflammable liquid not miscible with water. **Almonds, o. of.** 1. Fixed oil from sweet almonds. 2. Volatile o. from bitter almonds. **Amber, o. of,** antispasmodic and rubefacient. **Animal o.** 1. Any oil of animal origin. 2. Empyreumatic oil from bones. **Anise o.,** volatile o. from anise and star anise. **Bay, o. of,** volatile oil of *Myrcia acris;* also, of *Laurus nobilis.* **Ben, o. of,** fixed o. from nuts of *Moringa.* **Ben'ne, o. of,** fixed o. of sesamum seed. **Bergamot o.,** fragrant volatile o. of *Citrus medica.* **Birch, o. of.** 1. Tarry oil of white birch. 2. Volatile oil of black birch. **British o.,** a mixture of petroleum and of various oils. **Cade, o. of,** tarry oil of *Juniperus communis.* **Cajuput o.,** volatile o. of *Melaleuca cajuput.* **Camphorated o.,** liniment of olive-oil and camphor. **Caraway, o. of,** volatile o. from *Carum carui.* **Carron o.,** linseed oil mixed with lime-water: for burns. **Castor-o.,** purgative o. from seeds of *Ricinus communis.* **Citronella, o. of,** volatile oil of grasses, *Andropogon nardus,* etc. **Cloves, o. of,** stimulant volatile oil from cloves. **Cocoa-nut o.,** fixed oil of the cocoa-nut. **Cod-liver o.,** fixed oil of livers of cod-fish. **Cotton-o.,** fixed oil of seed of cotton-plant. **Croton o.,** vesicant purgative oil of seeds of *C. tiglium.* **Cubeb o.,** oil of cubebs. **Dead o.,** a petroleum derivative: antiseptic. **Essential o.** Same as *Volatile o.* **Eucalyptus-o.,** volatile oil of eucalyptus-leaves. **Eulachon, o. of,** fixed oil of candle-fish. **Fatty o.,** any solid or semisolid oil; a fat. **Fir, o. of,** volatile oil of pine-leaves. **Fusel o.,** amylic alcohol. **Haarlem o.,** a proprietary diuretic and stimulant oil. **Heavy o.,** oily product of action of sulphuric acid on alcohol. **Hemlock-o.,** volatile oil from leaves of hemlock-tree. **Herring-o.,** fixed o. of herrings. **Juniper-o.,** volatile oil of juniper-berries. **Lard-o.,** olein from hogs' lard. **Lavender-o.,** oil of various species of lavender. **Lemon-o.,** volatile oil from rind of lemons. **Linseed-o.,** fixed drying oil of flaxseed. **Male fern, o. of,** fixed oil from root of male fern. **Marjoram, o. of,** volatile o. of *Origanum majorana.* **Menhaden, o. of,** fixed o. from menhaden-fish. **Mirbane, o. of.** See *Nitrobenzene.* **Mustard, o. of,** volatile o. of mustard-seed. **Neat's-foot o.,** oil from feet of neat-cattle. **Neroli, o. of,** volatile oil of orange-flowers. **Olive-o.,** fixed oil from fruit of olive-tree. **Orange-o., Orange-berry o., Orange-flower o., Orange-leaf o., Orange-peel o.,** volatile oils derived from the orange. **Palm o.,** fixed oil from fruit of *Elæis guineensis.* **Paraffin-o.,** from coal, shale, or petroleum. **Patchouli, o. of,** volatile o. from patchouli-leaves. **Peanut-o.,** fixed o. from seeds of common peanut. **Pennyroyal, o. of,** volatile o. of pennyroyal. **Peppermint, o. of,** volatile o. of peppermint-leaves. **Petit-grain, o. of,** volatile o. of orange-leaves and shoots. **Poppy-seed, o. of,** fixed oil of poppy-seed. **Porpoise-o.,** fixed o. from blubber of porpoises. **Rape, o. of,** fixed oil from rape-seed. **Rhodium, o. of,** volatile oil from species of convolvulus; also, from *Amyris balsamifera;* also, a factitious mixture resembling the above. **Rock o.,** petroleum. **Rose-o.** See *Attar of roses.* **Rosemary o.,** volatile o. of common rosemary. **Rosin-o.,** volatile o. distilled from rosin. **Sandal-wood o.,** volatile o. of white sandal-wood. **Sassafras o.,** volatile o. of sassafras-root. **Savin o.,** volatile o. of savin-leaves. **Seal-o.,** fat of different species of seal. **Sesame o.,** fixed oil of sesamum-seeds. **Shale o.,** oil distilled from bituminous shales. **Shark o.,** fixed oil from sharks' livers.

Shore-o., variety of cod-liver o. **Sperm-o.**, fixed oil of sperm whale's blubber. **Spike, o. of**, o. of *Lavandula spica*. **Spruce-o.**, volatile o. from leaves and twigs of spruce-tree. **Straits o.**, a variety of cod-liver o. **O.-sugar.** Same as *Elæosaccharum*. **Sunflower-o.**, fixed drying o. from seeds of sunflower. **Sweet o.** See *Olive-o.* **Templin o.**, turpentine from pine-cones. **Turpentine, o. of**, from resinous juice of pine-trees. **Vitriol, o. of**, sulphuric acid. **Volatile o.**, any evaporable oil. **Walnut-o.**, fixed o. from walnut-kernels. **Walrus-o.**, from blubber of walruses. **Whale-o.**, from blubber of various kinds of whales. **Wintergreen, o. of**, from leaves of *Gaultheria procumbens*. **Wood-o.** Same as *Gurjun balsam*. **Ylang-Ylang, o. of**, volatile o. of flowers of *Cananga odorata*.

Oinoma'nia (oi-no-ma'ne-ah). Same as *Enomania*.

Oint'ment. A fatty medicated preparation for external use.

Old sight. Same as *Presbyopia*.

O'lea. 1. L. for *Olive*. 2. Pl. of *Oleum*.

Oleag'inous (o-le-aj'in-us). Oily; greasy.

O'leate. 1. Any salt of oleic acid. 2. A solution of a substance in oleic acid.

Olec'ranon. Curved process from the ulna at the elbow.

Olef'iant gas (o-lef'e-ant). Ethylen, C_2H_4.

Ole'ic acid. A yellow oily liquid from fats: its salts are oleates.

Ol'ein. Oleate of glyceryl; an oily constituent of oils and fats.

Oleobalsam'ic mixture. Alcoholic solution of balsam of Peru with volatile oils.

Oleocre'osote. A solution of creosote in oleic acid: used in phthisis.

Oleo-infu'sion. A preparation made by infusing a drug in oil.

Oleomar'garin. Artificial butter from tallow, lard, etc.

Oleores'in. Any natural combination of a resin and a volatile oil.

O'leum (o'le-um). L. for *Oil*.

Olfac'tion. The act of smelling; sense of smell.

Olfac'tory. Pertaining to the sense of smell. **O. center**, spot in cortex near front end of uncinate gyrus. **O. glomeruli**, coiling fibrillar structures in olfactory bulb.

Olib'anum. Frankincense; a gum-resin from species of *Boswellia*: stimulant emmenagogue.

Olige'mia, Oligæ'mia (ol-ig-e'me-ah). Deficiency in the volume of the blood.

Oligocho'lia (ol-ig-o-ko'le-ah). A lack of bile.

Oligochrome'mia. Insufficiency of hemoglobin in blood.

Oligocythe'mia. Scarcity of red corpuscles in blood.

Oligohe'mia (ol-ig-o-he'me-ah). See *Oligemia*.

Oligohydram'nios. Deficiency of the liquor amnii.

Oligoma'nia. Insanity on a few subjects; impairment of a few mental faculties.

Oligomenorrhe'a. Scantiness of the menstrual flow.

Oligosper'mia. Deficient secretion of semen.

Oligot'rophy (ol-ig-ot'rof-e). Insufficient nutrition.

Oligu'ria (ol-ig-u're-ah). Deficient secretion of urine.

Ol'ivary. Shaped like an olive.

Ol'ive. 1. The tree *Olea Europæa*; also its fruit, the latter affording a valuable oil. 2. Same as *Olivary body*.

Olopho'nia. Defective speech from malformed vocal organs.

Omag'ra. Gout in the shoulder-joint.

Omal'gia (o-mal'je-ah). Pain in the shoulder.

Omarthri'tis. Inflammation of the shoulder-joint.

Omen'tal. Pertaining to the omentum.

Omenti'tis. Inflammation of the omentum.

Omen'tum. A reduplication of the peritoneum going from the stomach to the adjacent organs. **Gastrohepatic o., Lesser**

o., fold joining the lesser curvature to the transverse fissure of the liver. **Great o., Gastrocolic o.,** a fold from the great curve of the stomach enfolding the transverse colon, etc.

Omniv'orous. Eating all kinds of food.

Omoceph'alus. Fetus with no arms and incomplete head.

Omodyn'ia (o-mo-din'e-ah). Rheumatic pain in the shoulder.

Omohy'oid (o-mo-hi'oid). See *Muscles, Table of.*

Omphalec'tomy. Excision of the umbilicus.

Omphal'ic (om-fal'ik). Pertaining to the navel.

Omphali'tis. Inflammation of the navel.

Omphal'ocele (om-fal'os-ēl). Same as *Umbilical hernia.*

Omphalomesenter'ic. Pertaining to umbilicus and mesentery.

Omphalop'agus. Same as *Monomphalus.*

Omphalophlebi'tis. Inflammation of umbilical veins.

Omphal'osite. Monster that cannot live after the navel-string is cut.

Omphalot'omy. The cutting of the navel-string.

On'anism. Masturbation; more correctly, incomplete sexual congress.

On'cograph. A recording instrument attached to the oncometer.

Oncol'ogy (on-kol'o-je). Sum of knowledge regarding tumors.

Oncom'eter. Instrument for measuring variations in size of viscera.

Oncot'omy (on-kot'o-me). The incision of an abscess or tumor.

Onioma'nia. Insane desire to buy or make purchases.

Onobai'o (on-o-bi'o). A deadly African arrow-poison.

Onto'geny (on-tod'jen-e). Development of an organism or ovum.

Onychatro'phia (o-nik-at-ro'fe-ah). Atrophy of the nails.

Onychau'xis (o-nik-awk'sis). Overgrowth of nails.

Onych'ia (o-nik'e-ah). 1. Same as *Paronychia.* 2. Ulceration of matrix of a nail.

Onychi'tis. Inflammation of the matrix of a nail.

Onych'ograph. Instrument for recording variations of blood-pressure in capillaries of finger-tips.

Onychographo'sis. Hooked or curved state of the nails.

Onychomyco'sis. Disease of nails arising from fungi.

Onychoph'agy (o-nik-of'aj-e). Biting or eating of the nails.

Onycho'sis. Disease or malformation of the nails.

O'nyx. A variety of hypopyon.

Onyxi'tis (o-nik-si'tis). Same as *Onychitis.*

O'oblast. A cell whence an ovum is developed.

Oophoral'gia (o-of-o-ral'je-ah). Pain in an ovary.

Oophorec'tomy. Surgical removal of an ovary.

Ooph'orin. An extract from the ovaries of cows.

Oophori'tis (o-of-o-ri'tis). Inflammation of an ovary.

Oophorocysto'sis. Formation of an ovarian cyst.

Oophoroma'nia. Insanity due to ovarian disease.

Oophorosalpingec'tomy. Removal of an oviduct and ovary.

Oophor'rhaphy (o-of-or'raf-e). Fixation by suture of a displaced ovary.

O'osperm (o'o-sperm). A fertilized ovum.

Opac'ity (o-pas'it-e). 1. Condition of being opaque. 2. Opaque spot or area.

Opaque (o-pāk'). Impervious to light-rays; not transparent.

O'pening contraction. A muscular contraction made on breaking the electric circuit.

Opera'tion. An act done with instruments or by the hands of a surgeon.

Op'erative. 1. Pertaining to an operation. 2. Effective; not inert.

Oper'cular (o-per'ku-lar). Pertaining to an operculum.

Oper'culum. 1. A lid or cover. 2. Part of cerebrum over the island of Reil.

O'phryon (o'fre-on). Middle point of transverse supra-orbital line.

Ophthalmec'tomy. Surgical removal of an eye.

Ophthal'mia (of-thal'me-ah). Severe inflammation of the eye. **Catarrhal o.,** simple conjunctivitis. **Caterpillar-o.,** inflammation of the conjunctiva and cornea from penetration by caterpillar's hairs. **Egyptian o.** See *Trachoma.* **Gonorrheal o.,** acute and severe purulent conjunctivitis from gonorrheal infection. **Granular o.,** acute and severe form of purulent conjunctivitis. **Jequirity-o.,** that produced by jequirity-poisoning. **Metastatic o.,** a kind due to metastasis or pyemia. **O. neonato'rum,** purulent ophthalmia of new-born. **Neuroparalytic o.** is due to lesion of branches of fifth nerve or Gasserian ganglion. **Phlyctenular o.,** a form with vesicles on epithelium of cornea or conjunctiva. **Purulent o.,** form with purulent discharge. **Spring o.,** a kind prevalent chiefly in the spring of the year. **Sympathetic o.,** iridocyclitis from disease or injury of fellow-eye. **Varicose o.** is associated with varicose veins of the conjunctiva.

Ophthal'mic. Pertaining to the eye.

Ophthalmi'tis. Inflammation of the eyeball.

Ophthalmoblennorrhe'a. Gonorrheal or purulent ophthalmia.

Ophthal'mocele. Same as *Exophthalmos.*

Ophthalmocó'pia. Fatigue of eyes; eye-strain.

Ophthalmodyn'ia. Neuralgic pain of the eye.

Ophthalmol'ogist. One who practises ophthalmology.

Ophthalmol'ogy. The study of the eye and its diseases.

Ophthalmomala'cia. Abnormal softness of the eyeball.

Ophthalmom'eter. Instrument for measuring the refractive power of the eye.

Ophthalmom'etry. Determination of refractive power of eye.

Ophthalmop'athy. Any disease of the eye.

Ophthalmophthi'sis. Shrivelling of the eye; phthisis bulbi.

Ophthal'moplasty. Plastic surgery of the eye or eyeball.

Ophthalmople'gia. Paralysis of the eye-muscles. **O. exter'na,** paralysis of external ocular muscles. **O. inter'na,** paralysis of iris and ciliary apparatus. **Nuclear o.,** that due to lesion of nuclei of motor-nerves of eye. **Partial o.,** form in which some of the eye-muscles are paralyzed. **Progressive o.,** gradual paralysis of all the eye-muscles. **Total o.** involves the eye-muscles proper, as well as the iris and ciliary body.

Ophthalmopto'sis (of-thal-mop-to'sis). Exophthalmos.

Ophthalmorrhex'is. Rupture of an eyeball.

Ophthal'moscope. An instrument for observing interior of eye.

Ophthalmos'copy. Examination of the eye by means of the ophthalmoscope. **Direct o.,** observation of an upright or erect mirrored image. **Indirect o.,** observation of an inverted image. **Medical o.,** that which is performed for diagnostic purposes. **Metric o.,** that performed for the measurement of refraction.

Ophthal'mostat. Same as *Blepharostat.*

Ophthalmostatom'eter. Instrument for measuring the degree of protrusion of the eyes.

Ophthalmotonom'eter. Instrument used in determining the amount of intra-ocular tension.

Ophthalmotonom'etry. Measurement of tension of eyeball.

Ophthal'motrope. An artificial eye that moves like a real eye.

Ophthalmotropom'eter. An instrument for measuring eye-movements.

Opi'anin (o-pi'an-in). An alkaloid from opium.

O'piate (o'pe-āt). A remedy containing opium.
Opioma'nia. Intense craving for opium.
Opioph'agism. The habitual use of opium.
Opis'thion (o-pis'the-on). Midpoint of lower border of foramen magnum.
Opisthoporei'a. Involuntary walking backward.
Opisthot'ic center (o-pis-thot'ik). The ossification center of petrous bone.
Opisthot'onos. Tetanic spasm which bends the head and feet backward.
O'pium. The dried latex or capsular juice of *Papaver somniferum*, or poppy: narcotic and poisonous. It contains morphin, codein, and many other alkaloids.
O'piumism. Habitual misuse of opium, and its consequences.
Opobal'samum. True balm of Gilead, or Mecca balsam.
Opoceph'alus (o-po-sef'al-us). Fetus with ears fused, one orbit, no mouth, and no nose.
Opodel'doc. Camphorated soap liniment.
Opodid'ymus, Opod'ymus. Fetus with two fused heads and sense-organs partly fused.
Op'pilative. Closing the pores; also, constipating.
Op'ponens. L. for *Opposing*. **O. min'imi dig'iti, O. pol'licis.** See *Muscles, Table of.*
Op'tic, Op'tical. Pertaining to, or subserving, vision. **O. chiasm, O. commissure.** See *Commissure.*
Opticocil'iary. Pertaining to the optic and ciliary nerves.
Opticopu'pillary. Pertaining to optic nerve and pupil.
Op'tics. The science of light and vision.
Op'togram. Visual image formed on the retina.
Optom'eter. Device for measuring power and range of vision.
Optomyom'eter (op-to-mi-om'et-er). Device used in measuring power of the ocular muscles.
Optostri'ate. Pertaining to thalamus opticus and corpus striatum.
O'ra serra'ta. The zigzag anterior edge of retina.
O'ral. Pertaining to the mouth.
Or'ange (or'enj). The tree *Citrus aurantium* and its fruit. **O.-root.** See *Hydrastis canadensis.*
Orbic'ular. Circular; rounded. **O. bone,** ossicle that usually becomes attached to the incus. **O. ligament,** circular ligament that surrounds neck of radius.
Orbicula'ris o'ris. See *Muscles, Table of.* **O. palpebra'rum.** See *Muscles, Table of.*
Or'bit. Bony socket that contains the eye.
Or'bital (or'bit-al). Pertaining to the orbit.
Orchec'tomy (or-kek'to-me). Excision of testicle.
Or'cheoplasty. Plastic surgery of scrotum.
Orchial'gia (or-ke-al'je-ah). Pain in testicle; orchiodynia.
Orchichore'a. Twitching or jerking of testicle.
Orchidec'tomy (or-kid-ek'to-me). Castration or semicastration.
Orchid'opexy (or-kid'o-pek-se). Suturation of a testicle.
Orchidot'omy. Same as *Orchotomy.*
Orchiepididymi'tis. Inflammation of testicle and epididymis.
Or'chiocele (or'ke-o-sēl). Hernial protrusion of a testicle.
Orchiococ'cus. A diplococcus from orchitis.
Orchiodyn'ia (or-ke-o-din'e-ah). Pain in the testicle.
Orchior'rhaphy (or-ke-or'af-e). Same as *Orchidopexy.*
Orchi'tis (or-ki'tis). Inflammation of the testicle.
Orchot'omy. Excision of one or both testicles.
Or'cin (or'sin). A poisonous antiseptic principle, $C_7H_8O_2$, mainly from lichens.
Or'deal bark. See *Casca.* **O. bean.** Same as *Calabar bean.*
Orex'in. A base, $C_{14}H_{12}N_2$: its hydrochlorate is stomachic.

Or'gan. Any part of the body with a special function. **O. of Corti.** Same as *Corti's organ.* **O. of Giraldès.** Same as *Paradidymis.* **O. of Rosenmüller.** Same as *Parovarium.* **O. of Ruffini,** end-organ in finger-tips.

Organ'ic. Pertaining to, or having, organs. **O. acid.** See *Acid.* **O. chemistry.** See *Chemistry.*

Or'ganism. Any individual animal or plant.

Organiza'tion. 1. The process of organizing or being organized. 2. Any organism or organized body.

Or'ganized. Possessing organs.

Organog'eny (or-gan-oj'en-e). The development of organs.

Organog'raphy (or-gan-og'raf-e). The description of organs.

Organolep'tic. Affecting the organism; also, affecting the organs of special sense.

Organol'ogy (or-gan-ol'oj-e). The sum of what is known regarding the organs.

Organopex'ia. Excision of uterine fibroid, in which the uterine wound is sewn to the abdominal wound.

Organother'apy (or-gan-o-ther'ap-e). The treatment of disease by administering animal organs or their extracts.

Or'gasm (or'gazm). Excitement attending venery.

Orien'tal sore. Any furuncular sore endemic in hot countries, as Aleppo boil, furunculus orientalis, and the like.

Orienta'tion. The determining of one's position with respect to surrounding objects.

Or'ifice. The entrance to any bodily cavity.

Orig'anum vulga're, O. majora'na. plants called marjoram: the volatile oil is stimulant and vulnerary.

Or'igin. The more fixed end of a muscle. The central (deep o.) origin of a nerve; also (superficial o.) the point of its emergence from the center.

Orolin'gual. Pertaining to the mouth and tongue.

Orona'sal (o-ro-na'zal). Pertaining to the mouth and nose.

Orophar'ynx. Part of pharynx below nasopharynx.

Or'phol. Betanaphtol-bismuth.

Or'piment. Arsenic trisulphid, As_2O_3; king's yellow.

Orrhorrhe'a (or-o-re'ah). A watery or serous discharge.

Orrhother'apy (or-o-ther'ap-e). Serum-therapy.

Or'ris. Rhizome or root of *Iris florentina:* used in dentifrices, etc.

Or'thin (or'thin). Compound of hydrazin and peroxybenzoic acid: antipyretic.

Orthocephal'ic, Orthoceph'alous. Having a head with a height-length index of from 70 to 75.

Orthochore'a. Choreic movements in the erect posture.

Orthodinitrocre'sol. Same as *Antinonnin.*

Orthodon'tia. Correction of dental irregularities.

Orthog'nathous. Having a gnathic index of less than 98.

Orthom'eter. Instrument for finding the relative protrusion of the two eyeballs.

Orthoped'ic. Pertaining to the correction of deformities.

Orthop'edist. An orthopedic surgeon.

Orthopho'ria. The proper or normal placement of organs.

Orthopne'a, Orthopnœ'a. Inability to breathe except in the upright position.

Or'thopraxy. The mechanical correction of deformities.

Orthop'tic. Correcting obliquity of one or both visual axes.

Or'thoscope. Apparatus which neutralizes the corneal refraction by means of a layer of water: used in ocular examinations.

Orthoscop'ic. Affording a correct and undistorted view.

Orthos'copy. Examination by means of an orthoscope.

Orthot'onos. Spasm which fixes the head, body, and limbs in a rigid straight line.

Ory'za sati'va. The plant that affords rice.

Os. Chemical symbol of *Osmium.*

Os, pl. *o'ra.* L. for *Mouth.* **O. exter'num,** external orifice of canal of cervix uteri. **O. inter'num,** internal orifice of canal of cervix uteri. **O. tin'cæ, O. u'teri,** the orifice of the womb.

Os, pl. *os'sa.* L. for *Bone.* **O. cal'cis,** calcaneum, or heel-bone. **O. cox'æ, O. innomina'tum,** the innominate bone. **O. hama'tum,** unciform bone. **O. mag'num,** the third bone in second row of the carpus. **O. orbicula're,** a bonelet of the ear which usually becomes joined to the incus. **O. pla'num,** a part of ethmoid bone. **O. pu'bis,** the pubes or pubic bone. **O. trique'trum,** a Wormian bone. **O. un'guis,** lacrimal bone.

O'sazone (o'sa-zōn). Any one of a series of compounds obtained by heating sugars with phenyl hydrazin and acetic acid.

Osce'do (os-se'do). The act of yawning.

Oschei'tis (os-ke-i'tis). Inflammation of the scrotum.

Os'cheocele (os'ke-o-sēl). A swelling or tumor of the scrotum.

Oscheohy'drocele. Hydrocele of the sac of scrotal hernia.

Os'cheoplasty. Plastic surgery of the scrotum.

Oschi'tis (os-ki'tis). Same as *Oscheitis.*

Oscita'tion (os-sit-a'shun). The act of yawning.

Os'culum. Any aperture or little opening.

Ö'se (a'zah). A loop of platinum wire inserted into a glass handle.

-osis. A termination signifying *disease* or *morbidity.*

Os'mazome (os'maz-ōm). An extraction from meat.

Os'mic acid. See *Acid.*

Osmidro'sis (os-mid-ro'sis). State in which the sweat has an abnormally strong odor.

Os'mium (oz'me-um). A hard metal; symbol Os.

Osmodyspho'ria. Intense and abnormal dislike of certain odors.

Osmom'eter. 1. Device for testing the sense of smell. 2. Instrument for measuring osmosis.

Osmo'sis. The passage of a fluid through a membrane.

Osmot'ic. Pertaining to osmosis.

Osphresiol'ogy. The science of odors and smells.

Os'sa. L. pl. of *os,* "bone." **O. innomina'ta,** innominate bones. **O. trique'tra,** Wormian bones.

Os'sagen. A calcium salt from red bone-marrow.

Os'sein. Animal matter of bone resembling callogen.

Os'seous. Composed of bone; bony.

Os'sicle (os'sik-l). A little or minute bone; any one of the auditory bonelets.

Ossic'ula (os-ik'u-lah). L. pl. of *Ossiculum.*

Ossiculec'tomy. Surgical removal of the ossicles of the ear.

Ossic'ulum (os-ik'u-lum). L. for *Ossicle.*

Ossif'erous (os-if'er-us). Producing bone.

Ossif'ic (os-if'ik). Forming or becoming bone.

Ossifica'tion (os-if-ik-a'shun). The formation of bone.

Ostal'gia (os-tal'je-ah). Pain in the bones.

Ostearthri'tis. Inflammation of bones and joints.

Ostearthrot'omy. Excision of an articular end of a bone.

Ostec'tomy (os-tek'to-me). Excision of a bone.

Os'tein (os'te-in). Animal matter of bone; ossein.

Ostei'tis. Inflammation of bone. **Condensing o.,** osteitis with hard deposits of earthy salts. **O. defor'mans,** osteitis with distortion of the bones affected. **Gummatous o.,** chronic form with syphilitic gummata. **Rarefying o.,** osteitis with absorption or diminution of earthy matter. **Sclerosing o.** Same as *Osteosclerosis.*

Osteo-an'eurysm. Aneurysm in a bone.

Osteo-arthri'tis. Same as *Ostearthritis.*

Osteo-arthrop'athy. Any disease of the joints and bones.

Osteo-arthrot'omy. Same as *Ostearthrotomy.*
Os'teoblast. Any one of the cells that are developed into bone.
Osteocarcino'ma. Osteoma combined with carcinoma.
Os'teocele. 1. Bony tumor of testis or scrotum. 2. Hernia containing bone.
Osteocephalo'ma. Encephaloid tumor of bone.
Osteochondri'tis. Inflammation of bone and cartilage.
Osteochondro'ma. Osteoma blended with chondroma.
Osteocla'sia, Osteoc'lasis. Surgical fracture or refracture of bone.
Os'teoclast. 1. An instrument for breaking bones. 2. A cell that assists in absorption of bone.
Os'teocope (os'te-ok-ōp). A severe pain in a bone.
Osteocop'ic. Of the nature of osteocope.
Osteocra'nium. Fetal cranium after its ossification.
Osteocysto'ma. A cystic tumor in bone.
Osteoden'tin. Dentin that resembles bone.
Osteoder'mia. A bony formation in the skin.
Osteodyn'ia. Pain in a bone.
Osteo-epiph'ysis (os-te-o-ep-if'is-is). A bony epiphysis.
Osteofibro'ma. Tumor composed of osseous and fibrous tissues.
Os'teogen. Soft material from which bone is formed.
Osteogen'esis, Osteog'eny. The development of the bones.
Osteog'raphy (os-te-og'raf-e). Description of the bones.
Os'teoid (os'te-oid). Resembling bone; bony.
Osteol'ogy. Sum of knowledge regarding bones.
Osteol'ysis. The decay or soft necrosis of bone.
Osteo'ma. A bony tumor; tumor on a bone. **O. denta'le,** dental exostosis. **O. du'rum, O. ebur'neum,** tumor of hard bony tissue. **O. medulla're,** o. containing marrow-spaces. **O. spongio'sum,** one containing cancellated bone.
Osteomala'cia (os-te-o-ma-la'she-ah). Softening of bones.
Osteomyeli'tis. Inflammation of bone-marrow.
Osteonecro'sis (os-te-o-nek-ro'sis). Necrosis of a bone.
Osteoneural'gia (os-te-o-nu-ral'je-ah). Neuralgia of a bone.
Osteop'athy (os-te-op'ath-e). Any disease of bone.
Osteoperiosti'tis. Inflammation of bone and periosteum.
Osteophlebi'tis. Inflammation of the veins of a bone.
Os'teophone (os'te-o-fōn). Same as *Audiphone.*
Osteoph'ony (os-te-of'o-ne). Same as *Bone-conduction.*
Osteophy'ma. Tumor or outgrowth of a bone.
Os'teophyte (os'te-of-it). Osseous tumor upon a bone.
Os'teoplast (os'te-o-plast). Same as *Osteoblast.*
Os'teoplasty (os'te-o-plas-te). Plastic surgery of bones.
Osteoporo'sis. Rarefaction of bone by enlargement of its cavities or formation of new spaces.
Osteopsathyro'sis. Same as *Fragilitas ossium.*
Osteor'rhaphy. The suturing or wiring of bones.
Osteosarco'ma. Sarcoma of a bone; also, sarcoma with bony contents.
Osteosclero'sis. Abnormal hardness of bone.
Osteosteato'ma. A fatty tumor of bone.
Os'teosuture (os'te-o-su-tūr). Same as *Osteorrhaphy.*
Os'teotome. Chisel or knife for cutting bone.
Osteot'omy. The surgical cutting of a bone. **Cuneiform o.,** removal of a wedge of bone. **Linear o.,** the sawing or simple cutting of a bone. **Macewen's o.,** supracondylar section of femur for genu valgum.
Os'teotrite. An instrument for rasping carious bone.
Os'tial (os'te-al). Pertaining to an orifice.
Osti'tis (os-ti'tis). Same as *Osteitis.*
Os'tium. A mouth or orifice. **O. abdomina'le,** fimbriated

end of oviduct. **O. inter'num,** uterine end of oviduct. **O. pharyn'geum,** nasopharyngeal end of Eustachian tube. **O. tympan'icum,** tympanic orifice of Eustachian tube. **O. vagi'næ,** external orifice of vagina.

Otacous'tic. Assisting the hearing.

Otal'gia (o-tal'je-ah). Pain in the ear.

O'taphone. An instrument to assist the hearing.

Othemato'ma. Same as *Hematoma auris.*

Otiat'rics. The therapeutics of ear-diseases.

O'tic. Of, or pertaining to, the ear.

Oticodin'ia (o-tik-o-din'e-ah). Vertigo from ear-disease.

Otit'ic (o-tit'ik). Pertaining to otitis.

Oti'tis. Inflammation of the ear: distinguished as *O. exter'na, inter'na,* or *me'dia,* according as it affects the external, internal, or middle ear. **Furuncular o.,** formation of furuncles in external meatus. **O. labyrin'thica** affects chiefly the labyrinth. **O. mastoid'ea,** o. which involves the mastoid spaces. **O. parasit'ica** is due to a micro-organism. **O. sclerot'ica** is marked by hardening of the ear-structures.

Otoceph'alus. Fetus lacking the lower jaw and having ears united below the face.

Otoclei'sis (o-to-kli'sis). Closure of auditory passages.

Otoco'nia. Collection of dust-like otoliths.

Otoc'onite (o-tok'o-nit). Same as *Otolith.*

O'tocrane (o'to-krān). The chamber in the petrous bone which lodges the internal ear.

O'tocyst (o'to-sist). Same as *Auditory vesicle.*

Otodyn'ia. Pain in the ear; earache.

Otogang'lion. Same as *Otic ganglion.*

Otog'raphy. Description of the ear.

O'tolith (o'to-lith). An ear-stone.

Otol'ogy. Sum of what is known regarding the ear.

Otomassage'. Massage of tympanic cavity and ossicles.

Otomy'ces (o-to-mi'sēz). Genus of fungi infesting the ear. **O. hage'ni** and **O. purpu'reus** have been described.

Otomyco'sis. Disease of ear due to presence of *Otomyces.*

Otoneural'gia. Pain in the ear.

Otoneurasthe'nia. Neurasthenia due to ear-disease.

Otop'athy (o-top'ath-e). Any disease of the ear.

Otopharyn'geal tube. Same as *Eustachian tube.*

O'tophone (o'to-fōn). Same as *Otaphone.*

Otopie'sis. Sinking in or depression of the membrana tympani.

O'toplasty. Surgical correction of deformity or defect of ear.

Otopol'ypus. Polypus in the ear.

Otopyorrhe'a, Otopyo'sis. Purulent discharge from ear.

Otorrha'gia (o-tor-ra'je-ah). Discharge of blood from the ear.

Otorrhe'a (o-tor-re'ah). A discharge from the ear.

Otoscleronec'tomy. Excision of ankylosed ear-ossicles.

O'toscope (o'tos-kōp). Instrument for inspecting or for auscultating the ear.

Otos'teal. Pertaining to the ear-bones or ossicles.

Otot'omy. Dissection or anatomy of the ear.

Otu'ria. The discharge of urine from the ear.

Onaba'in (wah-bah'in). A deadly glucosid, $C_{30}H_{46}O_{12}+7H_2O$, from an African arrow-poison: heart-stimulant and local anesthetic.

Ouli'tis. See *Ulitis,* etc.

Ounce. See *Weights and Measures, Table of.*

Ourol'ogy, etc. See *Urology,* etc.

Out-pa'tient. A hospital patient not treated within the walls.

O'va (o'vah). Pl. of *Ovum.*

O'val (o'val). Shaped like an egg. **O.-window.** Same as *Fenestra ovalis.*

Ovalbu'min. Albumin from the whites of eggs.
Ovar'aden. An extract from ovaries of cows.
Ovaral'gia, Ovarial'gia. Pain in an ovary.
Ova'rian. Pertaining to an ovary.
Ovariec'tomy (o-va-re-ek'tom-e). Excision of an ovary.
Ova'riocele (o-va're-o-sēl). Hernia of an ovary.
Ovariocente'sis. Surgical puncture of an ovary.
Ovariohysterec'tomy. Excision of ovaries and uterus.
Ovarios'tomy. The making of an opening into an ovarian cyst for drainage purposes.
Ovariot'omist. A surgeon who practises ovariotomy.
Ovariot'omy. Surgical removal of an ovary. **Normal o.,** the removal of a healthy ovary.
Ovari'tis. Inflammation of an ovary.
O'vary. The female gland in which ova are formed.
Overexten'sion. Extension beyond the normal limit.
O'verflow. Continuous escape of urine.
Overri'ding. The slipping of either part of a fractured bone past the other.
O'vi albu'men. White of egg.
O'viduct (o'vid-ukt). The canal that conveys ova from the ovary to the uterus.
Ovif'erous. Producing or conveying ova.
Ovifica'tion. Same as *Ovulation.*
O'vigerm. The cell which becomes an ovum.
Ovig'erous. Same as *Oviferous.*
Ovina'tion. Inoculation with sheep-pox.
Ovip'arous. Laying or producing eggs.
O'visac (o'vis-ak). A Graafian vesicle.
O'vi vitel'lus. The yolk of egg.
Ovomu'coid. A mucoid principle from egg-albumin.
Ovovivip'arous. Hatching the eggs within the body.
Ov'ular. Pertaining to an ovum.
Ovula'tion. The formation and discharge of the ovum from the ovary.
Ov'ule. The ovum in the ovary; any small egg-like structure. **Naboth's o.,** any one of the small cysts which result from the obstruction of ducts of glands in the cervix uteri. **Primitive o., Primordial o.,** a rudimentary ovum in the ovary.
O'vum. 1. L. for *Egg.* 2. Female reproductive cell. **Alecithal o.,** one which has no food-yolk, or very little. **Apoplectic o.,** one which is the seat of an extravasation of blood. **Blighted o.,** one in which development becomes arrested after impregnation. **Centrolithal o.,** one in which the formative yolk is arranged in a regular formation around the entire ovum. **Holoblastic o.,** one in which the food-yolk is scanty and is blended with the formative yolk. **Male o.,** a cell-form in diverticula of seminiferous tubules supposed to be an imperfect spermatozoon. **Mesoblastic o.,** one with a large and nearly inactive food-yolk. **Permanent o.,** a complete o. ready for fertilization. **Primordial o.,** any one of the egg-cells which eventually become ovules of the Graafian follicle. **Telolecithal o.,** one in which the food-yolk and formative yolk form each a hemisphere.
Oxac'id. Any acid that contains oxygen.
Ox'alate. Any salt of oxalic acid.
Oxaleth'ylin. A poisonous liquid, $C_6H_{10}N_2$.
Oxalic acid. A poisonous acid, $(COOH)_2$.
Oxalu'ria. Oxalic acid or oxalates in the urine.
Oxalylu'ria. A principle obtainable from uric acid.
Ox'id. Any compound of oxygen with an element or radical.
Oxida'tion. Act of oxidizing, or condition of being oxidized.
Ox'idize. To cause to combine with oxygen.

Ox'yacid (ok-se-as'id). Same as *Oxacid.*
Oxycepha'lia. Conical or sharp-pointed shape of head.
Oxyceph'alus. A head that is pointed or conical.
Oxychlo'rid. An oxid combined with its fellow chlorid.
Ox'ydum (ok'sid-um). L. for *Oxid.*
Oxyecoi'a. Morbid acuteness of the sense of hearing.
Oxyesthe'sia. Abnormal acuteness of the senses.
Ox'ygen. A gaseous element existing free in the air.
Oxygena'tion. Condition of being saturated with oxygen.
Oxyhemoglo'bin (ok-se-hem-o-glo'bin). Hemoglobin charged with oxygen in arterial blood.
Oxyi'odid. An oxid combined with its fellow iodid.
Ox'ymel. A medicated syrup of vinegar and honey.
Oxyn'tic. Secreting an acid substance.
Oxyo'pia. Abnormal acuteness of sight.
Ox'yphil, Oxyph'ilous. Stainable with an acid dye.
Oxyquin'olin. A principle, C_6H_7NO, from quinolin.
Ox'ysalt. Any salt of an oxacid.
Oxyspar'tein. Crystalline substance, $C_{15}H_{24}N_2O$, used hypodermically as a cardiac stimulant.
Oxyto'cic. Hastening childbirth ; also, a drug so acting.
Oxyu'ricide. A drug destructive to oxyuris.
Oxyu'ris vermicula'ris. The seat-worm or pin-worm ; an intestinal parasite.
Oxyvas'elin. Same as *Vasogene.*
Oz. An abbreviation for *Ounce.*
Oze'na, Ozæ'na. A disease with an offensive nasal discharge.
Ozo'cerit, Ozo'kerit. A mineral wax ; useful in skin-diseases.
O'zone (o'zōn). An allotropic form of oxygen : antiseptic and disinfectant.
Ozosto'mia. Foulness of the breath.

P.

P. Symbol of *Phosphorus.*
Pab'ulin. Albuminous substance in blood just after digestion.
Pab'ulum. L. for *Food.*
Pacchio'nian glands, P. bodies (pak-ke-o'ne-an). Small masses of the arachnoid substance in the cranial dura. **P. depressions,** depressions in the skull which lodge the p. glands.
Pachom'eter. Instrument for measuring thickness of body.
Pachya'cria, Pachya'kria (pa-ke-a'kre-ah). Same as *Acromegaly.*
Pachybleph'aron. Thickening of the eyelids.
Pachycephal'ic, Pachyceph'alous (pak-e-sef'al-us). Having thick head or skull.
Pachyceph'aly. Abnormal thickness of skull.
Pachydermat'ocele. Same as *Dermatolysis.*
Pachydermato'sis (pak-id-er-mat-o'sis). Chronic pachydermia ; hypertrophic rosacea.
Pachyder'mia (pak-id-er'me-ah). Hypertrophy of the skin.
Pachye'mia. Thick condition of the blood.
Pachylo'sis (pak-il-o'sis). A thickened, dry, and scaly state of the skin.
Pachymeningi'tis. Inflammation of the dura. **P. exter'na,** inflammation of the external layers of the dura. **P. inter'na,** inflammation of the inner layers of the dura. It is further qualified as *spinal, cranial, hemorrhagic,* etc.
Paci'ni's corpuscles (pah-che'nēz). Oval bodies surrounding certain nerve-endings in the skin.
Pack, Wet pack. A wet sheet to be wrapped about a patient : it is distinguished further as *hot* or *cold.*

Pacquelin's cautery (pahk-lanz'). Same as *Thermocautery.*

Pædiatrics and other words in **Pæ-.** See *Pediatrics*, etc.

Pag'enstecher's ointment. Yellow oxid of mercury in vaselin.

Pag'et's disease (pad'jets). 1. Inflammation of the nipple of a malignant type. 2. Same as *Osteitis deformans.*

Pain (pān). Distress or suffering. **After-p.,** expulsive contractions of the uterus which follow childbirth. **Bearing-down p.,** local pain in various diseases of the female pelvic organs. **False p.,** pains in the latter part of pregnancy which simulate those of labor. **Fulgurant p.,** intense shooting pains, as in locomotor ataxia. **Girdle-p.,** painful sensation as of cord about the waist. **Growing p.,** quasi-rheumatic pains peculiar to early youth. **P.-joy,** hysterical enjoyment of pain. **Lancinating p.,** sharp darting pain. **Osteocopic p.,** pain in bones peculiar to syphilis. **Starting p.,** pain and muscular spasm at the onset of sleep. **Terebrating p.. Boring p.,** a sensation as if a part were pierced with an awl.

Pain'ter's colic. Same as *Lead colic.*

Pal'atal. Pertaining to the palate.

Pal'ate. Roof of the mouth. **Artificial p.,** plate to close fissured palate. **Cleft p.,** congenital fissure of median line of palate. **Hard** or **bony p.,** anterior part of palate. **P.-bone,** bone of the palate and nares. **P.-hook,** hook for raising palate in rhinoscopy. **Soft p.,** part near the uvula.

Pal'atine (pal'at-in). Pertaining to the palate.

Palati'tis (pal-at-i'tis). Inflammation of the palate.

Palatoglos'sus. See *Muscles, Table of.*

Palatog'nathus. Congenital fissure of hard and soft palates.

Palatopharyn'geus. See *Muscles, Table of.*

Pal'atoplasty. Plastic surgery of the palate.

Palator'rhaphy. Same as *Staphylorrhaphy.*

Palatos'chisis (pal-at-os'kis-is). Fissure of palate.

Palatostaphyli'nus. Muscular slip to the uvula.

Palindro'mia. The recurrence of a disease.

Palingen'esis. 1. Regeneration or restoration. 2. Atavism, or reappearance of ancestral characters.

Pal'liative. 1. Affording relief, but not cure. 2. An alleviating medicine.

Pal'lor. Paleness; absence of skin-coloration.

Palm. 1. The hollow or flexor surface of the hand. 2. Any tree of the order *Palmaceæ.* **P.-oil,** fixed oil of *Elæis guineensis.*

Pal'mar. Pertaining to the palm.

Palma'ris. See *Muscles, Table of.*

Palmel'lin. A red pigment from *Palmella cruenta*, an alga.

Palmit'ic acid. See *Acid.*

Pal'mitin. A crystalline principle of fats and oils.

Pal'mos, Pal'mus. 1. Saltatory spasm; jumpers' disease. 2. A throb or leap.

Palpa'tion. The act of feeling with the hand.

Palpe'bra. An eyelid.

Pal'pebral. Pertaining to an eyelid. **P. cartilages.** Same as *Tarsal cartilages.*

Palpebra'lis. See *Muscles, Table of.*

Palpita'tion. Rapid beating of the heart.

Pal'sy (pawl'ze). See *Paralysis.* **Bell's p.,** facial paralysis. **Birth-p.,** palsy from injury received at time of birth. **Crutch-p.,** that due to the pressure of the crutch in the axilla. **Erb's p.,** palsy due to degenerative changes in pyramidal tract of spinal cord. **Hammer-p.,** variety caused by hard work with the hammer. **Lead-p.,** paralysis of arm-muscles from lead-poisoning. **Night-p.,** paresthesia of hands, worse at night. **Scriveners'**

p. Same as *Writers' cramp.* **Shaking p.,** paralysis agitans. **Wasting p.,** progressive muscular atrophy.
Pal'udal (pal'u-dal). Pertaining to, or arising from, marshes.
Pal'udism (pal'u-dizm). Malarial poisoning; impaludism.
Pampin'iform. Shaped like a tendril. **P. plexus.** See *Plexus.*
Pampin'ocele (pam-pin'os-ēl). Same as *Varicocele.*
Panace'a (pan-as-e'ah). A cure-all; a remedy for all diseases.
Panama fever (pah-nah-mah'). Same as *Chagres fever.*
Pan'aris. A whitlow; paronychia.
Panarthri'tis. Inflammation of all the joints.
Pa'nax. See *Ginseng.*
Pancardi'tis. General inflammation of the heart.
Pan'creas (pan'kre-as). A large gland below the stomach.
Pancreatec'tomy. Surgical removal of a pancreas.
Pancreat'ic (pan-kre-at'ik). Pertaining to the pancreas.
Pancreaticoduod'enal. Pertaining to pancreas and duodenum.
Pan'creatin (pan'kre-at-in). A ferment from the pancreas.
Pancreati'tis. Inflammation of the pancreas.
Pancreat'omy, Pancreatot'omy. Incision into pancreas.
Pancreaton'cus. Tumor of the pancreas.
Pandem'ic (pan-dem'ik). A widespread epidemic.
Pan'der's layers. The blastodermic layers.
Pandicula'tion (pan-dik-u-la'shun). The act of stretching and yawning.
Pangen'esis (pan-jen'es-is). The doctrine that in reproduction each cell of the parent body is represented by a particle.
Panhysterec'tomy. Complete extirpation of the uterus.
Pa'nis. L. for *Bread.*
Panneuri'tis. General or multiple neuritis. **P. epidem'ica,** beri-beri.
Pannic'ulus carno'sus. A muscular layer in superficial fascia.
Pan'nus. Abnormal membrane upon the cornea.
Panopep'tone. Proprietary invalid food containing bread and peptonized beef.
Panopho'bia (pan-of-o'be-ah). Vague and persistent dread of some unknown evil.
Panophthal'mia, Panophthalmi'tis (pan-of-thal-mi'tis). Inflammation of all the eye-structures.
Panostei'tis. Inflammation of every part of a bone.
Panoti'tis. Inflammation of internal and middle ear.
Pansper'mia (pan-sper'me-ah). 1. The doctrine that disease-germs are everywhere present. 2. Same as *Biogenesis.*
Pansphyg'mograph. A device that registers both heart- and pulse-movement.
Panthod'ic (pan-thod'ik). Radiating in every direction.
Pantopho'bia (pan-to-fo'be-ah). Same as *Panophobia.*
Pantoscop'ic glasses. Bifocal or Franklin spectacles.
Papa'in. A digestant remedy from papaw fruit.
Papa'ver. L. for *Poppy.*
Papav'erin. A white alkaloid from opium; hypnotic.
Papaw (pa-paw'). The tree *Carica papaya* of tropical America, or its fruit.
Papay'in (pa-pa'in). Same as *Papain.*
Papil'la (pap-il'lah). A small nipple-shaped elevation. **P. lacrima'lis,** a papilla at inner canthus pierced by lacrimal punctum. **P. spira'lis,** spiral ridge formed by Corti's organ.
Pap'illary (pap'il-er-e). Pertaining to a nipple or papilla. **P. muscles.** See *Musculi papillares.* **P. tumor.** See *Papilloma.*
Papilli'tis. Inflammation of optic papilla or disk.
Papillo'ma (pap-il-lo'mah). A tumor made up of hypertrophied papillæ.

Papillomato'sis (pap-il-o-mat-o'sis). Morbid state characterized by formation of papillæ.
Pa'poid. A ferment and digestant from papaw fruit.
Pap'ular (pap'u-lar). Of the nature of papules.
Papula'tion. The formation of papules.
Pap'ule (pap'yūl). A skin papilla; also, a pimple.
Papyra'ceous (pap-ir-a'shus). Like paper; chartaceous.
Paquelin's cautery. See *Cautery*.
Par. L. for *Pair*. **P. va'gum.** The two pneumogastric nerves.
Para-anesthe'sia. Anesthesia of the lower part of the body and of the legs.
Para-appendici'tis. Appendicitis involving nearby structures.
Par'ablast. Part of mesoblast from which blood-vessels are developed.
Parabu'lia (par-ah-bu'le-ah). Perversion of will.
Paracente'sis. Surgical puncture of a cavity; tapping.
Paracen'tral lobule. That convolution of the mesial surface of the brain which corresponds in position with the central convolution.
Paraceph'alus (par-as-ef'al-us). A fetus with defective head and imperfect sense-organs.
Parachlorphe'nol. A crystalline antiseptic and disinfectant.
Parachor'dal. Situated beside the notochord.
Parachro'ma, Parachromato'sis. Skin-discoloration.
Parachro'matin. The nucleoplasm of spindle in karyokinesis.
Paracine'sis (par-ah-sin-e'sis). Disease with perversion of motor powers.
Paracolpi'tis. Inflammation of parts adjoining the vagina.
Paracol'pium. The connective tissue around the vagina.
Paraco'to (par-ah-ko'to). An American bark resembling coto, but better and less pungent.
Paraco'toin. A crystalline principle from paracoto: astringent and antirheumatic.
Parac'risis. Any disease of the secretions.
Paracu'sis (par-ah-ku'sis). Depravement of the hearing. **P. duplica'ta.** Same as *Diplacusis*. **P. lo'ci,** inability to locate correctly the origin of sounds. **P. Willisia'na,** ability to hear best in a loud din.
Paracysti'tis. Inflammation of tissues around the bladder.
Paracys'tium. The connective tissue around the bladder.
Paradid'ymis (par-ah-did'im-is). A body on spermatic cord above the epididymis.
Paradox'ic contraction. Contraction of a muscle when its two ends are forcibly brought near each other.
Paræsthe'sia (par-es-the'se-ah). See *Paresthesia*.
Par'affin (par'af-in). A white waxy substance from petroleum and wood-tar.
Par'aform. White powder, $C_3H_6O_3$: an intestinal antiseptic.
Paragam'macism. Faulty utterance of *g*, *k*, and *ch* sounds.
Parageu'sia (par-ah-gu'zhe-ah). Perverted sense of taste.
Paraglob'ulin. A globulin from blood-serum, blood-cells, lymph, and various tissues.
Paraglobulinu'ria. Discharge of paraglobulin in the urine.
Paraglos'sa. Swelling of the tongue.
Paragra'phia (pah-rag-ra'fe-ah). Central disorder in which the patient writes one word in place of another.
Parahydro'pin. A proprietary diuretic containing theobromin.
Paralac'tic acid. Same as *Sarcolactic acid*.
Parala'lia (par-al-a'le-ah). A disorder of speech.
Paralam'bdacism. Inability to utter correctly the *l* sound.
Paralbu'min (par-ral-bu'min). An albumin from ovarian cysts.

Paral'dehyde (par-al'de-hid). A derivative, $C_6H_{12}O_3$, from aldehyde; hypnotic and anodyne.

Paralex'ia (par-ah-lek'se-ah). Impairment of the power of reading.

Paralge'sia, Paral'gia. Any abnormal and painful sensation.

Par'allax. Any apparent displacement of an object due to change in the observer's position.

Paralo'gia (pah-ral-o'je-ah). Disease of reasoning faculty.

Paral'ysis. Loss of power of voluntary motion or of sensation in a part from lesion of nerve-substance. **P. a'gitans**, shaking palsy; Parkinson's disease. **Alcoholic p.**, that caused by habitual drunkenness. **Ascending p.**, one which progresses cephalad. **Atrophic spinal p.**, poliomyelitis anterior. **Bell's p.**, **Facial p.**, affects the facial nerve. **Birth-p.** See *Birth-palsy*. **Brachial p.**, p. of an arm. **Brachiofacial p.** affects the face and arm. **Brown-Séquard's p.**, p. of motion on one side and of sensation on the other after hemisection of cord. **Bulbar p.**, due to changes in motor centers of oblongata. **Cerebral p.** is caused by some intracranial lesion. **Complete p.**, entire loss of power and function. **Crossed p.** affects one side of face and the other side of body. **Crural p.** affects chiefly the thigh or thighs. **Diphtheritic p.**, that which follows diphtheria. **Diver's p.**, caisson disease. **Duchenne's p.**, labioglossal p. **Erb's p.** See *Birth-palsy*. **Facial p.** See *Bell's p.* **General p.** See *Paresis*. **Glossolabial p.** See *Bulbar p.* **Hysterical p.** may simulate any form of p., and it appears to have no adequate causative lesion. **Incomplete p.**, partial p.; paresis. **Infantile p.**, poliomyelitis anterior. **Infantile spastic p.**, cerebral palsy of childhood. **Klumpke's p.**, atrophic paralysis of muscles of hand with anesthesia. **Kussmaul's p.**, **Landry's p.** See *Ascending p.* **Labial p.**, a form of bulbar p. **Lead-p.** is due to lead-poisoning. **Local p.**, p. of one muscle or one group of muscles. **Multiple p.**, a complication of local paralyses. **Nuclear p.**, one due to lesions in a nucleus of origin. **Obstetrical p.**, birth-palsy. **Ocular p.** See *Cycloplegia* and *Ophthalmoplegia*. **Oculomotor p.** affects the oculomotor nerve. **Periodic p.**, recurrent p., often due to malarial disease. **Pseudobulbar p.** is due to lesions in cerebral centers, and simulates bulbar p. **Pseudohypertrophic p.**, p. marked by enlargement and fatty degeneration of muscles. **Reflex p.**, one ascribable to peripheral irritation. **Spinal p.** See *Poliomyelitis anterior* and *Paraplegia*. **Wasting p.**, progressive muscular atrophy. **Writers' p.**, writers' cramp. For other varieties, see *Hemiplegia* and *Paraplegia*.

Paralyt'ic. 1. Pertaining to, or affected with, paralysis. 2. A person affected with paralysis. **P. dementia**, general paralysis.

Paral'yzant (par-ral'iz-ant). 1. Causing paralysis. 2. A drug that paralyzes.

Paramasti'tis (par-ah-mas-ti'tis). Inflammation of parts around the mammary gland.

Parame'nia (par-am-e'ne-ah). Disorder of menses.

Paramet'ric (par-am-et'rik). Situated near the womb.

Parametris'mus. Pain and spasm of muscle-fibers in the broad ligament.

Parametri'tis. Inflammation of parametrium.

Parame'trium. The tissues around the uterus.

Paramim'ia (par-ram-im'e-ah). Loss of power to make natural gestures and movements.

Parami'tome. Same as *Hyalomitome*.

Paramne'sia (par-ram-ne'zhe-ah). Derangement of the memory.

Paramne'sin. Same as *Thebain*.

Paramor'phia. Abnormality of form.

Paramu'sia (par-ah-mu'zhe-ah). Perversion of the musical faculties.

Paramyoc'lonus mul'tiplex. Paroxysmal clonic muscular contractions.

Paramyosin'ogen. A proteid like myosinogen, from muscle-plasm.

Paramyoto'nia. Impairment of muscular tonicity. **P. congenita'lis.** Same as *Thomsen's disease.*

Paranephri'tis. Inflammation of the suprarenal capsules.

Parane'phrus. A suprarenal capsule.

Paranesthe'sia (par-ran-es-the'ze-ah). Same as *Para-anesthesia.*

Paran'gi (par-rahn'gē). A Ceylonese endemic disease like yaws.

Paranoi'a. Perversion of will with mental eccentricity.

Paranoi'ac. A crank; an erratic person with tendency to insanity.

Paranu'clein. A substance like chromatin in nucleoli of cells.

Paranu'cleus. A body sometimes seen in cell-protoplasm near the nucleus.

Parapar'esis. Partial paralysis of lower limbs.

Parapep'tone. Same as *Antialbumate.*

Parapha'sia. Speech-disorder with misuse of words.

Para'phia (par-a'fe-ah). Disorder of the sense of touch.

Paraphimo'sis. Retraction of foreskin behind the glans penis.

Parapho'nia (par-ah-fo'ne-ah). Morbid alteration of voice.

Paraphra'sia (par-ah-fra'zhe-ah). Disorderly arrangement of spoken words.

Paraphreni'tis. Inflammation around the diaphragm.

Par'aplasm. 1. Any abnormal growth. 2. Same as *Hyaloplasm.*

Paraplas'tic. Having morbid formative power.

Paraplec'tic. Affected with paraplegia.

Paraple'gia (par-ah-ple'je-ah). Paralysis of legs and lower part of body. **Ataxic p.,** a kind due to lateral and posterior sclerosis of the cord. **Cerebral p.** is due to a bilateral cerebral lesion. **Cervical p.** affects especially both arms. **Ideal p.,** reflex p. from emotion. **P. doloro'sa,** with pain, due to neoplasms pressing on cord. **Peripheral p.,** painful variety, due to pressure of neoplasms on nerves. **Primary spastic p.** is said to be caused by degeneration in pyramidal tracts. **Spastic p., Tetanoid p.,** usually due to transverse lesions of the cord or anterolateral sclerosis.

Paraple'gic (par-ah-ple'jik). Pertaining to, or affected with, paraplegia.

Parapoph'ysis. Lower vertebral transverse process.

Parap'oplexy (par-ap'o-plek-se). Slight apoplexy.

Paraprocti'tis. Inflammation of tissues about the rectum.

Parap'sis (par-ap'sis). Morbid sense of touch.

Pararedu'cin. A leukomain from urine.

Pararho'tacism (par-ah-ro'tas-izm). Faulty enunciation of *r* sound.

Parar'thria. Imperfect utterance of words.

Parasalpingi'tis (par-ah-sal-pin-ji'tis). Inflammation of tissues around the oviduct.

Parasig'matism. Imperfect utterance of *s* sound.

Par'asite. A plant or animal living upon a living organism; also, a fetus that takes its sustenance from an autosite or twin fetus. **Facultative p.,** one normally parasitic, but capable of living alone.

Parasit'ic. Of the nature of, or pertaining to, a parasite.

Parasit'icide. A substance destructive to parasites.

Par'asitism. 1. The condition or state of being a parasite. 2. Infestation with parasites.

Parasitogen'ic (par-as-i-to-jen'ik). Due to parasites.

Parasitol'ogy. The sum of knowledge regarding parasites.
Paraspa'dia. Condition in which the urethra opens upon one side of the penis.
Parasynovi'tis. Inflammation of tissues about a synovial sac.
Parasyphilit'ic. Occurring with, but not due to, syphilis.
Parato'loid. Koch's lymph, or tuberculin.
Paratricho'sis. Growth of hair in abnormal situations.
Paratrim'ma. Intertrigo; skin-inflammation due to chafing.
Paratyphli'tis (pah-rat-if-li'tis). Same as *Para-appendicitis.*
Paraxan'thin. A leukomain from healthy urine.
Parax'ial. Situated alongside an axis.
Paregor'ic, P. elix'ir, camphorated tincture of opium.
Pare'ira (pah-ra'ir-ah). Root of *Chondodendron tomentosa:* diuretic and tonic.
Parencepha'lia. Congenital defect of brain.
Parencephali'tis. Inflammation of the cerebellum.
Parenceph'alous. Having a congenital deformity of brain.
Paren'chyma (par-en'kim-ah). The essential or functional elements of an organ as distinguished from its stroma or framework.
Parenchymati'tis. Inflammation of a parenchyma.
Parenchym'atous (par-en-kim'at-us). Of, or of the nature of, parenchyma. **P. pain,** pain at the peripheral end of a nerve.
Parepidid'ymis. Same as *Paradidymis.*
Par'esis. 1. General paralysis. 2. Slight or incomplete paralysis.
Pareso-analge'sia. Incomplete paralysis with analgesia.
Paresthe'sia (par-es-the'zhah). Morbid sensation.
Paret'ic. Affected with, or pertaining to, paresis.
Paridro'sis. Any disorder of the perspiration.
Pari'etal. Of, or pertaining to, the walls of a cavity. **P. bones,** bones which form the sides of the cranium. **P. lobe,** part of cerebrum above the horizontal branch of the fissure of Sylvius, and between the parieto-occipital and Rolandic fissures.
Pari'etes (pa-ri'et-ēz). The walls of a cavity or organ.
Par'is green. Aceto-arsenite of copper.
Park'inson's dis'ease. See *Paralysis agitans.*
Paroccip'ital. Situated beside the occipital bone.
Parol'ivary bodies. Gray masses on dorsal and mesial sides of corpus dentatum.
Paronych'ia (par-on-nik'e-ah). A felon or whitlow; abscess often with periostitis of finger. **P. tendino'sa,** septic inflammation of sheath of tendon of a finger.
Paro-oph'oron (par-o-of'or-on). A relic in the broad ligament of urinary portion of a Wolffian body.
Parop'sis. A disorder of vision.
Paros'mia, Parosphre'sis. Perversion of sense of smell.
Parostei'tis. Inflammation of tissues around a bone.
Parosto'sis. Ossification of tissues outside of the periosteum.
Parot'id. Situated near the ear. **P. duct,** efferent duct of parotid gland; Stenson's duct. **P. gland,** the largest of the salivary glands.
Parotidi'tis, Paroti'tis. Same as *Mumps.*
Parova'rian. Situated near the ovary.
Parovariot'omy. Removal of a cyst of the parovarium.
Parova'rium (par-o-va're-um). A tubular structure of the broad ligament: with the paro-ophoron it represents the embryonic Wolffian body.
Par'oxysm (par'ox-izm). A sudden recurrence or intensification of symptoms.
Paroxys'mal. Recurring in paroxysms.
Parrot-disease, gray. A fatal disease of parrots, due to *Micrococcus psittaci.*

Par'rot's disease. Pseudoparalysis syphilitica. **P.'s nodes,** bony knobs on cranium in infantile syphilis.

Pars'ley. The plant *Apium petroselinum:* diuretic and sedative.

Parthen'icin. Antipyretic alkaloid from *Parthenium Hysterophorus,* a plant of North America.

Par'thenin (par'the-nin). Antipyretic alkaloid from *Parthenium Hysterophorus.*

Parthenogen'esis. Asexual or virginal reproduction.

Partu'rient (par-tu're-ent). Giving birth; pertaining to childbirth. **P. canal,** passage through which fetus is expelled.

Parturifa'cient. A medicine which facilitates childbirth.

Parturiom'eter. Device used in measuring expulsive power of the uterus.

Parturi'tion (par-tu-rish'un). The act of bearing children.

Par'tus. Labor; childbirth; parturition. **P. agrippi'nus,** breech delivery. **P. Cæsa'reus,** delivery by Cesarean operation.

Paru'lis (par-u'lis). Same as *Gum-boil.*

Paru'ria. Discharge of urine from an unusual part.

Par'volin. A ptomain, $C_9H_{13}N$, from decaying fish or horse-flesh.

Par'vule (parv'ūl). A medicinal pellet or granule.

Pas'sion (pash'un). 1. Suffering; pain. 2. Strong emotion. **Iliac p.,** ileus.

Pas'sive. Neither spontaneous nor active. **P. congestion,** congestion due either to lack of vital power or to obstruction.

Pas'sivism. Sexual perversion with subjection of the will to another's.

Pas'sulæ (pash'u-le). L. for *Raisins.*

Paste (pāst). A soft viscid substance; often an escharotic mixture. **Arsenical p.,** caustic p. containing arsenic. **Canquoin's p.,** zinc chlorid mixed with flour and water. **Flour-p.,** flour and water paste used in surgery. **Fruit-p.,** inspissated fruit-juice used in pharmacy. **Jujube-p.,** a fruit-paste originally made of jujubes. **London p.,** caustic soda and quicklime paste. **Phosphorus-p.,** phosphorus made into a paste with flour: a rat poison. **Vienna p.,** caustic paste of potash and lime.

Pasteuriza'tion. The checking of fermentation by heating.

Pas'til, Pas'tille. A troche or lozenge; also, an aromatic mass to be burnt as a fumigant.

Patch. An area differing from the rest of a surface. **Drab-colored p.,** peculiar spot on liver after certain tropical hepatic diseases. **Mucous p.,** a lesion characteristic of syphilis; condyloma latum. **Opaline p.,** a mucous p. of the mouth sometimes seen in syphilis. **Peyer's p.** See *Peyer's patches.*

Patel'la. The knee-cap or knee-pan.

Patel'lar. Of, or pertaining to, the patella.

Pa'tency (pa'ten-se). The condition of being wide open.

Pa'tent (pa'tent). Wide open; patulous.

Pathet'ic (pa-thet'ik). Pertaining to the feelings. **P. muscle.** See *Obliquus muscle,* in *Muscles, Table of.* **P. nerve.** See *Patheticus,* in *Nerves, Table of.*

Pathet'icus. Either nerve of the 4th pair.

Path'etism (path'et-izm). Hypnotism or mesmerism.

Path'finder. Device for locating strictures of the urethra.

Path'ic (path'ik). Pertaining to disease.

Patho-anat'omy. Pathological anatomy.

Path'ogen (path'o-jen). Any disease-producing micro-organism.

Pathogen'esis. The development of morbid conditions or of disease.

Pathogenet'ic, Pathogen'ic. Causing disease; morbific.

Pathog'eny. Same as *Pathogenesis.*

Pathognomon'ic (pa-thog-no-mon'ik). Pointing out the nature of a disease or illness.

Patholog'ic, Patholog'ical. Pertaining to pathology. **P. histology,** histology of diseased tissues.

Pathol'ogy. The sum of what is known regarding diseases. **Cellular p.,** that which regards the cell as the basis of vital phenomena. **Comparative p.,** that which considers human disease-processes in comparison with those of the lower animals. **Experimental p.,** the study of artificially-induced pathologic processes. **General p.** takes cognizance of processes which may occur in various diseases and in different organs. **Humoral p.,** opinion that disease is due to abnormal conditions of the fluids of the body. **Special p.,** study of the pathology of particular diseases or organs. **Surgical p.,** pathology of such diseases as receive surgical treatment.

Pathol'ysis. Dissolution of tissues by disease.

Pathoma'nia (path-o-ma'ne-ah). Moral insanity.

Pathon'omy. Science of the laws of disease.

Pathopho'bia. Morbid fear of disease.

Pa'tient. A person who is undergoing treatment for disease.

Pat'ulous (pat'u-lus). Open; wide open.

Paullin'ia. Same as *Guarana.*

Paulocar'dia (paw-lo-kar'de-ah). Abnormal slowness of heart-beat.

Pave'ment epithelium. Epithelium made up of flattened cells in layers.

Pavil'ion (pav-il'yun). A dilated or flaring expansion at the end of a canal.

Pa'vor noctur'nus. Night-terrors.

Pa'vy's disease. Same as *Cyclic albuminuria.* **P.'s solution,** solution of copper sulphate and Rochelle salt in ammonia water.

Paw'olin. Ptomain, $C_9H_{13}N$, from rotten mackerel.

Paw'paw. 1. Same as *Papaw.* 2. The shrub *Asimina triloba,* and its fruit.

Pb. Symbol of lead (*plumbum*).

P. D. Abbreviation for *Prism-diopter.*

Pearl. A small medicated granule; also, a glass globule with a single dose of volatile medicine. **Epithelial p.** Same as *Pearly body.* **P.-disease,** tuberculosis of lower animals. **Laennec's p.'s,** round masses of sputum in bronchial asthma. **P.-tumor.** Same as *Cholesteatoma.*

Pearl'ash. Impure potassium carbonate in crystals.

Pear'ly body. A form of granule found in epithelioma.

Peat (pēt). Carbonized vegetable matter found in bogs.

Pebrine (peb-rēn'). A bacterial disease of silkworms.

Pec'cant. Unhealthy; causing ill health.

Pecil'oblast (pe-sil'ob-last). Same as *Pecilocyte.*

Pecil'ocyte (pe-sil'os-īt). A malformed blood-corpuscle.

Pecilocyto'sis. Presence of pecilocytes in the blood.

Pecilother'mal. Having cold blood.

Pec'quet's cistern (pek'kāz). Same as *Receptaculum chyli.*

Pec'ten. Same as *Os pubis.* **P. pu'bis.** See *Pectineal line.*

Pec'tic acid. An acid, $C_{32}H_{48}O_{32}$, from pectin.

Pec'tin. One of the carbohydrates of fruits and vegetables.

Pectin'eal. Pertaining to the os pubis. **P. line,** the portion of the ileopectineal line found on os pubis. **P. muscle.** See *Pectineus,* in *Muscles, Table of.* **P. ridge,** anterior or external bicipital ridge of humerus.

Pectine'us (pek-tin-e'us). See *Muscles, Table of.*

Pectin'iform. Shaped like a comb.

Pec'toral. Of, or pertaining to, the chest or breast; good in diseases of the chest. **P. species, P. tea,** a mixture of expectorant and demulcent herbs and aromatics.

Pectora'lis (pek-to-ra'lis). See *Muscles, Table of.*

Pectoril'oquy. Transmission of the sound of spoken words through chest-wall.

Pec'tose (pek'tōs). A principle in unripe fruits which in ripening becomes converted into pectin.

Pec'tus. The breast, chest, or thorax. **P. carina'tum,** chicken-breast or pigeon-breast; undue prominence of sternum.

Ped'al. Pertaining to the foot or feet.

Ped'erast (ped'er-ast). A practiser of pederasty.

Ped'erasty (ped'er-as-te). Unnatural association with boys.

Pediat'rics (pe-de-at'rix). The sum of knowledge regarding children's diseases.

Ped'icle (ped'ik-l). 1. The stem of a tumor. 2. The process which connects the lamina of a vertebra with the centrum.

Pedic'ulate (pe-dik'u-lāt). Provided with a pedicle.

Pedicula'tion. 1. The process of forming a pedicle. 2. Infestation with lice.

Pediculopho'bia (pe-dik-u-lo-fo'be-ah). Insane dread of lice.

Pediculo'sis. Infestation with lice; lousiness.

Pedic'ulus. 1. Same as *Pedicle.* 2. See *Louse.*

Ped'icure (ped'ik-ūr). A chiropodist, or corn-doctor.

Pedilu'vium. L. for *Foot-bath.*

Pediococ'cus. A genus or form of coccus of various species.

Pedobaromacrom'eter. Instrument for measuring and weighing infants.

Pedobarom'eter. Instrument for weighing infants.

Pe'duncle (pe'dung-kl). A stem or supporting part. **Callosal p.,** band which goes on either side from under the callosum to the fissure of Sylvius. **Cerebellar p.'s** (inferior, middle, posterior, and superior), bands of white substance which join the pons and cerebellum. **Cerebral p.** Same as *Crus cerebri.* **Pineal p.,** slender band going forward on either side from pineal body.

Pedun'cular (pe-dung'ku-lar). Pertaining to a peduncle.

Pedun'culate, Pedun'culated. Having a stalk or peduncle.

Peinother'apy. The hunger or starvation cure.

Pela'da, Pelade (pel-ahd'). Same as *Alopecia areata.*

Pelage (pe-lahzh'). The hairy system of the body.

Pelio'ma. A livid patch on the skin in typhoid.

Pelio'sis (pe-le-o'sis). Same as *Purpura.*

Pellag'ra. An endemic disease of Southern Europe, probably caused by eating damaged maize.

Pellagra'zein, Pellagro'cein. Poisonous ptomain from damaged maize.

Pel'let (pel'et). A small pill or granule.

Pelleti'erin (pel-let-e'ar-in). An alkaloid from pomegranate bark: it is destructive to tenia.

Pel'licle (pel'ik-l). A thin scum forming on the surface of liquids.

Pel'litory (pel'lit-or-e). 1. See *Pyrethrum.* 2. A plant of the genus *Parietaria.*

Pel'lotin. A hypnotic alkaloid, $C_{13}H_{19}NO$, from *Echinocactus.*

Pelveoperitoni'tis. Same as *Pelviperitonitis.*

Pel'vic (pel'vik). Pertaining to the pelvis. **P. girdle,** the girdle formed by the innominate bones.

Pelvim'eter. Instrument for measuring the pelvis.

Pelvim'etry. Measurement of capacity and diameter of pelvis.

Pelviot'omy. Cutting of the pelvic bones.

Pel'viotripsy. Crushing of the pelvis.

Pelviperitoni'tis. Inflammation of the pelvic peritoneum.

Pel'vis. 1. The basin formed by the innominate bones, sacrum, and coccyx. 2. The sac in the kidney of which the ureter is the outlet. **P. æquabil'iter jus'to ma'jor,** one unusually but symmetrically large in all directions. **P. æquabil'iter jus'to mi'nor,** one with all its diameters equally reduced. **P., axis of,** the perpendicular to anteroposterior diameter at either inlet or outlet. **Beaked p.**, one with the pubic bones laterally compressed and pushed forward. **Brim of p.**, upper entrance to pelvic space; the inlet, isthmus, margin, or superior strait. **Cordiform p.**, one somewhat heart-shaped. **Diameters of p.**, at brim, are the conjugate, anteroposterior, transverse, and right and left oblique; at outlet, anteroposterior, transverse, and oblique. **False p.**, the part above the iliopectineal line. **Floor of p.**, non-bony material forming lower boundary of pelvis. **Inclination of p., Obliquity of p.**, angle between axis of body and that of pelvis. **Kyphotic p.**, one marked by increase of conjugate diameter at brim with decrease of transverse diameter at outlet. **Malacosteon p.** Same as *Rachitic p.* **Masculine p.**, a woman's pelvis shaped like that of a man. **Nägele's p., Oblique p.**, one with diameters so distorted that the conjugate takes an oblique direction. **Osteomalacic p.**, one affected with osteomalacia. **Planes of p.**, imaginary surfaces which touch all points of the circumference, viz., plane of pelvic expansion and that of p. contraction. **Rachitic p.**, one affected with rickets. **Roberts's p.**, one with a rudimentary sacrum and great narrowing of the transverse and oblique diameters. **Rostrate p.**, one which is simply contracted. **Simple flat p.**, one with shortened anteroposterior diameter. **P. spino'sa**, a rachitic pelvis with the crest of the pubis very sharp. **Split p.**, one with congenital separation at the symphysis pubis. **True p.**, the part below the iliopectineal line.

Pem'phigoid. Like, or resembling, pemphigus.

Pem'phigus (pem'fig-us). A disease marked by formation of bullæ which, after absorption, leave pigmented spots. **P. benig'nus**, a very mild or slight form. **P. circina'tus** has the bullæ arranged in circles. **P. dissemina'tus**, one with scattered bullæ. **P. folia'ceus**, a variety with flaccid scabby bullæ. **P. hyster'icus**, a form ascribed to hysteria, gestation, or disease of sexual organs. **P. malig'nus**, a severe and sometimes fatal type. **P. neonato'rum**, a form occurring in young infants and ascribed to a microbic origin. **P. prurigino'sus**, a kind with severe itching. **P. solita'rius**, a variety with only one bulla. **P. syphilit'icus**, syphilitic eruption of bullæ. **P. veg'etans**, form in which the bullæ are followed by fungoid growths. **P. vulga'ris**, ordinary and uncomplicated p.

Pend'ulous (pend'yu-lus). Hanging loosely; drooping.

Pen'etrating. Piercing; entering deeply. **P. power.** Same as *Focal depth.* **P. wound**, a wound which reaches a natural cavity.

Pe'nial (pe'ne-al). Pertaining to the penis.

Penicil'lium (pen-is-il'e-um). A genus of mould-fungi.

Pe'nile (pe'nil). Pertaining to the penis.

Pe'nis. Male organ of copulation.

Peni'tis (pe-ni'tis). Inflammation of penis.

Penj'deh sore. An ulcer endemic in Asia: probably a kind of oriental boil.

Pen'niform (pen'if-orm). Shaped like a feather.

Pennyroy'al. Plants of the genera *Mentha* and *Hedeoma:* carminative and emmenagogue.

Pen'nyweight. Twenty-four grains Troy weight.

Pen'tad. Any element or radical with a value of five.

Pen'tal. An anesthetic hydrocarbon, C_5H_{10}. See *Amylen.*

Pentamethylendiam'in. Same as *Cadaverin.*

Pen'tane. An anesthetic hydrocarbon, C_5H_{12}.

Pentav'alent (pen-tav'al-ent). Same as *Quinquivalent.*

Pen'tene (pen'tēn). Same as *Amylen.*

Pentos'azon. An abnormal substance occurring in urine.

Pen′tose. Any sugar or hydrocarbon of formula $C_5H_{10}O_5$.
Pentosu′ria. Pentoses in the urine.
Pe′onin. A dye, $C_{19}H_{14}O_3$, used as a test for alkalies and acids.
Peot′omy. Surgical removal of penis.
Pe′po. The pumpkin and its seeds: teniacide and diuretic.
Pep′per (pep′er). Dried fruit of *Piper nigrum*.
Pep′permint. An herb, *Mentha piperita*: leaves carminative and stimulant.
Pep′sic (pep′sik). See *Peptic*.
Pep′sin. A ferment of the gastric juice: used as a remedy for dyspepsia.
Pepsin′ogen. A zymogen from gastric cells which changes into pepsin.
Peptar′nis. Peptone of beef: used as invalid food.
Pepten′zyme. A proprietary antidyspeptic enzyme.
Pep′tic. Pertaining to pepsin or to digestion.
Pepto′genous. Producing pepsin or peptones.
Peptoman′gan. A proprietary preparation of peptone with iron and manganese.
Pep′tone. Any proteid formed by the action of pepsin.
Peptone′mia. Presence of peptones in the blood.
Pep′tonized (pep′ton-īzed). Digested by pepsin.
Pep′tonoid. Any substance resembling a peptone.
Peptonu′ria. Peptones in the urine.
Peptotox′in. Any toxin or poisonous base from peptones.
Peracid′ity (per-as-id′it-e). Excessive acidity.
Peracute (per-ak-ūt′). Very acute.
Per a′num. L. for "by the anus."
Percep′tion. Reception of an impression through the senses.
Perceptiv′ity. Ability to receive sense-impressions.
Per′cerin. White alkaloid from bark of *Geissospermum læve*: tonic and antipyretic.
Perchlo′ric acid (per-klo′rik). An irritant acid, $HClO_4$: it forms perchlorates.
Per′colate (per′ko-lāt). 1. To submit to percolation. 2. Any liquid that has been percolated.
Percola′tion. The extraction of soluble parts of a drug by means of a liquid solvent.
Per′colator. Vessel used in percolation.
Percuss′. To subject to percussion.
Percus′sion. The act of striking a part as an aid in diagnosis. **Auscultatory p.**, p. combined with auscultation. **Immediate p.**, p. in which no pleximeter is used. **Instrumental p.**, that in which a plexor or hammer is used. **Mediate p.**, that in which a pleximeter is employed. **P.-note**, the sound made by percussion. **P.-wave**, principal ascending curve of the sphygmogram.
Percus′sor. An instrument for performing percussion.
Percuta′neous. Performed through the skin.
Perfla′tion (per-fla′shun). The act of blowing air into a space in order to force secretions out.
Per′forans. Any nerve or muscle perforating a part.
Perfora′tion. 1. An act of piercing. 2. A hole through a part.
Per′forator. An instrument for boring the fetal skull.
Perfrica′tion (per-fri-ka′shun). Rubbing with an ointment or embrocation.
Perinac′inous (per-e-as′in-us). Around an acinus.
Periappendici′tis. Inflammation of appendix with its surrounding peritoneum.
Periarteri′tis. Inflammation of tissues about a joint.
Periarthri′tis. Inflammation around a joint.
Periartic′ular (per-e-ar-tik′u-lar). Surrounding a joint.

Periax'ial (per-e-ak'se-al). Situated around an axis.
Periaxil'lary. Around the axilla.
Per'iblast. Protoplasm of a cell outside a nucleus.
Peribronchi'tis. Inflammation of the investment of a bronchus.
Pericar'diac, Pericar'dial. Relating to the pericardium.
Pericardicente'sis. The tapping of the pericardium.
Pericardiot'omy. Surgical incision of pericardium.
Pericardi'tis. Inflammation of the pericardium. **Adhesive p.,** that in which the two layers of pericardium adhere to each other. **Carcinomatous p.,** that associated with malignant disease of the pericardium. **Dry p.,** that without effusion. **External p.,** that which chiefly affects the outer surface of the pericardium. **Fibrinous p., Hemorrhagic p.,** variety in which there is a bloody exudate. **Localized p.,** form with white or milky spots. **Purulent p.,** spots with effusion of purulent fluid. **Serofibrinous p.,** form with serous fluid effusion with a little fibrin. **Tuberculous p.,** that caused by tuberculous disease.
Pericar'dium. Membranous bag which contains the heart. **Bread-and-butter p.,** peculiar appearance in fibrinous pericarditis produced by the rubbing together of two surfaces of pericardial membrane. **Parietal p.,** that fold of p. which is not in contact with the heart. **Shaggy p.,** p. with a shaggy coat of fibrinous exudate. **Visceral p.,** the portion in contact with the heart; epicardium.
Perice'cal (per-es-e'kal). Surrounding the cecum.
Pericementi'tis. Same as *Periodontitis.*
Pericemen'tum. A bony layer surrounding the fang of a tooth.
Perichondri'tis. Inflammation of perichondrium.
Perichon'drium (per-e-kon'dre-um). The membrane which covers the surface of a cartilage.
Perichor'dal. Surrounding the notochord.
Perichoroid'al. Surrounding the choroid coat.
Pericoloni'tis. Inflammation around the colon.
Pericolpi'tis. Inflammation of tissues around the vagina.
Pericon'chal (per-e-kong'kal). Around the concha.
Pericor'neal. Situated around the cornea.
Pericrani'tis (per-ik-ra-ni'tis). Inflammation of pericranium.
Pericra'nium. The periosteum of the skull.
Pericysti'tis. Inflammation of tissues about the bladder.
Periden'tal (per-e-den'tal). Same as *Periodontal.*
Peridesmi'tis. Inflammation of the peridesmium.
Perides'mium. The membrane which invests a ligament.
Peridias'tole (per-e-di-as'to-le). Time between the diastole and systole.
Perid'ymis. The tunica vaginalis testis.
Peridid'ymi'tis. Inflammation of tunica vaginalis of the testis.
Perifis'tular. Situated around a fistula.
Perifollicul'i'tis. Inflammation around the hair-follicles.
Periglot'tis. The mucosa of the tongue.
Perihepati'tis. Inflammation of peritoneum around the liver.
Perilaryngi'tis. Inflammation of tissues around the larynx.
Per'ilymph (per'il-imf). Fluid in the space between the membranous and osseous labyrinths of the ear.
Perimeningi'tis. See *Pachymeningitis.*
Perim'eter. Instrument for measuring the visual field.
Perimetri'tis. Inflammation of perimetrium.
Perime'trium. The peritoneum that enfolds the womb.
Perim'etry (pe-rim'et-re). Measurement of the visual field.
Perimyeli'tis. Inflammation of the pia of the spinal cord.
Perimysi'tis. Inflammation of the perimysium.
Perimys'ium. The tissue that envelops each primary bundle of muscle-fiber.

Perine'al (per-in-e'al). Pertaining to the perineum.
Perine'ocele. Hernia into the perineum; perineal hernia.
Perine'oplasty. Plastic surgery of the perineum.
Perineor'rhaphy. Suturation of the peritoneum.
Perineosyn'thesis. Repair of a lacerated peritoneum by suture and by a flap from wall of vagina.
Perineot'omy. Surgical incision through the perineum.
Perineph'ric (per-e-nef'rik). Around or about the kidney.
Perinephri'tis. Inflammation of peritoneal envelop of kidney.
Perineph'rium. The membrane surrounding the kidney.
Perine'um. Space or area between anus and genitalia.
Perineuri'tis. Inflammation of perineurium.
Perineu'rium. The sheath of a funiculus of nerve-fibers.
Perioc'ular (per-e-ok'u-lar). Around or about the eye.
Pe'riod (pe're-od). An interval or division of time. **Incubation-p.**, time between the implanting of a disease and its appearance. **Monthly p.**, time of menstruation. **Reaction-p.**, stage of rallying from shock after trauma.
Period'ic (pe-re-od'ik). Recurring at certain intervals.
Periodon'tal (per-e-o-don'tal). Around or about a tooth.
Periodonti'tis. Inflammation of periodontium.
Periodon'tium. Fibrous tissue that covers tooth-cement.
Period'oscope (per-e-od'os-kōp). Calendar or dial indicating probable date of parturition.
Peri-oöphori'tis. Inflammation of peritoneum about the ovary.
Perioptom'etry. Measurement of peripheral acuity of vision or of the limits of the visual field.
Perior'bita (per-e-or'bit-ah). Periosteum of the eye-socket.
Perior'bital (per-e-or'bit-al). Around or about the eye-socket.
Periorbi'tis (per-e-or-bi'tis). Inflammation of the periorbita.
Periorchi'tis. Inflammation of the tunica vaginalis of a testis.
Perios'teal (per-e-os'te-al). Pertaining to the periosteum.
Perios'teophyte. Bony growth on periosteum.
Perios'teotome. Instrument for dividing periosteum.
Periosteot'omy. Surgical incision of the periosteum.
Perios'teum. Fibrous sheath of bone.
Periosti'tis. Inflammation of periosteum. **Albuminous p.**, a form accompanied by the exudation of a clear albuminous liquid. **Dental p.** See *Periodontitis.* **Diffuse p.**, p. of the long bones not circumscribed. **Hemorrhagic p.**, that in which blood is extravasated under the periosteum.
Periosto'ma. A bony growth around bone.
Periostomedulli'tis. Inflammation of periosteum and marrow.
Periosto'sis. A bony growth around a bone.
Periostot'omy. Same as *Periosteotomy.*
Periot'ic (per-e-ot'ik). Situated around the ear. **P. bone**, the mastoid and petrous bones together.
Peripachymeningi'tis. Inflammation of substance between the dura and the bone.
Peripancreati'tis. Inflammation of tissues about pancreas.
Periph'erad (per-if'er-ad). Toward the periphery.
Periph'eral. Peripher'ic. Pertaining to the periphery.
Periph'ery (per-if'er-e). An outward part or surface.
Periphlebi'tis. Inflammation of external coat of a vein.
Peri'plast. Protoplasm of a cell outside of the nucleus.
Peripleuri'tis. Inflammation of tissue between pleura and chest-wall.
Peripneumo'nia. Pneumonia; also pleuropneumonia.
Periprocti'tis. Inflammation of tissues outside of rectum.
Periprostati'tis. Inflammation of substance around prostate.
Perirec'tal. Around or about the rectum.
Perire'nal. Around or about the kidney.

Perisalpingi'tis. Inflammation of peritoneum about oviduct.
Periscop'ic (per-is-kop'ik). Affording a wide range of vision.
Perisinui'tis. Inflammation of substance about a sinus.
Perispermati'tis. Inflammation of tissues about spermatic cord.
Perispleni'tis. Inflammation of peritoneal surface of spleen.
Peris'sad. Any element or radical with an odd-numbered valence.
Peristal'sis. Worm-like movement by which the alimentary canal propels its contents.
Peristal'tic (per-is-tal'tik). Of the nature of peristalsis.
Peristaph'yline (per-i-staf'il-in). Situated around the uvula.
Perisys'tole (per-is-is'tol-e). Time between a systole and diastole.
Peritendin'eum. The sheath of a tendon.
Perithe'lium (per-e-the'le-um). Fibrous layer around the capillaries.
Perithyroidi'tis. Inflammation of capsule of the thyroid.
Perit'omy (per-it'o-me). Treatment of pannus by removing a strip of conjunctiva.
Perito'neal. Pertaining to the peritoneum.
Peritone'um. Serous membrane which lines the abdominal walls (*parietal p.*) and the contained viscera (*visceral p.*).
Per'itonism. A condition of shock simulating peritonitis.
Peritoni'tis (per-it-o-ni'tis). Inflammation of the peritoneum. **Adhesive p.,** p. with adhesions between visceral and parietal layers. **Diffuse p.,** that which is not localized. **Puerperal p.,** that which occurs in childbed. **Septic p.,** that due to pyogenic micro-organism. **Serous p.,** that which is attended with copious liquid exudation. **Traumatic p.,** simple acute p. due to traumatism. **Tuberculous p.,** that which accompanies tuberculosis of the peritoneum.
Periton'sillar. Situated around a tonsil.
Peritonsilli'tis. Inflammation of peritonsillar tissues.
Perityphli'tis. Inflammation of tissues around the cecum.
Peri-ureteri'tis. Inflammation of tissues around the ureter.
Peri-u'terine. Surrounding or about the uterus.
Perivagini'tis. Inflammation of tissues around the vagina.
Perivas'cular. Situated or occurring around a vessel.
Perivasculi'tis. Inflammation of a perivascular sheath.
Per'kinism. An obsolete form of metallotherapy.
Perlèche (pâr-lāsh'). Contagious bacterial disease of the mouths of young children.
Per'manent teeth. Teeth of the second dentition.
Perman'ganate. Any salt of permanganic acid.
Per'meable. Not impassable; that may be traversed; pervious.
Perni'cious (per-nish'us). Tending to a fatal issue.
Per'nio. Same as *Chilblain.*
Perobra'chius (per-o-bra'ke-us). Fetus with deformity of feet and arms.
Perocepb'alus. Monster with a deformed head.
Perochi'rus (per-o-ki'rus). Fetus with malformation of hands.
Perome'lus. Fetus with malformed limbs.
Perone'us. See *Muscles, Table of.*
Per'onin. A proprietary anodyne remedy.
Peronos'pora Ferra'ni. A fungus said to cause yellow fever.
Per'opus (per'o-pus). Fetus with malformation of limbs.
Per os. L. for *by the mouth.*
Perox'id. An oxid with more than the normal proportion of oxygen.
Perplica'tion. Closure of a divided vessel by drawing its free end through an incision in its own wall.
Per rec'tum. L. for *by the rectum.*
Per'sonal equation. Difference between time-result of observations made by two different persons.

Perspira'tion. Sweat; also, the function of sweating.

Per tu'bam. Through a tube; especially used of the Eustachian tube.

Pertus'sis (per-tus'sis). Same as *Whooping-cough.*

Peru'vian bark. Same as *Cinchona.*

Pervigil'ium. Sleeplessness; abnormal wakefulness.

Per'vious. Same as *Permeable.*

Pes. 1. L. for *Foot.* 2. Lower or anterior part of crus cerebri. **P. accesso'rius.** Same as *Eminentia collateralis.* **P. anseri'-nus,** the goose's foot; terminal radiation of facial nerve. **P. corvi'nus,** crow's foot; wrinkles at outer canthus of eye. **P. hippocam'pi,** lower end of hippocampus major.

Pes'sary. 1. An instrument placed in vagina to support the uterus or rectum. 2. A medicated vaginal suppository.

Pes'sima. A skin-disease marked by papules and bordered with inflammatory patches.

Pest-house. Hospital for contagious diseases.

Pestif'erous (pes-tif'er-us). Causing a pestilence.

Pes'tilence (pes'til-ens). Any virulent epidemic contagious disease; also, an epidemic of such a disease.

Pestilen'tial. Of the nature of a pestilence.

Pes'tle (pes'sl). An instrument for pounding drugs in a mortar.

Pete'chia (pe-te'ke-ah). A small spot formed by effusion of blood.

Pete'chial (pe-te'ke-al). Characterized by petechiæ.

Petit mal (ptē mahl). Relatively mild form of epilepsy.

Petit's canal (ptēz). Circular channel around the lens. **P.'s operation,** division of the stricture for strangulated hernia. **P.'s triangle,** space between crest of ilium and the latissimus dorsi and external oblique muscles.

Petrifac'tion. Conversion into a stone-like substance.

Pétrissage (pa-três-sahzh'). Kneading action in massage.

Petrola'tum. Same as *Vaselin.*

Petro'leum. A natural oil obtained from wells and springs. **P. ointment,** soft petrolatum.

Pet'rolin (pet'rol in). Same as *Paraffin.*

Petromast'oid. 1. The periotic bone. 2. Pertaining to petrous and mastoid bones.

Petro'sal (pe-tro'sal). Pertaining to the petrous bone.

Petrosalpingostaphyli'nus. The levator palati muscle.

Petroseli'num. Parsley.

Pet'rous (pet'rus). Resembling rock or stone. **P. bone,** the conical hard under part of temporal bone.

Peyer's glands, P.'s patches (pi'erz). Whitish patches of lymph-follicles in mucous and submucous layers of small intestine.

Phaci'tis (fas-i'tis). Inflammation of the eye-lens.

Phacoi'doscope (fa-koi'dos-kōp). Same as *Phacoscope.*

Phacomala'cia (fak-o-mal-a'she-ah). Soft cataract.

Phacosclero'sis. Hardening of the eye-lens.

Pha'coscope. Instrument for viewing accommodative changes of the eye-lens.

Phagede'na (faj-e-de'nah). Rapidly spreading and sloughing ulcer.

Phageden'ic (faj-e-den'ik). Of the nature of phagedena.

Pha'gocyte (fa'go-sit). Any cell that destroys micro-organisms or harmful cells.

Phagocyto'sis. Destruction of injurious cells by phagocytes.

Phaki'tis (fak-i'tis). Same as *Phacitis.*

Phalacro'sis. Same as *Alopecia.*

Phalan'geal (fal-an'je-al). Pertaining to a phalanx.

Phalan'ges. Pl. of *Phalanx.*

Pha'lanx. Any bone of a finger or toe.

Phal'lic (fal'ik). Pertaining to the penis.

Phalli'tis (fal-i'tis). Inflammation of the penis.

Phallon'cus. Tumor or swelling of the penis.

Phal'lus (fal'us). The penis.

Phaner'oscope (fan-er'os-kōp). Instrument for illuminating the skin and rendering it translucent.

Phaneros'copy. Observation of skin by phaneroscope.

Phan'tasm (fan'tazm). An optical illusion; vision resulting from disease.

Phan'tom (fan'tum). 1. A phantasm. 2. A model of body or part thereof.

Phar'macal (far'mak-al). Pertaining to pharmacy.

Pharmaceu'tical (far-ma-su'tik-al). Pertaining to drugs.

Pharmaceu'tics (far-mah-su'tiks). The apothecary's art.

Phar'macist (far'mas-ist). An apothecary or druggist.

Pharmacodynam'ics. The study of the action of drugs.

Pharmacog'nosy, Pharmacog'raphy. The study or science of crude medicines.

Pharmacol'ogy. A treatise on drugs.

Pharmacope'ia. An authoritative treatise on drugs and their preparations.

Phar'macy. 1. The art of preparing and compounding medicines. 2. An apothecary's shop.

Pharyngal'gia. Pain in the pharynx.

Pharyn'geal. Pertaining to the pharynx. **P. arches.** Same as *Visceral arches.*

Pharyngec'tomy. Surgical removal of part of pharynx.

Pharyngis'mus. Muscular spasm of pharynx.

Pharyngi'tis. Inflammation of the pharynx. **Acute p., Catarrhal p.,** that which is due to cold and exposure. **Atrophic p.,** chronic p. which results in wasting of mucous membrane. **Chronic p.,** that which results from repeated acute attacks. **Croupous p.,** that which has the false membrane of true croup. **Diphtheritic p.,** sore throat with the general symptoms of diphtheria. **Granular p.,** a chronic variety in which the mucous membrane becomes granular. **Hypertrophic p.,** that which results in hypertrophy of mucous membrane. **P. sic'ca,** atrophic p. in which the throat becomes dry.

Pharyn'gocele. Hernia of esophagus and pharynx through pharyngeal wall.

Pharyngolaryngi'tis. Inflammation of pharynx and larynx.

Pharyngol'ogy. Scientific study of pharynx.

Pharyngomyco'sis. Bacterial disease of pharynx.

Pharyngople'gia. Paralysis of pharyngeal muscles.

Pharyn'goscope. Instrument for inspecting the pharynx.

Pharyngos'copy. Examination of pharynx.

Pharyngother'apy. Irrigation of nasopharynx in infectious diseases.

Pharyn'gotome (fa-ring'go-tōm). An instrument used in scarifying tonsils, etc.

Pharyngot'omy. Surgical incision of pharynx.

Phar'ynx (far'inx). The musculomembranous sac between the mouth and nares and the esophagus.

Phediure'tin (fe-di-u-re'tin). A diuretic and anodyne phenol preparation.

Phena'cetin (fen-as'et-in). An antipyretic and antirheumatic crystalline remedy, $C_{10}H_{13}NO_2$.

Phenantipy'rin. A phenol antipyretic.

Phe'nate (fe'nāt). A carbolate.

Phen'azone (fen'az-ōn). Same as *Antipyrin.*

Phengopho'bia (fen-go-fo'be-ah). Intolerance or dread of light.

Phen'ic acid. Same as *Carbolic acid.*

Phen'ocoll (fen'o-kol). An antipyretic and analgesic principle, $C_{10}H_{12}(NH_2)NO_2$, from coal-tar.
Phe'nol. Carbolic acid, or any of its homologues.
Phe'nolin. Antiseptic solution of cresol in potassium soap.
Phenolphtha'lein. A yellowish crystalline principle from coal-tar.
Phenosal'yl (fe-no-sal'il). A proprietary mixture of various antiseptic principles.
Phenosuc'cin. An antipyretic and analgesic principle.
Phe'nyl (fe'nil). The radical of carbolic acid, C_6H_5.
Phenylal'anin. An acid decomposition product, $C_9H_{11}NO_2$.
Phenylchi'nolin. A quinin-derivative more active than quinin.
Phenylhy'drazin. A principle, $C_6H_8N_2$: a good test for glucose.
Phenylmeth'ane. An antipyretic and analgesic substance, $(CH_2C_6H_5)_2$.
Phen'ylon (fen'il-on). Antipyrin.
Phenylu'rethan (fen-il-u'reth-ăn). Same as *Euphorin.*
Phi'al (fi'al or vi'al). A small bottle; vial.
Phimo'sis (fi-mo'sis). Tightness of the foreskin, which cannot be drawn back from over the glans.
Phlebec'tasis. Dilatation of a vein or of veins.
Phlebec'tomy (fle-bek'tom-e). Excision of a part of a vein.
Phlebecto'pia. Displacement of a vein.
Phlebi'tis (fle-bi'tis). Inflammation of a vein.
Phleb'ogram (fleb'o-gram). Sphygmographic record of a pulsating vein.
Phleb'olite, Phleb'olith. A venous calculus or concretion.
Phlebol'ogy (fleb-ol'o-je). A treatise on veins.
Phlebosclero'sis. Hardening of the coats of a vein.
Phlebothrombo'sis. Thrombosis of a vein.
Phleb'otome (fleb'o-tōm). A fleam or lancet for venesection.
Phlebot'omist. One who performs a venesection.
Phlebot'omy. Venesection for letting blood.
Phlegm (flem). 1. Mucus. 2. An old name for a supposed bodily humor.
Phlegma'sia (fleg-ma'zhe-ah). Inflammation with fever. **P. al'ba do'lens,** phlebitis of femoral vein in puerperal women.
Phlegmat'ic (fleg-mat'ik). Of dull and sluggish temperament.
Phleg'mon (fleg'mon). Inflammation of connective tissue, leading to ulcer or abscess. **Gas p.,** p. in which gas is formed.
Phleg'monous (fleg'mon-us). Of the nature of, or marked by, phlegmons.
Phlogogen'ic (flog-o-jen'ik). Producing inflammation.
Phlogo'sin (flo-go'sin). Substance, from cultures of *Staphylococcus aureus*, producing abscesses.
Phlogo'sis (flo-go'sis). Inflammation; also, erysipelas.
Phlorid'zin, Phlor'izin. Bitter glucosid, $C_{21}H_{24}O_{10}$, from bark of apple-trees: tonic and antiperiodic.
Phlorogin'cin. A crystalline principle, $C_6H_3(OH)_3$; used as a test for hydrochloric acid.
Phlyctæ'na, Phlycte'na. Vesicle containing a thin ichor or lymph.
Phlyctæn'ula, Phlyc'tenule. A minute vesicle; ulcerated nodule of cornea or conjunctiva.
Phlyc'tenoid. Resembling a phlyctæna.
Phlycten'ular. Associated with the formation of vesicles. See *Conjunctivitis, Keratitis.*
Phlyza'cium (fli-za'she-um). A little pustule.
Phocom'elos. Fetus with hands and feet, but not legs or arms.
Phona'tion (fo-na'shun). The utterance of vocal sounds.
Pho'natory bands. Same as *Vocal cords.*

Phonau'tograph (fo-naw'to-graf). Apparatus for registering vibrations caused by voice.

Phonen'doscope (fo-nen'do-skōp). A stethoscope that intensifies auscultatory sounds.

Phonet'ics (fo-net'iks). Science of vocal sounds.

Phon'ic (fon'ik). Pertaining to the voice.

Phon'ograph (fon'o-graf). Instrument by which sounds can be reproduced.

Phonol'ogy (fo-nol'o-je). Same as *Phonetics.*

Phonom'eter (fo-nom'et-er). Device for measuring intensity of vocal sounds.

Phonop'sia (fo-nop'se-ah). Perception, as of colors, caused by the hearing of sounds.

Pho'rotone. Instrument for exercising muscles of eye.

Phose (fōz). A subjective light-sensation.

Phos'phate (fos'fāt). Any salt of a phosphoric acid. **Acid p.**, any p. in which one or two hydrogen atoms are substituted by metals. **Ammoniomagnesium p.**, **Triple p.**, double salt of magnesium, ammonium, and orthophosphoric acid. **Bone p.**, normal calcium orthophosphate, $Ca_3(PO_4)_2$, of bone. **Earthy p.**, any p. of an alkaline earth. **Normal p.**, one in which three or six hydrogen atoms are replaced by a metal or metals.

Phosphat'ic (fos-fat'ik). Pertaining to, or containing, phosphates. **P. diabetes.** Same as *Diabetes mellitus.*

Phosphatu'ria. Excess of phosphates in the urine.

Phos'phene. A luminous sensation caused by pressing on the eyeball.

Phos'phid (fos'fid). A binary compound of phosphorus.

Phos'phin (fos'fin). Phosphoretted hydrogen, PH_3, a gas and radical.

Phos'phite (fos'fit). Any salt of phosphorous acid.

Phos'phorated (fos'fo-ra-ted), **Phos'phoretted.** Charged with phosphorus.

Phosphores'cence (fos-fo-res'ens). Emission of light without heat.

Phosphorhidro'sis. See *Phosphoridrosis.*

Phosphor'ic acid. See *Acid.*

Phosphoridro'sis. Excretion of luminous sweat.

Phos'phorism (fos'for-izm). Poisoning by phosphorus.

Phos'phorous acid (fos'for-us). See *Acid.*

Phosphoru'ria. Occurrence of phosphorus in the urine.

Phos'phorus (fos'for-us). A non-metallic translucent element, poisonous and very inflammable. **Amorphous p.**, **Red p.**, p. in a dark-red powder, not poisonous. **Metallic p.**, **Rhombohedral p.**, an allotropic form produced by heating ordinary p. **Ordinary p.**, a waxy solid, exceedingly poisonous.

Phosphu'ria (fos-fu're-ah). Same as *Phosphaturia.*

Photal'gia (fo-tal'je-ah). Pain, as in the eye, caused by light.

Photobiot'ic (fo-to-bi-ot'ik). Living only in the light.

Photochem'istry. Science of chemical action of light-rays.

Photo-electric'ity. Electricity developed by the action of light.

Pho'togene (fo'to-jēn). Same as *After-image.*

Photohematachom'eter. A device for making a photographic record of the speed of the blood-current.

Pho'tolyte (pho'to-lit). A substance decomposed by light.

Photom'eter. A device for measuring the intensity of light.

Photom'etry. Measurement of the intensity of light.

Photomic'rograph. Photograph of an object as magnified by the microscope.

Photon'osus. Disease due to too much sunlight.

Photopho'bia (fo-to-fo'be-ah). Abnormal intolerance of light.

Physiog'nomy (fiz-e-og'no-me). Determination of mental or moral character and qualities by the face.

Physiolog'ical. Pertaining to physiology or to the functions of the body.

Physiol'ogy (fiz-e-ol'o-je). Science of the functions of organisms and of organs.

Phy'socele (fi'so-sēl). A tumor containing gas.

Physohydrome'tra. Air or gas and serum in the uterine cavity.

Physome'tra (fi-so-me'trah). Air or gas in the uterine cavity.

Physostig'ma veneno'sum. Poisonous African plant: produces Calabar bean.

Physostig'min. A mydriatic alkaloid from Calabar bean.

Phytal'bumose. Albumose of vegetable origin.

Phytog'enous (fi-toj'en-us). Derived from plants.

Phytolac'ca decan'dra. An American plant; poke: antirheumatic and poisonous.

Phytopathol'ogy. 1. The pathology of plants. 2. Pathology of diseases caused by schizomycetes.

Phy'toplasm (fi'to-plasm). Protoplasm of plants.

Phyto'sis (fi-to'sis). Any disease of bacterial origin.

Phytozo'on (fi-to-zo'on). A zoophyte.

Pi'a, Pi'a ma'ter (pi'ah). The innermost membrane of the brain and cord.

Pia-arachni'tis (pi-ah-ar-ak-ni'tis). Same as *Leptomeningitis*.

Pi'al (pi'al). Pertaining to the pia.

Pi'alyn (pi'al-in). Same as *Steapsin*.

Pi'an (pe'an). Frambœsia, or yaws.

Pian'ists' cramp. Spasm of hand-muscles from continued piano-playing.

Piarrhe'mia (pe-ar-he'me-ah). Lipemia.

Pi'ca (pi'kah). Craving for unnatural articles as food.

Pi'ceous (pi'se-us). Of the nature of pitch.

Pi'chi (pe'tsche). The wood of *Fabiana imbricata*, a South American plant: used in cystitis.

Pic'olin (pik'o-lin). A basic liquid, C_6H_7N, from coal-tar, etc.

Pic'rate (pik'rāt). Any salt of picric acid.

Pic'ric acid (pik'rik). A crystalline dye and fixing agent.

Picrocar'min (pik-ro-kar'min). Compound of carmin and picric acid; a stain.

Pic'rol (pik'rol). A crystalline substitute for iodoform.

Picrotox'in. Poisonous principle from *Cocculus indicus*.

Pie'bald, or Pied, skin. Skin as it appears in leukoderma.

Pie'dra (pe-a'drah). Hair-disease in which nodules form on the shafts.

Pies'meter, Piesom'eter. Instrument for testing the sensitiveness of the skin to pressure.

Pig'ment. A coloring-matter or dyestuff.

Pig'mentary. Pertaining to, or of the nature of, a pigment.

Pigmenta'tion. Deposition of pigmentary matter.

Pil. Abbreviation of *pilula*, pill, or *pilulæ*, pills.

Pil'ary. Pertaining to the hair.

Pilast'ered femur. A fluted state of the femur.

Pil'eous (pil'e-us). Hairy.

Piles (pilz). See *Hemorrhoids*.

Pilig'anin (pi-lig'an-in). Poisonous alkaloid from *Lycopodium saururus*.

Pill. A small, roundish, medicated mass. See *Bland's*, *Blue*, *Cochia*, *Dinner p.*, etc.

Pil'lar. A supporting structure. **P. of the abdominal ring,** a column on either side of abdominal ring. **P's. of the fauces,** folds of mucous membrane at sides of fauces.

in the sphenoid bone in which the p. body is lodged. **P. membrane.** Same as *Schneiderian membrane.*

Pit'urin. Alkaloid, $C_{12}H_{16}N_2$, resembling nicotin.

Pityri'asis. A skin-disease with forming of branny scales. **P. cap'itis.** Same as *Alopecia furfuracea.* **P. circina'ta et margina'ta,** a variety of parasitic origin. **P. circina'ta, P. ro'sea,** p. with reddish scaly patches. **P. gravida'rum,** skin-discoloration peculiar to pregnancy. **P. ru'bra,** p. in which the skin throughout becomes red and scaly. **P. versic'olor,** tinea versicolor.

Pit'yroid. Like bran; branny.

Pix. L. for *Pitch.* **P. Burgun'dica,** resinous exudate of *Abies excelsa;* rubefacient. **P. Canaden'sis,** Canada pitch. See *Pitch.* **P. liq'uida,** L. for *Tar.*

Pix'ol. Disinfectant compound of tar, potash, and soap.

Place'bo. A medicine given to gratify or please a patient.

Placen'ta. The organ within the uterus which establishes a communication between mother and child. **Adherent p.,** one which adheres abnormally to the uterine wall after childbirth. **Annular p.,** one which extends around the interior of uterus like a belt or ring. **Battledore p.,** one with a marginal attachment of the cord. **P. cirsoi'des,** one in which the vessels appear to be varicose. **Duplex p.,** one which is divided into two parts. **Fundal p.,** a normally situated placenta. **Horseshoe p.,** a peculiar form of p. in some cases of twin pregnancy. **Incarcerated p.,** p. retained by irregular uterine contraction. **Maternal p.,** that part of the p. which comes next to the uterine wall: rarely adherent when the rest of the placenta is expelled. **P. membrana'cea,** abnormally thin form of p. **P. præ'via,** p. which intervenes between the intra-uterine cavity and cervical canal; it may lead to a fatal hemorrhage. **Retained p.,** one which is not expelled after childbirth. **Succenturiate p.,** an accessory or subsidiary placenta.

Placen'tal (pla-sen'tal). Of, or pertaining to, the placenta. **P. bruit, P. souffle,** auscultatory sound heard over the placenta in pregnancy.

Placenta'tion (pla-sen-ta'shun). The formation or attachment of placenta.

Placenti'tis (pla-sen-ti'tis). Inflammation of placenta.

Pla'cido's disk (plas'id-ōz). A keratoscopic disk marked with circles.

Pladaro'sis. A soft tumor on the eyelid.

Plagiocephal'ic (pla-je-o-sef-al'ik). Characterized by plagiocephaly.

Plagioceph'alism, Plagioceph'aly. State of having the head asymmetrical and twisted.

Plague (plāg). A highly contagious and fatal fever.

Planocel'lular. Composed of flat cells.

Plan'ta (plan'tah). The sole of the foot.

Plan'tar (plan'tar). Pertaining to the sole.

Planta'ris. See *Muscles, Table of.*

Planu'ria (pla-nu're-ah). The voiding of urine from an abnormal place.

Plaque (plahk). A flat area or plate; also, a blood-platelet.

Plas'ma (plaz'mah). 1. The serum and fibrinogen of the blood. 2. A glycerite of starch. **P. rhex'is,** the bursting of a cell from pressure exerted from within.

Plasmat'ic (plaz-mat'ik). Pertaining to plasma. **P. layer,** layer of blood-plasma next to the walls of a capillary.

Plas'min. A proteid from blood-plasma.

Plasmo'dium mala'riæ. A micro-organism parasitic within the cells of patients having malarial fever.

Plas'mogen (plaz'mo-jen). Bioplasm.

Plasmos'chisis (plaz-mos'kis-is). The splitting up of the plasma of the blood.

Pla'some. Hypothetical unit of living protoplasm.

Plas'son. Protoplasm of a non-nucleated cell or cytode.

Plas'ter. A tenacious preparation applied to the surface of the body. **Adhesive p.,** plaster of resin. **P.-bandage,** bandage stiffened with gypsum. **Blistering p.,** cerate of cantharides. **Court-p.,** plaster of isinglass on silk. **Diachylon p.,** lead-plaster. **P.-jacket,** a thoracic or trunk-bandage stiffened with plaster of Paris. **Lead-p.,** plaster containing lead monoxid; emplastrum plumbi. **Mustard p.,** paste of powdered mustard. **P. of Paris,** calcined gypsum or calcium sulphate. **Strengthening p.,** plaster containing ferric hydrate, pitch, and lead-plaster. **Warming p.,** a pitch-plaster containing cantharides or capsicum.

Plas'tic (plas'tik). Tending to build up tissues. **P. force,** the natural force that builds up tissues. **P. surgery,** surgery that restores lost or defective parts.

Plastic'ity (plas-tis'it-e). The quality of being plastic.

Plas'tid. Any cell or constructive unit.

Plas'tidule (plas'tid-ūl). Smallest unit of living protoplasm.

Plas'tin. One of the proteids of the cell-nucleus.

Plate. A flattened process, chiefly of bone. **Approximation p.,** a plate of bone, or the like, used in intestinal surgery. **Auditory p.,** bony roof of auditory meatus. **Axial p.,** the primitive streak of embryo. **Blood-p.** See *Blood-plaque*. **P.-culture,** bacterial culture in agar or gelatin on a glass plate. **Dorsal p.,** lengthwise ridge on either side on the dorsum of embryo. **End-p.** See *End-plate*. **Foot-p.,** flat portion of stapes. **Medullary** or **Neural p.,** plate of epiblast in embryo developing into neural canal. **Palate-p.,** that part of the palate-bone which forms a lateral half of roof of mouth. **Tarsal p.,** the quasi-cartilaginous substance which gives firmness to an eyelid. **Tympanic p.,** bony plate forming floor and sides of meatus auditorius.

Plat'iculture. Same as *Plate-culture*.

Plat'inode (plat'in-ōd). Collecting plate of an electric battery.

Plat'inum (plat'in-um). Heavy whitish metal; symbol Pt: its chlorids are medicinal.

Platycœ'lous, Platycœ'lous. Having vertebræ distally concave and proximally flat.

Platyceph'alous (plat-is-ef'al-us). Having a wide flat head.

Platycne'mia, Platycne'mism. Flatness of the tibiæ.

Platycne'mic. Having flattened tibiæ.

Plat'ycyte (plat'is-īt). A form of cell seen in tuberculous nodules.

Platyhier'ic (plat-e-hi-er'ik). Having a very wide sacrum.

Platypel'lic, Platypel'vic. Having the pelvis laterally very wide.

Platypo'dia (plat-e-po'de-ah). Flatness of the sole.

Plat'yrrhine. Having a very wide nose.

Platys'ma myoid'es. See *Muscles, Table of*.

Pled'get. A small compress or tuft.

Pleochro'ic, Pleochromat'ic. Showing various colors in varying circumstances.

Pleomas'tia, Pleoma'zia. The condition of having many mammæ.

Pleomor'phic. Occurring in various distinct forms.

Pleomor'phism. Quality of being pleomorphous.

Ple'onasm. An excess of parts.

Plesiomor'phous. Of like or similar form.

Plessim'eter (ples-sim'et-er). Same as *Pleximeter*.

Ples'sor (ples'or). Same as *Plexor*.

Pleth'ora (pleth'o-rah). Vascular turgescence, excess of blood, and fulness of habit.

Plethor'ic (pleth-or'ik). Characterized by plethora.

Plethys'mograph. Instrument for recording variations of parts in size and in blood-supply.

Pleu'ra. The serous membrane investing lungs and lining the thorax.

Pleu'ral. Pertaining to the pleura.

Pleural'gia (plu-ral'je-ah). Pain in the pleura, or in the side.

Pleurapoph'ysis (plu-rah-pof'is-is). A rib, or its homologue.

Pleu'risy (plu'ris-e). Inflammation of the pleura. **Acute p.** is marked by sharp, stabbing pain, fever, friction, fremitus, and to-and-fro friction-sounds. **Chronic p.** includes the dry and serofibrinous kinds. **Diaphragmatic p.** is limited to a spot near diaphragm. **Dry p.**, variety with a fibrinous exudate. **Encysted p.**, that whose effusion is circumscribed by adhesions. **Fibrinous p.** Same as *Plastic p.* **Hemorrhagic p.**, a variety in which there is a bloody exudate. **Ichorous p.**, empyema with with thin offensive pus. **Interlobular p.**, p. enclosed between lobules of the lung. **Latent p.**, that which causes little pain or inconvenience. **Mediastinal p.** affects the pleural folds about the mediastinum. **Metapneumonic p.**, that which depends upon a pneumonia. **Plastic p.** is characterized by deposition of a soft semisolid exudate in a layer. **Purulent p.** Same as *Empyema.* **Serofibrinous p.**, that whose watery exudate contains flocculi, while some fibrin is deposited. **Serous p.** is characterized by free exudation of serum.

Pleurit'ic (plu-rit'ik). Pertaining to, or of the nature of, pleurisy.

Pleuri'tis (plu-ri'tis). Same as *Pleurisy.*

Pleu'rocele (plu'ros-ēl). Hernia of lung-tissue, or of pleura.

Pleurodyn'ia (plu-ro-din'e-ah). Pain of intercostal muscles; also, pain of the pleural nerves.

Pleuroperitone'al cavity. Same as *Cœlom.*

Pleuropneumo'nia. Pleurisy complicated with pneumonia.

Pleurorrhe'a. A pleural effusion.

Pleuroso'mus. Fetus with protrusion of intestine at one side.

Pleurothot'onos. Tetanic bending of the body to one side.

Pleurot'omy. Surgical incision of the pleura.

Plex'iform (plek'sif-orm). Resembling a plexus.

Plexim'eter. 1. A plate to be struck in mediate percussion. 2. Glass plate used to show condition of skin under pressure.

Plex'or. Hammer used in diagnostic percussion.

Plex'us. A network or tangle, chiefly of veins or nerves. **Aortic p.**, nerve plexuses (1) on either side and in front of abdominal, and (2) around thoracic aorta. **Auerbach's p.**, between coats of intestine; sympathetic nerve. **Biliary p.**, network of bile-ducts, said to be sometimes observable in the liver. **Brachial p.**, great nerve-plexus of neck and axilla. **Cardiac p., anterior** or **superficial**, under arch of aorta. **Cardiac p., deep** or **great**, a plexus situated in front of the tracheal fork. **Carotid p., external**, around the external carotid artery. **Carotid p., internal**, on outer side of internal carotid. **Cavernous p.**, in the cavernous sinus. **Celiac p.**, on or near celiac axis. **Cervical p.**, opposite four upper vertebræ. **Cervical p., posterior**, in posterior cervical region. **Choroid p.**, fold of pia in third, fourth, and lateral ventricles. **Coccygeal p.**, near dorsum or coccyx. **Colic p's., right, middle**, and **ileo-**, parts of the superior mesenteric p. **Colic p., left**, part of the inferior mesenteric p. **Coronary p., anterior**, beneath the arch of aorta. **Coronary p., Gastric p.**, at lesser curve of stomach. **Coronary p., posterior**, at dorsum of heart. **Crural p.**, about upper part of femoral artery.

Cystic p., near gall-bladder. **Dental p., inferior,** around roots of teeth of lower jaw. **Diaphragmatic p.**, near phrenic artery. **Epigastric p.** Same as *Solar p.* **Esophageal p.**, about the esophagus. **Facial p.** surrounds part of facial artery. **Gangliform p.**, from roots of origin of inferior maxillary nerve. **Gastric p.**, one of the coronary plexuses of the trisplanchnic. **Gastroduodenal p.**, a branch of the celiac p. **Gastro-epiploic p.**, a portion of celiac p. **Gasto-epiploic p., left,** near convex border of stomach. **Hemorrhoidal p., inferior** and **superior**, near the rectum. **Hepatic p.**, near and in the liver. **Hypogastric p.**, before promontory of sacrum. **Hypogastric p., inferior.** Same as *Pelvic p.* **Ileo-colic p.** See above, under *Colic p.* **Infra-orbital p.**, under levator labii superioris. **Intestinal submucous p., Meissner's p.**, in submucosa of small intestine. **Lingual p.**, around lingual artery. **Lumbar p.**, in psoas muscle. **P. mag'nus profun'dus**, the deep cardiac p. **Mesenteric p., inferior,** around inferior mesenteric artery. **Mesenteric p., superior,** surrounds superior mesenteric artery. **Myenteric p.** Same as *Auerbach's p.* **Nasopalatine p.**, near incisor foramen. **Obturator p.**, around obturator nerve. **Occipital p.**, around occipital artery. **Ophthalmic p.**, about ophthalmic artery and optic nerve. **Ovar an p.** 1. Nerve-p. distributed to ovaries and uterine fundus. 2. Venous p. near ovary. **Pampiniform p.**, network of spermatic veins, or ovarian veins. **Pancreatic p.** supplies the pancreas. **Pancreaticoduodenal p.**, filaments to pancreas and duodenum. **Patellar p.** supplies region in front of knee. **Pelvic p., right** and **left,** supply viscera and other plexuses of pelvis. **Pharyngeal p.** 1. Nerve-p. which supplies the pharynx, etc. 2. Venous p. at side of pharynx. **Phrenic p.**, filaments to diaphragm and suprarenal capsules. **Prostatic p.** supplies the bladder. **Pterygoid p.**, venous p. near internal maxillary vein. **Pulmonary p., anterior** to root and substance of lungs, below and anteriorly. **Pulmonary p., posterior** to root of lungs, dorsal aspect, and lung-substance. **Pyloric p.** supplies region of pylorus. **Renal p.**, near renal artery. **Sacral p.** situated before the sacrum. **Solar p.**, great network on dorsal aspect of stomach. **Spermatic p.**, around spermatic vessels; supplies the testes. **Sphenoid p.**, upper part of internal carotid p. **Splenic p.**, situated around splenic artery. **Subsartorial p.**, at posterior border of sartorius muscle. **Subtrapezius p.**, situated under the trapezius. **Suprarenal p., right** and **left**, around suprarenal capsules. **Thyroid p., inferior** and **superior**, supply larynx, pharynx, and thyroid region. **Tonsillar p.**, to fauces, tonsil, and soft palate. **Tympanic p.** supplies the tympanum. **Uterine p.** 1. Nerve-p. supplies cervix and lower part of uterus. 2. Venous p., between layers of broad ligament. **Vaginal p.** 1. Nerve-p. supplies the vaginal walls. 2. Venous p., near orifice of vagina. **Vertebral p.**, around basilar and vertebral region. **Vesical p.** surrounds the vesical arteries. **Vidian p.** is made up of filaments from Vidian nerve.

Pli'ca (pli'kah), pl. *pli'cæ.* A plait or fold. **P. neuropath'ica,** curled state of the hair caused by nervous disorder. **P. palma'tæ,** folds of the arbor vitæ uterinus. **P. polon'ica,** a matting of the hair with crusts and vermin. **P. semiluna'ris,** fold of mucous membrane on outer canthus of the eye.

Pli'cate (pli'kāt). Plaited or folded.

Plicot'omy (pli-kot'om-e). Surgical division of the posterior fold of the tympanic membrane.

Plum'bic. Containing, or pertaining to, lead.

Plum'bism (plum'bizm). Lead-poisoning.

Plum'bum (plum'bum). L. for *Lead.*
Plum'mer's pills. Compound antimonial pills.
Plum'pers. Devices for extending sunken cheeks, as in artificial dentures.
Pluriloc'ular (plu-ril-ok'u-lar). Multilocular.
Plurip'ara. A woman who has borne several children.
Plurípar'ity. Fact or condition of having borne several children.
Plutoma'nia. Insane belief of the patient that he is very rich.
Pneodynam'ics (ne-o-di-nam'iks). Dynamics of respiration.
Pne'ograph (ne'og-raf). Device for registering respiratory movements.
Pneom'eter (ne-om'et-er). Same as *Spirometer.*
Pne'ophore (ne'o-fōr). Instrument to aid artificial respiration.
Pne'oscope (ne'os-kōp). Same as *Pneumograph.*
Pneumarthro'sis. Presence of gas or air in a joint.
Pneumathe'mia. Presence of air or gas in blood-vessels.
Pneumat'ic (nu-mat'ik). Of, or pertaining to, air or respiration. **P. cabinet,** a cabinet for enclosing a part for treatment with rarefied or compressed air.
Pneumat'ocele (nu-mat'o-sēl). 1. Hernia of lung-tissue. 2. A swelling containing a gas.
Pneumatodyspne'a. Dyspnea from emphysema.
Pneumat'ogram. A tracing made by a pneumatograph.
Pneumat'ograph. Device for registering movements of chest-wall.
Pneumatol'ogy. Science of gases and air and of their therapeutic use.
Pneumatom'eter (nu-mat-om'et-er). Same as *Spirometer.*
Pneumatom'etry. Measurement of respiratory movements.
Pneumat'oscope (nu-mat'os-kōp). Device for determining the absence or presence of pus in the air-cells of the mastoid.
Pneumato'sis (nu-mat-o'sis). Presence of air or gas in an abnormal situation.
Pneumatother'apy (nu-mat-o-ther'ap-e). Treatment by rarefied or compressed air.
Pneumatotho'rax (nu-mat-o-tho'rax). Same as *Pneumothorax.*
Pneumatu'ria (nu-mat-u're-ah). The presence of gas or air in urine.
Pneu'matype (nu'mat-īp). Deposit of moisture from the breath on glass in diagnosis.
Pneumec'tomy (nu-mek'tom-e). Excision of a piece of the lung.
Pneumobacil'lus. The bacillus of pneumonia.
Pneu'mocele (nu'mo-sēl). Protrusion of lung-tissue through chest-wall.
Pneumocente'sis (nu-mo-sen-te'sis). Surgical puncture of a lung.
Pneumococ'cus (nu-mo-kok'us). The diplococcus of pneumonia.
Pneumoconio'sis. Lung-disease due to inhaled dust.
Pneumoder'ma (nu-mo-der'mah). Subcutaneous emphysema.
Pneumoenteri'tis (nu-mo-en-ter-i'tis). Pneumonia and enteritis together.
Pneumogas'tric. Pertaining to the lungs and stomach. **P. lobe.** Same as *Flocculus.* **P. nerve.** See *Nerves, Table of.*
Pneu'mograph (nu'mo-graf). Same as *Pneumatograph.*
Pneumog'raphy (nu-mog'raf-e). Description of lungs.
Pneumohemorrha'gia. Apoplexy of the lungs.
Pneumohemotho'rax. Presence of gas or air and blood in pleural cavity.

Pneumohydropericar'dium. Presence of air or gas with effused serum in the pericardium.

Pneumohydrotho'rax. Presence of gas or air and liquid in the thoracic cavity.

Pneu'molith (nu'mo-lith). A pulmonary concretion.

Pneumomassage'. Air-massage of the tympanum.

Pneumomelano'sis. Melanosis of lung in pneumoconiosis.

Pneumom'eter (nu-mom'et-er). Same as *Spirometer.*

Pneumomyco'sis. See *Pneumonomycosis.*

Pneumonec'tasis (nu-mon-ek'tas-is). Emphysema of lungs.

Pneumonec'tomy. Same as *Pneumectomy.*

Pneumone'mia. Pulmonary congestion.

Pneumo'nia (nu-mo'ne-ah). Inflammation of lungs. **Abortive p.,** a form with a short and favorable course. **Acute p.,** lobar p. of bacterial origin. **Alcoholic p.,** lobar p. of drunkards. **Apex p., Apical p.,** p. limited to the apex of a lung. **Aspiration-p.,** p. due to inhalation of dust, food, or foreign body. **Bronchial p.** See *Bronchopneumonia.* **Catarrhal p.** Same as *Bronchial p.* **Central p.,** lobar p. beginning in the interior of the lobe of the lung. **Cerebral p.,** p. usually apical, with severe head-symptoms. **Cheesy p.,** when the alveoli become filled with necrosed cells and the cut surface looks like cheese. **Chronic fibrous p.,** p. with increase of interstitial and stromatic elements. **Contusion-p.,** p. following injury. **Croupous p.** Same as *Lobar p.* **Deglutition-p.,** p. from food-particles breathed into the lungs. **Desquamative p.** See *Cheesy p.* **Double p.** affects both lungs. **Embolic p.** is due to embolism. **Ephemeral p.,** simple congestion of lungs. **Fibrous p.** See *Chronic fibrous p.* **Gangrenous p.** See *Necropneumonia.* **Hypostatic p.,** that due to dorsal decubitus in weak or aged persons. **Interstitial p.,** chronic fibrous p. **Larval p.,** p. presenting the initial symptoms of the disease only. **Lobar p.** affects one or more lobes of a lung. **Lobular p.,** catarrhal or bronchial p. **Massive p.,** lobar p. with solidification of air-cells, bronchi, or even an entire lung. **Migratory p.,** p. gradually involving one lobe of the lung after another. **Pleuritic p.,** pleuropneumonia. **Pleurogenic p.** is secondary to pleural disease. **Purulent p.** is marked by formation of pus. **Septic p.** is due to septic poison, and is often lobular. **Superficial p.** affects only parts near the pleura. **Syphilitic p.** is due to syphilitic infection, and is of various types. **Typhoid p.,** an asthenic attack with typhoid symptoms. **Wandering p.** attacks various parts of the lung successively, and is probably of erysipelatous origin. **White p.,** infantile syphilitic p. with white fatty degeneration of lung.

Pneumon'ic (nu-mon'ik). Pertaining to the lung, or to pneumonia.

Pneumoni'tis (nu-mon-i'tis). Same as *Pneumonia.*

Pneumon'ocele (nu-mon'os-ēl). Same as *Pneumocele.*

Pneumonoconio'sis. Same as *Pneumoconiosis.*

Pneumonom'eter (nu-mon-om'et-er). Same as *Spirometer.*

Pneumonomyco'sis. Lung-disease caused by schizomycetes.

Pneumonop'athy (nu-mo-nop'ath-e). Any lung-disease.

Pneumono'sis (nu-mo-no'sis). Any lung-disease.

Pneumonot'omy. See *Pneumotomy.*

Pneumopal'udism. Malarial disease of the lungs.

Pneumopericar'dium. Air or gas in pericardium.

Pneumoperitone'um. Gas in the peritoneal cavity.

Pneumoperitoni'tis. Peritonitis with formation of gas.

Pneumopyopericar'dium. Air or gas and pus in the pericardium.

Pneumopyotho'rax. Presence of air and pus in the pleural cavity.

Pneumorrha'gia (nu-mor-ra'je-ah). Hemorrhage from the lungs.

Pneumoserotho'rax. Presence of gas and serum in pleural cavity.

Pneumother'apy (nu-mo-ther'ap-e). 1. Treatment of disease of lungs. 2. Same as *Pneumatotherapy.*

Pneumotho'rax (nu-mo-tho'rax). Gas or air in the pleural cavity.

Pneumot'omy (nu-mot'om-e). Surgical incision of a lung.

Pneumotox'in. A toxin produced by the bacteria of pneumonia.

Pneumoty'phus. Pneumonia concurrent with typhoid fever.

Pneumo-u'ria. Same as *Pneumaturia.*

Pock. A pustule, especially of smallpox. **P.-marked,** pitted or scarred, as a result of smallpox.

Pock'eting. Enclosure of the pedicle in ovariotomy within the edges of the external wound.

Podag'ra (pod-ag'rah). The gout.

Podal'gia (po-dal'je-ah). Pain in the feet.

Podal'ic version. Conversion of a more untoward presentation into a footling presentation.

Podarthri'tis (pod-ar-thri'tis). See *Podagra.*

Podelco'ma. Same as *Mycetoma.*

Podenceph'alus. Monster with the head held on by a mere pedicle.

Podobromidro'sis. Fetid perspiration of the feet.

Pododyn'ia (pod-od-in'e-ah). Pain in the feet.

Podophyl'lin (pod-of-il'in). The yellow purgative resin of podophyllum.

Podophyllotox'in. A poisonous principle from podophyllum.

Podophyl'lum pelta'tum. May-apple or mandrake: the root is purgative.

Pœ. For words thus beginning, see *Pe-.*

Pogoni'asis. Excessive or abnormal growth of the beard.

Pogo'nion. The anterior mid-point of the chin.

Poikil'ocyte (poi-kil'o-sit). A malformed blood-corpuscle.

Poikilocyto'sis. Presence of poikilocytes in the blood.

Poikilother'mal (poi-kil-o-ther'mal). Having cold blood.

Point, anterior focal, one of the cardinal points of the eye. **Cardinal p.,** any one of a set of six points of reference in the eye, or of four in pelvic inlet. **Craniometric p.,** any one of a set of points of reference used in craniometry. **Dew-p.,** temperature at which the dew begins to be deposited. **Disparate p's.,** points on the retinæ which are not paired exactly. **Far-p.** See *Far-p.* **Hysterogenic p.,** point on which if pressure be made a hysteric attack may be produced. **Lacrimal p's.** See *Puncta lacrimalia.* **McBurney's p's.,** points of special tenderness in appendicitis. **Malar p.,** point on external tubercle of malar bone. **Motor-p.** 1. Point at which a motor nerve enters a muscle. 2. Point whereon if galvanic stimulation be applied it will cause contraction of a corresponding muscle. **Near-p.** See *Near-p.* **Nodal p's.,** two cardinal points on posterior surface of lens. **P. of election,** point at which a certain operation is to be done by preference. **Posterior focal p.,** point on retina at which rays parallel to axis will converge. **Principal p's.,** two points on optic axis in anterior chamber of eye. **Valleix's p's.,** tender points on course of certain nerves in neuralgia.

Pointillage (pwahn-tel-yahz'). Massage with the points of the fingers.

Points douloureux (pwah doo-loo-ruh'). Same as *Valleix's points,* under *Point.*

Poiseuille's space (pwah-za-iz'). Space near the periphery of a blood-vessel entirely free from corpuscles.

Poi'son (poi'zn). Any substance which when applied to the body, or ingested, causes disease.

Poitrinaires (pwah-trin-ārz'). Patients with chronic chest-disease.

Poke. See *Phytolacca;* also *Veratrum viride.*

Po'lar. Of, or pertaining to, a pole. **P. bodies, P. cells, P. granules,** two cells which protrude from the unfertilized ovum, and later become detached. **P. stars,** the star-like figures of the diaster.

Polarim'eter (po-lar-im'et-er). Device for measuring the rotation of polarized light.

Polarim'etry (po-lar-im'et-re). Measurement of the rotation of polarized light.

Polar'iscope (po-lar'is-kōp). Instrument for the study of polarization.

Polar'ity (po-lar'it-e). Condition of having poles or of exhibiting opposite effects at the two extremities. **P. of a nerve,** a state in which a nerve exhibits both anelectrotonus and catelectrotonus.

Polariza'tion. The production of that condition in light by virtue of which its vibrations take place all in one plane, or else in circles and ellipses.

Po'larizer. An appliance for polarizing light.

Policlin'ic. A city hospital or infirmary.

Poliencephali'tis. Inflammation of gray substance of brain.

Poliomyelencephali'tis. Poliomyelitis combined with polioencephalitis.

Poliomyeli'tis (pol-e-o-mi-el-i'tis). Inflammation of gray substance of spinal cord. **Anterior p.,** acute inflammation of anterior horns of gray substance in spinal cord. **Ascending p.,** p. with a cephalad progression. **Chronic p.** Same as *Progressive muscular atrophy.*

Poliomyelop'athy. Any disorder of the gray matter of the myelon.

Po'lioplasm (po'le-o-plazm). See *Protoplasm.*

Polio'sis (pol-e-o'sis). Calvities; also premature grayness.

Po'lish plait. Same as *Plica polonica.*

Politzeriza'tion. Inflation of middle ear by means of Politzer's bag.

Pol'itzer's bag. Rubber bag for driving air through a Eustachian tube.

Pollakiu'ria (pol-la-ki-u're-ah). Unduly frequent passage of urine.

Pol'lex. L. for *Thumb.* **P. pe'dis.** great toe; hallux.

Pollu'tion. Discharge of semen without coition.

Polyade'nia (pol-e-ad-e'ne-ah). Same as *Pseudoleukemia.*

Polyad'enous (pol-e-ad'en-us). Having many glands.

Polyarthri'tis. Inflammation of several joints together.

Polyatom'ic (pol-e-at-om'ik). Made up of several atoms.

Polycho'lia (pol-ik-o'le-ah). Secretions of bile in excess.

Polychromat'ic. Many colored; variegated.

Polyclin'ic (pol-ik-lin'ik). Hospital or infirmary with many beds.

Polyco'ria (pol-e-ko're-ah). The presence of more than one pupil.

Polycrot'ic. Having several secondary pulse-waves.

Polyc'rotism (po-lik'rot-izm). Fact or quality of being polycrotic.

Polycye'sis (pol-e-si-e'sis). Multiple pregnancy.

Polycys'tic (pol-is-is'tik). Containing many cysts or cavities.

Polycythe'mia. Excess of red blood-corpuscles.

Polydac'tylism. Presence of supernumerary fingers.

Polydip'sia (pol-e-dip'se-ah). Extreme or abnormal thirst.

Polye'mia (pol-e-e'me-ah). Excessive amount of blood in the body. **P. hyperalbumino'sa,** excess of albumin in blood-plasma. **P. polycythe'mia,** an increase in red corpuscles of blood. **P. sero'sa,** condition in which amount of blood-serum is increased.

Polyesthe'sia (pol-e-es-the'zhe-ah). Condition in which a single object seems to be felt in several different places.

Polygalac'tia (pol-ig-al-ak'she-ah). Excessive secretion of milk without overflow.

Polyg'nathus (pol-ig'nath-us). Double monster united by the jaws.

Polygro'ma (pol-ig-ro'mah). A large hygroma.

Polygy'ria (pol-ij-ir'e-ah). Excess in the number of cerebral gyri.

Polyhæ'mia. Same as *Polyemia.*

Polyhe'dral. Having many sides or surfaces.

Polyhydram'nios. Excess of liquor amnii in pregnancy.

Polyidro'sis (pol-e-id-ro'sis). Excess in the secretion of sweat.

Polymas'tia (pol-im-as'te-ah). Presence of more than two mammæ.

Polym'elus (po-lim'el-us). Fetus with more than two legs.

Pol'ymer (pol'im-er). Any member of a series of polymeric substances.

Polyme'ria. Presence of supernumerary parts of the body.

Polymer'ic. Characterized by polymerism.

Polym'erism. 1. Excess in the number of parts present. 2. Isomerism in which the molecular weights of members of the series are in multiples of each other.

Polymor'phism. Quality of being polymorphous.

Polymor'phous (pol-im-or'fus). Occurring in various forms.

Polymyos'itis (pol-im-i-os-i'tis). Inflammation of many muscles at once.

Polyneuri'tis (pol-in-u-ri'tis). Inflammation of several nerves at once.

Polynu'clear. Possessing or affecting more than one nucleus.

Polyodon'tia. Presence of supernumerary teeth.

Polyo'pia (pol-e-o'pe-ah). State in which one object appears as two or more objects.

Polyor'chis (pol-e-or'kis). A person with more than two testes.

Polyo'tia (pol-e-o'she-ah). Presence of more than one ear on a side.

Pol'yp (pol'ip). Same as *Polypus.*

Polypar'esis. Condition of general paresis.

Polypha'gia (pol-e-fa'je-ah). Voracious or excessive feeding.

Polyphar'macy (pol-e-far'mas-e). Use of too many drugs together or of too much medicine.

Polyphra'sia (pol-e-fra'ze-ah). Morbid or insane volubility.

Polypif'erous (pol-ip-if'er-us). Producing a polyp.

Pol'yplast (pol'ip-last). Composed of many cells.

Polyplas'tic. Passing through great changes of form.

Polypne'a, Polypnœ'a (pol-ip-ne'ah). A rapid or panting respiration.

Pol'ypoid (pol'ip-oid). Resembling a polypus.

Polyp'orus officina'lis. Purging agaricus.

Polyp'otome (pol-ip'ot-ōm). Instrument for cutting off polypi.

Pol'ypus. Smooth and pedunculated growth from a mucous surface. **Blood-p.** Same as *Placental p.* **P. carno'sus,** a sarcoma. **Fibrinous p.,** intra-uterine p. made up of fibrin from retained blood. **Fibrous p.,** polypus made up mainly of fibrous tissue. **Mucous p.,** soft p. from local inflammatory hyperplasia of mucous membrane, or is a true myxoma. **Placental p.** is derived from a piece of retained placenta.

Polysar'cia (pol-is-ar'she-ah). Corpulence; obesity.

Polysar'cous (pol-is-ar'kus). Corpulent; too fleshy.

Polyscel'ia (pol-is-e'le-ah). Presence of more than two legs.

Pol'yscope (pol'is-kōp). Same as *Diaphanoscope.*

Polyso'mia. Condition of having several bodies.

Polyso'mus. A monster with double or triple body.

Polysper'mia, Polysper'mism. Excessive secretion of semen.

Polystich'ia (pol-is-tik'e-ah). Presence of two or more rows of eyelashes on a lid.

Polythe'lia (pol-e-the'le-ah). Two or more nipples on a mamma.

Polytrich'ia (pol-e-trik'e-ah). Same as *Hypertrichiasis.*

Polytro'phia (pol-it-ro'fe-ah). Over-nutrition.

Polyu'ria. Excess in the amount of urine discharged.

Po'made. Same as *Pomatum.*

Poma'tum. Ointment; chiefly for the hair.

Pomegran'ate (pum-gran'et). The tree *Punica granatum* and its astringent fruit: the root-bark destroys tapeworm.

Pom'pholyx (pom'fo-lix). 1. Any skin-disease marked by bullæ. 2. Same as *Cheiropompholyx.*

Pom'phus (pom'fus). A wheal.

Po'mum Ada'mi. Adam's apple; prominence on the throat caused by thyroid cartilage.

Pond's extract. A proprietary preparation of witch-hazel.

Pon'ogene (pon'o-jēn). Any waste material derived from the brain or nervous system.

Pons (ponz). 1. L. for *Bridge.* 2. Same as *Pons Varolii.* **P. hep'-atis,** a projection partially bridging the longitudinal fissure of the liver. **P. Tari'ni,** the floor of the posterior perforated space. **P. Varo'lii,** organ which connects the cerebrum, cerebellum, and oblongata.

Pon'tal, Pon'tile, Pon'tine. Pertaining to the pons Varolii.

Pop'lar (pop'lar). A genus (*Populus*) of trees the bark of which contains populin and salicin.

Poplitæ'us (pop-lit-e'us), **Poplite'us.** See *Muscles, Table of.*

Poplite'al (pop-lit-e'al). Pertaining to the ham or area behind the knee.

Pop'py. A plant. See *Papaver.*

Pop'ulin. Benzoyl-salicin, $C_{20}H_{22}O_8$, a sweet principle from poplar bark.

Por'cupine disease. Same as *Ichthyosis.*

Pore (pōr). A minute orifice, as of a sweat-gland.

Porencepha'lia (po-ren-sef-a'le-ah). Abnormal cavity, or cavities, in brain-tissue.

Porencephali'tis. Porencephalia with inflammation of brain.

Porenceph'alous (po-ren-sef'al-us). Characterized by porencephalia.

Pornog'raphy (por-nog'raf-e). The literature, or bibliography, of prostitution.

Poro'ma, Poro'sis. Inflammatory induration.

Poros'ity (po-ros'it-e). The condition of being porous.

Porot'omy (po-rot'o-me). Same as *Meatotomy.*

Po'rous. Filled with pores or open spaces.

Porphyriza'tion. Pulverization; reduction to a powder.

Porri'go. Ringworm or other disease of the scalp. **P. decal'-vans.** Same as *Alopecia areata.* **P. favo'sa.** Same as *Favus.* **P. larva'lis,** eczema with impetigo of scalp.

Por'ro's operation (por'rōz). Excision of pregnant uterus and ovaries by abdominal incision.

Por'ta hep'atis. The transverse fissure of the liver.

Por'tal. Pertaining to the porta hepatis.

Portcaus'tic, Portecaustique (port-kōs-teek'). A handle for holding a caustic substance.

Portenœud (port-ned'). Instrument for applying a ligature to pedicle of a tumor.

Por'tio du'ra. The facial nerve. **P. in'ter du'ram et mol'lem, P. interme'dia,** a fasciculus which joins the facial and acoustic nerves. **P. mol'lis.** acoustic nerve. **P. vagina'lis,** portion of uterus which projects into the vagina.

Port-wine stain. A form of nevus.

Po'rus. L. for *Pore.* **P. acus'ticus exter'nus,** outer end of external auditory meatus. **P. acus'ticus inter'nus,** opening of internal auditory canal into cranial cavity. **P. op'ticus,** opening in lamina cribrosa of the sclera for central retinal artery.

Posi'tion (po-zish'un). Attitude or posture of a patient. **Dorsal p.,** one with the patient lying on his back. **Edebohl's p., Simon's p.,** dorsal p., right knee and thigh drawn up, legs flexed on thighs, thighs on belly, hips elevated, thighs adducted. **Genucubital p., Knee-elbow p.,** the patient lies on the knees and elbows, the head on his hands. **Genupectoral p., Knee-chest p.,** patient on knees and chest, arms crossed above head. **Left lateral recumbent p., English p., Obstetric p.,** patient on left side, right thigh and knee drawn up. **Lithotomy p., Dorsosacral p.,** patient on the back, legs flexed on thighs, thighs flexed on belly and abducted. **Semiprone p., Sims's p.,** patient on left side and on chest, right knee and thigh drawn up, left arm along the back. **Trendelenburg's p.,** patient on back, on a plane inclined 45°, legs and feet hanging down over end of table.

Pos'itive electrode, P. pole. The electrode or pole connected with the negative element in a battery.

Posolog'ical (po-so-loj'ik-al). Pertaining to doses.

Posol'ogy (po-sol'o-je). Science or system of doses, or dosage.

Postax'ial. Situated or occurring behind an axis.

Postca'va. The ascending vena cava.

Postca'val. Pertaining to the postcava.

Postcen'tral. Situated or occurring behind a center.

Postci'bal (post-si'bal). Occurring after the taking of food.

Postclavic'ular. Situated or occurring behind the clavicle.

Postconnu'bial. Occurring or happening after marriage.

Postconvul'sive. Following after a convulsion.

Postdicrot'ic. Occurring after the dicrotic elevation of the sphygmogram.

Postepilep'tic. Following an epileptic attack.

Poste'rior (pos-te're-or). Situated behind or toward the rear. **P. chamber,** that part of the aqueous chamber of the eye situated behind the iris.

Postero-exter'nal. Situated on the outer side of a posterior aspect.

Posterome'dian. Situated on the middle of a posterior aspect.

Poster'ula (pos-ter'u-lah). Space between the turbinal bones and the posterior nares.

Post-feb'rile neuritis. See *Neuritis.*

Postgem'inum. The posterior corpora quadrigemina.

Postgenic'ulum. The internal geniculate body.

Posthet'omy (pos-thet'om-e). Same as *Circumcision.*

Pos'thioplasty (pos'thi-op-las-te). Plastic surgery of the foreskin.

Posthi'tis (pos-thi'tis). Inflammation of the foreskin.

Post'humous (post'u-mus). Occurring after death; born after father's death.

Postme'dian. Situated or occurring behind a median line or plane.

Post mor'tem. After death. **P.-m. wart,** warty growth on the hand of those who dissect dead bodies.

Postoblonga'ta. Part of oblongata below the pons.

Post-oc'ular neuritis. Inflammation of part of optic nerve behind the eyeball.

Postparalyt'ic (pōst-par-al-it'ik). Following an attack of paralysis.

Post-par'tum. Occurring after childbirth; after delivery.

Postpon'tile (pōst-pon'til). Situated behind the pons Varolii.

Postpyram'idal nucleus. Same as *Nucleus gracilis.*

Post'ural. Pertaining to posture or position.

Po'table (po'ta-bl). Drinkable; fit to drink.

Potamopho'bia. A dread of large bodies of water.

Pot'ash (pot'ash). 1. Potassium hydrate or hydroxid, KOH; caustic potash. 2. Potassium carbonate, K_2CO_3.

Potas'sa (po-tas'ah). Caustic potash.

Potas'sic (po-tas'ik). Containing potash.

Potas'sium. A metallic element whose salts are used in medicine.

Poten'tial (po-ten'shal). Existing and ready for action, but not yet active.

Po'tion (po'shun). A draft: a large dose of liquid medicine.

Pott's cur'vature. Curvature of spinal column following Pott's disease. **P.'s disease,** caries of the vertebræ. **P.'s fracture.** See *Fracture.*

Pouch (powtsh). Any pocket-like space or cavity.

Poul'tice (pōl'tis). Any soft pultaceous mass to be placed hot upon the skin.

Pound. See *Weights and Measures, Table of.*

Poupart's ligament (poo-parz'). See *Ligament.*

Pow'der. Aggregation of particles obtained by grinding or triturating a solid. **Aromatic p.,** powders of cinnamon, cardamom, and nutmeg. **Dover's p.,** powder of ipecac and opium. **Gray p.,** mercury with chalk. **Insect-p.,** powdered tops and flowers of various species of fleabane. **James's p.,** powder of antimonious oxid and calcium phosphate. **Seidlitz p.,** effervescent saline aperient powder. **Tully's p.,** powder of chalk, camphor, licorice, and morphin.

Pox. Any eruptive disease; chiefly used as a vulgar name of syphilis.

P. p. Abbreviation of *Punctum proximum,* near-point.

P. r. Abbreviation of *Punctum remotum,* far-point.

Prac'tice (prak'tis). Practical recognition and treatment of disease.

Practi'tioner (prak-tish'un-er). One who practices medicine.

Præ-. For words thus beginning, see *Pre-.*

Prax'inoscope. Instrument for studying the larynx.

Pre-atax'ic. Occurring before the advent of ataxia.

Pre-ax'ial (pre-ak'se-al). In front of the transverse axis of the body.

Precan'cerous. Occurring before the development of a cancer.

Preca'va. The descending vena cava.

Precen'tral. Situated in front of a center.

Prechor'dal. In front of the notochord.

Precip'itant. A substance that causes precipitation.

Precip'itate (pre-sip'it-āt). 1. To cause a substance in solution to settle down in solid particles. 2. A deposit made or substance thrown down by precipitation. **Red p.,** red oxid of mercury, HgO. **White p.,** ammoniated mercury, NH_2HgCl. **Yellow p.,** yellow oxid of mercury, HgO.

Precipita'tion. Act or process of precipitating.

Precor'dia (pre-kor'de-ah). Same as *Epigastrium*.

Precor'dial (pre-kor'de-al). Pertaining to the precordia; epigastric.

Precor'nu. Anterior cornu of lateral ventricle.

Precu'neus. The quadrate lobule of the cerebrum.

Prediastol'ic. Occurring before the diastole.

Predicrot'ic. Occurring before the dicrotic wave of the sphygmogram.

Prediges'tion (pre-dij-es'chun). Partial artificial digestion of food before its ingestion.

Predispo'sing. Conferring a tendency to disease.

Predisposi'tion. A diathesis or special tendency toward some disease.

Prefron'tal. The central part of the ethmoid bone. **P. lobe,** portion of central lobe in advance of the precentral fissure.

Pregenicula'tum. The external geniculate body.

Preglob'ulin (pre-glob'u-lin). A proteid derivable from cytoglobulin.

Preg'nancy. Condition of being with child; gestation. **Abdominal p.,** lodgement of ovum in abdominal cavity. **Extra-uterine p.,** development of ovum outside the walls of the uterus. **False p.,** apparent, but not real, pregnancy. **Hydatid p.,** p. with formation of hydatid mole. **Interstitial p.,** gestation in that part of oviduct which is within wall of uterus. **Molar p.,** conversion of ovum into a mole. **Multiple p.,** presence of more than one ovum in the uterus at same time. **Mural p.** Same as *Interstitial p.* **Ovarian p.,** pregnancy occurring in an ovary. **Phantom-p.,** abdominal enlargement in hysterical women, simulating pregnancy. **Tubal p.,** pregnancy within an oviduct.

Preg'nant. With child; gravid.

Prehemipleg'ic (pre-hem-ip-led'jik). Forerunning an attack of hemiplegia.

Prehen'sile. Capable of grasping or seizing.

Prehen'sion (pre-hen'shun). The act of grasping.

Prelim'bic (pre-lim'bik). Situated before a limbus.

Pre'lum abdomina'le. Squeezing of abdominal viscera between diaphragm and abdominal wall, as in defecation, etc.

Pre'mature labor. Labor before proper term, but after viability.

Premax'illary. Situated before the maxilla. **P. bone.** Same as *Incisive bone.*

Premo'lar. In front of the molar teeth.

Premon'itory (pre-mon'it-o-re). Giving a warning.

Prena'tal. Existing or occurring before birth.

Prepatel'lar. Situated in front of the patella.

Prephthi'sis (pre-thi'sis). The initial stages of pulmonary phthisis.

Pre'puce (pre'pūs). Cutaneous fold or cover of glans penis; foreskin.

Prepu'tial (pre-pu'shal). Of, or pertaining to, the prepuce.

Presbycu'sis (pres-be-ku'sis). Impairment of hearing due to old age.

Presbyo'pia (pres-be-o'pe-ah). Impairment of eyesight due to old age.

Prescrip'tion. A written direction for the preparation and administering of medicines.

Presenta'tion. The appearance at the os uteri of some particular part of the body of the fetus at birth.

Presphe'noid (pre-sfe'noid). Anterior portion of the body of the sphenoid bone.

Pres'sure-myelitis. See *Myelitis.* **P. point,** a point of extreme sensibility to pressure.

Prester'num. Same as *Manubrium.*

Presyl'vian fissure (pre-sil've-an). The anterior branch of the Sylvian fissure.

Presys'tole. Interval of time just before the systole.

Presystol'ic (pre-sis-tol'ik). Occurring before the systole.

Pretib'ial (pre-tib'e-al). Situated in front of the tibia.

Preven'tive. Same as *Prophylactic.*

Prever'tebral (pre-ver'te-bral). Situated in front of a vertebra.

Pri'apism (pri'ap-izm). Persistent abnormal erection of penis.

Prick'le-cell. A cell having fibrillary radiating processes connecting it with similar adjacent cells. **P.-layer.** Same as *Stratum granulosum.*

Prick'ly heat. Same as *Lichen tropicus.*

Pri'mæ vi'æ. The alimentary canal.

Pri'mary. First in order; principal.

Primip'ara. A woman who has had but one child.

Primipar'ity. Condition or fact of having borne only one child.

Primip'arous. Having borne one child only.

Prim'itive. First in point of time; original. **P. streak, P. trace,** opaque streak in the area pellucida in front of which the ovum is developed.

Primor'dial (pri-mor'de-al). Original or primitive.

Prin'ceps (prin'seps). A principal artery.

Prin'ciple. A definite essential constituent.

Pri'nos verticilla'tus. The tonic and astringent bark of the black alder.

Prism. A solid with a triangular or polygonal cross-section. **Enamel-p.,** any one of the columns which make up the enamel of teeth. **Nicol p.** See *Nicol prism.* **P.-diop'ter,** the unit of prismatic refraction; a deflection of one centimeter at the distance of one meter.

Prismoptom'eter. Instrument for testing the refraction of the eye by means of a revolving prism.

Pris'mosphere (priz'mo-sfēr). A prism combined with a globular lens.

Pri'vates. The external genitalia.

Pro-am'nion. That part of the embryonal area at front and sides of head which remains without mesoderm for some time.

Pro'bang. A flexible rod with a ball or sponge at the end; used in diseases of esophagus or larynx. **Ball-p.,** one with an ivory bulb at end. **Bristle p., Horse-hair p.,** one with an expansible tuft of horse-hairs or bristles at end. **Sponge-p.,** one which is tufted with sponge.

Proba'tionary ward. A ward for the temporary detention of patients suspected of having a contagious disease.

Probe. A long slender instrument for exploring wounds. **Anel's p.,** delicate probe for lacrimal puncta and canals. **Blunt p.,** one with a blunt point. **Bowman's p.,** one of a set of probes for use on nasal duct. **Drum-p.,** one with a reverberator to indicate contact with a foreign body. **Electric p.,** one which on contact with a foreign body completes an electric circuit. **Eyed p.,** one with a slit for a ligature or tape near one end. **Lacrimal p.,** one designed for use on the tear-passages. **Meerschaum p.,** a probe with meerschaum tip, which on contact with a leaden bullet becomes darkened. **Nélaton's p.,** a bullet-probe with an unglazed porcelain head. **Uterine p.,** a probe for uterine exploration. **Vertebrated p.,** flexible p. made up of small links. **Wire p.,** a probe of steel wire.

Proc'ess (pros'es). A long projecting point or prominence. **Acromion p.** See *Acromion.* **Alveolar p.** See *Alveo-*

lar border. **Auditory p.,** bony tube of auditory meatus. **Basilar p.,** forward process of occipital to articulate with sphenoid bone. **Ciliary p.,** fringe-like processes which encircle the margin of eye-lens. **Coracoid p.,** projection from anterior and upper edge of scapula. **Coronoid p.,** a process of lower jaw; also, one of ulna. **Deiters's p.,** axis-cylinder process of a nerve-cell. **Dendritic p.,** the branched p. of a nerve-cell. **Ensiform p.** Same as *Ensiform cartilage.* **Ethmoid p.,** projection from upper border of inferior turbinated bone. **Falciform p.** 1. Upper and outer border of saphenous opening. 2. The falx cerebri. **Funicular p.,** process of peritoneum descending along with the testicle. **Hamular p.,** hook-like process on lower extremity of internal pterygoid plate. **Jugular p.,** process of occipital bone touching jugular foramen. **Lacrimal p.,** process of inferior turbinated which joins with the lacrimal bone. **Lenticular p.** See *Processus lenticularis.* **Long p. of incus.** process which joins the orbiculare to incus proper. **Long p. of malleus.** Same as *Processus gracilis.* **Malar p.,** eminence by which the superior maxilla articulates with the malar bone. **Mammillary p.,** a tubercle on each superior articular process of a lumbar vertebra. **Mastoid p.,** conical projection at base of mastoid portion of temporal bone. **Maxillary p.,** bony plate which descends from ethmoid process of lower turbinated bone. **Nasal p.,** part of lateral wall of upper jaw-bone. **Odontoid p.,** tooth-like process of atlas which ascends and articulates with atlas. **Olecranon p.** See *Olecranon.* **Olivary p.,** small oval p. behind optic groove of sphenoid bone. **Orbital p.** 1. Process of palate-bone which passes upward and outward. 2. Process which goes inward from inner surface of upper jaw-bone, forming part of floor of nostril and roof of mouth. **Postglenoid p.,** tubercle which separates glenoid fossa from auditory process. **Protoplasmic p.,** any process of a nerve-cell not continued as an axis-cylinder. **Pterygoid p.,** a process of the palate-bone; also, one of the sphenoid. **Rau's p.,** the long process of the malleus. **Short p.** See *Processus brevis.* **Sphenoid p.,** one of the processes of palate-bone. **Spinous p.,** four processes of ilium, one of the sphenoid, and one of almost all the vertebræ. **Styloid p.,** a process each of the fibula, radius, temporal bone, and ulna. **Superior vermiform p.,** upper part of median lobe of the cerebellum. **Temporal p.,** posterior angle by which the malar bone articulates with the zygomatic process of temporal bone. **Transverse p.,** process on either side of a vertebra. **Unciform p.,** hooked projection from the ethmoid, and one from unciform bone; also, hook at anterior end of the gyrus of the hippocampus. **Vaginal p.,** a process of the peritoneum which forms the tunica vaginalis testis; also, a process of the sphenoid, and one of the temporal bone. **Xiphoid p.,** the ensiform cartilage. **Zygomatic p.,** an important p. of temporal bone, and also of the malar bone.

Process'us (pro-ses'us). L. for *Process*, or *Processes.* **P. bre'vis,** short p. of the malleus; also, short p. of incus. **P. clava'tus,** point on posterior pyramid of oblongata, near apex of fourth ventricle. **P. cochleariform'mis,** bony plate which divides the canal of Eustachian tube from that of tensor tympani. **P. e. cerebel'lo ad medul'lam,** the restiform bodies. **P. e. cerebel'lo ad pon'tem,** middle peduncles of cerebellum. **P. e. cerebel'lo ad tes'tes,** superior peduncles of cerebellum. **P. gra'cilis,** the long process of the malleus. **P. hama'tus,** the unciform process. **P. lenticula'ris,** lenticular process of malleus. Same as *Orbicular bone.* **P. lon'gus.** 1. Long process of incus. 2. Long process of malleus.

Prociden'tia (pro-sid-en'she-ah). A falling down or prolapse.

Procrea'tion (pro-kre-a'shun). The act of begetting or generating.

Proctag'ra. Pain in the rectum.

Proctalgia (prok-tal'je-ah). Pain in the rectum.

Proctatre'sia (prok-tat-re'ze-ah). Rectal stricture.

Proctec'tomy (prok-tek'tom-e). Surgical removal of the rectum.

Procten'clisis. Anal constriction.

Proctcuryn'ter. An instrument for stretching the anus.

Procti'tis. Inflammation of the rectum.

Proc'tocele (prok'to-sēl). A hernial protrusion of part of the rectum.

Proctococ'cypexy (prok-to-kok'sip-ek-se). The suturation of the rectum to the coccyx.

Proctocystot'omy. Removal of vesical stone through rectum.

Proctode'um, Proctodæ'um. A fold of epiblast that forms the cloaca, etc.

Proctodyn'ia (prok-to-din'e-ah). Pain in the rectum.

Proctoparal'ysis. Paralysis of the anal sphincter.

Proc'topexy (prok'to-pek-se). The fixation of the rectum by suture.

Proc'toplasty. Plastic surgery of the rectum.

Proctople'gia (prok-to-ple'je-ah). Same as *Proctoparalysis.*

Proctopto'sis. Prolapse or procidentia of the rectum.

Proctor'rhaphy. The sewing up of a wound or defect of the rectum.

Proctorrhe'a. A discharge from the anus.

Proc'toscope. A rectal speculum.

Proctos'copy. Rectal inspection.

Proc'totome (prok'to-tōm). A knife for making rectal incisions.

Proctot'omy (prok-tot'om-e). Incision of the rectum; division of a rectal stricture.

Prodigio'sus toxin. An antitoxin from *Bacillus prodigiosus:* it is used for malignant tumors.

Pro'drome (pro'drōm). A premonitory symptom.

Produc'tive inflammation. Inflammation attended with a new growth of connective tissue.

Pro-enceph'alus. A fetus with a protrusion of the brain through a frontal fissure.

Profes'sional (pro-fesh'un-al). Pertaining to one's profession or occupation.

Profun'da fem'oris. See *Arteries, Table of.*

Proglos'sis. The tip of the tongue.

Proglot'tis, pl. *proglottides.* A joint or segment of a tapeworm.

Prog'nathism. Projection of the jaws.

Prog'nathous (prog'nath-us). Having projecting jaws.

Progno'sis. A prediction as to the probable result of an attack of a disease.

Prognos'tic. Affording an indication as to prognosis.

Prognos'ticate. To state the probable outcome of an illness.

Progres'sive muscular atrophy. Atrophy of successive groups of muscles due to degenerations in the spinal cord. See *Atrophy.*

Prola'bium. The exposed red part of the lip.

Pro'lapse (pro'laps), **Prolap'sus.** The falling down or sinking of a part; procidentia.

Prolifera'tion. The formation and reproduction of cells.

Prolif'erous (pro-lif'er-us). Characterized by proliferation.

Prolif'ic (pro-lif'ik). Fruitful; productive.

Prolig'erous (pro-lij'er-us). Producing an ovum. See *Discus proligerus.*

Prom'ontory. A projecting process or eminence. **P. of the sacrum,** the upper or projecting part of the sacrum.

Prona'tion (pro-na'shun). The act of turning the palm downward.

Prona'tor muscles. See *Muscles, Table of.*

Prone (prōn). Lying with the face downward.

Proneph'ros (pro-nef'ros). The primordial kidney.

Pronu'cleus. Nucleus of the egg-element (*female p.*) or of the sperm-element (*male p.*) after the coalition of the spermatozoon with the ovum.

Proof spirit. Alcohol containing 42.5 to 49.24 per cent. of absolute alcohol.

Pro-ot'ic. Situated in front of the ear.

Prop'-cells. See *Hensen's cells.*

Propen'yl (pro-pen'il). Same as *Glyceryl.*

Propep'sin (pro-pep'sin). Same as *Pepsinogen.*

Propep'tone (pro-pep'tōn). Same as *Hemialbumose.*

Propeptonu'ria. Same as *Hemialbumosia.*

Properitone'al hernia. Hernia into the space in front in parietal peritoneum.

Prophylac'tic (pro-fil-ak'tik). Tending to ward off disease.

Prophylax'is (pro-fil-ak'sis). Prevention of disease; preventive treatment.

Propion'ic acid. A fatty acid, $C_3H_6O_2$, from chyme, sweat, etc.

Propri'etary medicine. A remedy owned or patented.

Propto'sis (prop-to'sis). Prolapse or procidentia.

Propul'sion (pro-pul'shun). A tendency to fall forward; also, festination.

Propylam'in. A base or ptomain, C_3H_9N: antirheumatic.

Prop'ylene (prop'il-ēn). A gaseous hydrocarbon, C_3H_6, from coal, etc.

Pro re na'ta. According to circumstances.

Pror'sad. In a forward direction.

Prosec'tor. One who dissects an anatomic subject for demonstration.

Prosenceph'alon. The forebrain; the anterior part of the anterior cerebral vesicle of the embryo.

Prosogas'ter (pros-o-gas'ter). Same as *Foregut.*

Prosopal'gia (pros-o-pal'je-ah). Neuralgia of the trifacial nerve.

Prosopantri'tis (pros-o-pan-tri'tis). Inflammation of the frontal sinuses.

Prosopecta'sia. Oversize of the face.

Prosoponeural'gia. Facial neuralgia.

Prosopos'chisis (pros-o-pos'kis-is). Congenital fissure of the face.

Prosoposternodym'ia (pros-o-po-ster-no-dim'e-ah). Double monster joined from face to sternum.

Prosopothoracop'agus (pros-o-po-thor-ak-op'ag-us). Twin fetuses joined in the thorax, face, and neck.

Prosopoto'cia. Face-presentation in labor.

Prostatal'gia. Pain in the prostate gland.

Prostataux'e (pros-tat-awks'e). Enlargement of the prostate gland.

Pros'tate. A gland surrounding the neck of the bladder and urethra in the male.

Prostatec'tomy. Surgical removal of the prostate or of a part of it.

Prostat'ic (pros-tat'ik). Pertaining to the prostate gland.

Prostati'tis (pros-tat-i'tis). Inflammation of the prostate gland.

Prostatorrhe'a. Gleety or catarrhal discharge from the prostate.

Prostatot'omy. Surgical cutting of the prostate.

Pros'thesis (pros'the-sis). 1. Replacement of an absent part by an artificial one. 2. An artificial organ, as an eye, leg, or denture.

Prosthet'ics (pros-thet'iks). Branch of surgery pertaining to artificial organs or parts.

Prostitu'tion. Indiscriminate sexual intercourse.

Prostra'tion. Extreme exhaustion or powerlessness.

Pro'tagon. A crystalline principle, $C_{160}H_{308}N_5PO_{35}$, from brain-substance, said to be a mixture of lecithin and cerebrin.

Protal'bumose. Same as *Protoalbumose.*

Protam'in. An amin or base, $C_{16}H_{32}N_9O_2$, from spermatozoa and fish-spawn.

Protec'tive. Oiled silk used in surgery for its waterproof qualities. **P. proteid.** See *Alexin, Sozin, Phylaxin.*

Pro'teid. An albuminoid constituent of the body.

Pro'tein. An old name for the supposed essential constituent of all proteids: it is probably identical with alkali-albumin.

Proteol'ysis. Conversion of proteids into peptones.

Proteolyt'ic. Effecting the digestion of proteids.

Pro'teose (pro'te-ōs). Any albumose or other substance intermediate between a proteid and a peptone.

Pro'teus. A genus of schizomycetes. **P. hom'inis** occurs in rag-sorters' disease. **P. mirab'ilis, sep'ticus, vulga'ris,** and **zen'keri,** are pathogenic.

Proth'esis (proth'es-is). Same as *Prosthesis.*

Prothrom'bin. Thrombin in an inactive earlier state.

Protoal'bumose. An albumose obtainable from cultures of the bacillus of anthrax.

Pro'toblast (pro'to-blast). A cell with no cell-wall.

Protochlo'rid (pro-to-klo'rid). That one of a series of chlorids of the same element which contains the least chlorin.

Protogas'ter (pro-to-gas'ter). Same as *Foregut.*

Protoglob'ulose. An albumose produced in the digestion of globulin.

Protomyos'inose. One of the two albumoses formed in the digestion of myosin.

Protoneph'ros (pro-to-nef'ros). Same as *Pronephros.*

Protonu'clein. A proprietary nuclein preparation, $C_{29}H_{49}N_{10}P_5O_{32}$.

Pro'tophyte (pro'to-fīt). Any unicellular plant or vegetable organism.

Pro'toplasm. A granular material, the essential constituent of the living cell.

Protoplas'mic. Pertaining to, or consisting of, protoplasm. **P. process,** a dendrite, or branching process, of a nerve-cell.

Pro'toplast. 1. Protoplasm. 2. An embryonic cell.

Pro'tospasm (pro'to-spazm). A spasm which begins in a limited area and extends to other parts.

Protover'tebra. Same as *Somite.*

Protox'id. That one of a series of oxids of the same element which contains the least amount of oxygen.

Protozo'a, pl. of *protozoōn.* A class of unicellular animal organisms.

Protozo'an. Any species or organism of the protozoa; used also adjectively.

Protrac'tor. Instrument for drawing bodies from wounds.

Protu'berance. A projecting part.

Proud flesh. Any redundant mass of granulations.

Prox'imad. In a proximal direction; toward the proximal end.

Prox'imal. Nearest the trunk, center, or median line.

Prox'imate (proks'im-āt). Immediate; nearest. **P. cause,** that cause of a disease which immediately precipitates the attack. **P. principle,** any one of the definite compounds into which a tissue may be directly or readily resolved.

Pru'nus Virginia'na. The bark of wild cherry: sedative and expectorant.

Prurig'inous (pru-rij'in-us). Of the nature of prurigo.

Pruri'go (pru-ri'go). Papular skin-disease with itching.

Pruri'tus (pru-ri'tus). Severe itching. **P. hiema'lis,** an itching skin-disease peculiar to cold climates.

Prus'sian-blue (proo'shan). Ferric ferrocyanid, $Fe.3Fe(C_6N_6)_2$.

Prus'siate (proo'she-āt). Same as *Cyanid.*

Prus'sic acid (proos'sik). Same as *Hydrocyanic acid.*

Psal'is (sal'is). Same as *Fornix.*

Psalte'rium (sal-te're-um). Same as *Lyra.*

Psammo'ma (sam-mo'mah). A fibrous tumor of the brain-tissue containing brain-sand.

Psammother'apy (sam-o-ther'ap-e). Same as *Ammotherapy.*

Psell'ism (sel'izm). Stuttering or stammering.

Pseudacon'itin. Crystalline alkaloid, $C_{27}H_{41}O_9$, from *Aconitum ferox.*

Pseudacous'mia, Pseudacu'sis. Condition in which sounds seem altered in quality of pitch.

Pseudarthri'tis. An hysteric joint-affection.

Pseudarthro'sis (seu-dar-thro'sis). A false joint following a fracture.

Pseudenceph'alus (seu-den-sef'al-us). A fetus with tumor in place of brain.

Pseudesthe'sia (pseu-des-the'zhe-ah). An imaginary sensation; sense as of pain in a lost part.

Pseudo-angi'na (seu-do-an-ji'nah). Nervous disorder resembling angina.

Pseudo-ap'oplexy. Condition like apoplexy, but without hemorrhage.

Pseudobacter'ium. A cell resembling a bacterium.

Pseudoblep'sis. Condition in which objects look different from what they really are.

Pseudobul'bar paralysis. Paralysis of the same regions as in bulbar paralysis, but due to some brain-lesion.

Pseu'docele (su'do-sēl). The fifth ventricle of the brain.

Pseudoceliot'omy. The pretended performance of abdominal section.

Pseudochromesthe'sia. A condition in which sounds induce a sensation as of color.

Pseudocri'sis (su-do-kri'sis). A false crisis.

Pseu'docroup (su'do-kroop). Same as *Laryngismus stridulus.*

Pseudocye'sis (su-do-si-e'sis). Spurious or false pregnancy.

Pseudo-ede'ma (su-do-e-de'mah). A puffy state resembling edema.

Pseudo-erysip'elas. An inflammatory subcutaneous disease resembling erysipelas.

Pseudo-esthe'sia. Same as *Pseudesthesia.*

Pseudogan'glion (su-do-gan'gle-on). An enlargement of a nerve not unlike a ganglia.

Pseudogeusesthe'sia (su-do-gūs-es-the'ze-ah). A condition in which sensations of taste are accompanied by sensations as of color.

Pseudoglio'ma (su-do-gli-o'mah). An exudate in the vitreous simulating glioma.

Pseudohermaphrod'itism. See *Hermaphrodism, spurious.*

Pseudoher'nia (su-do-her'ne-ah). An inflamed sac or gland simulating strangulated hernia.

Pseudohydropho'bia. Same as *Hydrophobophobia.*

Pseudohyoscyam'in. An alkaloid, $C_{17}H_{23}NO_3$, from *Duboisia myoporoides.*

Pseudohypertroph'ic paralysis. Paralysis with enlargement and fatty degeneration of the affected muscles.

Pseudohyper'trophy. Increase of size with loss of function.

Pseudoleuke'mia. Progressive and fatal anemia with lymphomata.

Pseudoleukocythe'mia. Same as *Pseudoleukemia*.

Pseudoma'nia (su-do-ma'ne-ah). Insanity in which the patient accuses himself of crimes which he has not committed.

Pseudomelano'sis. Pigmentation of tissues after death.

Pseudomem'brane (su-do-mem'brān). See *False membrane*.

Pseudomne'sia. A condition in which the patient seems to remember things which never occurred.

Pseudomu'cin (su-do-mu'sin). A variety of mucin from ovarian cysts.

Pseudoneuro'ma. A growth on a nerve simulating neuroma.

Pseudonu'clein. Same as *Paranuclein*.

Pseudoparal'ysis. A loss of muscular power with no real paralysis.

Pseudopar'asite. See *Facultative parasite*.

Pseudophthi'sis (su-dof-thi'sis). A wasting not due to tuberculosis.

Pseudople'gia (su-do-ple'je-ah). Hysteric paralysis.

Pseudopo'dium (su-do-po'de-um). A temporary protrusion, mainly of the ectosarc of an ameba, serving for purposes of locomotion.

Pseudop'sia (su-dop'se-ah). Same as *Pseudoblepsia*.

Pseudora'bies (su-do-ra'be-ez). Same as *Hydrophobophobia*.

Pseudoscarlati'na. Eruption with fever following wounds, childbirth, etc. It is a septic condition.

Pseudosclero'sis. A disease with the symptoms, but not the lesions, of sclerosis.

Pseudos'mia (su-doz'me-ah). A delusion as to smell.

Pseudos'toma. An apparent communication between stained endothelial cells.

Pseudota'bes. A disease simulating locomotor ataxia.

Pseudotuberculo'sis. Condition like tuberculosis, but without any tubercular bacilli.

Pseudoxan'thin. A leukomain, $C_4H_5N_5O$, from muscular tissue; also, an isomer of xanthin from uric acid.

Psilo'sis (si-lo'sis). Falling out, or removal, of the hair.

Pso'as muscles (so'as). See *Muscles, Table of*. **P. abscess**, abscess of the loin with vertebral disease.

Psod'ymus (sod'im-us). A sysomic monster with two heads and two trunks, but united below.

Psoi'tis (so-i'tis). Inflammation of a psoas muscle or its sheath.

Pso'ra (so'rah). Scabies; also, psoriasis.

Psorelco'sis. Ulceration due to scabies.

Psorenteri'tis. The condition of the bowels in Asiatic cholera.

Psori'asis. A skin-disease of many varieties, characterized by scaly red patches. **P. annula'ris**, p. in ring-shaped patches. **P. bucca'lis.** Same as *Leukoplakia buccalis*. **P. circina'ta.** Same as *P. annularis*. **P. diffu'sa**, form in which there is coalescence of large contiguous lesions. **P. gyra'ta**, a form with patches in serpentine arrangement. **P. palma'ris**, a syphiloderm of palms and soles. **P. puncta'ta**, form in which the lesions consist of minute red papules which become surmounted with pearly scales. **P. universa'lis**, a form with lesions over the whole body.

Psoroco'mium. An itch-hospital.

Psorophthal'mia. Ulcerative marginal blepharitis.

Pso'rosperm (so'ro-sperm). A vesicular parasitic organism.

Psorosper'miæ. The spores of parasitic myxosporidian animal organisms.

Psorospermo'sis. Morbid state due to presence of psorosperms.
Pso'rous (so'rus). Affected with itch.
Psychal'gia (si-kal'je-ah). Painful cerebration.
Psychi'atry, Psychiat'rics (sik-i'at-re, sik-e-at'riks). The treatment of mental disorders.
Psy'chic, Psy'chical (si'kik, si'kik-al). Pertaining to the mind. **P. blindness.** Same as *Mind-blindness*. **P. contagion,** transfer of nervous disorder by imitation. **P. deafness.** Same as *Mind-deafness*.
Psychocor'tical centers. Those centers in the cortex of the brain that are concerned in mental operations.
Psychogen'esis. Mental development.
Psychol'ogy (si-kol'o-je). Science of mind and of mental operations.
Psychom'etry (si-kom'et-re). Measurement of work done and of time consumed in mental operations.
Psychomo'tor (si-ko-mo'tor). Pertaining to, or causing, voluntary movement.
Psychoneuro'sis (si-ko-nu-ro'sis). A functional disorder of the mind and nerves.
Psychopathol'ogy. Psychology of mental diseases.
Psychop'athy (si-kop'ath-e). Any disease of the mind.
Psychophys'ics (si-ko-fiz'iks). Science of the relations of mental processes to their causation and manifestations.
Psychophysiol'ogy. Physiology of the mind.
Psychople'gic. An agent lessening cerebral excitability.
Psycho'sin. A cerebroside found in brain-tissue.
Psycho'sis (si-ko'sis). Any mental disease.
Psychother'apy (si-ko-ther'ap-e). 1. Psychiatry. 2. Mind-cure.
Psychropho'bia (si-kro-fo'be-ah). Insane or morbid dread of cold.
Psychrophore (si'kro-fōr). Device for applying cold to the urethra.
Psychrother'apy. Treatment of disease by applying cold.
Psydra'cium (si-dra'se-um). An obsolete name for certain skin-diseases.
Ptar'mic (tar'mik). Causing sneezing; sternutatory.
Pte'rion (te're-on). Point of junction of frontal, parietal, temporal, and sphenoid bones.
Pteryg'ium (ter-ij'e-um). Patch of thickened conjunctiva extending over a part of the cornea.
Pter'ygoid (ter'ig-oid). Shaped like a wing. **P. bones, P. processes,** two large processes of the sphenoid bone.
Pterygomax'illary. Pertaining to a pterygoid process and the upper jaw.
Pterygopal'atin (ter-ig-o-pal'at-in). Pertaining to a pterygoid process and the palate-bone.
Ptilo'sis (ti-lo'sis). Falling out, or loss, of the eyelashes.
Pti'san (ti'zan). Barley water or any similar preparation.
Ptoma'in (to-ma'in). Any alkaloidal or basic product of putrefaction.
Ptomaine'mia (to-ma-in-e'me-ah). The presence of ptomains in the blood.
Ptomat'ropin (to-mat'ro-pin). A ptomain from decaying sausages.
Pto'sis (to'sis). Paralytic drooping of the upper eyelid. **Abdominal p.** See *Splanchnoptosis*. **P. sympath'ica,** p. associated with myosis, vasomotor facial paralysis, and diseases of the cervical sympathetic system.
Ptyal'agogue (ti-al'ag-og). Same as *Sialagogue*.
Pty'alin (ti'al-in). A ferment found in saliva.
Pty'alism (ti'al-izm). Excessive secretion of spittle; salivation.

Ptyal'ocele (ti-al'o-sēl). See *Ranula*.
Pu'beral (pu'ber-al). Pertaining to puberty.
Pu'berty (pu'ber-te). The age at which the generative power becomes established.
Pu'bes (pu'bēz). 1. The hair on the external genitalia, or the region covered with it. 2. The pubic bone.
Pubes'cence (pu-bes'sens). 1. Puberty. 2. Lanugo.
Pu'bic (pu'bik). Relating to the pubes. **P. bone,** the lower front part of the innominate bone.
Pubiot'omy. Cutting through the pubic bone.
Pu'bis (pu'bis). The pubic bone.
Pubofem'oral. Pertaining to the pubis and femur.
Puboprostat'ic. Pertaining to the pubes and prostate.
Puboves'ical. Pertaining to the pubes and bladder.
Puden'da. The external genitalia (plural).
Pudendag'ra. Pain in the pudendum.
Puden'dal. Pertaining to the pudenda.
Puden'dum. The external genital parts.
Pu'dic (pu'dik). Same as *Pudendal*.
Pu'riculture. Art of raising and training children.
Pu'erile (pu'er-il). Pertaining to a child, or to children. **P. respiration,** exaggeration of breath-sounds, such as is normal in healthy childhood.
Puer'pera (pu-er'per-ah). A woman in childbed.
Puer'peral. Pertaining to childbirth. **P. convulsions,** convulsions in childbed. **P. fever, P. septicemia,** septicemic peritonitis and metritis occurring in childbed.
Puer'peralizm. Diseases incident to childbirth.
Puer'perant. A puerperal woman.
Puerpe'rium. The period or state of confinement; childbed.
Pu'gil, Pugil'lus (pu'jil). A handful.
Pu'lex. A genus of insects, including fleas and chigoes.
Pullula'tion. The act of sprouting, or of budding.
Pulmom'eter (pul-mom'et-er). An apparatus for measuring the lung-capacity.
Pulmom'etry (pul-mom'et-re). Measurement of lung-capacity.
Pul'monary. Pertaining to the lungs.
Pul'monec'tomy. Pneumonectomy.
Pulmon'ic (pul-mon'ik). Same as *Pulmonary*.
Pulmoni'tis (pul-mo-ni'tis). Inflammation of the lung.
Pulp. Any soft and juicy animal or vegetable tissue. **P.-cavity,** space within a tooth containing dental pulp. **Dental p.,** the soft vascular interior substance of a tooth. **Digital p.,** soft cushion on the palmar or plantar surface of the last phalanx of the finger or toe.
Pulpa'tion, Pul'ping. Reduction to a pulpy form.
Pulpi'tis. Inflammation of the dental pulp.
Pul'py. Soft; pultaceous.
Pul'satile (pul'sat-il). Characterized by a rhythmic pulsation.
Pulsatil'la. The herb *Anemone Pulsatilla:* alterative and depressant.
Pulsa'tion (pul-sa'shun). A throb, or rhythmic beat, as of the heart.
Pulse (puls). The expansion and contraction of an artery. **Anacrotic p.,** one with two or more expansions to a beat. **Bigeminal p.,** pulse in which two beats follow each other in rapid succession, each group of two being separated from the following by a longer interval. **Capillary p.,** an intermittent filling and emptying of the skin-capillaries. **Caprizant p.** See *Goat-leap pulse*. **Catacrotic p.,** one which makes a break in the line of descent of the sphygmogram. **Catadicrotic p.,** one with a primary and secondary expan-

sion. **P.-clock**, old device for determining pulse-rate. **Cordy p.**, a tense, firm pulse. **Corrigan's p.**, jerky pulse with full expansion and sudden collapse. **P.-curve.** Same as *Sphygmogram.* **Dicrotic p.**, one with exaggerated recoil wave. **Entoptic p.**, illumination of visual field at each heart-beat after violent exercise. **Full p.**, one with copious volume of blood. **Gaseous p.**, a very full soft pulse. **Goat-leap p.**, an irregular bounding p. **Hard p.**, one which is characterized by high tension. **Hyperdicrotic p.**, one whose sphygmogram shows an aortic notch below the base line: a sign of extreme exhaustion. **Infrequent p.**, abnormally slow p. **Intermittent p.**, one in which various beats are dropped. **Irregular p.**, one in which beats occur at irregular intervals. **Jerky p.**, pulse in which the artery is suddenly and markedly distended. **Jugular p.**, pulsation in jugular veins. **Paradoxic p.**, one that is weaker during inspiration, as in some cases of adherent pericardium. **Quick p.**, one which strikes the finger smartly and leaves it quickly. **Slow p.**, one of slow rate; also, one of prolonged systole and diastole. **Thready p.**, one that is very fine and scarcely perceptible. **Tricrotic p.**, one which is marked by three sphygmographic waves to the pulse-beat. **Venous p.**, that which occurs in a vein. **Water-hammer p.** Same as *Corrigan's p.* **Wiry p.**, a small tense pulse.

Pulsime'ter. Apparatus for measuring force of pulse.

Pul'sus. L. for *Pulse.* **P. bigem'inus**, pulse with the beats occurring in pairs. **P. ce'ler**, a swift abrupt pulse. **P. paradox'us.** See *Paradoxic pulse.* **P. tar'dus**, an abnormally slow pulse.

Pultaceous (pul-ta'sbus). Like a poultice; pulpy.

Pulv. Abbreviation of L. *Pulvis*, powder.

Pulveriza'tion. The reduction of any substance to powder.

Pulver'ulent (pul-ver'u-lent). Powdery; dusty.

Pulvi'nar. Posterior inner part of optic thalamus.

Pul'vis (pul'vis). L. for *Powder.*

Pump. Apparatus for drawing and removing liquid. **Air-p.**, one for exhausting or forcing in air. **Breast-p.**, p. for taking milk from the breast. **Dental p.**, device for removing saliva during dental operation. **Stomach-p.**, p. for removing poisons from stomach.

Punc'ta, pl. of *punctum.* **P. doloro'sa**, painful points in course of nerves affected with neuralgia. **P. lacrima'lia**, outlets of lacrimal canaliculi. **P. vascul'osa**, minute red spots which mark the cut surface of white substance of brain.

Punc'tate. Spotted; full of points, or of punctures.

Punc'tum. L. for *Point.* **P. cæ'cum.** Same as *Blind-spot.* **P. lachryma'le**, one of the puncta lacrimalia. **P. prox'imum.** Same as *Near-point.* **P. remo'tum.** Same as *Far-point.*

Punc'ture. An act of piercing; also, a wound made by a pointed instrument. **Lumbar p.** See *Quincke's puncture.*

Punc'tured wound. A wound made by a stab or prick.

Pun'gent. Penetrating or sharp; somewhat acrid.

Pu'pil. The opening in the center of the iris. **Argyll-Robertson p.**, one which is myotic and responds to accommodative effort, but not to light. **Artificial p.**, one made by iridectomy. **Cat's-eye p.**, one with a narrow vertical aperture. **Hutchinson's p.**, one dilated on one side. **Pin-hole p.**, one which is extremely contracted.

Pu'pillary. Pertaining to the pupil.

Pupillom'eter. Apparatus for measuring diameter of pupil.

Pupillos'copy. Same as *Skiascopy.*

Pupillostatom'eter. Instrument to measure distance between pupils.

Purga'tion (pur-ga'shun). Catharsis; purging effected by medicines.

Pur'gative (pur'gat-iv). 1. Effecting a purgation; cathartic. 2. A cathartic medicine.

Purge (purj). 1. A purgative medicine or dose. 2. To evacuate the bowels by means of a medicine.

Pu'riform. Like, or resembling, pus.

Pur'kinje's cells. Large branched cells of the cerebellar cortex. **P.'s fibers,** moniliform fibers in the subendocardial heart-tissue. **P.'s figures,** shadows of retinal blood-vessels. **P.'s vesicle.** Same as *Germinal vesicle.*

Purkinje-Sanson images (poor-kin'ya-sahn-sōn'). Three pairs of images of one object seen in observing the pupil.

Puromu'cous. Consisting of pus and mucus together.

Pur'pura. A disease characterized by formation of purple patches on the skin and in the mucous membranes. **P. ful'minans,** a fatal purpura of young children. **P. hæmorrha'gica,** severe purpura with copious hemorrhages. **P. rheumat'ica,** purpura with severe pains and fever. **P. sim'plex,** purpura with slight or trifling symptoms.

Purpu'ric. Pertaining to, or affected with, purpura.

Pur'purin. A red coloring-matter, $C_{14}H_5O_2(OH)_3$, of the urine.

Pur'ring thrill. Thrill comparable to a cat's purring, due to mitral stenosis.

Pu'rulence (pu'ru-lens). The condition of being purulent.

Pu'rulent. Containing or consisting of pus.

Pur'uloid. Resembling pus; pus-like.

Pus. A liquid inflammation-product made up of cells and a thin fluid called liquor puris. **Blue p.,** pus with a bluish tint produced by *Bacillus pyocyaneus.* **Curdy p.,** pus mixed with cheesy flakes. **Ichorous p.,** thin, acrid pus. **Laudable p., P. laudan'dum,** whitish inodorous pus, regarded as indicative of less danger than the other varieties. **P.-poultice.** a mass of pus formerly allowed to remain on the surface of a sore with the idea that it was the natural dressing for such a lesion. **Sanious p.,** bloody pus.

Pus'tulant (pus'chu-lant). Causing pustulation.

Pus'tular. Pertaining to, or of the nature of, a pustule.

Pustula'tion. The formation of pustules.

Pus'tule. An elevation of the cuticle filled with pus or lymph. **Malignant p.,** true anthrax.

Pustulo-crusta'ceous. Characterized by pustules and crusts.

Puta'men. The darker and outer portion of the lenticular nucleus.

Putrefac'tion. Decomposition of animal or vegetable matter, effected largely by the action of micro-organisms.

Putrefac'tive. Of the nature of, or pertaining to, putrefaction.

Putres'cent (pu-tres'sent). Rotting; undergoing putrefaction.

Putres'cin (pu-tres'in). A liquid ptomain from decaying matter.

Pu'trid. Characterized by putrefaction; rotten. **P. fever,** typhus or typhoid fever. **P. sore-throat,** cynanche maligna; gangrenous sore-throat.

Pu'trilage. Putrescent or putrid matter.

Pyæ'mia. See *Pyemia.*

Pyarthro'sis. The presence of pus in a joint-cavity.

Pyeli'tis. Inflammation of the pelvis of the kidney. **Calculous p.** is due to calculi. **Hemorrhagic p.** is attended with hemorrhage.

Pyelocysti'tis. Inflammation of renal pelvis and bladder.

Pyelom'eter (pi-el-om'et-er). A pelvimeter.

Pyelonephri'tis. Inflammation of the kidney and its pelvis.

Pyelot'omy. Incision of the pelvis of the kidney.

Pye'mia. Septic infection due to absorption of pyogenic germs.
Pye'sis, Pyo'sis. The formation of pus.
Pygodid'ymus. Fetus with double hips and pelvis.
Pygome'lus. Fetus with extra limbs on the buttocks.
Pygop'agus. Twin fetus joined at the buttocks.
Py'in. An albuminoid sometimes found in pus.
Pyknomor'phous. Having the stained portions of the cell-body compactly arranged.
Pykno'sis (pik-no'sis). Degeneration of a cell in which it becomes denser and smaller.
Py'la. Passage from the third ventricle to the Sylvian aqueduct.
Pylephlebi'tis. Inflammation of the portal vein.
Pylethrombo'sis. Obstruction of portal vein by a thrombus.
Pylom'eter. Apparatus for measuring obstructions at the entrance of the bladder.
Pyloral'gia (pi-lo-ral'je-ah). Pain and spasm of the pylorus.
Pylorec'tomy (pi-lo-rek'to-me). Removal of the pylorus.
Pylor'ic (pi-lor'ik). Pertaining to the pylorus.
Pylori'tis. Inflammation of the pylorus.
Pylor'oplasty. Plastic surgery of the pylorus.
Pylo'rus. The distal or duodenal aperture of the stomach.
Pyocol'pocele (pi-o-kol'po-sēl). A suppurating vaginal tumor.
Pyocol'pos. A collection of pus in the vagina.
Pyoc'tanin. Same as *Pyoktanin.*
Pyocy'anin (pi-o-si'an-in). A pigment, $C_{14}H_{14}NO_2$, from blue pus.
Py'ocyte (pi'o-sit). A pus-corpuscle: said to be a true leukocyte.
Pyogen'esis (pi-o-jen'es-is). The formation of pus.
Pyogen'ic (pi-o-jen'ik). Producing suppuration.
Pyohæ'mia, Pyohe'mia (pi-o-he'me-ah). Same as *Pyemia.*
Pyohemotho'rax. The presence of pus and blood in the cavity of the thorax.
Py'oid (pi'oid). Resembling or like pus.
Pyok'tanin blue. Methyl violet: a germicide and stain. **P. yellow,** an amin, used as a stain.
Pyome'tra (pi-o-me'trah). An accumulation of pus within the uterus.
Pyonephro'sis (pi-o-nef-ro'sis). A collection of pus within the kidney.
Pyo-ova'rium (pi-o-o-va're-um). An ovarian abscess.
Pyopericardi'tis. Suppurative pericarditis.
Pyopericar'dium (pi-o-per-ik-ar'de-um). The presence of pus in the pericardium.
Pyophthalmi'tis. Purulent inflammation of the eye.
Pyophylac'tic membrane. The lining membrane of an abscess cavity.
Pyophysome'tra. Presence of pus and gas in the uterus.
Pyopneumotho'rax. Pus and gas or air in the pleural cavity.
Pyopoie'sis (pi-o-poi-e'sis). Same as *Pyogenesis.*
Pyorrhe'a, Pyorrhœ'a. A copious discharge of pus. **P. alveola'ris,** purulent inflammation of the dental periosteum.
Pyosal'pinx. An accumulation of pus in an oviduct.
Pyosepthæ'mia, Pyosepthe'mia. Same as *Septicopyemia.*
Pyosepticе'mia. See *Septicopyemia.*
Pyostat'ic. Arresting suppuration.
Pyotho'rax. An accumulation of pus in the thorax.
Pyoxan'those. A yellow pigment from pus.
Pyr'amid (pir'am-id). Any cone-shaped eminence upon an organ. **P. of the cerebellum,** a conic projection, the central portion of the inferior vermiform process. **P. of Ferrein,** any one of the intracortical prolongations of the Malpighian pyramid. **Lalouette's p.** See *Pyramid of the thyroid gland.* **Malpig-**

hian p., any one of the conic masses of the medulla of the kidney. **P's. of the medulla**, two anterior and two posterior columns within the oblongata. **P. of the thyroid**, the third lobe of the thyroid body.

Pyram'idal. Shaped like a pyramid. **P. bone**, the cuneiform bone of the carpus. **P. tract**, a set of motor fibers going from the motor area and passing to the pyramids of the oblongata: they afterward become the p. tracts of the spinal cord.

Pyramida'lis. See *Muscles, Table of.*

Pyran'tin. An antipyretic substance, $C_{12}H_{13}NO_3$.

Pyrene'mia. The presence of nucleated red corpuscles in the blood.

Pyre'nin. The substance of a nucleolus.

Pyre'thrum. The root of *Anacyclus pyrethrum*, or pellitory: sialagogue and sedative.

Pyret'ic (pi-ret'ik). Pertaining to, or characterized by, fever.

Pyre'tin (pi-re'tin). An analgesic and antipyretic preparation.

Pyretogen'esis (pi-re-to-jen'es-is). The origination of fevers.

Pyretog'enin (pi-re-toj'en-in). A base from bacterial cultures.

Pyretog'enous (pi-re-toj'en-us). Producing or causing fever.

Pyretog'raphy (pi-ret-og'raf-e). Description of fevers.

Pyretol'ogy (pi-ret-ol'o-je). The sum of what is known regarding fevers.

Pyrex'ia (pi-rek'se-ah). Fever; elevation of temperature.

Pyrex'ial (pi-rek'se-al). Pertaining to fever.

Pyr'idin (pir'id-in). An antispasmodic, C_5H_5N, from coal-tar and tobacco.

Py'riform. Pear-shaped. **P. fascia**, the fascia covering the pyriformis muscle.

Pyrifor'mis (pir-if-or'mis). See *Muscles, Table of.*

Pyrobo'rate (pi-ro-bo'rāt). Any salt of pyroboric acid.

Pyrobo'ric acid. The acid, $H_2B_4O_7$, obtained by heating boric acid.

Pyrocat'echin (pi-ro-kat'e-chin). An antipyretic substance from catechu.

Pyrocatechinu'ria, Pyrocatechu'ria. The presence of pyrocatechin in the urine.

Pyr'odin (pir'o-din). A poisonous antipyretic: used in skin-diseases.

Pyrogal'lic acid, Pyrogal'lol. See *Acid.*

Pyrogen'ic (pi-ro-jen'ik). Inducing fever.

Pyrolig'neous (pi-ro-lig'ne-us). Obtained by the destructive distillation of wood.

Pyroma'nia (pi-ro-ma'ne-ah). An insane propensity to incendiarism.

Pyrom'eter (pi-rom'et-er). A device for measuring high degrees of heat.

Pyropho'bia (pi-ro-fo'be-ah). Insane dread of fire.

Pyrophos'phate. Any salt of pyrophosphoric acid.

Pyrophosphor'ic acid. See *Acid.*

Pyro'sis. Heartburn or water-brash.

Pyrot'ic (pi-rot'ik). Caustic.

Pyrotox'in (pi-ro-tok'sin). A toxin developed during a fever.

Pyrox'ylin (pi-roks'il-in). Gun-cotton; cotton treated with nitric and sulphuric acids.

Py'rozole. A proprietary coal-tar antipyretic.

Py'rozone (pi'roz-ōn). A proprietary preparation of hydrogen peroxid.

Pyr'rol. An oily base, C_4H_5N, from various animal matters.

Pythogen'esis. Production by means of filth.

Pythogen'ic (pi-tho-jen'ik). Caused by filth or putrefaction.

Pyu'ria (pi-u're-ah). Passage of urine containing pus.

Q.

Q. L. Abbreviation for *quan' tum li' bet:* "as much as you please."
Q. S. Abbreviation for *quan' tum suf' ficit:* "as much as will suffice."
Quack. A charlatan; an ignorant or fraudulent empiric.
Quack'ery. The practice or methods of a quack; charlatanry.
Quadrang'ular (kwod-rang'u-lar). Having four angles.
Quad'rate (kwod'rāt). Square or squared. **Q. lobe,** one of the smaller lobes of the liver. **Q. lobule,** the precuneus; a part of the parietal lobe of the cerebrum.
Quadra'tus lumbo'rum, etc. See *Muscles, Table of.*
Quad'riceps exten'sor. See *Muscles, Table of.*
Quadrigem'inal (kwod-rij-em'in-al). Fourfold; in four parts. **Q. bodies.** Same as *Corpora quadrigemina.*
Quadrilat'eral (kwod-ril-at'er-al). Having four sides.
Quadrip'ara. A woman who has born four children.
Quadriv'alent (kwod-riv'al-ent). Having a valence of four.
Quad'ruplet (kwod'ru-plet). Any one of four children born at one birth.
Qual'itative, Qual'itive. Pertaining to quality. **Q. analysis.** See under *Analysis.*
Quan'titative, Quan'titive. Pertaining to quantity. **Q. analysis.** See under *Analysis.* **Q. vision,** vision just sufficient to distinguish light from darkness.
Quantiv'alence (kwon-tiv'al-ens). Chemical valence; atomicity or combining power.
Quan'tum li'bet. L. for "as much as you please."
Quan'tum suf'ficit. L. for "as much as suffices."
Quar'antine (kwar'an-tēn). Place or period of detention of ships coming from infected or suspected ports.
Quar'tan (kwor'tan). Recurring every third (fourth) day.
Quartip'ara (kwor-tip'ar-ah). A woman who has had her fourth child.
Quassa'tion (kwas-sa'shun). The crushing or shattering.
Quass'ia (kwash'e-ah). Bitter tonic wood of *Picræna excelsa.*
Quas'sin (kwas'sin). Bitter principle, $C_{32}H_{44}O_{10}$, from quassia.
Quater'nary (kwah-ter'nar-e). Containing four elements; fourth.
Quat'uor pills. Pills of iron, quinin, nux vomica, and aloes.
Quebra'cho (kwe-brah'tsho). Bark of tree *Aspidosperma quebracho blanco* of Chili: antiperiodic and tonic.
Quer'cus al'ba. White oak; bark is a tonic astringent.
Quick'ening. The first recognizable movements of the fetus in the uterus.
Quick'lime. Caustic or unslacked lime.
Quick'silver. Mercury.
Qui'gila. An infectious disease resembling leprosy, occurring in Brazil.
Quilla'ia sapona'ria. Chilian tree: its bark (soap-bark) is used in catarrhs, bronchitis, etc.
Quil'led or **Quil'ted suture.** An interrupted suture with double thread, quill, and loops for lacerated intestine.
Quinal'gene (kwin-al'jēn). Same as *Analgene.*
Quinasep'tol (kwin-as-ep'tol). Same as *Diaphthol.*
Qui'nate (kwi'nāt). Any salt of quinic acid.
Quince. Fruit of *Cydonia vulgaris:* a demulcent.
Quinck'e's disease. Urticaria œdematosa. **Q.'s puncture,** the tapping of the spinal membranes to obtain cerebrospinal fluid for examination.
Quin'ia (kwin'e-ah). See *Quinin.*
Quin'ic acid (kwin'ik). An acid, $C_7H_{12}O_6$, from cinchona bark.
Quin'in (kwin'in). A bitter white alkaloid, $C_{20}H_{24}N_2O_2+3H_2O$,

from cinchona: used as a tonic and antiperiodic. **Q. fever,** fever with eruption on the skin from an overdose of quinin.
Quin'inism (kwin'in-izm). Same as *Cinchonism.*
Quin'oform. A compound of formaldehyd and cinchona.
Quinoi'din (kwin-oi'din). Same as *Chinoidin.*
Quin'olin (kwin'ol-in). An oily liquid, C_6H_7N, from quinin.
Quin'one (kwin'ōn). A principle, $C_6H_4O_2$, obtained by oxidizing quinic acid.
Quinopro'pylin. An antiperiodic homologue of quinin.
Quin'osol. An antiseptic oxyquinolin preparation.
Quino'vin. A glucosid, $C_{30}H_{48}O_8$, from cinchona.
Quinqui'na (kwin-kwi'nah). Same as *Cinchona.*
Quinquiv'alent. Same as *Pentavalent.*
Quin'sy (kwin'ze). Acute suppurative tonsillitis.
Quin'tan (kwin'tan). Recurring every fifth (fourth) day.
Quintip'ara. A woman who has born five children.
Quin'tuplet (kwin'tu-plet). One of five children born at one birth.
Quio'nin. Tasteless quinin.
Quiz. Instruction by questions and answers. **Q. class,** a class of students banded together for the purpose of being questioned by a teacher.
Quotid'ian. Recurring every day.

R.

R. Abbreviation for *Réaumur.*
R. Abbreviation for *Recipe:* "take."
Rab'id. Affected with hydrophobia or rabies.
Ra'bies (ra'be-ēz). The hydrophobia of animals.
Rac'emose (ras'e-mōs). Shaped like a bunch of grapes.
Rachial'gia (ra-ke-al'je-ah). Pain in the spinal column.
Rachid'ian. Pertaining to the spine.
Rachil'ysis (ra-kil'is-is). Correction of lateral curvature of spinal column by combined traction and pressure.
Rachiocamp'sis. Spinal curvature.
Rachioch'ysis. Dropsy of the spinal canal.
Rachiodyn'ia. Pain in the spinal cord.
Rachiom'eter. Apparatus for measuring spinal curvatures.
Rachiomyeli'tis. Myelitis.
Rachiople'gia. Spinal paralysis.
Ra'chiotome (ra'ke-ot-ōm). Instrument for cutting into the spinal column.
Rachiot'omy (ra-ke-ot'o-me). The cutting into, or through, the spinal column.
Ra'chis (ra'kis). The vertical or spinal column.
Rachis'chisis (ra-kis'kis-is). Congenital fissure of spinal column.
Rachit'ic (ra-kit'ik). Affected with, or pertaining to, rickets. **R. rosary,** a succession of bead-like prominences along costal cartilages.
Rachi'tis (rak-i'tis). See *Rickets.*
Radesy'ge (rah-da-se'geh). Ulcerative skin-disease formerly prevalent in Scandinavia.
Ra'diad. Toward the radial side or aspect.
Ra'dial (ra'de-al). Pertaining to the radius.
Ra'diant, Ra'diate. Diverging from a center.
Radia'tion. 1. Divergence from a center. 2. Structure made up of divergent elements. **Optic r.,** strand of fibers continuous with those of corona radiata, derived mainly from pulvinar, geniculate bodies, and optic tract. **Striothalamic r.,** fiber-system which links the thalamus to the subthalamic r. **Thalamic r.,** tracts of fibers from optic thalami radiating into hemisphere.
Rad'ical (rad'ik-al). 1. Directed to the cause; going to the root

or source of a morbid process. 2. Atom or group of atoms which may be combined with other atoms or groups. **R. operation,** one intended to effect a complete cure.

Rad'icle (rad'ik-l). One of the smallest branches of a vessel or nerve.

Radic'ular. Pertaining to a root or radicle. **R. fibers,** fibers connected with roots of spinal nerves. **R. vessels,** arterial branchlets which supply roots of cerebral and spinal nerves.

Radiocar'pal. Pertaining to the radius and carpus.

Ra'diograph (ra'de-o-graf). Same as *Skiagraph.*

Radiog'raphy (ra-de-og'raf-e). Same as *Skiagraphy.*

Radi'olus. A probe or sound.

Radio-ul'nar. Pertaining to the radius and ulna.

Ra'dius. The bone of the thumb side of the forearm. **R. fix'us,** straight line from hormion to inion.

Ra'dix, pl. *rad'ices.* L. for *Root.*

Rag-sor'ters' disease. A febrile disease of bacterial origin in persons who assort paper-rags.

Rail'way-kidney. A kidney-disease ascribed to the jar of railway travel. **R.-spine,** a complication of nervous and myelonic symptoms caused by injuries received in railway accidents.

Rai'sins (ra'zinz). Dried grapes; passulæ or uvæ passæ.

Râle (rahl). Any abnormal respiratory sound heard in auscultation. [See *Table of the Râles,* pp. 384, 385.]

Ramifica'tion. Distribution in branches.

Ramollisement (ra-mol-lees-maw'). Fr. for *Softening.*

Ra'mus. A branch, as of a nerve, vein, or artery. **R. commun'icans,** a branch which connects a spinal nerve with a sympathetic ganglion.

Ran'cid. Having a musty rank taste or smell.

Range of accommodation. Difference in diopters between the accommodation of the eye at its near-point and at its far-point.

Ra'nine (ra'nin). Pertaining to a ranula or to the lower surface of the tongue.

Ran'ula. A cystic tumor beneath the tongue.

Ranvier's nodes (rah-ve-āz'). Constrictions on nerve-fibers at about the interval of one millimeter.

Rape. Coitus without the consent of the woman.

Rapha'nia (raf-a'ne-ah). 1. Nervous disease said to be caused by eating wild or black radishes. 2. Pellagra. 3. Ergotism.

Ra'phe (ra'fe). Ridge that marks the line of union of the halves of a symmetric organ.

Rarefac'tion. Condition of being or becoming less dense.

Rar'efying osteitis. See under *Osteitis.*

Rash. A temporary eruption on the skin, as in urticaria or strophulus. **Canker-r.,** popular name for *Scarlatina.* **Caterpillar-r.,** local eruption attributed to poisoning by hairs of caterpillars. **Drug r., Medicinal r.,** one caused by medication. **Mulberry r.,** peculiar eruption of typhus fever looking like the eruption of measles. **Nettle-r.** See *Urticaria.* **Rose-r.** See *Roseola.* **Tooth-r.** See *Strophulus.*

Ras'patory. A file or rasp for surgeons' use; xyster.

Rasu'ra. Filings or scrapings.

Ratan'hia (rat-an'he-ah). See *Krameria.*

Rath'ke's pouch (raht'kiz). Diverticulum from embryonic buccal cavity whence the anterior lobe of the pituitary body is developed.

Rat'ion (rash'un). Fixed daily allowance of food granted to a soldier or sailor.

Ra'tional (rash'un-al). Accordant with reason. **R. symptom.** Same as *Subjective symptom.*

A TABLE OF THE PRINCIPAL RÂLES.

NAME.	HEARD IN.	HOW PRODUCED.	QUALITIES.	SIGNIFICANCE.
Amphoric.	Expiration and inspiration.	By air in cavity communicating with a bronchus.	Musical, large, tinkling.	Shows a cavity from tubercle or abscess.
Bubbling, large.	Expiration and inspiration.	Passage of air through mucus in a bronchus or trachea.	Large and moist.	Lung-congestion and bronchitis.
Bubbling, medium.	Expiration and inspiration.	Air passing through mucus in the bronchia.	Smaller than in next above; moist.	Capillary and other bronchitis.
Bubbling, small.	Expiration and inspiration.	Air passing through mucus in bronchioles.	Moist, small, and almost crepitant.	Capillary bronchitis of children.
Cavernous.	Expiration and inspiration.	Air passing through small cavities which collapse in expiration.	Metallic and hollow.	Third stage of tuberculosis.
Clicking.	In inspiration.	Air passing through soft material in the small bronchi.	Sticky and small.	Early stages of tuberculosis.
Consonating.	Expiration and inspiration.	Air passing through.	Clear and ringing.	Tuberculous pneumonia.
Crackling, dry.	Inspiration.	By broken-down lung-tissue.	Short, sharp, and loud.	Second stage of tuberculosis; gangrene of lungs.
Crackling, medium.	Mainly in inspiration.	By fluids in smaller bronchi.	Dry and somewhat small.	Softening of a pulmonary exudate or of a tuberculous deposit.
Crackling, small.	Mainly in inspiration.	By fluids in smaller bronchi.	Dry, small, and almost crepitant.	Softening of a pulmonary exudate or of a tuberculous deposit.
Crepitant.	End of inspiration.	Entrance of air into collapsed vesicles, usually near base of lung.	Small; sounds like hair rubbed between the fingers.	Early pneumonia; hypostatic pneumonia; edema of lungs; local deposit of tubercle.

Dry.	Inspiration and expiration.	Narrowing of bronchial tubes by thickening of the mucous lining; spasm of the muscular coat; mucus within or without; pressure from outside.	Large and sonorous; sometimes small and hissing, or whistling.	In asthma, bronchitis, and in localized incipient tuberculosis.
Extra-thoracic.		In larynx or trachea.		
Friction.	Expiration and inspiration; chiefly near end of inspiration.	By the rubbing together of serous surfaces, roughened or dried by inflammation.	Crackling, breaking, grating, grazing, rubbing.	Pericarditis and pleurisy.
Gurgling.	Expiration and inspiration.	Passage of air through fluid in cavities on coughing.	Large and moist like the bursting of large bubbles.	Advanced stages of tuberculosis.
Guttural.		In the throat.		
Moist.		Air going through fluids in a bronchus [illegible].		
Mucous.	Expiration and inspiration.	Bursting of viscid bubbles in the bronchia.	A variety of subcrepitant.	Emphysema of lungs.
Redux.	Expiration and inspiration.	Air going through [illegible] fluid in a bronchial tube.	Unequal and crackling.	Stage of resolution in pneumonia.
Sibilant.	Expiration and inspiration.	Narrowing of bronchia [illegible] adherent mucus, by spastic contraction or thickening of the lining membrane.	High-pitched, piping, or hissing.	Asthma, bronchitis, and local in incipient tuberculosis.
Sonorous.	Expiration and inspiration.	From reduced caliber [illegible] a bronchus, from spasm, [illegible]ternal pressure, or tumefacti[illegible] its substance.	Snoring; low in pitch.	Frequent in asthma and in bronchitis.
Subcrepitant.	Expiration and inspiration.	Air passing through mu[illegible]n bronchioles.	Moist and small.	Capillary bronchitis.

Rats'bane. Arsenic trioxid or arsenous anhydrid, As_2O_3.
Rat'tle. A râle. See also *Death-rattle.*
Rat'tlesnake. See *Crotalus.*
Rat-tooth forceps. Forceps with teeth that interlock.
Rau's apophysis (rawz). Same as *Processus gracilis.*
Ray. A line of light or heat. **Actinic r.,** a light-ray which produces chemical changes. **R.-fungus.** Same as *Actinomyces.* **Medullary r.,** any cortical extension of a bundle of tubules from a Malpighian pyramid of the kidney. **Röntgen r., X-ray.** See *Röntgen ray.*
Raynaud's disease (ra-nōz'). Same as *Acroasphyxia.*
Rb. Symbol for *Rubidium.*
R. D. A. The right dorso-anterior position of the fetus.
R. D. P. The right dorsoposterior position of the fetus.
Reac'tion. 1. Opposite action or counter-action. 2. Phenomena caused by chemical action of substances on each other. **Amphoteric r.,** alteration of color of both blue and red litmus. **R. of degeneration,** loss of response to faradic stimulus in a muscle, and to galvanic and faradic stimulus in a nerve. **Electric r.,** response to electric stimulation. **Hemiopic pupillary r.,** reaction in some cases of hemianopia in which the stimulus of light thrown upon one side of the retina causes the iris to contract, while light thrown upon the other side arouses no response. **Myotonic r.,** increase in faradic excitability, as in Thomsen's dis[illegible]se. **R.-period, R.-time,** time elapsing between [illegible] [illegible]tion.
[illegible] [illegible]ployed to produce a chemical [illegible]
[illegible] [illegible]usulphid, As_2S_2.
[illegible]tion [illegible] performance of an amputation.
Reap[illegible] [illegible]rai[illegible] [illegible] in harvesters produced by awns and dust from grai[illegible]. [illegible]
Réaumur's scale (ra-[illegible]). Thermom[illegible]ter-scale with melting-point of ice at 0° and boiling point of water at 80°.
Recei'ver. A vessel for collect[illegible]g a gas or a distillate.
Receptac'ulum chy'li. Expansion at lower end of thoracic duct.
Reces'sus. A cavity or recess. **R. pharyn'geus,** fossa in nasopharynx on either side of the Eustachian tubes.
Rec'ipe (res'ip-e). 1. L. for *Take.* 2. A prescription or formula.
Recip'rocal reception. Articulation in which each surface is convex in one way and concave in another.
Reclination. The turning of the eye-lens over on its back for the cure of cataract.
Reclus's disease (rek'lūz). A cystic disease of the mammary gland.
Rec'rement (rek'rim-ent). Saliva or other secretion which is reabsorbed into the blood.
Recrementi'tious. Of the nature of a recrement.
Recrudes'cence (re-kru-des'ens). Recurrence of symptoms after temporary abatement.
Recrudes'cent (re-kru-des'ent). Breaking out anew.
Rec'tal (rek'tal). Pertaining to the rectum. **R. crisis,** severe pains of the rectum in locomotor ataxia. **R. reflex,** the reflex by which the accumulation of feces in rectum excites defecation.
Rectal'gia (rek-tal'je-ah). Pain in the rectum.
Rectifica'tion. The process of purifying or correcting.
Rect'ified. Brought to an established standard of purity. **R. spirit,** alcohol freed from fusel oil and containing but 16 per cent. of water.
Recti'tis. Inflammation of the rectum.
Rec'tocele (rek'to-sēl). Hernia of the rectum through the vagina.

Rectococ'cypexy (rek-to-kok'sip-ek-se). Fixation of rectum to the coccyx.

Rectocystot'omy. Vesical incision through the rectum.

Rec'topexy (rek'to-pek-se). Surgical fixation of rectum.

Rectopho'bia (rek-to-fo'be-ah). Morbid foreboding in patients with rectal disease.

Rec'toscope (rek'tos-kōp). Speculum for rectal examination.

Rectosteno'sis. Stricture or narrowing of rectum.

Rectot'omy (rek-tot'om-e). Same as *Proctotomy.*

Recto-ure'thral. Pertaining to the rectum and urethra.

Recto-u'terine. Pertaining to rectum and uterus.

Rectovag'inal (rek-to-vaj'in-al). Pertaining to rectum and vagina.

Rectoves'ical (rek-to-ves'ik-al). Pertaining to rectum and bladder.

Rec'tum. Distal portion of large intestine.

Rec'tus muscles. See *Muscles, Table of.*

Recupera'tion. Recovery of health and energy.

Recur'rence (re-ker'ens). The return of symptoms after a remission.

Recur'rent. Returning after a remission. **R. sensibility,** sensibility remaining in a nerve after its section.

Recurved (re-kervd'). Bent backward.

Red blindness. Inability to discern red tints. **R. gum.** Same as *Strophulus.* **R. lead,** lead tetroxid, Pb_3O_4; [illegible]nium. **R. nucleus,** a mass of gray matt[illegible] [illegible]er. See *Capsicum.* **R. soften**[illegible], [illegible] [illegible]orm [illegible] [illegible] of [illegible] the brain and cord.

Redintegra'tion (red-in-teg-ra'shun). Restitution [illegible]

Redressement force'. Forcibl[illegible] [illegible]rrection of kn[illegible] [illegible]

Reduce (re-dūs'). To replace [illegible] [illegible]al position [illegible]

Redu'cible. Sus[illegible] [illegible] of bei[illegible] [illegible]educed.

Redu'cin (re-du'sin). A leukomain[illegible] $H_{36}N_6O_9$, from urochrome.

Reduc'tion (re-duk'shun). C[illegible]rrection of a fracture, luxation, or hernia.

Redu'plicated. Doubled; bent back.

Reduplica'tion. A doubling back.

Refine (re-fīn'). To purify or free from foreign matter.

Reflec'tion (re-flek'shun). A turning or bending back.

Reflec'tor (re-flek'tor). A device for reflecting light or sound.

Reflex (re-fleks'). 1. Reflected. 2. A reflected action or movement. **Abdominal r.,** contractions about navel on downward friction of abdominal wall. **Ankle-clonus, Ankle-r.,** pressure on sole with flexion of foot causes clonic contraction of tendo Achillis. **R. arc,** an afferent nerve, a nerve-center, an efferent nerve, and a muscle. **Biceps r.,** tap on tendon of biceps of arm causes it to contract. **Bulbocavernous r.,** tap on dorsum of penis retracts the bulbocavernous portion. **R.-center,** nerve-center where sensory impressions give rise to involuntary motor impulses. **Chin-r., Jaw-jerk,** stroke on lower jaw causes clonic movement. **Ciliospinal r.,** stimulus of skin of neck dilates pupil. **Corneal r., Eyelid-closure,** irritation of conjunctiva closes lids. **Cranial r.,** any reflex whose paths are connected with the brain. **Cremasteric r.,** stimulation of skin of thigh retracts testis. **Crossed r.,** stimulation of one side of body makes a reflex on other side. **Davidsohn's r.,** light seen through pupil when electric light is held in mouth. **Deep r.,** any reflex elicited by irritating a deep structure. **Dorsal r.,** stimulation of skin along erector spinæ contracts muscles of back. **Elbow-jerk.** See *Biceps r.* **Epigastric r.,** stimulation in fifth and sixth intercostal spaces near axilla dimples the epigastrium. **Faucial r.,** irritation of fauces causes vomiting. **Femoral r.**, irritation of skin on upper anterior aspect of thigh flexes foot and first three toes and extends knee. **Front-tap r., Tendo Achillis r.**, tap on shin-muscles of extended leg contracts gastrocnemius. **Gluteal r.**, stroke over skin of buttock contracts the glutæl muscles. **Interscapular r., Scapular r.**, stimulus between scapulæ contracts scapular muscles. **Jaw-jerk.** See *Chin-r.* **Knee-jerk, Patellar r., Westphal's sign**, stroke on tense patellar tendon contracts the quadriceps and jerks the foot. **Laryngeal r.**, irritation of fauces and larynx causes cough. **Lumbar r.** Same as *Dorsal r.* **Nasal r.**, irritation of Schneiderian membrane provokes sneezing. **Obliquus r.**, stimulus of skin below Poupart's ligament contracts part of external oblique. **Palatal r.**, stimulation of palate causes swallowing. **Palmar r.**, tickling of palm flexes fingers. **Paradoxic patellar r.**, stroke on patellar tendon, the patient lying on his back, contracts the adductor muscles; also, forcible flexion and sudden relaxation of leg contracts anterior muscles. **Paradoxic pupillary r.**, stimulation of retina by light dilates pupil. **Patellar r.** See *Knee-jerk.* **Penis-r.** Same as *Bulbocavernous r.* **Periosteal r.**, tap on bones of leg or forearm causes muscular contraction. **Peroneal r.**, stroke on tense peroneal muscles or when foot is turned in causes reflex movements. **Pharyngeal r.**, stimulus to pharynx causes swallowing. **Plantar r.**, irritation of sole contracts the toes. **Platysmal r.**, nipping the platysma myoides contracts pupil. **Pupillary r.**, stimulus of light contracts pupil. **Scapular r.** Same as *Interscapular r.* **Skin-r.** See *Platysmal r.* **Sole-r.** See *Plantar r.* **Spinal r.**, any reflex emanating from a center in spinal cord. **Superficial r.**, any reflex provoked by a superficial stimulation. **Tendo Achillis r.** See *Front-tap r.* **Toe-r.**, strong flexion of great toe flexes all muscles of lower extremity. **Virile r.** Same as *Bulbocavernous r.* **Wrist-clonus r.**, extreme extension of hand causes local jerking movements.

Re'flux (re'flux). A return flow.

Refract'. To ascertain errors of ocular refraction.

Refrac'ta do'si. In repeated and divided doses.

Refrac'tion (re-frak'shun). The deviation of light in traversing obliquely a medium of differing density. **Double r.**, refraction in which incident rays are divided into two refracted rays. **Dynamic r.**, refraction of the eye when at rest. **R.-index**, refringent power of any body as compared with air. **Static r.**, refraction of the eye when its accommodation is paralyzed.

Refrac'tionist. One skilled in correcting errors of refraction of the eye.

Refrac'tive (re-frak'tiv). Pertaining to refraction.

Refractom'eter. Apparatus for measuring refraction.

Refrac'tory. Not readily yielding to treatment.

Refrac'ture. Operation of breaking again an improperly treated fracture.

Refran'gible (re-fran'jib-l). Susceptible of being refracted.

Refresh (re-fresh'). To freshen or make raw again.

Refrig'erant (re-frij'er-ant). Relieving fever and thirst.

Refrigera'tion (re-frij-er-a'shun). Therapeutic reduction of a high temperature.

Refu'sion (re-fu'zhun). The returning of blood to the vessels.

Regenera'tion (re-jen-er-a'shun). Renewal; repair of injured tissue.

Reg'imen (rej'im-en). Methodical system of diet and habits.

Re'gion (re'jun). Any particular part of the body. **Axillary r.**, the axilla and its borders. **Ciliary r.**, part of eye occupied by ciliary body and its adjuncts. **Clavicular r's., right and left,**

regions of the clavicles. **Epigastric r.,** median region of abdomen between hypochondriac regions. **Hypochondriac r's., right** and **left,** regions of abdomen on either side below ribs. **Hypogastric r.,** lowest median abdominal region between inguinal regions. **Infra-axillary r.,** situated below axilla. **Infraclavicular r.,** space on either side of chest below clavicle. **Inframammary r.,** below the mamma and above lower border of twelfth rib. **Infrascapular r.,** below scapula on either side of vertebral column. **Infraspinous r.,** below spine of scapula. **Inguinal r.,** the groin. **Inguinal r's., right** and **left,** lowest abdominal on either side below lumbar regions. **Interscapular r.,** space between scapulæ. **Ischiorectal r.,** region between ischium and rectum. **Lumbar r's., right** and **left,** on either side of umbilical region. **Mammary r.,** on either side of chest between third and sixth ribs. **Motor r., Rolandic r.,** ascending frontal and parietal convolutions. **Precordial r.,** region of heart and pit of stomach. **Scapular r.,** region of the back over the scapula. **Sensory r.,** a parietotemporal region of cortex. **Supraclavicular r.,** space above clavicle. **Supraspinous r.,** above spine of scapula. **Umbilical r.,** medial abdominal region between lumbar regions.

Re'gional (re'jun-al). Pertaining to a region.

Regres'sive (re-gres'siv). Going back; retreating.

Reg'ular. Normal; conforming to rule. **R. practitioner,** a physician of the scientific and more generally recognized school. **R. school,** system of medicine based upon scientific facts and the knowledge gained by experience.

Regur'gitant (re-gur'jit-ant). Flowing back.

Regurgita'tion. 1. The casting up of undigested food. 2. A flowing backward of the blood.

Rei'chart's cartilage (ri'karts). The cartilage of the hyoid arch of the embryo whence the styloid process, stylohyoid ligaments, etc., are developed.

Reich'mann's disease (rik'mahnz). Same as *Gastrorrhea.*

Reid's base-line (reedz). See *Base-line*, under *Line.*

Reil's island (rilz). See *Island of Reil.*

Re-implanta'tion. Replacement of what has been taken out.

Re-infec'tion. A second infection by a similar agent.

Re-inocula'tion. An inoculation that follows a previous one.

Reinsch's test (rinsh'ez). Test for arsenic with copper and hydrochloric acid.

Re-inver'sion. Restoration to normal place of an inverted organ.

Reiss'ner's canal (ris'nerz). Same as *Cochlear canal.* **R.'s membrane,** thin membrane between R.'s canal and scala vestibuli.

Rejuvenes'cence. A return to youth.

Relapse (re-laps'). Return of a disease after its apparent cessation.

Relap'sing fever. See *Fever.*

Rel'ative near-point. See *Near-point.*

Relax'ant (re-lak'sant). Causing a relaxation.

Relaxa'tion. A lessening of tension.

Relief' incision. A cut made to relieve tension or congestion.

Remak's fiber (re-maks'). A non-medullated nerve-fiber. **R.'s ganglion,** a ganglion in the wall of the right auricle. **R.'s symptom,** abnormal lapse of time before a painful sensation is perceived.

Reme'dial (re-me'de-al). Curative; acting as a remedy.

Rem'edy (rem'ed-e). Anything that cures, palliates, or prevents disease.

Remis'sion (re-mish'un). A diminution or abatement of symptoms.

Remit'tent (re-mit'ent). Having periods of abatement and of exacerbation, as a certain form of malarial fever.

Ren. L. for *Kidney*.

Ren'aden. A proprietary extract of the kidney; used in Bright's disease.

Re'nal (re'nal). Pertaining to the kidney.

Ren'culin. An albuminoid said to exist in the suprarenal bodies.

Renicap'sule. The suprarenal body.

Ren'iform. Shaped like a kidney.

Ren'in. An extract prepared from the kidneys.

Renipor'tal. Pertaining to the portal system of the kidney.

Ren'ipuncture. Surgical incision of capsule of kidney.

Ren'net. Preparation of calf's stomach which coagulates milk.

Ren'nin. A ferment from gastric juice.

Ren'nogen. A substance from which rennin is developed.

Repel'lant. Capable of dispersing a swelling.

Repercola'tion. Second or repeated percolation with same materials.

Repercus'sion (re-per-kush'un). 1. The driving in of an eruption or scattering of a swelling. 2. Ballottement.

Reple'tion (re-ple'shun). Condition of being full.

Reposi'tion. Replacement in the normal position.

Repos'itor (re-poz'it-or). Instrument for replacing displaced parts.

Reproduc'tion. Production of offspring by organized bodies.

Reproduc'tive. Serving for purposes of reproduction.

Resal'gin (re-sal'jin). A compound of antipyrin and resorcin.

Resec'tion. Excision of a part of an organ.

Reserve' air. Air left in the lungs at end of expiration that may be partly expelled by forced expiration.

Res'ervoir of Pecquet. Same as *Receptaculum chyli*.

Resid'ual. Remaining; left behind. **R. air,** air that cannot be expelled from the lungs by forced respiration.

Resid'uum (re-zid'u-um). A residue or remainder.

Resil'ience (re-sil'e-ens). Elasticity; quality of rebounding.

Resil'ient (re-sil'e-ent). Elastic; inclined to contract after dilatation.

Res'in (rez'in). 1. An inflammable amorphous substance of many kinds, obtained from plants and trees. 2. Same as *Rosin*. **R.-plaster.** See *Plaster*.

Res'inol (rez'in-ol). Same as *Retinol*.

Res'inous (rez'in-us). Of the nature of a resin.

Resis'tance coil. A coil of wire introduced into an electric circuit to increase the resistance.

Re'sol. Antiseptic solution of wood-tar and soap.

Resolu'tion (rez-o-lu'shun). Subsidence of inflammation; softening and disappearance of a swelling.

Resol'vent. Promoting resolution.

Res'onance (rez'on-ans). Sound elicited by percussion. **Amphoric r.,** sound as of blowing over an empty bottle. **Cracked-pot r.,** a peculiar sound elicited over a pulmonary cavity by percussion. **Hydatid r.,** peculiar sound in combined auscultation and percussion of a hydatid cyst. **Skodaic r.,** increased percussion resonance at upper part of chest with flatness below it. **Tympanic r.,** drum-like reverberation of a cavity filled with air. **Tympanitic r.,** peculiar sound elicited by percussing a tympanitic abdomen. **Vesicular r.,** normal pulmonary resonance. **Vesiculo-tympanic r.,** resonance partly vesicular and partly tympanic. **Vocal r.,** sound of ordinary speech as heard through the chest-wall. **Whispering r.,** auscultatory sound of whispered words heard through chest-wall.

Res'onant (rez'on-ant). Giving a vibrant sound on percussion.

Resopy'rin. A mixture of resorcin and antipyrin.

Resor'bin. Mixture of oil, wax, soap, gelatin, and lanolin.

Resor'cin. A crystalline principle, $C_6H_4(OH)_2$: antiseptic and antipyretic.

Resor'cinism. Chronic poisoning by resorcin.

Resorcylal'gin. A combination of resorcin and antipyrin.

Resorp'tion (re-sorp'shun). Removal by absorption of excreted matter.

Res'pirable (res'pir-a-bl). Suitable for respiration.

Respira'tion (res-pir-a'shun). The act or function of breathing. **Abdominal r.** is chiefly kept up by abdominal muscles and diaphragm. **Absent r.**, that in which respiratory sounds are suppressed. **Accelerated r.** is that which exceeds 25 respirations a minute. **Amphoric r.** is characterized by amphoric resonance. **Artificial r.** is maintained by artificial means. **Bronchial r.** Same as *Tubular r.* **Bronchocavernous r.**, that which is both cavernous and tubular. **Bronchovesicular r.**, intermediate between bronchial and vesicular r. **Cavernous r.**, marked by a peculiar resonance, usually due to cavity in lung. **Cheyne-Stokes r.** is characterized by rhythmic alterations of intensity. **Cog-wheel r.** has peculiarly broken or jerky inspiration. **Costal r.**, performed mainly by rib-muscles. **Cutaneous r.**, exhalation of vapors and absorption of oxygen by skin. **Forced r.** takes in more air than is needed. **Interrupted r.**, breathing in which the sounds are not continuous. **Labored r.**, that which is performed with difficulty. **Metamorphosing r.** Same as *Bronchocavernous r.* **Puerile r.**, breathing-sounds too intense, or like those of children. **Rude r.**, bronchovesicular respiration. **Slow r.**, less than 12 respirations per minute. **Stertorous r.** is accompanied by abnormal snoring sounds. **Tubular r.** has high-pitched sounds, as if made by blowing through a tube. **Vesicular r.**, the natural breathing of a sound and healthy person. **Vesiculocavernous r.**, cavernous r. with a vesicular quality.

Res'pirator. Apparatus to qualify the air that is breathed through it.

Res'piratory (res'pir-at-o-re). Pertaining to respiration. **R. bundle, R. column.** See *Solitary fasciculus.* **R. quotient**, quotient obtained by dividing quantity of carbon dioxid exhaled by quantity of oxygen inhaled in breathing.

Respirom'eter. Instrument for determining the character of the respiration.

Restibra'chium. Inferior peduncle of cerebellum.

Res'tiform. Shaped like a rope. **R. body**, lateral column of the oblongata passing to the cerebellum.

Res'tis (res'tis). Same as *Restiform body.*

Restitu'tion. Rotation of presenting part of fetus outside the vagina.

Restor'ative. 1. Promoting a return of health. 2. A remedy that aids in restoring the health.

Resuscita'tion. Restoration to life of one apparently dead.

Ret'ching (ret'ching). Strong involuntary effort to vomit.

Re'te. A network or net. **R. Malpig'hii, R. muco'sum**, the innermost stratum of epidermis. **R. mirab'ile**, a network of small anastomosing blood-vessels, chiefly from a single trunk. **R. muco'sum**, the lower epidermic layer. **R. tes'tis**, the network formed in the mediastinum of the testis by the vasa recta.

Reten'tion (re-ten'shun). The persistent keeping within the body of matters normally excreted. **R.-cyst**, a tumor-like accumulation of secretion whose natural outlet is blocked.

Retic'ular (re-tik'u-lar). Resembling a network. **R. formation**, a network of fibers in the oblongata passing into the pons.

R. lamina, R. membrane, the membrane which covers the organ of Corti.

Retic'ulum (re-tik'u-lum). L. for *Network.*

Re'tiform (re'tif-orm). Same as *Reticular.*

Ret'ina. The innermost tunic and perceptive structure of the eye, formed by the expansion of the optic nerve.

Retinac'ulum. A band or cord holding any organ in its place. **R. ligamen'ti arcua'ti,** short external lateral ligament of knee-joint. **R. Morgag'ni,** ridge formed by the coming together of segments of ileocecal valve. **R. peroneo'rum infe'rius,** band across peroneal tendons on outside of calcaneum. **R. peroneo'rum supe'rius,** external annular ligament of ankle. **R. ten'dinum,** an annular ligament of ankle or wrist. **R. of Weibrecht.** See *Weibrecht's retinacula.*

Ret'inal. Pertaining to the retina.

Retini'tis. Inflammation of the retina. **R. pigmento'sa,** retinal sclerosis with pigmentation and atrophy.

Retinochoroidi'tis. Inflammation of the retina and choroid.

Ret'inol. A hydrocarbon, $C_{32}H_{16}$, obtainable from rosin: solvent.

Retinos'copy (ret-in-os'kop-e). Same as *Skiascopy.*

Retort'. A globular long-necked vessel used in distillation.

Retrac'tile (re-trak'til). Susceptible of being drawn back.

Retrac'tion. The act of drawing back; condition of being drawn back.

Retrac'tor. Instrument for drawing apart the lips of a wound.

Ret'rahens au'rem. See *Muscles, Table of.*

Retrobul'bar. Situated or occurring behind the eyeball.

Retroce'dent. Going back; coming back or returning. **R. gout,** gout of which the outward symptoms disappear and are replaced by severe visceral affections.

Retroces'sion (re-tro-sesh'un). A going back or return.

Retroclu'sion. Acupressure by means of a pin passed over, back of, and under a vessel.

Retrocol'lic. Pertaining to the back of the neck.

Re'troflexed. Bent back; sharply recurved.

Retroflex'ion (re-tro-flek'shun). The bending of an organ so that its top is thrust back.

Ret'rograde (ret'ro-grād). Going backward; retracing a former course. **R. metamorphosis.** Same as *Catabolism.*

Retrog'raphy (re-trog'raf-e). Writing looking like ordinary writing seen in a mirror: it is seen in certain brain-diseases.

Retro-in'sular. Behind the island of Reil.

Retromam'mary. Situated behind the mammary gland.

Retrona'sal. Pertaining to the back part of the nose.

Retro-oc'ular (re-tro-ok'u-lar). Situated behind the eye.

Retroperitone'al. Situated behind the peritoneum.

Retroperitoni'tis. Inflammation in the space behind the peritoneum.

Retropharyn'geal (re-tro-far-in'je-al). Occurring behind the pharynx.

Retropul'sion (re-tro-pul'shun). 1. A driving back, as of the fetal head in labor. 2. Tendency to walk backward, as in some cases of locomotor ataxia.

Retroster'nal pulse. Venous pulse felt over the suprasternal notch.

Retrotar'sal (re-tro-tar'sal). Situated behind tarsus of the eye.

Retro-u'terine. Occurring behind the uterus.

Retrovaccina'tion. Inoculation of cow with human vaccine virus.

Retrover'sion. The tipping of an entire organ backward.

Ret'zius, lines of. Brownish lines in the enamel of a tooth. **R., space of,** succession of areolar spaces in front of bladder. **R.,**

veins of, veins which connect the branches of the portal vein with the postcava.

Reuss's test (rois'ez). Test for atropin with sulphuric acid and an oxidizing agent.

Revel'lent (re-vel'ent). Causing revulsion.

Revivifica'tion. The refreshing of a wound.

Revul'sant. An agent causing revulsion.

Revul'sion (re-vul'shun). Derivation of blood from a diseased part to another part.

Revul'sive. 1. Effecting a revulsion. 2. A derivative agent.

Rhabdi'tis (rab-di'tis). A genus of parasitic nematode worms.

Rhabdomyo'ma. Myoma of striated muscular elements.

Rhachial'gia and other words in **Rhach-.** See *Rachialgia*, etc.

Rhaco'ma. 1. Excoriation. 2. A pendulous scrotum.

Rhag'ades (rag'ad-ēz). Painful fissures in the skin.

Rham'nus. Genus of trees; buckthorns. See *Cascara sagrada* and *Frangula*.

Rhapha'nia (raf-a'ne-ah). Same as *Raphania*.

Rha'phe (ra'fe). Same as *Raphe*.

Rhat'any (rat'an-e). See *Krameria*.

Rhe'ochord (re'o-kord). Same as *Rheostat*.

Rheom'eter (re-om'et-er). 1. Same as *Galvanometer*. 2. Instrument for measuring rapidity of the blood-current.

Rhe'ophore (re'of-ōr). Same as *Electrode*.

Rhe'oscope (re'os-kōp). Device indicating the presence of an electric current.

Rhe'ostat. Appliance for regulating the resistance in an electric circuit.

Rhe'otome (re'ot-ōm). A device for breaking an electric circuit.

Rhe'otrope. An instrument for reversing a current.

Rhestocythe'mia. Occurrence of degenerated red blood-corpuscles in the blood.

Rhe'um (re'um). See *Rhubarb*.

Rheum (rūm). A watery discharge from the nose, eyes, or sores.

Rheumarthro'sis. Articular rheumatism.

Rheumatal'gia. Rheumatic pain.

Rheumat'ic. Pertaining to, or affected with, rheumatism. **R. fever,** acute inflammatory rheumatism.

Rheu'matism (ru'mat-izm). A constitutional disease marked by pain in joints or muscles, usually recurrent, and often due to exposure. **Gonorrheal r.,** arthritis associated with gonorrheal urethritis. **Inflammatory r.,** acute rheumatism with fever and a marked tendency to heart-complications. **Muscular r.,** rheumatism of voluntary muscles and their fibrous structures.

Rheumatis'mal edema. Rheumatism with painful subcutaneous swellings.

Rheu'matoid arthritis. See *Arthritis*.

Rheumatop'yra (ru-mat-op'ir-ah). Rheumatic fever.

Rheum'ic diathesis. Same as *Dartrous diathesis*.

Rhex'is (rek'sis). The rupture of a blood-vessel.

Rhig'olene (rig'ol-ēn). An inflammable liquid: used as a local freezing anesthetic.

Rhi'nal (ri'nal). Pertaining to the nose.

Rhinal'gia (ri-nal'je-ah). Pain in the nose.

Rhinal'gin. Compound of alumnol, oil of valerian, menthol, and cocoa-butter: used in rhinal and lacrimal inflammations.

Rhinenceph'alon (ri-nen-sef'al-on). The olfactory lobe of the brain.

Rhi'neurynter (ri'nu-rin-ter). Dilatable bag for plugging a nostril.

Rhin'ion (rin'e-on). Lower end of the suture between nasal bones.

Rhini'tis. Inflammation of nasal mucous membrane. **Acute r.,** coryza or cold in the head. **Atrophic r.** is marked by wasting of mucous membrane and glands. **R. caseo'sa.** rhinitis with gelatinous and fetid discharge. **Fibrinous r.,** a form with development of false membrane. **Hypertrophic r.,** that in which mucous membrane thickens and swells. **Vasomotor r.,** hay-fever.

Rhino'byon. A nasal tampon.

Rhinoceph'alus. Fetus with a nose like a proboscis.

Rhinoclei'sis. Obstruction of the nasal passages.

Rhinodyn'ia. Pain in the nose.

Rhinola'lia (ri-no-la'le-ah). Nasal twang from defect or disease of nasal passages. **R. aper'ta** is due to excessive patulousness of posterior nares. **R. clau'sa** is due to too great closure of the same.

Rhin'olin. A proprietary antipyretic and antiseptic.

Rhi'nolite, Rhi'nolith. Nasal calculus or concretion.

Rhinolithi'asis. The formation of rhinolites.

Rhinol'ogist (ri-nol'o-jist). An expert in diseases of the nose.

Rhinol'ogy (ri-nol'o-je). The sum of knowledge regarding the nose and its diseases.

Rhinomec'tomy (ri-nom-ek'to-me). Excision of the inner canthus.

Rhinom'eter (ri-nom'et-er). Apparatus for measuring the nose.

Rhinonecro'sis. Necrosis of the nasal bones.

Rhinopho'nia (ri-no-fo'ne-ah). Nasal twang or quality of voice.

Rhinophy'ma (ri-no-fi'mah). Nodular congestion and swelling of the nose.

Rhi'noplasty (ri'no-plas-te). The forming of a new nose from tissue from some other part.

Rhinopol'ypus (ri-no-pol'ip-us). Nasal polypus.

Rhinorrha'gia (ri-no-ra'je-ah). Copious hemorrhage from nose.

Rhinorrhe'a. A nasal mucous discharge.

Rhinoscle'rin. A preparation of the bacillus of rhinoscleroma used in treating that disease.

Rhinosclero'ma. A hard growth in the nasal mucous membrane.

Rhi'noscope (ri'no-skōp). Speculum for nasal examination.

Rhinos'copy. Specular examination of the nose.

Rhinostegno'sis. Obstruction of the nasal passages.

Rhizodon'tropy. Fixing an artificial crown to a natural root of tooth.

Rhizodon'trypy. Perforation of root of a tooth for the escape of morbid matter.

Rhizo'ma, Rhi'zome (ri-zo'mah, rhi'zōm). Subterranean root-stem of a plant.

Rho'dallin (ro'dal-in). Same as *Thiosinamin.*

Rhodogen'esis (ro-do-jen'es-is). Regeneration of rhodopsin after its bleaching by the light.

Rho'dophane (ro'do-fān). A red pigment from retinal cones.

Rhodophylax'is (ro-do-fil-ak'sis). Same as *Rhodogenesis.*

Rhodop'sin (ro-dop'sin). Visual purple; pigment of outer segment of retinal rods.

Rhom'boid. Shaped like a rhomb or kite. **R. fossa, R. sinus.** Same as *Fourth ventricle.*

Rhomboi'deus (rom-boi'de-us). See *Muscles, Table of.*

Rhon'chial (rong'ke-al). Pertaining to a rhonchus.

Rhon'chus (rong'kus). A coarse dry râle in the bronchial tubes.

Rho'tacism (ro'tas-ism). Incorrect utterance of *r* sounds.

Rhu'barb (roo'barb). Root of *Rheum officinale:* purgative and astringent.

Rhus toxicoden'dron. Poison sumac: antirheumatic.

Rhypopho'bia (ri-po-fo'be-ah). Morbid fear of filth.

Rhythm (rith'um). A measured movement.

Rhytido'sis (rit-id-o'sis). A wrinkling, as of the cornea.

Rib. Any one of the twenty-four bones of the sides of the chest. **False r's.**, the ribs not attached directly to the sternum. **Floating r's.**, the last two pairs of ribs. **True r's.**, the ribs that are attached to the sternum.

Ribes's ganglion (rēbz). Supposed cephalic end of the sympathetic nervous system.

Rice. The cereal plant *Oryza sativa;* also, its seed or grain.

Rice-water stools. Stools of cholera which look like water in which rice has been boiled.

Rich'ter's hernia (rik'terz). Hernia which involves only a part of the lumen of the gut.

Ri'cin (ri'sin). A poisonous principle from the seed of castor-oil plant.

Ric'inin (ris'in-in). Alkaloid from castor-oil plant.

Ric'inus commu'nis. Plant whose seeds afford castor-oil.

Rick'ets. Disease of childhood in which the bones become crooked and deformed and their earthy salts are diminished; rachitis.

Rick'ety. Affected with rickets; rachitic.

Ri'ders' bone (ri'derz). Same as *Cavalry bone.* **R.s' leg, R.s' sprain,** sprain of the adductor leg-muscles which takes place in riding on horseback.

Ridg'ling. A man or animal with one testicle removed.

Ri'ga's disease (re'gahz). Cachectic aphthæ, a fatal inherited and microbic disease.

Rigg's disease (rigz). Alveolodental periostitis.

Ri'gor (ri'gor). 1. A chill; rigidity. **R. mor'tis,** rigidity or stiffening after death.

Ri'ma. A crack or chink. **R. glot'tidis,** the chink between the vocal cords. **R. respirato'ria,** the space behind the arytenoid cartilages.

Ri'mous. Full of cracks or fissures.

Rim'ula. A minute fissure of the cord or brain.

Rin'derpest. The cattle-plague, a contagious disease of cattle.

Ring, external abdominal. Opening in aponeurosis of external oblique for spermatic cord or for round ligament. **Internal abdominal r.,** aperture in transversal fascia for spermatic cord or for round ligament. **Löwe's r.,** ring in visual field caused by macula lutea. **Maxwell's r.,** a ring resembling Löwe's, but smaller and fainter. **Müller's r.,** muscular ring surrounding cervical canal and body of uterus at an advanced stage of pregnancy. **Spermatorrheal r.,** a ring worn on the penis to prevent erections.

Ring'worm. Parasitic skin-disease in circular patches.

Ri'nolite (ri'no-lit). See *Rhinolite.*

Ri'olan's bouquet (re'o-lanz). Cluster of ligaments and muscles attached to styloid process. **R.'s muscle,** ciliary part of orbicularis palpebrarum.

Ri'pa (ri'pah). The line of reflection of the ependyma of the ventricles of the brain over a plexus.

Ripault's sign (re-pōz'). Change in shape of pupil on pressure upon the eye, transitory during life, but permanent after death.

Riso'rius (ri-so're-us). See *Muscles, Table of.*

Ris'us sardon'icus. Grinning expression produced by spasm of facial muscles.

Rit'ter-Valli law. See *Law.*

Rit'ter's disease. See *Disease.*

Ri'valry stripe. A flickering sensation in the eyes when the fields of vision are too different to be combined in one visual image.

Rive'rius's draft. The solution of sodium citrate.
Rivin'ius, ducts of. Ducts of sublingual gland. **Ligament of R.** Same as *Shrapnell's membrane.*
Riz'iform (riz'if-orm). Resembling grains of rice.
Rob. A jelly or confection, as of mulberries, etc.
Rob'ertson's pupil. Same as *Argyll-Robertson pupil.*
Rob'orant. Conferring strength.
Rochelle salt (ro-shel'). Sodium and potassium tartrate.
Rock-crystal. A variety of quartz used in making spectacle lenses. **R.-fever.** Same as *Mediterranean fever.*
Ro'dent ulcer. A spreading sluggish sore, chiefly of the face.
Roent'gen rays (rent'gen). See *Röntgen rays.*
Rokitan'sky's disease. Acute yellow atrophy of the liver.
Rolan'dic. Described by, or named in honor of, Rolando. **R. area,** excitomotor area of the cerebrum. **R. fissure.** See *Fissure.* Cleft between ascending frontal and ascending parietal convolutions.
Roll'er. A cylinder of cotton, linen, or flannel rolled up for surgeon's use.
Rom'berg's symptom. Difficulty in standing when the eyes are shut: a sign of locomotor ataxia.
Rougeur (roh-zher'). Gouge-forceps or nippers.
Rönt'gen rays (rent'gen). Species of energy generated by an electric current, Ruhmkorff coil, and vacuum tube, and used in taking photographs through the flesh and through opaque objects.
Rönt'genism. Disease induced by injudicious use of Röntgen rays.
Röntog'raphy (ren-tog'raf-e). Same as *Skiagraphy.*
Roof-nu'cleus. A nucleus of the middle lobe of the cerebellum above the roof of the fourth ventricle.
Root-ar'teries. Same as *Radicular vessels.*
Root-zone. That part of the white matter of the myelon connected with the anterior and posterior nerve-roots.
Ro'sa. L. for *Rose.*
Rosa'cea (ro-za'se-ah). Same as *Acne rosacea.*
Rosan'ilin (ro-zan'il-in). A substance, $C_{20}H_{19}N_3$, from coal-tar: from it dyes and stains are prepared.
Rose. A plant of the genus *Rosa.* **R.-catarrh. R.-cold.** a variety of hay-fever occurring when roses bloom. **R.-rash.** Same as *Roseola.*
Rose'mary. The plant *Rosmarinus officinalis:* its oil is emmenagogue, anodyne, and stimulant.
Ro'senmüller's body. Same as *Parovarium.* **R.'s cavity. R.'s fossa.** fossa on either side of nasopharyngeal orifice of Eustachian tubes.
Rose'ola. A non-contagious rose-rash; rubeola. **R. choler'ica,** eruption sometimes seen in cholera. **Syphilitic r.,** eruption of rose-colored spots in early secondary syphilis. **R. typho'sa.** the eruption of typhoid or typhus fever. **R. vacci'na,** a rash sometimes occurring after vaccination.
Ro'ser's method, R.'s position. The position of the patient with head downward in operations on the air-passages.
Ros'in. The product that remains after the distillation of oil of turpentine.
Rosmari'nus. See *Rosemary.*
Roso'lic acid (ro-sol'ik). See *Acid.*
Ross'bach's disease (ros'bahks). Same as *Hyperchlorydria.*
Rostel'lum. The hook-bearing part of the head of worms.
Ros'trate. Beaked; having a beak.
Ros'trum. A beak-shaped process. **R. of the corpus callosum,** the anterior part of the callosum.
Rot. 1. Decay. 2. A disease of sheep.

Rota'tion. Process of turning around an axis. **R.-joint,** a variety of ginglymus.
Rotato'res spinæ. See *Muscles, Table of.*
Rö'theln (rö'teln). Same as *Rubeola.*
Rot'ula (rot'u-lah). 1. The patella. 2. A lozenge or troche.
Rot'ular (rot'u-lar). Pertaining to the patella.
Rouget du porc (roo-zha duh pork'). Same as *Swine-erysipelas.*
Rouleau (roo-lo'). A roll of red blood-corpuscles resembling a pile of coins.
Round ligament. See *Ligament.* **R. worm,** a parasite of the genus *Ascaris.*
Roup (roop). An infecting disease of fowls.
Rub'ber-dam. Sheet of India-rubber used by dentists in mouth-work.
Rub'ber-tissue. Gutta percha in sheets.
Rube'do (ru-be'do). Redness of the skin.
Rubefa'cient. 1. Reddening the skin. 2. An agent that reddens the skin.
Rubel'la, Rube'ola. 1. A disease not unlike measles, but much milder; German or French measles. 2. Measles.
Rubes'cent (ru-bes'ent). Growing red.
Ru'bia (ru'be-ah). See *Madder.*
Rubid'ium. Rare metal, not unlike potassium: its bromid, RbBr, and iodid, RbI, are medicinal.
Rubi'go (ru-bi'go). L. for *Rust.*
Ru'bus. A genus of plants: *R. villosus,* and other species called blackberry, have astringent root-bark.
Ruc'tus. Belching of wind; eructation.
Rude respiration. See *Respiration.*
Rudimen'tary (ru-dim-en'tar-e). Incompletely developed.
Rue. The herb *Ruta graveolens:* abortifacient and emmenagogue, and having a poisonous oil.
Ru'ga (ru'gah). A ridge or fold.
Ru'gose (ru'gōs), **Ru'gous.** Ridgy; wrinkled.
Rugos'ity. 1. Condition of being rugose; roughness. 2. A ridge or ruga.
Ruhm'korff coil (room'korf). A powerful form of induction-coil.
Rum. Alcoholic spirit from the refuse of sugar-making.
Ru'men. The first stomach of a cud-chewing mammal.
Ru'mex cris'pus. A plant—yellow dock: root tonic and astringent.
Ru'mination. See *Merycism.*
Rump. The buttock or gluteal region.
Run. To discharge pus or mucus.
Run'round. Superficial felon or whitlow seated at the edge of the nail.
Ru'pia. Condition in tertiary syphilis marked by the formation of bullæ.
Rupopho'bia. Insane dislike for dirt.
Rup'ture. 1. Hernia. 2. The bursting or breaking of a part.
Rus'sian bath. See *Bath.*
Rust's disease. A form of Pott's disease.
Rus'ty sputum. Sputum colored with blood, seen in pneumonia.
Rut. The state of being in heat.
Ru'ta. L. for *Rue.*
Rutido'sis. Same as *Rytidosis.*
Ru'tin. A crystalline substance from rue.
Ruys'chian membrane, R. tunic. Same as *Entochoroidea.*
Rye. The cereal plant *Secale cereale,* and its nutritious seed.
Rytido'sis. Wrinkling of the cornea after death.

S.

S. Abbreviation for *Sigma*, mark; *sinister*, left; and symbol of *sulphur*.

S. angle. Angle between radius fixus and a line joining basion and staphylion.

Sabadil'la. The poisonous seed of *Veratrum sabadilla:* used to destroy parasites.

Sabatier's suture (sab-at-e-āz'). See *Suture*.

Sabi'na (sab-I'nah). L. for *Savin*.

Sab'ulous (sab'u-lus). Gritty or sandy.

Sabur'ral. Gritty; gravelly.

Sac. A bag-like organ. **Hernial s.,** peritoneal pouch which encloses protruding intestine. **Lacrimal s.,** dilated upper end of the lacrimal duct. **Yolk s.,** the umbilical vesicle.

Sac'cate (sak'āt). 1. Shaped like a sac. 2. Contained in a sac.

Sac'charated. Sugary; charged with sugar.

Saccharephidro'sis (sak-ar-ef-id-ro'sis). Sweet perspiration.

Sacchari'ferous (sak-ar-if'er-us). Containing sugar.

Saccharifica'tion. Changed into sugar.

Saccharim'eter. Same as *Saccharometer*.

Sac'charin (sak'ar-in). Very sweet coal-tar product, $C_7H_5SO_3N$.

Sac'charine (sak'ar-in). Sugary; sweet.

Saccharogalactorrhe'a. Secretion of milk containing an excess of sugar.

Saccharom'eter. Polarimeter or other device for measuring proportion of sugar in a solution.

Saccharomy'ces. A genus of protophytes, the yeast fungi.

Saccharorrhe'a (sak-ar-o-re'ah). Glycosuria.

Sac'charose (sak'ar-ōs). Ordinary cane- or beet-sugar.

Sac'charum (sak'ar-um). L. for *Sugar*. **S. lac'tis,** milk-sugar or lactose.

Saccholac'tin (sak-o-lak'tin). Sugar of milk.

Sac'ciform (sak'sif-orm). Shaped like a bag or sac.

Sac'culated (sak'u-la-ted). Containing saccules.

Sac'cule (sak'ūl). 1. A small sac. 2. Part of the membranous labyrinth of the vestibule communicating with the ductus communis.

Sacculococh'lear canal. Canal connecting saccule and cochlea.

Sac'culus (sak'u-lus). A saccule. **S. laryn'gis,** fovea on outside of either false vocal cord.

Sac'cus (sak'us). A sac. **S. endolymphat'icus,** sac of dura in the aqueduct of the vestibule. **S. lacrima'lis.** See *Lacrimal sac*.

Sachs'se's solution. Solution of potassium iodid, potassium hydrate, and red iodid of mercury in water.

Sa'cra me'dia. Middle sacral artery.

Sa'crad. Toward the sacrum.

Sa'cral. Pertaining to the sacrum. **S. canal,** extension of the vertebral canal through the sacrum. **S. grooves,** extensions of the vertebral grooves on the back of the sacrum. **S. nerves,** spinal nerves which emerge from the sacral foramina.

Sacral'gia (sa-kral'je-ah). Pain in the sacrum.

Sacrifi'cial operation. Operation by which some organ is sacrificed for the good of the patient.

Sacro-ante'rior. Having the sacrum directed forward.

Sacrococcyg'eal. Pertaining to the sacrum and coccyx.

Sacrocoxi'tis. Inflammation of the sacro-iliac joint.

Sacro-il'iac. Pertaining to the sacrum and ilium. **S.-i. disease,** painful tuberculous inflammation of sacro-iliac articulation.

Sacrolumba'lis. See *Muscles, Table of*.

Sacrolum'bar. Of, or pertaining to, the sacrum and loins.
Sacroposte'rior. Having the sacrum directed backward.
Sacrosciat'ic (sa-kro-si-at'ik). Pertaining to the sacrum and ischium.
Sacrospi'nal. Pertaining to the sacrum and the spinal column.
Sacro-u'terine. Pertaining to the sacrum and uterus.
Sacrover'tebral. Pertaining to the sacrum and the vertebræ.
Sa'crum. The triangular bone between and behind the two ilia.
Sad'dle-joint. Articulation in which the articulating surfaces are convex in one direction and concave in the other. **S.-nose,** a nose with a sunken bridge.
Sa'dism. Sexual perversion in which satisfaction is derived from the infliction of cruelty upon another.
Sae'misch's ulcer (sa'mish-ez). Infectious corneal ulcer.
Sæp'tum (sep'tum). See *Septum.*
Safe'ty tube. Open part of the Eustachian tube.
Saff'lower (saf'low-er). See *Carthamus.*
Saf'fron. See *Crocus.* **American s.** See *Carthamus.*
Saf'ranin (saf'ran-in). A poisonous substance, $C_{18}H_{18}N_4$: used as a pink stain.
Safran'ophil (saf-ran'o-fil). Readily stained with safranin.
Saf'rol. Anodyne, $C_{10}H_{10}O_2$, from sassafras oil.
Sagape'num. Fetid gum-resin much like galbanum.
Sage (sāj). *Salvia officinalis,* a labiate plant: aromatic, astringent, and stimulant.
Sag'ittal (saj'it-al). Like an arrow. **S. section,** anteroposterior vertical section of the head. **S. suture,** suture between the two parietal bones.
Sa'go. Starch from pith of various palm-trees. **S.-spleen,** spleen with amyloid degeneration, in which the Malpighian corpuscles look like grains of sago.
Sagra'din. A proprietary extract from *Cascara sagrada.*
Saint An'thony's fire. Erysipelas; also, contagious anthrax. **S. Gothard's' disease.** See *Ankylostomiasis.* **S. Vitus's dance.** See *Chorea.*
Sal. L. for *Salt.* **S. aera'tus,** sodium bicarbonate. **S. alem'-broth.** See *Alembroth.* **S. ammoni'acus,** ammonium chlorid. **S. commu'nis,** common salt; sodium chlorid. **S. de duo'bus,** potassium sulphate. **S. enix'um,** potassium bisulphate. **S. pol'ychrest,** potassium sulphate with sulphur. **S. prunel'la,** potassium nitrate in balls. **S. so'dæ,** sodium carbonate. **S. volat'ilis,** ammonium carbonate.
Salaam convulsion (sa-lahm'). Same as *Nodding spasm.*
Salace'tol. A crystalline compound of acetone and salicylic acid: antirheumatic.
Sala'cious (sal-a'shus). Full of lust.
Salac'tol. A compound of sodium salicylate, sodium lactate, and hydrogen peroxid; useful in diphtheria.
Salamand'erin. Poisonous base from skin of a salamander.
Salan'tol. A proprietary compound of acetone and salicylic acid.
Sal'danin. A locally anesthetic alkaloid from *Datura arboreum.*
Sa'lep. Tubers of various orchids: nutritious and demulcent.
Sal'icin (sal'is-in). Tonic and antiperiodic glucosid, $C_{13}H_{18}O_7$, from willow and poplar.
Salicylac'etol (sal-is-il-as'et-ol). Same as *Salacetol.*
Salicylam'id. A yellow germicidal principle, $C_7H_7NO_2$.
Salic'ylate (sal-is'il-āt). Any salt of salicylic acid.
Salic'ylated. Impregnated or charged with salicylic acid.
Salicyl'ic acid (sal-is-il'ik). See *Acid.*
Salic'ylid (sal-is'il-id). An anhydrid of salicylic acid.
Salicylsulpho'nic acid. See *Acid.*

Salicylu'ric acid. Compound of glycol and salicylic acid, obtained from urine after administration of salicylic acid.

Salife'brin. Acetanilid salicylate, $C_{13}H_{11}NO_2$: anodyne and antipyretic.

Sal'ifiable. Capable of combining with an acid to form a salt.

Salifor'min. Salicylate of formin: a uric-acid solvent.

Salig'enin (sal-ij'e-nin). A principle, $C_7H_8O_2$, obtainable from salicin.

Salim'eter. A hydrometer for determining the strength of saline solutions.

Sa'line (sa'lin). Salty; of the nature of a salt.

Sal'iphen. Salicyl-phenetidin, a colorless antipyretic substance.

Salipy'rin (sal-ip-i'rin). Antipyrin salicylate, $C_{18}H_{18}N_2O_4$: anodyne and antipyretic.

Salire'tin. Resinous substance, $C_{14}H_{14}O_3$.

Salis'bury treatment (sawlz'ber-e). Treatment of obesity by use of large amounts of beef, codfish, and hot water.

Salithy'mol (sal-ith-i'mol). Thymol salicylate: anodyne and antipyretic.

Sali'va (sa-li'vah). The fluid secreted by the salivary glands; spittle.

Sal'ivant, Sal'ivatory. Causing an excessive flow of saliva.

Sal'ivary (sal'iv-er-e). Pertaining to the saliva.

Saliva'tion. Excessive discharge of saliva; ptyalism.

Sa'lix (sa'lix). L. for *Willow.*

Salmon patch (sam'un). Dull red patch formed in cornea in interstitial keratitis.

Sal'mon's operation (sah'munz). See *Back cut of Salmon.*

Sal'ocoll. Phenocoll salicylate: antipyretic and anodyne.

Sal'ol. Phenyl salicylate, $C_{13}H_{10}O_3$: antirheumatic and antipyretic.

Sal'ophene. Acetylparamidol, $C_{14}H_{13}NO_4$: useful in rheumatism.

Salpingec'tomy (sal-pin-jek'to-me). Removal of an oviduct or Eustachian tube.

Salpin'gian (sal-pin'je-an). Pertaining to an oviduct.

Salpin'gion (sal-pin'je-on). A point at the apex of the petrous bone on lower surface.

Salpingi'tis (sal-pin-ji'tis). Inflammation of an oviduct or Eustachian tube.

Salpingocath'eterism. Catheterization of the Eustachian tube.

Salpingocye'sis. Pregnancy in an oviduct.

Salpingo-oöphorec'tomy. Surgical removal of an oviduct and ovary.

Salpingo-oöphori'tis, Salpingo-ovari'tis. Inflammation of an ovary and oviduct.

Salpingopharyn'geus. The levator palati muscle.

Salpingor'rhaphy. Suture of oviduct to ovary after excision of a portion of the ovary.

Salpingostaphyli'nus. The tensor palati muscle.

Salpingos'tomy (sal-ping-gos'to-me). Formation of an opening to the oviduct.

Salpingot'omy (sal-ping-got'om-e). Surgical incision of an oviduct.

Sal'pinx. 1. An oviduct. 2. A Eustachian tube.

Salpy'rin (sal-pi'rin). Same as *Salipyrin.*

Salt (sawlt). 1. Sodium chlorid. 2. Any compound of a base or radical and acid; any compound of an acid only a part of whose replaceable hydrogen atoms have been substituted. **Basic s.,** any salt with more than the normal proportion of the basic element. **Bay-s.,** common salt from sea-water. **Common s.,** sodium chlorid. **Double s.,** any salt in which the hydrogen atoms of the acid have been replaced by two metals. **Epsom s.**, magnesium sulphate. **S. frog**, Cohnheim's frog; frog from whose vessels all blood has been artificially removed and replaced by a salt solution. **Glauber's s.**, sodium sulphate. **Haloid s.**, any binary compound of a halogen—*i. e.*, of chlorin, iodin, bromin, fluorin, or cyanogen. **Monsel's s.**, iron subsulphate: chiefly used as a styptic. **Neutral s., Normal s.**, one which is neither acid nor basic. **Normal** or **physiologic s. solution**, sodium chlorid (0.6 to 0.75 per cent.) dissolved in water: restorative, and used in physiologic experiments. **Preston s.** See *Smelling s.* **S.-rheum**, chronic eczema. **Rochelle s.**, potassium and sodium tartrate. **Smelling s.**, aromatized ammonium carbonate.

Salta'tion (sal-ta'shun). Dancing.

Sal'tatory spasm. See *Palmus.*

Sal'ter's swing (sawl'terz). A form of sling or swing for suspending a fractured leg.

Saltpe'ter. Potassium nitrate, KNO_3.

Salts. See *Epsom salts, Glauber's salts, Rochelle salts*, under *Salt.*

Sal'ubrin. A proprietary antiseptic substance.

Salu'brious. Conducive to health; wholesome.

Sal'ubrol. An iodoform substitute made by action of bromin on a compound of methylene and antipyrin.

Sal'ufer. Sodium silicofluorid: antiseptic and germicide.

Sal'umin. Aluminum salicylate: astringent and disinfectant.

Sal'utary (sal'u-ta-re). Healthful.

Salvatel'la. A small vein of the dorsum of the hand.

Salve (sahv). A thick ointment or cerate.

Sal'via (sal've-ah). See *Sage.*

Sambu'cin. A diuretic preparation from sambucus.

Sambu'cus. A genus of shrubs; elder: flowers of various species are sudorific.

Samshin (sam-shiu'). Chinese spirit distilled from the fermented liquor of boiled rice.

San'ative (san'at-iv). Curative; healing.

San'atol. Thick, brown liquid from carbolic and sulphuric acids: disinfectant and antiseptic.

Sanato'rium. 1. A sanitarium. 2. A health-station; chiefly a health-resort in a hot region.

San'atory (san'at-o-re). Conducive of health.

Sand-bath. 1. Use of sand in heating glass vessels. 2. Therapeutic application of hot sand.

Sand-flea. See *Chigre.*

Sand-tumor. Same as *Psammoma.*

San'dal-wood. 1. Wood of *Santalum album*; white sandal-wood: its oil is used like copaiba. 2. The wood of *Pterocarpus santalinus*; red saunders.

San'darac. The resin of *Callitris quadrivalvis*, an African tree.

Sane (sān). Sound in mind.

Säng'er's operation (sāng'erz). A form of Cesarean section.

Sanguic'olous (sang-gwik'o-lus). Living in the blood.

Sanguifica'tion. The conversion of food materials into blood.

San'guinal. A blood-preparation used in anemia.

Sanguina'ria Canaden'sis. A plant, blood-root: the rhizome is used in bronchitis, etc.

Sanguina'rin. An alkaloid from sanguinaria.

San'guine. 1. Abounding in blood. 2. Ardent, hopeful.

Sanguin'eous (san-gwin'e-us). Bloody; abounding in blood.

Sanguin'olent (san-gwin'o-lent). Of a bloody tinge.

San'guis (sang'gwis). L. for *Blood.*

Sanguisu'ga (sang-gwis-u'gah). A leech.

Sa'nies (sa'ne-ēz). A fetid ichorous discharge containing serum, pus, and blood.
Sa'nious (sa'ne-us). Of the nature of sanies.
Sanita'rium. An establishment for the treatment of disease.
San'itary. Promoting, or pertaining to, health.
Sanita'tion. The establishment of conditions favorable to health.
San'ity (san'it-e). Soundness; especially soundness of mind.
Sanmet'to. Proprietary compound of saw-palmetto and santal-oil; used for bladder affections.
San'oform. Colorless crystalline substance, di-iodomethyl salicylate: used as a substitute for iodoform.
San'talum (san'tal-um). See *Sandal-wood.*
Santon'ica. Dried flowers of *Artemisia maritima*, levantine wormseed or cina: vermifugal, etc.
San'tonin. A poisonous active principle, $C_{15}H_{18}O_3$, from santonica.
Santori'ni's cartilage. The corniculum laryngis. **S.'s duct,** an accessory pancreatic duct. **S.'s fissures,** clefts in the fibro-cartilage of the pinna. **S.'s muscle,** the risorius. **S.'s veins,** emissary veins of the head.
Saphe'na (sa-fe'nah). A saphenous vein
Saphe'nous nerves. Two nerves that accompany each s. vein. **S. opening,** passage in fascia lata for long saphena **S. veins,** two important veins (long and short s.) of the thigh.
Sap'id (sap'id). Having taste or flavor.
Sa'po (sa'po). L. for *Soap.*
Sapocar'bol. Antiseptic solution of cresol in potassium soap.
Sapona'ceous (sa-po-na'shus). Soapy; of soap-like feel or quality.
Saponifica'tion. The conversion of a fat or oil into a soap.
Sapo'nin. A poisonous glucosid, $C_{32}H_{54}O_{18}$, from various plants.
Saporif'ic. Producing taste or flavor
Sapotox'in. Poisonous glucosid found in quillaia bark.
Sap'phism (saf'fizm). Sexual perversion between women; tribadism.
Sapræ'mia, Sapre'mia. Poisoning of blood from entrance of septic products.
Sa'prin. A ptomain, $C_5H_{14}N_2$, of decaying viscera
Saprodon'tia (sap-ro-don'she-ah). Caries of the teeth.
Saprogen'ic, Saprog'enous (sa-proj'en-us). 1. Causing putrefaction. 2. Arising from putrefaction.
Sap'rol. Antiseptic mixture of crude cresols in hydrocarbons.
Saproph'ilous. Living on dead matter.
Sap'rophyte (sap'rof-it). A plant organism that grows upon decaying matter.
Saprophyt'ic (sap-rof-it'ik). Of the nature of a saprophyte.
Sapropy'ra, Saproty'phus. Typhus fever.
Sar'cin (sar'sin). Same as *Hypoxanthin.*
Sar'cina (sar'sin-ah). A genus of schizomycetes. **S. ventric'uli,** a variety found in stomach of man and animals.
Sarci'tis (sar-si'tis). Inflammation of muscle-tissue.
Sarco-adeno'ma. Same as *Adenosarcoma.*
Sar'cocele (sar'ko-sēl). A fleshy swelling of the testis.
Sar'cocoll, Sarcocol'la. A gum from Africa and another from Asia: now discarded as medicines.
Sar'code (sar'kōd). Same as *Protoplasm.*
Sarco-enchondro'ma. Sarcoma blended with enchondroma.
Sarcog'lia (sar-kog'le-ah). Matter composing the eminences of Doyère.
Sar'coid (sar'koid). Resembling flesh.
Sarcolac'tic acid. See *Acid.*

Sarcolem'ma. Elastic sheath that encloses each fiber of striated muscle.

Sarcol'ogy. The science of the soft tissues of the body.

Sarco'ma (sar-ko'mah), pl. *sarco'mata.* A tumor made up of a substance like the embryonic connective tissue; often highly malignant. **Adipose s.** contains a copious element of fat. **Alveolar s.,** that in which groups of sarcoma-cells are enclosed in alveolar spaces. **Angiolithic s.** Same as *Psammoma.* **Chondrosarcoma,** one which contains cartilaginous elements. **Fibrosarcoma** contains also fibrous tissue. **Giant-celled s.,** a variety named from its containing large multinucleated cells. **Lymphosarcoma,** round-celled s., with the cells in a reticulum. **Melanotic s.,** variety with cells containing melanin. **Myeloid s.** See *Giant-celled s.* **Myxosarcoma,** that which has partly undergone a mucous degeneration. **Osteosarcoma,** a sarcoma involving a bone, or containing bony elements. **Round-celled s.,** a variety named from the form of its cells. **Spindle-celled s.,** a form with spindle-shaped cells; recurrent fibroid.

Sarcomato'sis. Condition characterized by development of sarcomata.

Sarcom'atous. Of the nature of, or resembling, a sarcoma.

Sar'comere (sar'ko-mēr). Any one of the segments into which the lines of Krause divide a muscular fibrilla.

Sar'coplasm. Interfibrillary matter of striated muscles.

Sar'coplast. An interfibrillar cell of a muscle itself capable of being developed into a muscle.

Sarcop'tes. A genus of itch-mites or acarides. **S. hom'inis.** Same as *Acarus scabiei.*

Sarco'sin. A substance, $C_3H_7NO_2$, from the decomposition of caffein and creatin.

Sarcosporid'ia. Minute parasites in the muscles of cattle, sheep, and other animals.

Sarcosto'sis (sar-kos-to'sis). Ossification of fleshy tissue.

Sar'costyle (sar'kos-til). Any one of the fibrillæ of an elementary muscle-fiber.

Sarcot'ic (sar-kot'ik). Producing blood.

Sar'cous (sar'kus). Pertaining to flesh or muscle-tissue. **S. element,** any one of the minute elements into which a sarcostyle may be divided. **S. substance,** porous material of a sarcous element.

Sardon'ic laugh. Same as *Risus sardonicus.*

Sar'kine (sar'kin). Same as *Hypoxanthin.*

Sarsaparil'la. Root of *Smilax officinalis:* alterative and diuretic.

Sar'tian disease (sar'shun). Infectious disease of Turkestan, like oriental boil.

Sarto'rius (sar-to're-us). See *Muscles, Table of.*

Sas'safras varifo'lium. Tree of North America: bark of root is an aromatic astringent.

Sat'ellite veins. The veins that accompany certain arteries.

Sat'urated compound. A compound that has all the chemical affinities of its elements satisfied.

Satura'tion. The state of a solvent when it holds in solution all it can possibly contain.

Sat'urnine. Pertaining to, or produced by, lead.

Sat'urnism (sat'ern-izm). Lead-poisoning.

Satyri'asis. Excessive venereal impulse in the male.

Saun'ders, red (sahn'derz). Wood of *Santalum rubrum:* a staining agent.

Saurider'ma. A variety of ichthyosis.

Sau'ridon. A disinfectant substance distilled from fossil shale.

Sau'sage poison (saw'sej). Same as *Allantotoxicon.*

Sa'vill's disease. An epidemic skin-disease with papular rash.

Sa'vin. The shrub *Juniperus sabina,* whose oil is a poisonous emmenagogue.

Saviot'ti's canals. Artificially formed slits between glandular cells of pancreas.

Sa'vory. Having an agreeable taste or odor.

Saw. Cutting instrument with a toothed or serrated edge. **Adam's s.,** a small saw for osteotomy. **Butcher's s.,** one in which the blade can be set at various angles. **Chain-saw,** one in which the teeth are set in links, the saw being moved by pulling upon one or another handle. **Crown s.,** a form of trephine. **Hemp s.,** a hempen cord used in cutting soft tissues. **Hey's s.,** a very small saw for enlarging orifices in bones. **S.-palmetto,** the palm *Serenoa serrulata:* diuretic, sedative, analeptic.

Sayre's jacket (sairz). A plaster-of-Paris jacket worn in Pott's disease.

Scab. The crust of a superficial sore.

Sca'bies. Itch; contagious skin-disease due to the itch-mite *Sarcoptes scabiei.*

Scabri'ties (ska-brish'e-ez). Scabby or rough state.

Sca'la (ska'lah). L. for *Staircase; ladder.* **S. me'dia,** space in ear between membrane of Reissner and membrana basilaris. **S. tym'pani,** part of spiral canal below the lamina spiralis. **S. vestib'uli,** part of spiral canal below lamina spiralis.

Scald (skawld). A burn caused by a hot liquid or hot moist vapor. **S.-head,** a crusty disease of the scalp, as favus.

Sca'lene tubercle (ska'lēn). Same as *Lisfranc's tubercle.*

Scale'nus. See *Muscles, Table of.*

Scall (skawl). A crusty disease, as of the scalp.

Scalp. The hairy part of the head.

Scal'pel. A straight knife with convex edge.

Scal'prum (skal'prum). A raspatory or xyster.

Sca'ly (ska'le). Characterized by scales.

Scam'mony. Resinous exudate from root of *Convolvulus scammoniæ; scammonia:* purgative.

Scan'ning utterance. Separation of spoken syllables by decided pauses.

Scaphocephal'ic, Scaphoceph'alous. Having a boat-shaped or keeled head.

Sca'phoid. Shaped like a boat. **S. abdomen.** See *Abdomen.* **S. bone,** a boat-shaped bone of the carpus and of the tarsus.

Scap'ula. The shoulder; flat triangular bone behind the shoulder.

Scapulal'gia (skap-u-lal'je-ah). Pain in the scapula.

Scap'ular. Of, or pertaining to, the scapula.

Scap'ulary. A shoulder-bandage bifurcated in front.

Scapuloclavic'ular. Pertaining to the scapula and the clavicle.

Scar (skahr). Same as *Cicatrix.*

Scarf-skin. The epidermis or cuticle.

Scarifica'tion. The making of small superficial incisions.

Scar'ificator. An instrument for scarifying.

Scarlati'na. Acute contagious fever with scarlet erythema; scarlet fever. **S. angino'sa,** s. with severe throat-symptoms.

Scarlat'inal. Pertaining to, or due to, scarlatina.

Scarlatin'iform, Scarlat'inoid. Resembling scarlatina.

Scar'let fever. Same as *Scarlatina.*

Scar'pa's fascia. Part of deep layer of superficial abdominal fascia crossing Poupart's ligament. **S.'s foramen,** passage in upper jaw-bone for nasopalatine nerve. **S.'s liquor.** Same as *Endolymph.* **S.'s membrane,** membrane that closes the fenestra rotunda. **S.'s triangle,** triangle bounded by inner edge of sartorius, Poupart's ligament, and outer edge of adductor longus.

Scav'enger-cells. Lymph-cells of neuroglia believed to aid in removing effete matter.
Scha'cher's ganglion (shah'kerz). The ciliary ganglion.
Schacho'wa's spiral tube (shah-ko'vahz). Spiral part of a uriniferous tubule.
Schede's method (shēdz'). Treatment of necrosis of bone by removing dead bone and keeping the cavity filled with an aseptic clot.
Schee'le's green (ska'lez). Copper arsenite, $Cu_2As_2O_5$.
Schemat'ic eye (ske-mat'ik). A diagram or model of the eye.
Scherlie'vo (skār-le-a'vo). A contagious disorder formerly prevalent in Austria.
Scheur'len's bacillus (shur'lenz). A bacillus of carcinoma.
Schindyle'sis (skin-dil-e'sis). An articulation in which one bone is received into a cleft in another.
Schistoceph'alus. A fetus born with a cleft head.
Schis'tocyte. A blood-corpuscle undergoing segmentation.
Schistocyto'sis. Accumulation of schistocytes in the blood.
Schistoglos'sia (skis-to-glos'e-ah). Cleft tongue.
Schistoproso'pia. Congenital fissure of the face.
Schistoproso'pus. Fetus born with a cleft face.
Schistor'rhachis. Same as *Spina bifida.*
Schistoso'mus. A fetus with a fissured abdomen.
Schistotho'rax. Fissure of the chest or sternum.
Schizomyce'tes. Group of plant micro-organisms to which the bacteria or microbes belong.
Schizomyco'sis. Any disease due to the presence of schizomycetes.
Schlemm's canal. A minute annular vein at junction of sclera and cornea. **S.'s ligament**, two ligamentous bands of the capsule of the shoulder-joint.
Schneider'ian membrane. The mucous membrane that lines the nasal cavity.
Schön'lein's disease. *Purpura rheumatica.*
Schott treatment. Treatment of heart-disease by medicated baths and exercise.
Schrä'ger's lines (shra'gerz). Lines on the dentin of the teeth.
Schuel'ler's glands. The urethral glands.
Schultze's granule masses. Collections of blood-plaques in the blood. **S.'s primitive fibrillæ**, minute fibrillæ into which the axis-cylinder of a nerve sometimes divides.
Schwann's sheath. Same as *Neurilemma.* **S.'s white substance.** Same as *Myelin*, first definition.
Schweinfurth's green. Copper aceto-arsenite.
Schwelle (shwel'eh). Ger. for *Threshold.*
Sciage (se-ahzh'). A sawing process in massage.
Sciat'ic (si-at'ik). Pertaining to the ischium.
Sciat'ica (si-at'ik-ah). Neuralgia and neuritis of the sciatic nerve.
Scil'la (sil'lah). L. for *Squill.*
Scintilla'tion. Sensation of sparks before the eyes.
Scir'rhoid. Like, or resembling, scirrhus.
Scirrho'ma. Same as *Scirrhus.*
Scirrhosar'ca (skir-o-sar'kah). Same as *Scleroderma.*
Scir'rhous (skir'rus). Of the nature of scirrhus.
Scir'rhus (skir'rus). Hard cancer with predominance of connective tissue.
Scis'sor-leg (siz'zer). A crossing of the legs from deformity.
Scle'ra (skle'rah). Same as *Sclerotic coat.*
Scle'ral (skle'ral). Pertaining to the sclera.
Sclerecta'sia. A bulging state of the sclera.
Sclerec'tomy. Excision of a portion of the sclera.

Sclere'ma. Same as *Scleroderma.* **S. neonato'rum**, a disease of early infancy with hardening and tightness of the skin.

Scleri'asis (skle-ri'as-is). Same as *Scleroderma.*

Scleririt'omy. Incision of the sclera and iris in anterior staphyloma.

Scleri'tis (skle-ri'tis). Inflammation of the sclera.

Sclerochoroidi'tis. Inflammation of the sclera and choroid.

Sclerocor'nea. The sclera and choroid considered as one.

Sclerodactyl'ia. Scleroderma of the fingers and toes.

Scleroder'ma. Disease in which the skin or a part of it becomes hard, rigid, and thickened. **S. neonato'rum.** Same as *Sclerema neonatorum.*

Sclerog'enous. Producing a hard tissue or material.

Scleroiri'tis. Inflammation of the sclera and iris.

Sclerokerati'tis. Inflammation of the sclera and cornea.

Sclerokeratoiri'tis. Inflammation of the sclera, cornea, and iris.

Sclero'ma (skle-ro'mah). See *Sclerosis.*

Scleromu'cin. A slimy, active principle from ergot.

Scleronyx'is. Paracentesis, or puncture of the sclera.

Sclerophthal'mia. State in which sclera encroaches upon the cornea, so that only a portion of the latter remains clear.

Sclerosarco'ma. A firm, fleshy variety of epulis.

Scle'rosed. Affected with sclerosis; hardened.

Sclero'sing. Undergoing or causing sclerosis.

Sclero'sis. Induration with hypertrophy of connective tissue. **Amyotrophic lateral s.,** disease which affects lateral columns and anterior gray matter of cord. **Diffuse s.,** that which extends through a large part of brain and cord. **Disseminated s.,** form with many sclerotic patches dispersed through brain and cord. **Insular s.,** that occurring in separate patches. **Lateral s., primary,** affects especially the crossed pyramidal tracts. **Multiple s.,** sclerosis of brain and cord occurring in scattered patches. **Vascular s.** See *Arteriosclerosis.*

Scleroskel'eton. Part of bony skeleton formed by ossification in ligaments, fasciæ, and tendons.

Sclerosteno'sis (skle-ro-sten-o'sis). Hardening with contraction.

Sclerot'ic. Hard; affected with sclerosis. **S. acid,** one of the active principles of ergot. **S. coat,** the membrane which, with the cornea, forms the external coat of the eye.

Sclerot'ica (skle-rot'ik-ah). Same as *Sclerotic coat.*

Sclerotiece'tomy. Excision of a part of the sclera.

Scleroticochoroidi'tis. Same as *Sclerochoroiditis.*

Scleroticonyx'is (skle-rot-ik-o-nik'sis). Same as *Scleronyxsis.*

Scleroticot'omy (skle-rot-ik-ot'om-e). Incision of the sclera.

Scleroti'tis (skle-ro-ti'tis). Same as *Scleritis.*

Sclero'tium. Hard mass formed by certain fungi, as ergot.

Scle'rotome. An instrument used in sclerotomy.

Sclerot'omy (skle-rot'o-me). Surgical incision of the sclera.

Scolecol'ogy. Same as *Helminthology.*

Sco'lex, pl. *sco'lices.* A larval stage of cestode parasites.

Scoliom'eter. Apparatus for measuring curves.

Scoliorhachit'ic. Both scoliotic and rhachitic.

Scoliosiom'etry. Measurement of spinal curvature.

Scolio'sis. Lateral curvature of spinal column.

Scoliot'ic. Pertaining to, or affected with, scoliosis.

Scoop. Kind of spoon for clearing out cavities.

Scopa'rius. Tops of *Cytisus scoparius,* or broom: diuretic and cathartic.

Scopolam'in, Scopo'lein. Poisonous mydriatic alkaloid from plants of the genus *Scopolia,* etc.

Scoracra'tia (sko-rak-ra'she-ah). Involuntary defecation.

Scorbu'tic. Pertaining to, or affected with, scurvy.

Scor'butus (skor'bu-tus). L. for *Scurvy.*

Scotodinia. Vertigo with headache and dimness of vision.

Scot'ogram, Scot'ograph. Same as *Skiagram.*

Scotog'raphy. Same as *Skiagraphy.*

Scoto'ma. 1. A blind or partly blind area in the visual field. 2. Appearance as of dark, vanishing, cloudy patches before the eyes. **Absolute s.,** area in the visual field as to which the eye is absolutely blind. **Annular s., Ring-s.,** zone of scotoma which surrounds the center of the visual field. **Central s.,** limited to a part of visual field corresponding to macula lutea. **Color-s.,** color-blindness as to a part of the visual field. **Flittering s.,** variety with serrate margins, and usually producing an extensive defect. Same as *Teichopsia.* **Negative s.,** one due to lesion of retina, and not perceptible to the patient. **Positive s.,** one which appears to the patient as a dark spot. **Relative s.,** scotoma in which perception of light is impaired, but not lost. **Scintillating s.** See *Teichopsia.*

Scotom'eter. Instrument for measuring scotomata.

Screa'tus. Paroxysmal attacks of hawking.

Scriv'eners' palsy. Same as *Writers' Cramp.*

Scrobic'ulate. Marked with pits; pitted.

Scrobic'ulus cor'dis. Pit of the stomach; precordial depression.

Scrof'ula. Tuberculous disease of lymphatic glands and of bone, with slowly suppurating abscesses.

Scrof'ulide, Scrof'uloderm. Any skin-disease of scrofulous nature.

Scrofulo'sis (skrof-u-lo'sis). The scrofulous diathesis.

Scrof'ulous. Affected with, or of the nature of, scrofula.

Scro'tal (skro'tal). Pertaining to the scrotum.

Scroti'tis (skro-ti'tis). Inflammation of the scrotum.

Scro'tocele (skro'to-sēl). Scrotal hernia.

Scro'tum. The pouch which contains the testicles.

Scru'ple. Twenty grains apothecaries' weight; symbol, ℈.

Sculte'tus's bandage. A many-tailed bandage with overlapping flaps.

Scurf. Dandruff; branny substance of epidermic origin.

Scur'vy. A disease like purpura, due to improper food. **S. of the Alps,** pellagra.

Scute. A bony plate separating the upper part of the tympanic cavity from the mastoid cells.

Scutella'ria. A genus of labiate herbs. **S. laterifo'lia,** or Skull-cap, is a safe nervine.

Scu'tiform (sku'tif-orm). Shaped like a shield.

Scu'tulum (sku'chu-lum), pl. *scu'tula.* A favus crust.

Scu'tum. The thyroid cartilage.

Scyb'ala (sib'al-ah). Plural of *scybalum.*

Scyb'alous (sib'al-us). Of the nature of a scybalum.

Scyb'alum (sib'al-um), pl. *scyb'ala.* A hard mass of fecal matter.

Scy'phoid (si'foid). Shaped like a cup or goblet.

Scyth'ian disease (sith'e-an). Male sexual perversion, with atrophy of external genitalia.

Scyti'tis (si-ti'tis). Same as *Dermatitis.*

Scytoblaste'ma. The rudimentary skin.

Scytoblaste'sis. The condition of having a rudimentary skin.

Seam'stresses' cramp. Neurosis caused by hard work with the needle.

Search'er. A sound used in searching for stone in the bladder.

Seasick'ness. Nausea and malaise caused by the motion of a vessel.

Sea-tangle. Sea-weed, *Laminaria,* used as a tent.

Seat-worm. Same as *Oxyuris.*

Seba'ceous (se-ba'shus). Pertaining to, or secreting, sebum.
Sebip'arous. Secreting or producing sebum.
Seb'olite, Seb'olith. Calculus in a sebaceous gland.
Seborrha'gia (seb-o-ra'je-ah). Same as *Seborrhea.*
Seborrhe'a, Seborrhœ'a. Disease marked by excessive discharge from the sebaceous glands, forming greasy scales on the body. **S. capilit'ii,** s. of the scalp. **S. congesti'va.** Same as *Lupus erythematosus.* **S. cor'poris,** that which affects the trunk. **S. fa'ciei,** affects the face. **S. ni'gra, S. ni'gricans,** s. with dark-colored crusts. **S. oleo'sa,** form marked with excessive oiliness of the skin, chiefly about the nose and forehead. **S. sic'ca,** commonest form of s., characterized by formation of brownish-gray scales.
Seborrhe'ic, Seborrhœ'ic. Affected with seborrhea.
Se'bum. 1. A greasy secretion which lubricates the skin. 2. Suet.
Seca'le. L. for *Rye.* **S. cornu'tum.** Same as *Ergot.*
Secer'nent. An organ which separates matter from the blood.
Seclu'sion of the pupil. Posterior annular synechia.
Second intention. See under *Healing.*
Second pair of nerves. The optic nerves.
Sec'ondary. Following another; not first in order or importance.
Secre'ta. The secretions.
Secre'tion (se-kre'shun). The process of separating various substances from the blood; also, any substance thus separated.
Secretodermato'sis. Derangement of secreting function of the skin.
Sec'retory. Pertaining to secretion.
Sec'tion. 1. An act of cutting. 2. A cut surface.
Sec'tioning (sek'shun-ing). The cutting of thin sections of tissue for the microscope.
Sec'tor. The area of a circle included between an arc and the radii bounding it.
Secundagrav'ida. A woman with child the second time.
Secun'dines (se-kun'dinz). Same as *Afterbirth.*
Secundip'ara. A woman who has born two children.
Secun'dum ar'tem. In an approved or professional manner.
Sed'atin. 1. Valerylphenetidin. 2. Antipyrin.
Seda'tion. The production of a sedative effect.
Sed'ative. 1. Allaying activity and excitement. 2. A remedy that allays excitement. **Cardiac s.,** a drug that decreases the force of the heart. **Nervous s.,** a hypnotic.
Sed'entary. Sitting; of inactive habits.
Sed'iment. A precipitate formed spontaneously.
Sed'litz powders. See *Seidlitz powders.*
Seed (sēd). See *Semen.*
Seg'ment. A part cut off or demarcated.
Segmen'tal. Forming a segment; undergoing segmentation.
Segmenta'tion. Division into similar parts. **S.-cavity.** Same as *Blastocele.* **S.-nucleus,** nucleus of one fertilized ovum formed by the blending of sperm-nucleus and egg-nucleus. **S.-sphere.** Same as *Blastomere.*
Se'guin's signal symptom. Involuntary contraction of muscles occurring just before an epileptic attack.
Seid'litz powders. Aperient effervescing powders.
Sei'zure (se'zhur). A sudden attack of a disease.
Self-abuse'. Masturbation.
Self-diges'tion. Same as *Auto-digestion.*
Self-infec'tion. Same as *Auto-infection.*
Self-lim'ited disease. Any disease that runs a limited and definite course.
Self-pollu'tion. Masturbation.

Self-suspen'sion. Suspension of the body by the head and axillæ for the purpose of stretching the vertebral column.
Sel'la tur'cica. Same as *Pituitary fossa.*
Sel'ters water, Seltz'er water. An effervescent mineral water.
Semeiog'raphy, Semeiol'ogy. Same as *Symptomatology.*
Semeiot'ic. Pertaining to symptoms.
Semeiot'ics (se-mi-ot'iks). Same as *Symptomatology.*
Sem'el (sem'el). L. for *Once.*
Semelin'cident. Affecting a person only once.
Se'men. 1. A seed. 2. Liquid secreted by the testes and discharged in copulation. **S. con'tra.** Same as *Santonica.*
Semenu'ria. Discharge of semen in the urine.
Semicanal'. A trench or furrow open at one side.
Semicir'cular canals. The three passages forming back part of the ear.
Semiflex'ion. Position of a limb midway between flexion and extension.
Semilu'nar. Of a half-moon shape. **S. bone,** the second bone of the first row of wrist, counting from the thumb side. **S. ganglion,** a large nerve-ganglion of the abdominal cavity. **S. lobe,** the most backward of the two lobes on the upper cerebellar surface. **S. valve,** the valve of the aorta and pulmonary artery.
Semimembrano'sus. See *Muscles, Table of.*
Sem'inal. Pertaining to the semen.
Semina'tion. Introduction of semen into the uterus.
Seminif'erous. Producing or carrying semen.
Seminor'mal solution. One having half as much of a reagent as the normal solution.
Semiprone' posture. Same as *Sims's position.*
Se'mis. L. for *Half;* abbreviated to *ss.*
Semispina'lis muscles. See *Muscles, Table of.*
Semisul'cus. A depression which, with an adjacent one, forms a sulcus.
Semitendino'sus. See *Muscles, Table of.*
Sen'ecin. An alkaloid from *Senecio.*
Sene'cio. A genus of plants used in medicine.
Sen'ega. Root of *Polygala senega:* diuretic and expectorant.
Sen'egin. The active principle of senega.
Senes'cence (sen-es'ens). Condition of growing old.
Se'nile. Pertaining to old age. **S. gangrene.** See *Gangrene.*
Senil'ity. Feebleness of body and mind incident to old age.
Sen'na. Leaflets of various species of *Cassia:* cathartic.
Senn's bone-plates. Disks of decalcified bone: used in intestinal surgery.
Sensa'tion. An impression conveyed by an afferent nerve to the sensorium commune.
Sense. A faculty by which conditions or properties of things are perceived. **S.-body,** a peripheral sense-organ. **S.-capsule,** a cup-like receptacle of a peripheral sense-organ. **S.-epithelium,** epithelium with specialized function of sensation. **Muscular s.,** sense by which muscular movement is perceived. **S.-organ,** the peripheral termination of a sensory nerve. **S.-shock,** condition like effect of a blow in hysteric persons on awaking from sleep.
Sensibil'ity. Capacity for perception or feeling.
Sen'sible. Appreciable by the senses; perceptible.
Sen'sitive. Able to receive or transmit a sensation; capable of feeling, or of responding to, a stimulus.
Sen'sitized (sen'sit-īzd). Rendered sensitive.
Senso'rial. Pertaining to the sensorium.
Sensorimo'tor. Both sensory and motor.
Senso'rium. Any sensory nerve-center. **S. commu'ne,** part

of cerebral cortex that receives and co-ordinates all the impulses sent to individual nerve-centers.

Sen'sory (sen'so-re). Pertaining to, or subserving, sensation. **S. amusia.** See *Amusia*. **S. aphasia.** See *Aphasia*. **S. crossway**, posterior portion of internal capsule of the brain. **S. decussation,** the superior pyramidal decussation in the oblongata. **S. epilepsy,** epilepsy in which the convulsions are replaced by delusions of sense and by hallucinations.

Sen'tient (sen'she-ent). Able to feel; sensitive.

Sep'arator, Sep'aratory. A device for effecting a separation.

Se'pium (se'pe-um). Cuttle-fish bone.

Sep'sin. A poisonous ptomain from animal matter and decaying yeast.

Sep'sis. Poisoning by putrefying material.

Septæ'mia, Septe'mia (sep-te'me-ah). Same as *Septicemia*.

Sep'tal (sep'tal). Pertaining to a septum.

Sep'tan. Recurring every seventh (sixth) day.

Sep'tic. Produced by, or due to, putrefaction.

Septicæ'mia, Septice'mia. A morbid condition due to presence of pathogenic bacteria and the associated poisons in the blood. **Sputum-s.,** s. caused by inoculations of some bacterium of the sputum.

Septice'mic. Pertaining to, or of the nature of, septicemia.

Sep'ticin. Mixture of hexylamin and amylamin from putrid flesh.

Septicopye'mia. Septicemia combined with pyemia.

Septip'ara. A woman pregnant for the seventh time.

Septiv'alent. Able to combine with or replace seven hydrogen atoms.

Septom'eter. 1. Apparatus for measuring the thickness of the nasal septum. 2. Instrument for ascertaining amount of septic matter in the air.

Sep'tone. A pathogenic ferment from septic matter.

Septopye'mia. Same as *Septicopyemia*.

Sep'tum, pl. *sep'ta*. A dividing wall or partition. **S. atrio'rum, S. auricula'rum,** wall that separates the auricles of the heart. **Crural s.,** the layer that closes the femoral ring. **S. lu'cidum.** 1. Partition between the lateral ventricles of the brain. 2. The stratum corneum of the epidermis. **Nasal s.,** the boundary between the two nasal cavities. **S. pectinifor'me,** the wall that separates the corpora cavernosa. **Rectovaginal s.,** tissues between rectum and vagina. **S. scro'ti** divides the two chambers of the scrotum. **S. ventriculo'rum,** the partition between the ventricles of the heart.

Sep'tuplet. Any one of seven children born at one birth.

Séquar'din. Sterilized testicular extract.

Sequel'a, pl. *sequel'æ*. Lesion or affection following and caused by an attack of disease.

Seques'ter (se-kwes'ter). A sequestrum.

Sequestra'tion. 1. Formation of sequestra. 2. Isolation of patients.

Sequestrec'tomy, Sequestrot'omy. Excision of a sequestrum.

Seques'trum, pl. *seques'tra*. Piece of dead bone that has become separated from the sound in necrosis.

Seralbu'min. The albumin of the blood.

Se'rial (se're-al). Arranged in, or forming, a series.

Ser'iceps. A silken bag used in making traction on fetal head.

Se'riflux (se'rif-lux). A watery discharge.

Seriscis'sion (ser-is-izh'un). Cutting through soft tissues with a silk ligature.

Serocoli'tis. Inflammation of the peritoneum of the colon.

Serofib'rinous. Both serous and fibrinous.
Serohepati'tis. Inflammation of the peritoneum of the liver.
Serolem'ma. Membrane whence the false amnion is developed.
Ser'olin. A neutral crystalline principle from blood-serum.
Seromu'cous. Both serous and mucous.
Seropneumotho'rax. Pneumothorax with serous effusion.
Seropuru'lent. Both serous and purulent.
Seropus' (se-ro-pus'). Serum mingled with pus.
Sero'sa (se-ro'sah). Any serous membrane.
Serose'rous. Connecting two serous surfaces.
Seros'ity. The quality of serous fluids.
Serosynovi'tis. Synovitis with effusion of serum.
Serother'apy. Therapeutic use of animal serums.
Seroti'na (ser-o-te'nah). The decidua serotina.
Se'rous. Pertaining to, or like, serum. **S. cavity,** any one of the larger lymph-spaces. **S. fluid,** normal lymph of a serous cavity. **S. gland.** See *Gland.* **S. inflammation,** inflammation with an exudation of serum. **S. membrane.** See *Membrane.*
Serpenta'ria. The rhizome of *Aristolochia serpentaria,* or Virginia snakeroot: tonic, diaphoretic, and stimulant.
Serpig'inous. Creeping from part to part.
Serpi'go (ser-pi'go). Any creeping eruption.
Serpyl'lum. L. for *Thyme.*
Ser'rate, Ser'rated. Having a saw-like edge or border.
Serra'tion. A notch like that between two saw-teeth.
Serra'tus muscles (ser-a'tus). See *Muscles, Table of.*
Serrefine (sār-fēn'). A forceps for compressing a bleeding vessel.
Serrenœud (sār-nuhd'). An appliance for tightening a ligature.
Ser'rulate. Characterized by minute serrations.
Serto'li's cells (sar-to'lēz). Cells whence spermatoblasts are developed. **S.'s column,** a long cell in a seminiferous tubule supporting spermatogenic cells.
Se'rum. A clear liquid which may be separated from the coagulum and corpuscles of the blood. **S.-albumin,** albumin of the blood. **S.-globulin.** Same as *Paraglobulin.* **S.-lutein,** a yellow coloring-matter from serum. **S.-test for typhoid fever.** See *Widal's reaction.* **S.-therapy.** Same as *Serotherapy.*
Seru'mal calculus. See *Calculus.*
Serumu'ria (se-rum-u're-ah). Same as *Albuminia.*
Ses'ame. The plants *Sesamum indicum* and *S. orientale,* with oil-bearing seeds.
Ses'amoid. Shaped like a sesame seed. **S. bone,** a small flat bone formed in a tendon. **S. cartilages.** See *Cartilage.*
Sesqui-. A prefix meaning one and a half.
Sesquiox'id. A compound of three parts of oxygen with two of another element.
Ses'quisalt. A salt containing three parts of an acid with two of a base.
Ses'sile. Not pedunculated; having a broad base.
Seta'ceous (se-ta'she-us). Like a bristle.
Se'ton. A strip or skein of linen drawn through a wound in the skin to make an issue.
Setsch'enow's centers. Reflex inhibitory centers in the spinal cord and oblongata.
Seven-day fever. Same as *Relapsing fever.*
Seventh pair of nerves. The facial nerves.
Se'vum (se'vum). L. for *Suet.*
Sewer-gas. Poisonous emanation from foul sewers.
Sex. The distinctive generative character.
Sexdig'ital. Having six digits.

Sex'tan. Recurring every sixth (fifth) day.
Sextip'ara. A woman pregnant for the sixth time.
Sex'tuplet. Any one of six children born at the same birth.
Sex'ual (sex'u-al). Pertaining to sex.
Sexual'ity. The characteristic of the male and female reproductive elements.
Sex'valent. Having a chemical valence of six.
Shad'owgram, Shad'owgraph. Same as *Skiagraph.*
Sha'king palsy. Same as *Paralysis agitans.*
Shank. The tibia or shin.
Shar'pey's fibers. Fibers that unite the lamellæ of bone.
Sheath (shēth). A tubular case or envelop. **Arachnoid s.,** delicate membrane between pial sheath and dural sheath of optic nerve. **Dentinal s.,** the structure lining the dentinal canals. **Dural s.,** external investment of the optic nerve. **Femoral s.,** fascial sheath of the femoral vessels. **S. of Henle.** See *Henle's sheath.* **Lamellar s.,** the perineurium. **Medullary s.,** the sheath of myelin surrounding the axis-cylinder. **Nerve-s.,** the perineurium. **Perivascular s.,** wide lymphatic tube around the smallest blood-vessels. **Pial s.,** extension of pia partly intersecting the optic nerve. **S. of Schwann,** the neurilemma. **Synovial s.,** synovial membrane lining the cavity of a bone through which a tendon moves.
Sheep-pox. A disease of sheep analogous to small-pox or to kine-pox.
Shin. The prominent anterior edge of tibia and leg. **S.-bone,** the tibia.
Shin'gles (shing'glz). Same as *Herpes zoster.*
Ship-fever. Same as *Typhus.*
Shock. Sudden vital depression due to injury or emotion.
Shod'dy-fever. Febrile disorder among workers in shoddy mills, due to the inhalation of dust.
Shoe'makers' cramp. Spasm of muscles of hand and arm in shoemakers.
Short-sight. Same as *Myopia.*
Shot-gun prescription. A prescription of many medicines at once, given with hope that some of them may prove effective.
Shoul'der (shōl'der). The junction of the arm and trunk, and of clavicle and scapula. **S.-blade,** the scapula.
Show. Appearance of blood forerunning labor or menstruation.
Shrap'nell's membrane. The flaccid upper segment of the membrana tympani.
Si. Symbol of *Silicon.*
Siala'den. A salivary gland.
Sialadeni'tis. Inflammation of a salivary gland.
Sialadenon'cus. A tumor of a salivary gland.
Sial'agogue. 1. Producing a flow of saliva. 2. A drug which increases the flow of saliva.
Sia'line (si'al-in). Pertaining to the saliva.
Sialis'mus (si-al-iz'mus). Salivation.
Sial'olith (si-al'o-lith). A salivary calculus.
Sialolithia'sis. The formation of salivary calculi.
Sialon'cus (si-al-ong'kus). A tumor of a salivary gland.
Sialorrhe'a. Salivation; ptyalism.
Sialos'chesis. Suppression of secretion of saliva.
Sib'bens. A disease formerly prevalent in Scotland, probably syphilitic.
Sib'ilant. Of a shrill, whistling, or hissing character.
Sib'ilus. A sibilant or whistling râle.
Sick. 1. Not well; not in good health. 2. Affected with nausea. 3. Menstruating. **S.-headache,** migraine.
Sick'ness. State of being sick; illness. **African s.** See *African*

lethargy. **Car-s.**, nausea and malaise from railway travel. **Falling s.**, epilepsy. **Green s.**, chlorosis. **Monthly s.**, menstruation. **Morning s.**, nausea of early pregnancy. **Mountain-s.**, nausea and dyspnea at great elevations. **Sea-s.**, See *Seasickness.* **Sweating s.** See *Anglicus sudor.*

Siderodromopho'bia. Morbid dread of railway travel.

Sideroph'ilous. Tending to absorb iron.

Sider'oscope. Apparatus for detecting the presence of iron.

Sidero'sis. 1. Pneumonia due to inhalation of iron particles. 2. Excess of iron in the blood.

Sigaul'tian operation (se-go'she-an). See *Symphyseotomy.*

Sight (sit). Act or faculty of seeing.

Sig'matism. Excessive or incorrect use of *s* sounds in speaking.

Sig'moid. Shaped like the letter C or S. **S. flexure,** distal S-shaped part of colon. **S. fossa,** curved fossa on the mastoid process.

Sigmoidi'tis. Inflammation of the sigmoid flexure.

Sigmoidoprocto'tomy. Establishment of artificial passage from sigmoid flexure to the rectum.

Sigmoid'oscope. Speculum for examining the sigmoid flexure.

Sigmoidos'copy. Specular examination of the sigmoid flexure.

Sigmoidos'tomy. Creation of artificial anus in sigmoid flexure.

Sign (sin). An objective evidence of disease. **Abadie's s.**, spasm of levator palpebræ superioris muscle: a sign of exophthalmic goiter. **Allis's s.**, relaxation of fascia between crest of ilium and greater trochanter: sign of fracture of neck of femur. **Argyll-Robertson pupil s.** See *Pupil s.* **Baccelli's s.**, reverberation of the patient's whispered voice heard on auscultation through the chest-wall: sign of pleural effusion. **Baruch's s.**, resistance of temperature in rectum to a bath of 75° for fifteen minutes: sign of typhoid fever. **Bernhardt's s.**, perverted and painful sensations on outer and anterior surfaces of thigh: seen in displacement of external cutaneous nerve. **Biermer's s.** See *Gerhardt's s.*, second def. **Biernaski's s.**, analgesia of ulnar nerve. **Bouilland's s.**, peculiar tinkling at right of apex-beat of heart in hypertrophy of heart. **Brach-Romberg s.** See *Romberg's s.* **Burton's s.**, blue line at junction of teeth with gums in chronic lead-poisoning. **Cardarelli's s.**, lateral movements of trachea, symptomatic of aneurysm of aorta. **Cheyne-Stokes s.** See under *Respiration.* **Chvostek's s.**, sudden spasm on tapping one side of face: seen in post-operative tetany. **Clark's s.**, obliteration of hepatic dulness from tympanitic distention of the abdomen. **Corrigan's s.** 1. Purple line at junction of teeth with gums in chronic copper-poisoning. 2. Corrigan's pulse. See *Pulse.* **Dalrymple's s.**, abnormal widening of palpebral opening in exophthalmic goiter. **Dance's s.**, depression in the right iliac region in intussusception. **Davidsohn's s.**, reflection of light through the pupil in transillumination: seen in health. **Drummond's s.**, whiff heard at the open mouth during respiration in cases of aortic aneurysm. **Duroziez's s.** See *Duroziez's murmur.* **Filipovitch's s.**, yellow discoloration of prominent parts of palms and soles in typhoid fever. **Flint's s.**, Flint's murmur. See *Murmur.* **Friedreich's s.**, diastolic collapse of the cervical veins, due to adherent pericardium. **Garel's s.**, absence of light-perception on affected side of antrum of Highmore on electric transillumination: seen in disease of antrum of Highmore. **Gerhardt's s.** 1. Absence of movement of larynx in dyspnea from aneurysm of aorta. 2. Change of percussion-sound on change of patient's position: seen in pneumothorax and pulmonary tuberculosis. **Glasgow's s.**, systolic sound in brachial artery in latent aneurysm of aorta. **Grancher's s.**, equality in pitch between expiratory and inspiratory murmurs: sign of obstruction to expiration. **Gubler's s.** See *Gubler's tumor.* **Guyon's s.,** renal ballottement, indicative of floating kidney. **Heberden's s.** See *Heberden's nodosities.* **Hegar's s.,** softening of lower uterine segment, indicative of pregnancy. **Hick's s.,** intermittent uterine contraction, apparent after end of third month of pregnancy: it may also be caused by a tumor of the uterus. **Hutchinson's s.** 1. Dull red discoloration of cornea in syphilis. 2. Notched teeth, interstitial keratitis, and otitis occurring together: indicative of syphilis; called also *Hutchinson's trio.* **Jaccoud's s.,** prominence of the aorta at the suprasternal notch in leukemia. **Jacquemin's s.,** violet color of mucous membrane of vagina after fourth week of pregnancy. **Jadelot's s.** See *Jadelot's lines.* **Jorisenne's s.,** non-acceleration of pulse on changing from horizontal to erect position: significant of pregnancy. **Josseraud's s.,** loud metallic second sound over pulmonic area in acute pericarditis. **Keene's s.,** increased diameter of leg at malleoli in Pott's fracture of fibula. **Küster's s.,** cystic tumor in median line anterior to uterus in cases of ovarian dermoids. **Laennec's s.** 1. Rounded gelatinous masses in sputum of bronchial asthma: called also *Laennec's perles.* 2. A modified subcrepitant râle heard in pulmonary emphysema: called also *Laennec's râle.* **Litten's s.,** the diaphragm phenomenon; the shadow rising and falling with respiration seen through the thoracic walls and indicating the movements of the diaphragm. **Mannkopf's s.,** increase in frequency of pulse in pain: not present in simulated pain. **Oliver's s.,** tracheal tugging in aneurysm of the aorta. **Palmoplantar s.** See *Filipovitch's s.* **Parkinson's s.,** immobile, mask-like expression in paralysis agitans. **Parrot's s.** 1. Dilatation of the pupil on pinching the skin of the neck: seen in meningitis. 2. See *Parrot's nodes.* **Paul's s.,** feeble apex-beat with strong impulse over the body of the heart in pericarditis. **Porter's s.** Same as *Oliver's s.* **Quincke's s.,** blanching of the finger-nails at each diastole of the heart: seen in aortic insufficiency. **Raynaud's s.,** cold state of the fingers alternating with burning head and redness: seen in Raynaud's disease. **Ritter-Rolet s.,** flexion of the foot on gentle electric stimulation; extension on energetic stimulation. **Romberg's s.,** swaying of the body on standing with feet close together and eyes closed: sign of locomotor ataxia. **Rosenbach's s.,** loss of abdominal reflex in inflammatory disease of intestines. **Seguin's s.,** contraction of muscles preceding and giving warning of an epileptic attack. **Skeer's s.,** small circle in iris near pupil in both eyes: seen in tuberculous meningitis. **Skoda's s.,** tympanic sound on percussion of chest above a large pleural effusion or above consolidation of pneumonia. **Stairs-s.** See *Stairs.* **Stellwag's s.,** apparent widening of palpebral opening in exophthalmic goiter. **Stokes's s.,** severe throbbing in abdomen at right of umbilicus in acute enteritis. **Tarnier's s.,** effacement of angle between upper and lower uterine segments in pregnancy: indicative of inevitable abortion. **Trousseau's s.,** muscular spasm on pressure over large arteries or nerves: seen in tetany. **Vigouroux's s.,** diminished electric resistance of the skin in exophthalmic goiter. **Von Graefe's s.,** failure of upper lid to move downward with the eyeball in glancing downward: seen in exophthalmic goiter. **Weber's s.,** paralysis of oculomotor nerve of one side and hemiplegia of opposite side. **Wernicke's s.,** the hemiopic pupillary reaction. See *Reaction.* **Westphal's s.,** loss of knee-jerk in locomotor ataxia. **Wintrich's s.,** change in pitch of percussion-note when mouth is opened and closed, indicative of a cavity in the lung.

Sig'na. Latin for "*Mark*" or "*Write*"; written *S.* or *Sig.* on prescriptions.

Sig'nal symptom. Peculiar sensation or movement announcing an approaching attack of Jacksonian epilepsy.

Sig'nature. The part of a prescription which gives directions as to taking the medicine.

Sig'natures, doctrine of. Obsolete doctrine that the uses of a medicine are shown by its appearance or by some other visible indication.

Sik'imin. Poison principle of *Ilicium religiosum.*

Sil'lea. Silicon dioxid, SiO_2; also, its homeopathic preparations.

Sili'cate. Any compound of silicic acid with a base.

Silic'ic acid (sil-is'ik). An acid, H_4SiO_4, forming silicate.

Sil'icon. A non-metallic tetrad element; symbol Si.

Sil'ver. A white metal; symbol Ag.

Sil'ver-fork deformity or **fracture.** Fracture of distal end of radius, causing a peculiar deformity.

Si'mon's position. Position of the patient flat on the back, with the thighs and legs flexed and abducted, and hips elevated.

Sim'ple fracture. See *Fracture.* **S. inflammation,** inflammation without pus or other specific inflammatory product.

Sim'pler, Sim'plist. An herb-doctor.

Sim'ples (sim'plz). Medicinal plants.

Sims's depressor. A wire loop for depressing anterior vaginal wall. **S.'s position,** patient lying on left side and front of left chest with right thigh strongly flexed. **S.'s speculum,** a speculum which raises the posterior vaginal wall while the anterior is pushed down by a depressor.

Simul. Latin word meaning "together."

Simu'lation. 1. The act of counterfeiting an illness. 2. Imitation of one disease by another.

Sin'albin. A crystalline principle, $C_{30}H_{44}N_2S_2O_{16}$, from white mustard.

Sin'apin. An alkaloid, $C_{16}H_{23}NO_5$, from white mustard.

Sin'apis (sin'ap-is). L. for *Mustard.*

Sin'apism (sin'ap-izm). A mustard-plaster or paste.

Sin'apized. Mixed with or containing mustard.

Sincip'ital. Pertaining to the sinciput.

Sin'ciput. The upper and front part of the head.

Sin'ew (sin'u). A tendon or fibrous cord.

Sing. Abbreviation of L. *Singulo'rum,* "of each."

Sin'ger's node or **nodule.** A swelling sometimes developed between the arytenoid cartilages of singers.

Singul'tus (sin-gul'tus). Hiccup.

Sinis'trad (sin-is'trad). To or toward the left.

Sinis'tral. Pertaining to the left side.

Sinis'trin. A sugar, $C_6H_{10}O_5$, found in squills, etc.

Sink'alin. An alkaloid from mustard. Same as *Cholin.*

Sin'uous (sin'u-us). Bending in and out; winding.

Si'nus. 1. A recess, cavity, or hollow space. 2. A dilated channel for venous blood. **Air-s.,** cavity in a bone containing air. **Aortic s., S. of Valsalva,** a pouch-like dilatation of aorta or pulmonary artery opposite segment of semilunar valve. **Cavernous s.,** venous s. extending from sphenoid fissure to apex of petrous portion of temporal bone, communicating behind with the inferior and superior petrosal sinuses. **Circular s.,** venous s. around pituitary body. **S. circula'ris i'ridis.** Same as *Schlemm's canal.* **Coronary s.,** venous s. in the groove between left cardiac auricle and left ventricle. **Frontal s.,** large air-s. above either eye. **Inferior longitudinal s.,** venous s. along lower border of falx cerebri. **Inferior petrosal s.,** venous s. arising from cavernous s. running along lower edge of petrous bone to internal jugular vein. **S. of kidney,** inward extension of hilum of kidney. **S. of larynx,** ventricle of larynx.

Lateral s., venous s. which begins at torcular Herophili and goes to internal jugular. **Lymph s.**, a lymph-channel; space which conveys lymph. **Mastoid s's.**, cells within mastoid portion of temporal bone. **Maxillary s.**, the antrum of Highmore. **S. of Morgagni**, space between basilar process of occipital and superior constrictor muscle. **Occipital s.**, a small venous s. in attached margin of falx cerebelli opening into torcular Herophili. **S.-phlebitis**, inflammation of a venous s. **Placental s.**, venous channel around edge of placenta. **S. pocula'ris**, lacuna in prostatic portion of urethra. See *Uterus masculinus*. **Prostatic s.** See *Uterus masculinus*. **Rhomboid s.**, the fourth ventricle. **Sphenoid s.**, an air-space in the sphenoid bone. **Straight s.**, venous s. going from inferior longitudinal to lateral s. **Superior longitudinal s.** goes along upper edge of falx cerebri and ends at the torcular. **Superior petrosal s.** runs in a groove in petrous bone from posterior part of cavernous s. to lateral s. **Terminal s.**, vein which encircles the vascular area of the blastoderm. **S.-thrombosis**, thrombosis of a venous s. **Transverse s.** unites the two inferior petrosal sinuses. **Urogenital s.**, duct into which in the embryo the Wolffian ducts and bladder empty, and which goes to the cloaca. **Valsalva, s. of.** See *Aortic s.*

Sinusi'tis (sin-u-si'tis). Inflammation of a sinus, especially the maxillary sinus.

Sinusoid'al current. Alternating faradic current whose potential repeatedly rises from zero to a maximum, and then declines to zero again.

Si'phon. A bent pipe with arms of unequal lengths for drawing liquid from one receptacle to another.

Siphono'ma. A tumor made up of a series of tubes.

Sirenom'elus. A monster with blended legs and no feet.

Sitieir'gia. Hysteric anorexia.

Sitiol'ogy (sit-e-ol'o-je). See *Sitology*.

Sitiopho'bia, Sitopho'bia. Insane dread of taking food.

Sitol'ogy. The science of food and nourishment.

Sitoma'nia. 1. Sitophobia. 2. Periodic bulimia.

Si'tus inver'sus vis'cerum. Lateral transposition of the viscera of the thorax and pelvis.

Sitz-bath. A hip-bath.

Sixth nerve. See *Abducens*, in *Nerves, Table of*.

Ska'tol. A crystalline substance, C_9H_9N, from feces.

Skein (skān). The thread-like figure seen in the earlier stages of karyokinesis.

Skel'etal. Pertaining to the skeleton. **S. muscle**, a muscle attached to or moving some part of the skeleton. **S. tissue**, a general name for bony, ligamentous, fibrous, and cartilaginous tissues.

Skeletiza'tion. 1. Extreme emaciation. 2. Removal of soft parts from the skeleton.

Skeleto'genous. Producing skeletal structures or tissues.

Skeletol'ogy. Sum of knowledge regarding the skeleton.

Skel'eton. The bony framework of the body.

Ski'agram, Ski'agraph. A picture made by the Röntgen rays.

Skiag'raphy. The art of producing skiagraphs.

Ski'ascope. 1. A fluoroscope. 2. Instrument used in skiascopy.

Skias'copy. Same as *Pupilloscopy* or *Retinoscopy*.

Skin. The outer integument composed of epidermis and corium. **S.-bound**, hide-bound; sclerodermatous. **S.-bound disease.** Same as *Scleroderma*. **S.-grafting**, implantation of bits of healthy skin to form centers of cicatrization.

Skleri'asis (skle-ri'as-is). See *Scleroderma*.

Sklero-. For words beginning thus, see those beginning *Sclero-*.

Skoda'ic resonance, S. tympany. Tympanic resonance in upper part of chest with flatness below.
Sko'da's sign. Same as *Skodaic resonance.*
Sko'togram, Skot'ograph. Same as *Skiagram.*
Skotog'raphy (sko-tog'raf-e). See *Skiagraphy.*
Skull. The cranium; bony framework of the head. **S.-cap.** 1. The sinciput or calvarium. 2. See *Scutellaria.*
Sleep-epilepsy. Same as *Narcolepsy.* **S.-walking.** Same as *Somnambulism.*
Sleep'ing-dropsy, S.-sickness. See *African lethargy.*
Slen'der column, S. fasciculus. Same as *Funiculus gracilis.* **S. lobe,** a lobule on the lower aspect of the cerebellum.
Slide. A glass plate on which objects are placed for microscopic examination.
Sling. A bandage or suspensory for supporting a part.
Slough. A mass of dead tissue in, or cast out from, living tissue.
Slough'ing. The formation or separation of a slough.
Small-pox. See *Variola.*
Smear-culture. Bacterial culture in which the infective matter is smeared over the surface of the medium.
Smee cell. A form of galvanic cell.
Smeg'ma. Thick cheesy secretion under the prepuce.
Smel'ling salts. Aromatized ammonium carbonate.
Smi'lax (smi'lax). See *Sarsaparilla.*
Smiths' cramp. Spasm of the arm and hand occurring in blacksmiths.
Sn. Symbol of tin (L. *Stannum*).
Snake'root. See *Cimicifuga, Senega,* and *Serpentaria.*
Snare. A wire loop for removing polypi and tumors.
Sneeze. To expel air forcibly through the nose and mouth.
Snel'len's types. A variety of test-types for oculists' use.
Snore. Noisy breathing in sleep or coma; stertor.
Sno'ring râle. A sonorous râle.
Snow-blindness. Same as *Niphablepsia.*
Snuf'fles. Catarrhal discharge from the nasal mucous membrane in infants, chiefly in syphilis.
Soap. A compound of fatty acid with an alkali. **S.-bark.** See *Quillaia.*
So'cia parot'idis. A detached part or exclave of the parotid gland.
Sock'et. A hollow part into which a corresponding part fits.
So'da. Sodium hydrate, NaOH.; also sodium carbonate or bicarbonate. **S.-water,** water charged with gaseous carbon dioxid.
So'dic. Containing soda or sodium.
So'dium. A soft alkali metal; symbol Na. **S. bicarbonate,** a white powder, $NaHCO_3$: antacid. **S. carbonate,** an alkaline irritant, $Na_2CO_3 + 10H_2O$. **S. chlorid,** NaCl; common salt. **S. hydrate,** NaOH, caustic soda. **S. iodid,** NaI.: used like potassium iodid. **S. phosphate,** $Na_2HPO_4 + 12H_2O$: cathartic. **S. sulphate,** Glauber's salt: purgative.
Sod'omy. Copulation between males.
Soem'mering's foramen. See *Fovea centralis.* **S.'s spot,** the macula lutea of the retina.
Sof'tening. Process of becoming soft. **S. of the brain,** progressive dementia with general paresis: it may be *yellow* or *red* when the products of disintegration of the blood mingle with the brain-matter, or *white* when there is no hemorrhage.
Soft palate. The soft posterior portion of the palate.
Sola'nin. Alkaloid, $C_{42}H_{75}NO_{15}$, from *Solanum nigrum:* poisonous and narcotic.
Sola'num nig'rum. A genus of plants including potato, black night-shade, etc.

So'lar plexus. A plexus of ganglia and nerves for the abdominal viscera. See *Plexus.*

Sole. The bottom of the foot. **S.-reflex,** muscular contraction on stimulating the sole.

So'leus. See *Muscles, Table of.*

Sol'idism, Solidis'tic pathology. Obsolete doctrine that all diseases are due to condensation or expansion of the solid tissues.

Sol'itary fasciculus. See *Fasciculus.* **S. glands,** lymphoid nodules in mucous membrane of large and small intestines.

So'lium (so'le-um). A variety of tapeworm.

Solubil'ity (sol-u-bil'it-e). Quality of being soluble.

Solu'tion. 1. Process of dissolving. 2. Liquid containing dissolved matter. See also *Contiguity, Solution of,* and *Continuity, Solution of.*

Solu'tol. Antiseptic solution of cresol and sodium creosotate.

Solv. Abbreviation of L. *Solve,* "dissolve."

Sol'vent. 1. Effecting a solution. 2. A liquid that dissolves.

Sol'veol. Antiseptic solution of sodium creosotate in cresol.

Sol'vin. A liquid preparation capable of destroying red blood-corpuscles.

So'macule. The smallest possible particle of protoplasm.

Somat'ic (so-mat'ik). Pertaining to the body. **S. death,** death of the entire body.

Somat'oblasts. Cytoblasts aggregated in the protoplasm of the cell outside the nucleus.

Somat'ochrome. A nerve-cell whose cell-body stains readily.

Somatodym'ia. Teratic union of the bodies of twin fetus.

Somatol'ogy. The sum of what is known regarding the body.

Som'atome. 1. An appliance for cutting the body of a fetus. 2. A somite.

Somat'oplasm (so-mat'o-plazm). The body-substance.

Somat'opleure. 1. The somatic mesoblast. 2. Layer formed by union of the somatic mesoblast and the epiblast.

So'matose. A concentrated proprietary meat-food.

Somatot'omy. Human anatomy.

Somatotrid'ymus. A fetal monster with three trunks.

So'mite (so'mit). Same as *Protovertebra.*

Som'nal. A hypnotic and diuretic compound of chloral hydrate and urethan, $C_7H_{12}NO_3Cl$.

Somnam'bulism. Habitual walking in sleep.

Somnifa'cient. Hypnotic; causing sleep.

Somnif'erous. Producing sleep.

Somnil'oquism, Somnil'oquy. The habit of talking in one's sleep.

Som'nolence (som'no-lens). Sleepiness.

Somnolen'tia. 1. Incomplete sleep; drowsiness. 2. Drunken sleep.

Sonde coudée (sond koo-da'). Catheter with an elbow.

Son'itus (son'it-us). See *Tinnitus.*

Sonom'eter. An apparatus for testing acuteness of hearing.

Sono'rous. Resonant; sounding. **S. râle,** snoring respiration-sound from narrowing of the bronchi.

Soor. Ger. for *Thrush.*

Soot-cancer, Soot-wart. Cancer of the scrotum.

Sophistica'tion. Adulteration of food or medicine.

So'por. Coma or deep sleep.

Soporif'ic. Producing deep sleep.

So'porose. Associated with coma or with deep sleep.

Sorbefa'cient. A remedy that favors absorption.

Sor'des. Foul matter collected on lips and teeth in low fevers. **S. gas'trica,** food lying undigested in the stomach.

Sore throat. See *Tonsillitis* and *Pharyngitis.*

Sorghum (sor′gum). A variety of cane-sugar.

Souffle (soofl). A soft, blowing auscultatory sound. **Fetal s.,** murmur sometimes heard over pregnant uterus, supposed to be due to compression of umbilical cord. **Funic s., Funicular s.,** hissing s. synchronous with fetal heart-sounds, probably from umbilical cord. **Placental s., Uterine s.,** sound made by blood in arteries of gravid uterus. **Splenic s.,** sound said to be sometimes heard over diseased spleen.

Sound. 1. Sensation produced on auditory nerve by vibrations of the air. 2. Instrument to be introduced into cavities, so as to detect foreign bodies or to dilate strictures.

South′ernwood. See *Abrotanum.*

So′zal. Aluminum sulphocarbolate: antiseptic.

So′zin. Any proteid naturally occurring in the body which acts as a protector against disease.

Sozo-i′odol. An antiseptic substance, $C_6H_4SO_4I_2$.

Space (spās). A region or area of the body. **S.-nerves,** fibers of the auditory nerve going to the semicircular canals. **Nuel's s.,** space in organ of Corti between outer hair-cells and outer rods. **Perforated s.,** space at base of brain pierced by blood-vessels. **S.-sense,** faculty by which the position and space-relations of objects are perceived.

Spagyr′ic. Pertaining to the obsolete alchemistic practice of medicine.

Spane′mia. Anemia; thinness of the blood.

Span′ish fly. See *Cantharis.*

Spanopne′a, Spanopnœ′a. Nervous affection with slow, deep breathing and subjective feeling of dyspnea.

Spar′adrap. A medicated adhesive.

Spargo′sis. 1. Distention of mamma with milk. 2. Elephantiasis.

Spar′tein. Alkaloid, $C_{15}H_{26}N_2$, from broom: its sulphate acts like digitalin.

Spasm. A sudden violent involuntary contraction, as of the muscles. **Clonic s.,** spasm in which rigidity is followed immediately by relaxation. **Habit s.,** spasm acquired by habit. **Handicraft s.,** any occupation-neurosis. **Myopathic s.** accompanies a disease of muscles. **Saltatory s.** See *Palmus.* **Tetanic s.,** emprosthotonos, pleurothotonos, or opisthotonos. **Tonic s.,** spasm in which rigidity persists for a considerable time. **Toxic s.** is due to a poison.

Spasmat′ic, Spasmod′ic. Of the nature of spasm.

Spas′modism. A spasmodic condition due to medullary excitation.

Spasmol′ogy (spaz-mol′o-je). The science of spasms.

Spasmophil′ia. Abnormal tendency to convulsions.

Spasmo′tin. A poisonous principle from ergot.

Spasmotox′in. A poisonous ptomain from bacillus of tetanus.

Spas′mous (spaz′mus). Like a spasm.

Spas′mus nu′tans. Nodding spasm.

Spas′tic. Of the nature of, or characterized by, spasms. **S. hemiplegia.** See *Hemiplegia.* **S. paraplegia.** See *Paraplegia.*

Spat′ula. A flat blunt instrument used for spreading plasters, mixing ointments, etc.

Spay. To deprive of the ovaries.

Spear′mint. The herb *Mentha viridis:* it is carminative.

Special′ist. A practitioner who treats a special class of diseases.

Spe′cies. 1. Primary subdivision of a genus. 2. A mixture of powdered simples for infusion.

Speci′fic. 1. Pertaining to a species. 2. A remedy specially indicated for any particular disease. **S. gravity,** weight of a substance as compared with that of another assumed as a standard. **S. remedy.** Same as *Specific,* 2d def.

Speci'lum. A bougie, probe, or sound.
Spec'tacles. Pair of lenses in a frame to assist vision.
Spec'tral. Performed by means of the spectrum.
Spectrom'etry. Determination of the place of lines in a spectrum.
Spectrophotom'eter. Apparatus for measuring light-sense by means of a spectrum.
Spectrophotom'etry. The use of the spectrophotometer.
Spec'troscope. Instrument for developing and analyzing the spectrum of a body.
Spec'trum. Variously colored band into which light is decomposed in passing through a prism or grating of glass.
Spec'ulum. Appliance for opening to view a passage or cavity of the body.
Speech-center. Center in the third left frontal convolution which regulates speech.
Spend. To ejaculate semen in coitus.
Sperm (sperm). Semen. **S.-cell,** a spermatozoön; more correctly, a spermatid. **S.-nucleus,** nucleus or head of a spermatozoön.
Spermace'ti. A white crystalline fat from the head of the sperm-whale.
Spermacra'sia. A weak state of the semen.
Spermat'ic. Pertaining to the semen. **S. artery,** a branch of the abdominal aorta in the spermatic cord. **S. canal.** See *Canal.* **S. cord,** cord containing vas deferens, and the arteries, veins, and nerves of the testicle. **S. plexus.** See *Plexus.*
Sper'matid. A cell derived from a secondary spermatocyte by division and developing into a spermatozoön.
Sperm'atin. An albuminoid substance from the semen.
Sper'matism (sper'mat-izm). Emission of semen.
Spermati'tis (sper-mat-i'tis). Same as *Deferentitis.*
Spermat'oblast (sper-mat'o-blast). Same as *Spermatid.*
Spermat'ocele. A scrotal cyst containing spermatozoa.
Spermat'ocyst (sper-mat'o-sist). A seminal vesicle.
Spermatocysti'tis. Inflammation of a seminal vesicle.
Spermat'ocyte, primary. A cell derived from a spermatogonium. **Secondary s.,** one of the two cells into which a primary spermatocyte divides, and which in turn gives origin to spermatids.
Spermatogem'ma. A mass of spermatocytes.
Spermatogen'esis, Spermatog'eny. The development or production of spermatozoa.
Spermatogo'nium. A cell originating in a seminal tubule and dividing into two spermatocytes.
Sper'matoid (sper'mat-oid). Resembling semen.
Spermatol'ogy. A treatise on semen.
Spermatopath'ia. Diseased state of the semen.
Spermatopho'bia. Morbid dread of spermatorrhea.
Spermat'ophore. A capsule containing several spermatozoa.
Spermatopoiet'ic. Promoting the secretion of semen.
Spermatorrhe'a. Involuntary and excessive discharge of semen.
Spermatosche'sis. Suppression of the semen.
Spermat'ospore. A spermatogonium.
Spermato'vum. A fecundated ovum.
Spermat'ozoid, Spermatozo'ön. The male generative cell, consisting of a head or nucleus and a flagellum or tail.
Spermatu'ria. Presence or discharge of semen in the urine.
Sper'min. 1. A therapeutic preparation of the testes of animals. 2. A leukomain, C_2H_5N, from semen and various other animal substances.

Sper'moblast. Same as *Spermatoblast* or *Spermatid.*
Sper'molith. A stone in the spermatic duct.
Sper'moplasm. The protoplasm of the spermatids.
Sper'mosphere. Group or mass of spermatoblasts formed by division of a spermatogonium.
Sper'mospore. See *Spermatogonium.*
Sp. gr. Abbreviation of *Specific gravity.*
Spha'celate (sfas'el-āt). To become gangrenous.
Sphacela'tion (sfas-el-a'shun). Mortification or gangrene.
Sphac'elism (sfas'el-izm). Gangrenous state or process.
Sphaceloder'ma. Symmetric gangrene of the skin.
Sphacelotox'in. Same as *Spasmotin.*
Sphac'elous (sfas'el-us). Gangrenous; sloughing.
Spha'celus (sfas'el-us). A slough; a mass of gangrenous tissue.
Sphæræsthe'sia, Spheresthe'sia. Morbid sensation, as of contact with a ball.
Sphærobac'teria, Spherobac'teria. A group of bacterial forms to which the micrococci belong.
Sphærococ'cus, Spherococ'cus. A genus or form of microbic coccus.
Sphe'nion. The cranial point at the sphenoid angle of the parietal bone.
Sphenoceph'alus. A monster fetus with wedge-like head.
Spheno-eth'moid bone. Curved plate of bone in front of each lesser wing of the sphenoid bone. **S. recess,** a groove back of the roof of the nasal fossa.
Sphe'noid. Wedge-shaped. **S. bone,** a small cranial bone. **S. fissure,** the cleft between the great and small wings of sphenoid.
Sphenomax'illary. Pertaining to the sphenoid and maxilla.
Sphenotre'sia. A breaking up of the base of the fetal skull.
Sphe'notribe. An instrument used in sphenotresia.
Sphenotur'binal bone. A thin curved bone anterior to either small wing of the sphenoid.
Sphe'roid (sfe'roid). A sphere-like body.
Sphero'ma (sfe-ro'mah). A spheric tumor.
Spherom'eter. Apparatus for measuring the curvature of a surface.
Sphinc'ter. A ring-like muscle which closes a natural orifice.
Sphincteral'gia (sfink-ter-al'je-ah). Pain in the sphincter ani.
Sphinc'teroplasty. An operation for restoring a defective sphincter.
Sphincterot'omy. The cutting of a sphincter.
Sphingo'in (sfing-o'in). A leukomain, $C_{17}H_{35}NO_2$, from brain-substance.
Sphyg'mic (sfig'mik). Pertaining to the pulse.
Sphygmochro'nograph. A self-registering sphygmograph.
Sphygmoge'nin. Substance derived from the suprarenal body, believed to increase arterial tension.
Sphyg'mogram. Record or tracing made by a sphygmograph.
Sphyg'mograph. Apparatus for registering the movements of the arterial pulse.
Sphyg'moid (sfig'moid). Resembling the pulse.
Sphygmol'ogy. Sum of what is known regarding the pulse.
Sphygmom'eter. An instrument to measure the pulse.
Sphyg'mophone. Device for rendering the pulse-beat audible.
Sphyg'moscope. Device for rendering the pulse-beat visible.
Sphygmosys'tole. The part of the sphygmogram that corresponds to the systole of the heart.
Sphygmotonom'eter. An instrument to measure elasticity of arterial walls.
Sphyrot'omy (sfĭr-ot'om-e). Surgical removal of a part of the malleus.

Spi'ca. Figure-of-eight bandage with turns crossing each other.

Spic'ula, Spic'ulum. A sharp, needle-like body or spica.

Spi'der-cells. Same as *Deiters's cells.*

Spige'lia marilaud'ica. Pinkroot, a plant whose rhizome is anthelmintic.

Spige'lian lobe. A small lobe below and behind the right lobe of the liver.

Spige'lin. The active alkaloid of *Spigelia.*

Spilo'ma, Spi'lus. A nevus or birth-mark.

Spiloplax'ia. A red spot occurring in leprosy.

Spi'na. A spine. **S. bif'ida,** congenital cleft of vertebral column with meningeal protrusion. **S. vento'sa,** enlargement and thinning of a vertebra in cancer or caries, with an appearance as if it were puffed full of air.

Spi'nal. Pertaining to a spine or to the vertebral column. **S. canal,** canal in vertebral column which lodges the spinal cord. **S. cord,** the myelon; cord of nerve-substance lodged in the spinal canal. **S. epilepsy,** a condition in spastic paraplegia in which clonic and tonic spasms succeed each other. **S. hemiplegia.** See *Hemiplegia.* **S. irritation,** a nervous disturbance with tenderness along the spinal column. **S. marrow,** the spinal cord. **S. nerves,** the thirty-one pairs of nerves derived from the spinal cord. **S. paralysis,** anterior poliomyelitis; also paraplegia. **S. reflex,** any reflex of which the center is in the spinal cord.

Spina'lis. See *Muscles, Table of.*

Spi'nant. Any agent which acts directly upon the spinal cord.

Spi'nate (spi'nāt). Having thorns; shaped like a thorn.

Spin'dle-celled. Having slender fusiform cells.

Spin'dle, nuclear. Spindle-shaped figure of achromatin in the cell-nucleus during karyokinesis.

Spine. 1. A slender thorn-like process of bone. 2. The vertebral column.

Spinoglen'oid ligament. Ligament which joins the spine of the scapula to the lip of the glenoid cavity.

Spinomus'cular segment. Motor cells in the medulla and cord and the nerves which originate in them.

Spinoneu'ral. Pertaining to the myelon and the peripheral nerves.

Spi'nous. Pertaining to, or like, a spine. **S. point,** a point over a spinous process abnormally sensitive to pressure. **S. process,** apophysis going backward from each vertebra.

Spin'therism, Spinthero'pia. Photopsy; sparks before the eyes.

Spi'ral. Winding like the thread of a screw. **S. bandage,** roller bandage applied spirally. **S. canal,** canal which encloses the scala tympani, scala media, and scala vestibuli. **S. lamina,** the lamina spiralis.

Spi'rem. Wreath of chromatin fibrils in karyokinesis.

Spiril'lum. A genus of schizomycetes. **S. an'serum,** a species from blood of diseased geese. **S. bucca'le,** a species from the tartar of teeth. **S. chol'eræ Asiat'icæ,** the comma-bacillus; from stools of patients with epidemic cholera. **S. of Finckler-Prior,** also from cholera stools. **S. Metschniko'wi,** a species from blood of diseased fowls. **S. Mil'leri,** a species from carious teeth. **S. Obermei'eri,** the bacillus of relapsing fever. **S. sputi'genum,** a species found in saliva. **S. tyro'genum,** a species found in cheese, resembling cholera spirillum.

Spir'it. Any volatile or distilled liquid; also, a solution of a volatile material in alcohol. **Corn-s.,** whiskey distilled from maize. **Mindererus, S. of,** liquor ammoniæ acetatis. **Niter, S. of,** spiritus ætheri nitrosi. **Potato-s.,** whiskey distilled from potatoes. **Proof-s.**, dilute alcohol with 40 to 50 per cent. of pure alcohol. **Rectified s.**, alcohol with 16 per cent. of water.

Spir'ituous (spir'it-u-us). Alcoholic; containing a considerable proportion of alcohol.

Spir'itus. L. for *Spirit.* **S. frumen'ti,** whiskey. **S. junip'eri,** gin. **S. myr'cic,** bay rum, a preparation of oil of myrcia, oil of orange-peel, oil of pimenta, and alcohol. **S. odora'tus,** cologne water. **S. vi'ni gal'lici,** brandy.

Spirobacte'ria. A group of spiral microbes or schizomycetes.

Spiroche'ta. A genus of spirobacteria. **S. Obermei'eri,** a species found in blood of patients with relapsing fever.

Spi'rograph. Apparatus for recording respiratory movements.

Spirom'eter. An instrument for measuring the air taken into and expelled from the lungs.

Spirom'etry. Measurement of breathing capacity of lungs.

Spi'rophore. Device for artificial breathing.

Spiruli'na. A micro-organism occurring in coiled filaments.

Spis'sated. Inspissated; thickened by drying.

Spis'situde. Quality of being inspissated.

Spit'tle. Saliva; digestive fluid of the mouth.

Splanchnapoph'ysis. A skeletal element, like the lower jaw, connected with the alimentary canal.

Splanchnecto'pia. Misplacement of a viscus or of the viscera.

Splanch'nic (splank'nik). Of, or pertaining to, the viscera. **S. nerves,** branches from the sympathetic to viscera.

Splanch'nocele. Portion of the celom whence the visceral cavities are formed.

Splanchnog'raphy. Descriptive anatomy of the viscera.

Splanch'nolith (splank'no-lith). Intestinal calculus.

Splanchnol'ogy. Sum of knowledge regarding the viscera.

Splanchnopath'ia. Disease of the viscera.

Splanch'nopleure. The inner lamina of the mesoblast; also, the layer formed by the union of that lamina with the hypoblast.

Splanchnopto'sis. Prolapse or falling down of viscera.

Splanchnos'copy. See *Transillumination.*

Splanchnoskel'eton. Skeletal structures connected with viscera.

Splanchnot'omy (splank-not'om-e). Anatomy or dissection of the viscera.

Splay-foot. Flat-foot; pes planus.

Spleen. A viscus in the left hypochondriac region, close to the cardiac end of the stomach. **S.-pulp,** soft parenchyma of the spleen.

Splenadeno'ma. Hyperplasia of the spleen-pulp.

Splenal'gia (sple-nal'je-ah). Pain in the spleen.

Splen'culus. An accessory spleen, or splenic exclave.

Splen'did line. Same as *Linea splendens.*

Splenec'tasis. Enlargement of the spleen.

Splenec'tomy. Excision of the spleen.

Splenec'topy. Displacement or wandering of the spleen.

Splenelco'sis. Ulceration of the spleen.

Splene'mia. Leukemia with splenic disease.

Splen'ic. Pertaining to the spleen. **S. apoplexy, S. fever,** true or malignant anthrax. **S. vein,** a vein which carries the blood from the spleen to the portal vein.

Splenifica'tion. Same as *Splenization.*

Spleni'tis. Inflammation of the spleen.

Sple'nium. 1. A compress or bandage. 2. The posterior end of the callosum.

Sple'nius. See *Muscles, Table of.*

Spleniza'tion. The condition of a tissue, as of the lung, when it has the appearance of splenic tissue.

Splen'ocele. A hernia of the spleen.

Splenocol'ic. Pertaining to the spleen and colon.
Splenodyn'ia. Pain in the spleen.
Splenog'raphy. A description of the spleen.
Splenohe'mia. Splenic congestion.
Sple'noid (sple'noid). Resembling the spleen.
Spleno'ma (sple-no'mah). A splenic tumor.
Splenomala'cia. Abnormal softness of the spleen.
Splenomega'lia. Enlargement of the spleen.
Splenon'cus (sple-nong'kus). See *Splenoma.*
Splenop'athy. Any disease of the spleen.
Splenopex'ia, Sple'nopexy. Surgical fixation of a wandering spleen.
Splenophren'ic ligament. Peritoneal fold which suspends the spleen.
Splenopneumo'nia. Pneumonia and splenization of the lung; or splenization and congestion of lung from heart-disease.
Splenot'omy. Surgical incision of the spleen.
Splint. A rigid or flexible appliance for the fixation of displaced or movable parts.
Splin'ter. A fragment of fractured bone.
Split pelvis. Congenital separation of pubic bones at the symphysis.
Spondylal'gia (spon-dil-al'je-ah). Pain in the vertebræ.
Spondylarthri'tis. Inflammation of one or more vertebral joints.
Spondyli'tis. Inflammation of vertebræ. **S. defor'mans,** arthritis deformans of vertebral joints. **S. tuberculo'sa,** vertebral caries; Pott's disease.
Spondylize'ma. Downward displacement of a vertebra in consequence of the destruction of the one below it.
Spondylodyn'ia. Pain in a vertebra.
Spondylolisthe'sis. Forward displacement of the lumbar vertebræ, with consequent pelvic deformity.
Spondylop'athy. Any disease of the vertebræ.
Spondylos'chisis. Congenital fissure of a vertebral arch.
Spondylot'omy. Same as *Rhachitomy.*
Sponge. Elastic fibrous skeleton of *Euspongia officinalis:* used mainly as an absorbent. **S.-bath,** application of water to the body with a sponge. **S.-graft,** bit of sponge inserted in an ulcer to promote granulation. **S.-tent,** tent of compressed and waxed sponge.
Spon'gia us'ta. Burnt sponge; alterative.
Spon'giform. Having the form or quality of a sponge.
Spon'gin (spun'jin). Tough substance forming the basis of sponge.
Spon'gioblast. One of the embryonic cells whose processes form the network whence neuroglia is formed.
Spon'gioid (spun'je-oid). Resembling a sponge in structure.
Spongiopi'line. Cotton fabric containing bits of sponge and made waterproof on one side.
Spon'gioplasm. Network of fibrils pervading the cell-substance.
Spon'gy. Of sponge-like appearance or texture. **S. body.** See *Corpus spongiosum.* **S. portion,** part of urethra contained in the corpus spongiosum.
Sponta'neous. Self-originated; originated within the organism. **S. abortion.** See under *Abortion.*
Spoon-nail. A nail with a concave outer surface.
Sporad'ic. Not widely diffused; occurring here and there.
Sporad'oneure. An isolated nerve-cell in any tissue.
Sporan'gia (spo-ran'je-ah). Round vesicles containing conidiaspores: seen in certain mould-fungi.

Spore. A reproductive cell of a protozoön or cryptogamic plant.
Sporif'erous. Producing or bearing spores.
Sporogen'ic (spo-ro-jen'ik). Capable of developing into spores.
Sporog'ony. Development from an unfertilized spore.
Spo'rophore. Part of an organism bearing the spores.
Sporozo'a. A class of endoparasitic protozoans.
Sport. A lusus naturæ, or freak of Nature.
Sporula'tion. Formation of spores.
Spor'ule (spor'ūl). A small spore.
Spot'ted fever. Cerebrospinal meningitis.
Sprain. Wrenching of a joint, with partial rupture of its attachments. **S.-fracture**, separation of a tendon or ligament from its insertion, taking with it a piece of bone.
Spray. A liquid minutely divided, as by a jet of air or steam.
Sprew, Sprue. Same as *Thrush*.
Spring conjunctivitis. See *Vernal catarrh*. **S. ligament**, the ligament which joins the os calcis to the scaphoid bone.
Spunk. Surgeon's agaric charged with potassium nitrate.
Spur. A projecting piece of bone.
Spu'rious. Simulated; false.
Spur'red rye. Ergot or ergotized rye.
Spu'tum. Matter ejected from the mouth. **S.-septicemia**, septicemia from inoculation with sputum or saliva.
Squa'ma. A scale or scale-like plate of bone.
Squamopari'etal, Squamosopari'etal. Pertaining to the squamous and parietal bones.
Squamo'sal. The squamous portion of temporal bone.
Squa'mous. Scaly or plate-like. **S. bone, S. portion**, upper fore part of temporal bone forming an upright plate. **S. epithelium**, epithelium made up of flat thin scales. **S. suture**, the squamoparietal suture.
Square lobe. 1. The quadrate lobe of the liver. 2. Quadrate lobe of cerebrum. 3. Anterior lobe of cerebellum.
Squar'rous. Scurvy or scabby.
Squill. *Scilla maritima*, a diuretic and expectorant plant.
Squint. Same as *Strabismus*.
Squir'ting cucumber. See *Elaterium*.
Sr. Symbol of *Strontium*.
Ss. Abbreviation for L. *Semis*, half.
Stab-culture. Bacterial culture into which the germs are introduced by thrusting a point into the medium.
Sta'bile current. Therapeutic electric current applied by stationary electrodes.
Stacca'to speech or **utterance.** Same as *Scanning speech*.
Stactom'eter. Device for measuring drops.
Sta'dium. L. for *Stage*. **S. decremen'ti**, the stage of defervescence. **S. incremen'ti**, the stage of increase of fever.
Staff. An instrument introduced into the urethra as a guide in cutting.
Stage. 1. A period or distinct phase of a disease. 2. The plate or platform of a microscope. **Algid s.**, a condition marked by flickering pulse, subnormal temperature, and varied nervous symptoms. **Amphibolic s.**, stage which intervenes between acme and decline of an attack. **Asphyxial s.**, preliminary stage of epidemic cholera, marked by cramps, severe pain, and great thirst. **Cold s.**, chill or rigor of a malarial attack. **Eruptive s.**, period during which an exanthem is making its appearance. **Expulsive s.**, stage during which the child is expelled from uterus. **First s.**, the time when the fetal head is being moulded and the cervix dilated. **Hot s.**, period of pyrexia in a malarial paroxysm. **S. of invasion**, time during which the system is coming under a morbific influence. **S. of latency**,

incubation-period of any infectious disorder. **Pre-eruptive s.,** stage after infection and before eruption. **Pyrogenetic s.,** stage of invasion of a febrile attack.

Stagna'tion. A stoppage, as of a current of blood.

Stain. A material used in coloring tissues.

Stairs sign. Difficulty in descending a stairway in locomotor ataxia.

Stam'ina (stam'in-ah). Vigor.

Stam'mering. Faltering and interrupted speech. **S. bladder,** a bladder with muscles that act spasmodically.

Stand'ard solution. A solution containing a fixed amount of a reagent.

Stan'nic acid. A vitreous acid of tin, H_2SnO_3, forming stannates. **S. chlorid,** a colorless liquid, $SnCl_4$.

Stan'num. L. for *Tin*.

Stapedec'tomy. Excision of the stapes.

Stape'dial. Pertaining to the stapes.

Stapediovestib'ular. Pertaining to the stapes and vestibule.

Stape'dius. A muscle of the middle ear.

Sta'pes. Stirrup-shaped ossicle of the ear.

Staphyl'ion (sta-fil'e-on). Cranial point at median line of posterior edge of hard palate.

Staphyli'tis. Inflammation of the uvula.

Staphylococce'mia (staf-il-o-kok-se'me-ah). The occurrence of staphylococcus in the blood.

Staphylococ'cus. A genus or form of bacterial coccus. **S. pyo'genes,** the micro-organism of suppuration : there are several varieties. **S. pyo'genes al'bus** has white cultures. **S. pyo'genes au'reus** is most frequently found and has golden-yellow cultures. **S. pyo'genes cit'reus** forms citron-yellow cultures.

Staphylohe'mia. The presence of staphylococci in the blood.

Staphylo'ma. Protrusion of the sclera or cornea. **Anterior s.** See *Keratoglobus*. **S. cor'neæ,** bulging and thinning of cornea. **Posterior s., S. posti'cum,** backward bulging of sclera at backward pole of eye.

Staphylomyco'sis (staf-il-o-mi-ko'sis). The systemic condition due to staphylococci.

Staphylon'cus. A tumor of the uvula.

Staphylopharyn'geus. The palatopharyngeus muscle.

Staph'yloplasty. Plastic surgery of the uvula.

Staphylopto'sis. Relaxation of the uvula.

Staphylor'rhaphy. The suturation of a cleft palate.

Staphylot'omy. Excision or incision of the uvula, or of a staphyloma.

Staphysa'gria. Poisonous seeds of *Delphinium staphysagria*: parasiticide.

Staphysa'grin. Poisonous alkaloid, $C_{22}H_{33}NO_5$, from staphysagria.

Star-an'ise. See *Illicium*.

Starch. The carbohydrate, $C_6H_{10}O_5$, from various plant-tissues. **Animal s.** See *Glycogen*. **Corn-s.,** nutritive s. from maize. **S.-enema,** enema of starchy water. **Iodized s.,** starch that has been treated with iodin.

Stars of Verheyen. The venæ stellatæ; rosettes of venous radicles beneath the capsule of the kidney.

Starva'tion. Long-continued deprival of food. **S.-cure,** treatment of disease by restricted diet.

Sta'sis. A stoppage of the circulation.

Stasopho'bia. Dread of standing upright.

Stat'ic, Stat'ical. Not in motion; at rest. **S. breeze,** current of air passing from a static electrical machine when in operation. **S. electricity,** electricity evolved by friction or which does not move in currents. **S. machine,** apparatus for generating static electricity. **S. reflex spasm,** solitary spasm or palmus.

Stat'ics. Science of matter in equilibrium or at rest.

Sta'tim (sta'tim). L. for "at once."

Sta'tionary air. Air left in the lungs after a normal expiration.

Statom'eter. Apparatus for measuring degree of exophthalmia.

Sta'tus. Condition or state. **S. arthrit'icus,** disturbance which foreruns a gouty attack. **S. epilep'ticus,** condition in which epileptic spasms rapidly succeed each other. **S. præs'ens,** condition of a patient at the time of observation. **S. typho'sus,** typhoid state or condition.

Stauraple'gia. Crossed hemiplegia.

Staves'acre. Same as *Staphysagria.*

Steap'sin. A pancreatic ferment saponifying fats and oils.

Stear'ic acid. A solid acid, $C_{18}H_{36}O_2$, of fats and oils forming stearates.

Ste'arin. A white solid crystalline substance in fat, $C_3H_5(C_{18}H_{35}O_2)_3$.

Stearop'tene. The solid constituent of a volatile oil.

Stearrhe'a. Same as *Seborrhea.*

Ste'atite. Same as *Talcum.*

Steat'ocele. Fatty swelling of the scrotum.

Steato'ma. 1. Same as *Lipoma.* 2. A sebaceous cyst.

Steatopyg'ia (ste-at-o-pij'e-ah). Excessive fatness of the buttocks; Hottentot deformity.

Steatorrhe'a (ste-at-or-rhe'ah). Same as *Seborrhea.*

Steato'sis. 1. Disease of sebaceous glands. 2. Fatty degeneration.

Steatozo'ön. Same as *Demodex folliculorum.*

Stel'late. Star-shaped; arranged in rosettes. **S. ligament,** anterior costovertebral ligament. **S. veins, Stellulæ Verheyen'ii.** See *Stars of Verheyen.*

Stell'wag's sign. Elevation of upper lid in exophthalmic goiter.

Sten'ion. Cranial point at either end of the smallest transverse diameter in the temporal region.

Stenocar'dia (ste-no-kar'de-ah). Angina pectoris.

Stenoceph'aly (ste-no-sef'al-e). Narrowness of the head or cranium.

Stenocho'ria (ste-no-ko're-ah). Same as *Stenosis.*

Stenopæ'ic, Stenope'ic. Having a narrow opening or slit.

Ste'no's duct. Same as *Stenson's duct.*

Sten'osed (sten'ost). Narrowed; constricted.

Steno'sis. Narrowing or contraction of a duct or canal. **Aortic s.,** narrowing of aortic orifice of heart or of the aorta itself. **Cardiac s.,** narrowing or diminution of any heart-passage or cavity. **Cicatricial s.,** stenosis caused by a contracted cicatrix. **Mitral s.,** stenosis of left auriculoventricular orifice.

Stenotho'rax. An abnormally straight, short, or narrow thorax.

Stenot'ic (sten-ot'ik). Marked by narrowing or constriction.

Sten'son's duct. The duct of parotid gland. **S.'s foramina,** two incisive foramina of superior maxillary bone.

Stepha'nion. Cranial point at intersection of temporal ridge and coronal suture.

Stercobi'lin. Hydrobilirubin from fecal matter.

Stercora'ceous. Consisting of, or containing, feces.

Stercoræ'mia. See *Stercoremia.*

Ster'coral. Pertaining to, or caused by, feces.

Stercore'mia. Toxic state occasioned by poisons absorbed from retained feces.

Ster'corin. Crystallizable material from feces.

Ster'cus. L. for *dung* or *feces.*

Stere (stăr). Same as *Kiloliter*.
Stereogno'sis (ster-e-og-no'sis). The sense by which the form of objects is perceived.
Stereom'etry (ster-e-om'et-re). The measurement of the contents of a solid or hollow body.
Ster'eoplasm. The more solid portion of protoplasm.
Stereoscop'ic vision. Vision in which objects appear to have their solid form, or are not seen as flat pictures.
Ster'esol. A proprietary antiseptic application for skin-diseases.
Sterig'mata. Radially arranged outgrowths, crowded together on the upper half of the sphere into which the conidia bearers of the aspergillus expand.
Ster'ile. 1. Not producing young; unproductive; barren. 2. Aseptic; not containing micro-organisms.
Steril'ity. Barrenness; inability to produce young.
Steriliza'tion. Process of freeing a substance from septic germs.
Ster'ilizer. A mechanism used in sterilizing objects.
Ster'nal. Pertaining to the sternum.
Sternal'gia (ster-nal'je-ah). Pain in the sternum.
Ster'nebra (ster'ne-brah). Any one of the segments of the sternum.
Sternoclavic'ular. Pertaining to the sternum and clavicle.
Sternocleidomas'toid. See *Muscles, Table of*.
Sternocos'tal. Of, or pertaining to, sternum and ribs.
Sternohy'oid. See *Muscles, Table of*.
Ster'noid (ster'noid). Resembling the sternum.
Sternomas'toid. Same as *Sternocleidomastoid*.
Sternop'agus. Twin fetuses united at sternum.
Sternothy'roid. See *Muscles, Table of*.
Ster'num. Breast-bone; bone in median line of thorax in front.
Sternuta'tio convulsi'va. Paroxysmal sneezing.
Sternu'tatory. 1. Causing sneezing. 2. Drug that causes sneezing.
Ster'tor. Snoring; sonorous respiration.
Ster'torous. Of the nature of stertor.
Steth'ograph (steth'o-graf). Apparatus to record chest movements.
Stethokyr'tograph. Apparatus for measuring amount of expansion of chest.
Stethom'eter. An instrument to measure chest expansion.
Stethophonom'eter. An instrument for measuring the intensity of auscultatory sounds.
Steth'oscope. Instrument for performing mediate auscultation.
Stethos'copy. Examination with the stethoscope.
Sthen'ic. Characterized by overaction; strong. **S. fever,** fever marked by high temperature and strong pulse.
Stib'ialism. Antimonial poisoning.
Stib'ium. L. for *Antimony*.
Stick'ing plaster. Rosin or adhesive plaster.
Stiff-neck. 1. Rigidity of neck from rheumatism. 2. Torticollis or wry-neck. **S. fever,** cerebrospinal meningitis.
Stig'ma. 1. A spot, dot, or impression upon the skin. 2. Any space between the cells of the endothelium of a capillary. 3. A readily stainable area in epithelium at the points of union of groups of cells. 4. That part of the pistil of a flower which receives the pollen.
Stig'mata may'dis. The silk of maize; corn-silk; it is diuretic.
Stigmat'ic. Pertaining to a stigma.
Stigmatiza'tion. The formation of impressions on the skin.
Stil'let, Stil'lette. 1. A delicate probe. 2. A wire used to stiffen or clear a catheter.
Still'born. Dead at or before birth.

Stillicid'ium. 1. A dribbling or flowing by drops. 2. Epiphora.

Stillin'gia silvat'ica. Queensroot, an alterative plant.

Stil'ling's canal. The hyaloid canal of the vitreous. **S.'s. nucleus.** Same as *Red nucleus.*

Stim'ulant. 1. Producing stimulation. 2. An agent which stimulates. **Alcoholic s.,** one with ethyl alcohol as its basis. **Cardiac s.,** one which increases the heart's action. **Cerebral s.,** one which exalts action of the brain. **Diffusible s., Diffusive s.,** one which acts promptly, but transiently. **General s.,** one which acts upon the whole body. **Hepatic s.,** one which arouses the functions of the liver. **Spinal s.,** one which acts upon or through the spinal cord. **Stomachic s.,** one which assists stomach-digestion. **Vascular s.,** one which appeals to vasomotor nerves.

Stim'ulate. To excite functional activity in a part.

Stim'ulus. Any agent producing reaction in an irritable tissue. **Adequate s., Homologous s.,** one which acts upon end-organs. **Chemical s.,** one that acts by a chemical process. **Electric s.,** application of electricity. **Heterologous s.** acts upon all the nerve-elements of the sensory apparatus. **Mechanical s.,** one which acts by mechanical means. **Thermal s.,** a stimulant application of heat.

Stir'rup, Stir'rup-bone. The stapes.

Stitch. 1. A sudden cutting pain. 2. A loop made in sewing or suturing. **S.-abscess,** an abscess formed about a stitch.

Stokes's lenses. Apparatus used in diagnosis of astigmatism.

Sto'ma, pl. *sto'mata.* A minute pore, orifice, or stigma on a free surface.

Stom'ach. The ovoid musculomembranous digestive pouch below the esophagus. **S.-bucket,** a little cup for taking out samples of the stomach's contents. **S.-cough,** reflex cough excited by stomach-irritation. **S.-pump,** a pump for clearing out the contents of the stomach. **S.-tooth,** a lower canine tooth. **S.-tube,** 1. A siphon used in washing out the stomach. 2. A feeding-tube.

Stom'achal. Stomach'ic. A gastric stimulant.

Stomati'tis. Inflammation of the mouth. **S. aphtho'sa, Aphthous s.,** one characterized by aphthæ. **Catarrhal s.,** simple stomatitis. **Epidemic s.,** foot-and-mouth disease. **Gangrenous s.** See *Cancrum oris.* **Mercurial s.,** that arising from mercury-poisoning. **Mycotic s.,** that which is due to a micro-organism. **Scorbutic s.,** a form due to scurvy. **Ulcerative s.,** stomatitis with shallow ulcers.

Stomatol'ogy. Sum of what is known regarding the mouth.

Stomatomyco'sis. Any mouth-disease due to schizomycetes.

Stomatonecro'sis, Stomatono'ma. Same as *Noma.*

Stomatop'athy. Any disorder of the mouth.

Stomat'oplasty. Plastic surgery of the mouth or of the os uteri.

Stomatorrha'gia. Hemorrhage from the mouth.

Stomat'oscope. Instrument for inspecting the mouth.

Stomoceph'alus. Fetus with rudimentary jaws and mouth.

Stomodæ'um, Stomode'um. An invagination of the embryonic ectoderm whence the mouth-cavity is formed.

Stomox'ydæ (sto-mok'sid-e). Common flies.

Stone. A calculus or concretion.

Stool. A fecal discharge.

Stop-needle. A needle with a disk to prevent deep penetration.

Sto'rage battery. Apparatus for storing electricity.

Sto'rax. Balsam from *Liquidambar orientalis:* diuretic and anticatarrhal.

Strabis'mic (stra-biz'mik). Pertaining to, or of the nature of, strabismus.

Strabismom'eter. Apparatus for measuring strabismus.

Strabis'mus. A squint; deviation of one or both of the eyes. **Accommodative s.**, s. due to defect or excess of ocular accommodation. **Alternating s., Bilateral s.**, one in which either eye is alternately fixed. **Concomitant s.**, that in which the affected eye accompanies the other in its movements. **Convergent s.**, one eye, or both, turned inward; cross-eye. **Divergent s.**, strabismus with outward deviation. **Intermittent s.**, that which recurs at intervals. **Paralytic s.** is due to paralysis of one or more muscles. **Spastic s.** is due to spastic contraction of an ocular muscle.

Strabom'eter. The strabismometer.

Strabot'omy. The cutting of an ocular tendon for strabismus.

Straight arterioles. See *Arteriolæ rectæ*. **S. sinus**, a venous sinus along the tentorium and falx cerebri. **S. jacket.** Same as *Camisole*.

Strain (strān). 1. Injury from overuse. 2. To filter or perform a colation.

Straits of the pelvis. The openings of the true pelvis, distinguished as superior and inferior.

Stramo'nium. The jimson-weed, *Datura stramonium*; seeds and leaves are narcotic and antispasmodic.

Strangalesthe'sia. Same as *Zonesthesia*.

Stran'gles. Infectious disease of horses with mucopurulent inflammation of the respiratory mucous membrane.

Stran'gulated. Congested by reason of constriction or hernial protrusion.

Strangula'tion. Congestion due to constriction or stricture.

Stran'gury. Slow and painful discharge of urine.

Strap'ping. The dressing of a wound or part with strips of adhesive plaster.

Strat'ified epithelium. See *Epithelium*.

Strat'iform (strat'if-orm). Having the form of a layer.

Stra'tum. A layer. **S. cor'neum**, the outer or horny layer of the epidermis. **S. granulo'sum.** 1. The layer of epidermis next to the stratum corneum. 2. One of the layers of the retina. 3. A layer of the cortex of the cerebellum. **S. lu'cidum**, the stratum corneum of the epidermis. **S. Malpig'hii, S. muco'sum, S. spino'sum**, the rete mucosum, or innermost layer of the epidermis.

Straw'berry tongue. A tongue with enlarged and reddened fungiform papillæ.

Streak (strēk). A line, stripe, or trace. **S.-culture**, a bacterial culture in which matter is implanted in streaks. **Medullary s.** Same as *Medullary groove*. **Meningitic s.** See *Tache cérébrale*. **Primitive s.**, faint white trace at aftermost end of germinal area.

Streng'thening plaster. Plaster of iron hydrate.

Streph'otome. Instrument for invaginating the hernial sac.

Streptobacte'ria. Those bacteria which are linked into chains.

Streptococce'mia. Occurrence of streptococci in the blood.

Streptococ'cus. A genus or form of bacterial coccus. **S.-antitoxin**, an antitoxin used against erysipelas, etc. **S. aphthic'ola**, species from foot-and-mouth disease of cattle. **S. articulo'rum**, species from diphtheritic mucous membranes. **S. Charri'ni**, a pathogenic species from true anthrax. **S. Dis'sei**, a species from blood of certain cases of syphilis. **S. enteri'tis**, enteritis due to streptococci. **S. e'qui**, a species from contagious coryza of horses. **S. erysipel'atis**, the species that causes erysipelas; Loeffler's bacillus. **S. hydrophobo'rum**, a species from the brain of animals with rabies. **S. Lu'cæ**, a species from soft chancer or chancroid. **S. Manfre'dii**, a species which causes lobar pneumonia. **S. meningit'idis**, a species from cerebrospinal meningitis. **S. morbillo'sus,** a species from measles. **S. pyo'genes,** a species from erysipelatoid suppurations. **S. pyo'genes malig'nus,** a species from leukemic spleen. **S. sep'ticus,** a pathogenic species from foul soil. **S. sep'ticus liquefa'ciens,** a species from the blood of septic poisoning after scarlatina. **S. toxica'tus,** a species said to afford one of the poisons of *Rhus toxicodendron.*

Strep'tothrix. A genus of schizomycetes.

Stret'cher. A litter for conveying the sick or wounded.

Stri'a, pl. *stri'æ.* L. for *Streak.*

Stri'æ acus'ticæ. The striæ medullares. **S. atroph'icæ,** white streaks due to skin-atrophy. **S. longitudina'les latera'les,** two white lines across upper surface of the callosum. **S. medulla'res,** white lines across the floor of fourth ventricle. **S. pinea'lis,** the anterior peduncle of pineal gland. **S. termina'lis.** Same as *Tænia semicircularis.*

Stri'ate, Stri'ated. Having streaks or striæ. **S. bodies,** the corpora striata.

Stria'tion. 1. Quality of being streaked. 2. A streak or scratch, or a series of streaks.

Stria'tum (stri-a'tum). The corpus striatum.

Stric'ture. An abnormal narrowing of a duct or passage. **Cicatricial s.,** one which follows a wound or sore. **Functional s.** Same as *Spasmodic s.* **Impermeable s.,** one which closes the lumen of a passage. **Irritable s.,** one the passage of which causes pain. **Organic s.,** one due to structural changes in or about a canal. **Spasmodic s.** is due to muscular spasm.

Stric'turotome. Instrument for cutting strictures.

Stricturot'omy. Surgical division of a stricture.

Stri'dor. A shrill harsh sound. **S. den'tium,** noise made by grinding the teeth. **S. serrat'icus,** sound like that caused by filing a saw, caused by respiration through a tracheotomy-tube.

Strid'ulent, Strid'ulous. Attended with stridor; making a harsh noise.

Strobi'la, Strobi'lus. An adult tapeworm; adult stage of a tapeworm.

Stro'boscope. Apparatus on the principle of a zoetrope for exhibiting the successive phases of animal movements.

Stroke. A sudden and severe attack. **S.-culture.** See *Culture.*

Stro'ma. Tissue which forms the ground-substance, framework, or matrix of an organ. **S.-plexus,** network formed by ramifications of the nerves of the cornea within the substantia propria.

Stro'meyer's splint. A splint consisting of two hinged portions which can be fixed at any angle.

Stron'gylus (stron'jil-us). A genus of parasitic nematode worms.

Stron'tium (stron'she-um). A yellowish metal, some of whose salts are medicinal.

Strophan'thin (stro-fan'thin). A poisonous glucosid from strophanthus.

Strophan'thus his'pidus. An African shrub: the seeds are used like digitalis.

Stroph'ulus (strof'u-lus). Tooth-rash; a papular infantile eruption. **S. al'bidus.** Same as *Milium.* **S. infan'tum,** the urticaria of infants. **S. prurigino'sus,** a variety attended with severe itching.

Struc'tural disease. A disease attended with anatomic or histologic change in tissues.

Stru'ma. Goiter or scrofula. **S. malig'na,** carcinoma of the thyroid body. **S. suprarena'lis,** a kind of fatty tumor of the suprarenal capsules.

Strumec'tomy. Removal of scrofulous glands.

Strumipri'val cachexia. See *Cachexia.*
Strumi'tis (stru-mi'tis). Same as *Thyroiditis.*
Strumoder'ma (stru-mo-der'mah). Same as *Scrofuloderma.*
Stru'mous (stru'mus). Same as *Scrofulous.*
Strych'nia (strik'ne-ah). Same as *Strychnin.*
Strych'nin (strik'nin). Poisonous bitter alkaloid, $C_{21}H_{22}N_2O_2$ from nux vomica.
Strychninoma'nia. Insanity caused by strychnin.
Strych'nism (strik'nizm). Poisoning by strychnin.
Strych'nos (strik'nos). Genus of poisonous trees. See *Nux vomica, Ignatia, Hoang-nan.*
Stu'dent's placenta. Placenta retained in consequence of unskilful manipulation.
Stump. Distal end of the part of limb left in amputation.
Stupe. A cloth, sponge, or the like charged with hot water and medicated for external application.
Stupefa'cient (stu-pe-fa'shent). Narcotic; soporific.
Stupema'nia (stu-pe-ma'ne-ah). Stuporous insanity.
Stu'por. Partial or nearly complete unconsciousness.
Stupra'tion, Stu'prum. Rape.
Stut'tering. Difficulty in speech due to a kind of habit-spasm.
Sty, Stye. Inflammation of a sebaceous gland of the eyelid; hordeolum. **Meibomian s.,** inflammation of a Meibomian gland. **Zeissian's s.,** inflammation of a Zeissian gland.
Style, Sty'let. Same as *Stilet.*
Stylis'cus. A slender cylindric tent.
Styloglos'sus (sti-lo-glos'us). See *Muscles, Table of.*
Stylohyoi'deus. See *Muscles, Table of.*
Sty'loid. Shaped like a pen or stylus; long and pointed.
Stylomas'toid. Pertaining to the styloid and mastoid processes of the temporal bone.
Stylomax'illary. Pertaining to the styloid process of the temporal bone and to a maxillary bone.
Stylopharyn'geus. See *Muscles, Table of.*
Sty'lus. A stilet; also a pencil or stick, as of caustic.
Stype. A tampon or pledget of cotton.
Styp'sis (stip'sis). Employment of styptics.
Styp'tic. 1. Arresting hemorrhage by means of an astringent quality. 2. A markedly astringent remedy. **S. collodion,** a preparation of collodion and tannin. **S. cotton,** cotton charged with iron subsulphate.
Styp'ticin. Cotarnin hydrochlorid, $C_{12}H_{13}NO_3H_2O.HCl$: an internal styptic.
Sty'racin. A crystalline substance, $C_{18}H_{16}O_2$, from styrax.
Styr'acol. Cinnamyl guaiacol, $C_6H_4(OC_9H_7O.OCH_3)$: antiseptic.
Sty'rax. Same as *Storax.*
Sty'rol. A fragrant oily hydrocarbon, C_8H_8, from storax, etc.
Sty'rone (sti'rōn). Cinnamic alcohol, $C_9H_{10}O$.
Subabdom'inal. Situated below the abdomen.
Subac'etate (sub-as'et-āt). Any basic acetate.
Subac'id (sub-as'id). Somewhat acid.
Subacro'mial. Below or beneath the acromion.
Suba'cute. Somewhat acute; between acute and chronic.
Subanco'neus (sub-an-ko'ne-us). See *Muscles, Table of.*
Subaponeurot'ic. Situated beneath an aponeurosis.
Subarach'noid. Situated beneath the arachnoid. **S. space,** the space between the pia and arachnoid.
Subar'cuate fossa. A pit on the posterior internal surface of the petrous bone.
Subastrag'alar. Situated under the astragalus.
Subastrin'gent. Moderately astringent.
Subau'ral (sub-aw'ral). Beneath the ear.

Subcap'sular. Below a capsule, especially the capsule of the cerebrum.

Subcar'bonate. Any basic carbonate.

Subcartilag'inous. 1. Situated beneath cartilage. 2. Partly cartilaginous.

Subchron'ic (sub-kron'ik). Between chronic and subacute.

Subcla'vian. Situated under the clavicle. **S. artery.** See *Arteries, Table of.* **S. triangle,** the triangle of the neck bounded by the clavicle, sternomastoid, and omohyoid.

Subclavic'ular. Same as *Subclavian.*

Subcla'vius. See *Muscles, Table of.*

Subconjuncti'val. Situated beneath the conjunctiva.

Subcontin'uous fever. Remittent fever.

Subcor'acoid. Situated under the coracoid process.

Subcor'tical. Situated beneath the cerebral cortex.

Subcos'tal. Beneath a rib or the ribs.

Subcra'nial. Beneath the cranium.

Subcrep'itant. Somewhat crepitant in character.

Subcrura'us, Subcrure'us. See *Muscles, Table of.*

Subcul'ture. Culture of bacteria derived from another culture.

Subcuta'neous. Situated or occurring beneath the skin. **S. surgery,** surgery performed through a small opening in the skin. **S. wound,** a wound having a very small opening through the skin.

Subcutic'ular. Beneath the cuticle.

Subdelir'ium. A partial or mild delirium.

Subdiaphragmat'ic. Situated under the diaphragm.

Subdu'ral. Situated beneath the dura. **S. space,** space between the arachnoid and dura.

Subenceph'alon. The pons, oblongata, crura, and corpora quadrigemina.

Subendocar'dial. Situated beneath the endocardium.

Subendothe'lial. Beneath an endothelial structure.

Subendothe'lium. See *Debove's membrane.*

Subepider'mal. Situated beneath the epidermis.

Subepithe'lial. Situated beneath the epithelium.

Su'berin. Variety of cellulose obtained from cork.

Subfas'cial (sub-fas'shal). Situated beneath a fascia.

Subfeb'rile (sub-feb'ril). Somewhat febrile.

Subfla'vous ligament. Yellowish ligament between the laminæ of a vertebra.

Subfron'tal. Beneath a frontal lobe or convolution.

Subgle'noid. Situated under the glenoid fossa.

Subglos'sal. Situated under the tongue.

Subglossi'tis. Inflammation of the under surface of the tongue.

Subgrunda'tion (sub-grun-da'shun). Depression of one fragment of bone beneath another.

Subhy'oid. Situated beneath the hyoid bone.

Subic'ulum. Same as *Uncinate convolution.*

Subinflamma'tion. Slight or mild inflammation.

Subinflam'matory. Marked by subacute inflammation.

Subin'trant fever. Intermittent fever in which the paroxysms follow one another so closely that they overlap.

Subinvolu'tion. Incomplete involution.

Subi'odid. That iodid of any series which contains the least iodin.

Sub'ject. 1. A person or animal subjected to treatment or experiment. 2. A body for dissection.

Subjec'tive. Pertaining to, or perceived only by, the individual; not perceptible to the senses of another person. **S. sensation,** a sensation that originates within the organism, and is not a response to an external stimulus. **S. symptom,** a symptom perceived by the patient alone.

Subju'gal (sub-ju'gal). Below the malar bone.
Subla'tio ret'inæ. Detachment of the retina of the eye.
Sub'limate. A substance obtained or prepared by sublimation.
Sublima'tion. Process of vaporizing and condensing a solid substance without melting it.
Sublim'inal. Below the limen or threshold of sensation. See *Threshold.*
Sublin'gual. Situated under the tongue. **S. gland,** a salivary gland beneath and on either side of the tongue.
Sublingui'tis. Inflammation of the sublingual gland.
Subluxa'tion. Incomplete or partial dislocation.
Submam'mary. Beneath the mammary gland.
Submaxil'la (sub-mak-sil'ah). The inferior maxilla.
Submax'illary. Situated beneath a maxilla. **S. gland,** a salivary gland on the inner side of each ramus of the lower jaw.
Submaxilli'tis. Inflammation of submaxillary gland.
Submen'tal. Situated beneath the chin.
Submor'phous. Neither amorphous nor perfectly crystalline.
Submuco'sa. The layer of areolar tissue situated beneath the mucous membrane.
Submu'cous. Situated beneath or under the mucous membrane.
Subnarcot'ic. Moderately narcotic.
Subna'sal point. Central point at base of nasal spine.
Subneu'ral (sub-nu'ral). Beneath a nerve or the neural axis.
Subnor'mal. Below or less than normal.
Subnu'cleus. A partial or secondary nucleus.
Suboccip'ital. Situated below or under the occiput. **S. nerve,** the first cervical or spinal nerve.
Suboper'culum. Portion of occipital gyrus overlying the insula.
Subor'bital (sub-or'bit-al). Beneath the orbit.
Subox'id. That oxid in any series which contains the least oxygen.
Subpap'ular (sub-pap'u-lar). Indistinctly papular.
Subpatel'lar. Beneath or below the patella.
Subpedun'cular lobe. Same as *Flocculus.*
Subpericar'dial. Situated beneath the pericardium.
Subperios'teal. Situated or performed beneath the periosteum. **S. operation,** an operation upon a bone without removal of the periosteum.
Subperitone'al. Situated or occurring beneath the peritoneum.
Subpharyn'geal (sub-far-in'je-al). Beneath the pharynx.
Subphren'ic. Beneath or under the diaphragm.
Subplacen'ta (sub-pla-sen'tah). The decidua vera.
Subpleu'ral. Situated beneath the pleura.
Subpon'tine. Situated below the pons.
Subprepu'tial. Situated beneath the prepuce.
Subpu'bic. Situated beneath the pubic bone.
Subpul'monary. Situated beneath the lung.
Subret'inal. Situated beneath the retina.
Sub'salt. Any basic salt.
Subscap'ular. Situated below or under the scapula.
Subscapula'ris. See *Muscles, Table of.*
Subscrip'tion. The part of a prescription which gives directions for compounding the ingredients.
Subse'rous. Situated beneath a serous membrane.
Subspi'nous dislocation. Dislocation of the head of the humerus into space below the spine of the scapula.
Sub'stage. Part of the microscope underneath the stage.
Substan'tia. L. for *Substance.* **S. cine'rea,** the gray substance of the brain and spinal cord. **S. ferrugin'ea,** pigmented nerve-cell substance of the locus cœruleus. **S. gelatino'sa,** substance sheathing posterior horn of spinal cord and lining the central canal. **S. gris'ea,** gray matter, especially of the spinal cord. **S. ni'-**

gra. Same as *Locus niger*. **S. perfora'ta,** a posterior embryonic structure on the floor of the third ventricle. **S. pro'pria.** Same as *Lamina propria*.

Subster'nal. Situated below the sternum.

Substitu'tion. Chemical replacement of one substance by another.

Sub'stitutive. Effecting a change or substitution of symptoms.

Subsul'tus ten'dinum. Twitching movement of muscles and tendons in typhoid condition.

Subsyl'vian. Situated under the fissure of Sylvius.

Subtar'sal. Situated below the tarsus.

Subthalam'ic. Situated below the thalamus.

Subthal'amus. Yellowish node situated below the thalamus.

Sub'tle (sut'tl). 1. Very fine, as a subtle powder. 2. Very acute, as a subtle pain.

Subtrochanter'ic. Situated below the trochanter.

Subtu'beral. Situated under a tuber.

Subtympan'ic. Having a somewhat tympanic quality.

Subu'beres. Latin for unweaned or suckling children.

Subumbil'ical space. Somewhat triangular space within the body-cavity just below the navel.

Subun'gual, Subun'guial. Situated beneath a nail.

Subure'thral. Situated or occurring beneath the urethra.

Subvag'inal (sub-vaj'in-al). Situated under a sheath or below the vagina.

Subver'tebral (sub-ver'te-bral). Situated on ventral side of vertebral column.

Subvi'rile. Having deficient virility.

Subvitri'nal (sub-vit-ri'nal). Situated beneath the vitreous.

Subvolu'tion (sub-vo-lu'shun). The turning over of a flap.

Subzo'nal (sub-zo'nal). Situated below the zona pellucida.

Succeda'neous. Of the nature of a substitute.

Succeda'neum (suk-se-da'ne-um). A substitute for something else.

Succentu'riate. Accessory; serving as a substitute. **S. placenta.** See *Placenta*.

Succin'ic acid (suk-sin'ik). See *Acid*. An acid, $C_4H_6O_4$, from amber: it forms succinates.

Suc'cinum. L. for *Amber*.

Succiru'bra bark. Red cinchona bark.

Suc'cus. L. for *Juice*. **S. enter'icus,** intestinal or enteric juice. **S. gas'tricus,** the gastric juice.

Succus'sion (suk-kush'un). The act of shaking a patient so as to detect the presence of liquid in the cavities of the body.

Sucholo-albu'min. A poisonous proteid characteristic of hog-cholera.

Sucholotox'in. A toxin from hog-cholera.

Suck. To feed from the breast.

Suck'ing-pad. The buccal fat-pad of a young child.

Su'crol. A sweet crystalline substitute for sugar, $CH_3N_2O(C_6H_4\text{-}OC_2H_5)$.

Su'crose (su'krōs). Same as *Saccharose*.

Sudam'ina. Whitish vesicles from retained sweat.

Suda'tion. 1. The process of sweating. 2. Excessive sweat.

Sudato'ria (su-dat-o're-ah). Same as *Ephidrosis*.

Sudato'rium. A hot-air bath or sweat-bath.

Su'dor. Sweat; perspiration. **S. Ang'licus.** See *Anglicus sudor*. **S. cruen'tus,** the sweating of blood; hematidrosis.

Su'doral (su'dor-al). Characterized by profuse sweating.

Sudor'ic acid. An acid which exists in suint.

Sudorif'erous, Sudorip'arous. Secreting or producing sweat.

Sudorif'ic (su-dor-if'ik). An agent causing sweating.

Su'et. Fat from abdominal cavity of ox or sheep; sevum.

Suffoca'tion. Stoppage of respiration or asphyxia due to it.

Suffumiga'tion. Fumigation; also, a substance burnt in fumigation.

Suffu'sion. State of being blood-shot or of being moistened.

Sug'ar (shŭg'ar). A sweet carbohydrate of various kinds and of both animal and vegetable origin. **Beet-s.,** saccharose from root of beet. **Cane-s.,** saccharose from sugar-cane. **Diabetic s.,** glucose. **Fruit-s.** See *Levulose*. **Invert s.,** a natural mixture of dextrose and levulose. **Liver-s.,** glucose. **Maple-s.,** saccharose from maple-sap. **Milk-s.** See *Lactose*. **Muscle-s.** See *Inosite*.

Sugges'tible. Liable to be so acted upon as to be made to act automatically.

Sugges'tion. The production of a condition or state in a person by imparting to him an idea from without.

Sugges'tionize. To treat a patient by suggestion.

Sugilla'tion. An ecchymosis or bruise.

Suint (swint). The fatty natural soap which exists in sheep's wool: lanolin is prepared from it.

Sul'cate, Sul'cated. Furrowed or marked with sulci.

Sul'cus. A fissure, chiefly of the brain. **Intraparietal s.,** that which divides the superior from inferior parietal bones. **S. præcentra'lis,** a sulcus situated in front of fissure of Rolando. **S. pulmona'lis,** groove on the back along either side of the vertebral column. **S. spira'lis,** grooved extremity of the lamina spiralis of the cochlea. **S. tympan'icus,** groove into which the membrana tympani fits. **Vertical s.** Same as *S. præcentralis*.

Sul'fonal. Same as *Sulphonal*.

Sulphal'dehyd. An ill-smelling oily hypnotic.

Sulpham'inol. A yellowish absorbent and antiseptic powder, $C_{12}H_9NO_2S$.

Sulphanil'ic acid. An anilin preparation, useful in otitis, laryngitis, etc.

Sul'phate. Any salt of sulphuric acid.

Sul'phid. Any binary compound of sulphur.

Sulphindigot'ic acid. An acid, $C_8H_5NO.SO_3$, whose salts of potassium and sodium constitute indigo-carmin.

Sul'phite (sul'fīt). Any salt of sulphurous acid.

Sulphocar'bol, Sulphocarbol'ic acid. An antipyretic and antiseptic remedy, $C_6H_6SO_4$.

Sul'phonal (sul'fo-nal). A crystalline somnifacient, $C_7H_{16}S_2O_4$.

Sul'phonalism. The symptoms produced by sulphonal-poisoning.

Sulphonaph'tol. A proprietary antiseptic: called also *milk oil*.

Sulphophe'nol. Same as *Sulphocarbol*.

Sulphoricin'ic acid. An acid prepared from castor oil: antiseptic and disinfectant.

Sul'phugator. A roll of muslin charged with sulphur to be burnt for a fumigation.

Sul'phume. A proprietary depurant said to be pure sulphur in a liquid form.

Sul'phur (sul'fur). A non-metallic element; said by some to be a compound: symbol S.

Sul'phurated, Sul'phuretted. Combined or charged with sulphur. **S. hydrogen.** See *Hydrosulphuric acid*, under *Acid*.

Sul'phuret. Same as *Sulphid*.

Sulphu'ric acid. See *Acid*.

Sul'phurous acid. See *Acid*.

Su'mac, Su'mach (su'mak). See *Rhus*.

Sum'bul. The root of *Ferula sumbul:* nervine and antispasmodic.

Sum'mer cholera, S. complaint, S. diarrhea. Relatively mild form of gastro-enteritis. **S. rash,** lichen tropicus, or prickly heat.

Sun'burn. Dermatitis with burning and redness due to exposure to sun's rays.

Sun'day-morn'ing paralysis. A musculospiral paralysis due to alcoholic debauch.

Sun'stroke. Insolation or thermic fever.

Superalimenta'tion. Therapeutic treatment by excessive feeding.

Supercil'iary. Pertaining to the region of an eyebrow.

Supercil'ium (su-per-sil'e-um). L. for *Eyebrow.*

Superexcita'tion. Extreme or excessive excitation.

Superfecunda'tion. Successive fertilization of two ova formed at the same menstrual period.

Superfeta'tion. Fertilization of two ova formed at different menstrual periods.

Superfic'ial (su-per-fish'al). Situated on or near the surface. **S. fascia.** thin tough membrane that covers the muscles immediately under the skin.

Superficia'lis. Superficial; also a superficial artery.

Superimpregna'tion. Superfecundation; also superfetation.

Superinvolu'tion of the uterus. Excessive involution by which the organ is reduced to less than its normal size.

Supe'rior. Having a higher situation.

Superlacta'tion (su-per-lak-ta'shun). Over-secretion of milk.

Supermotil'ity. An excess of motility in any part.

Superna'tant. Floating upon the surface of a liquid.

Supernu'merary. In excess of the regular number.

Superphos'phate (su-per-fos'fāt). Any acid phosphate.

Su'persalt. Any salt with excess of acid; a persalt.

Supersat'urated solution. A solution made in a heated condition and thus containing a greater quantity of the solid than it could absorb at its normal temperature.

Superscrip'tion. The sign ℞ before a prescription.

Supersecre'tion. Excess of any secretory function.

Supina'tion. The turning of the palm of the hand upward.

Su'pinator. See *Muscles, Table of.* **S. lon'gus reflex,** tapping the tendon of the supinator longus produces flexion of the forearm.

Su'pine (su'pin). Lying on the dorsum.

Suplago-al'bumin. An albumose characteristic of swine-plague.

Suplagotox'in. A ptomain of swine-plague.

Supplemen'tal air. That part of the residual air of the lung which, after the tidal air is expelled, may be driven out by forced respiration.

Suppos'itory. A solid, easily fusible, medicated mass to be introduced into the vagina or rectum.

Suppres'sion. Sudden stoppage of a secretion, excretion, or normal discharge.

Sup'purant. An agent causing suppuration.

Suppura'tion. Formation of, conversion into, or discharge of pus.

Sup'purative. Associated with, or favoring, suppuration. **S. fever,** pyemia.

Supra-acro'mial. Situated above the acromion.

Supra-auric'ular. Situated above an auricle.

Supracho'roid. Situated above or upon the choroid.

Suprachoroi'dea. The outermost layer of the choroid.

Supraclavic'ular. Situated above the clavicle. **S. point,** point above clavicle at which stimulation produces contraction of the muscles of the arm.

Supracon'dylar. Situated above a condyle or condyles.

Supracos'tal. Situated above or outside of the ribs.

Supracot'yloid. Situated above the acetabulum.

Supra-epicon'dylar. Situated or occurring above the epicondyle.

Supragle'noid tubercle. The tubercle which attaches the long head of the biceps to head of scapula.

Suprahy'oid (su-prah-hi'oid). Situated above the hyoid bone. **S. muscles,** the digastricus, stylohyoid, mylohyoid, and geniohyoid muscles.

Supra-in'guinal region. Region bounded by the rectus abdominis, Poupart's ligament, and the line through the crest of ilium.

Supralum'bar. Situated or occurring above the loin.

Supramalle'olar. Situated above a malleolus.

Supramar'ginal convolution. A convolution above the posterior limb of the fissure of Sylvius.

Supramas'toid crest. A ridge on the temporal bone continuing backward to the posterior root of the zygoma.

Supramaxil'la. The upper jaw-bone.

Supramax'illary. Pertaining to the upper jaw.

Suprames'tal triangle. Triangle formed by the posterior root of the zygoma above, the upper and posterior segment of the osseous external meatus below, and by a line drawn from the posterior portion of the external osseous meatus to the zygomatic root.

Supra-occip'ital bone. That part of the occipital bone behind the foramen magnum: it is distinct in early childhood.

Supra-or'bital. Situated above the orbit.

Suprapel'vic (su-prah-pel'vik). Situated above the pelvis.

Suprapon'tine. Situated above or in upper part of the pons.

Suprapu'bic. Situated or performed above the pubes.

Supraren'aden. A proprietary preparation made from the suprarenal bodies.

Suprare'nal. Above a kidney. **S. body, S. capsule,** a triangular organ above either kidney. **S. extract,** an organotherapeutic remedy for Addison's disease.

Suprascap'ular. Situated above the scapula. **S. nerve.** See *Nerves, Table of.*

Supraspi'nal (su-prah-spi'nal). Situated on the spine.

Supraspina'lis. See *Muscles, Table of.*

Supraspina'tus. See *Muscles, Table of.*

Supraspi'nous fossa. A depression above the spine of the scapula.

Supraster'nal. Situated above the sternum.

Suprasyl'vian convolution. Same as *Supramarginal convolution.*

Supratroch'lear. Situated above the trochlea.

Supravag'inal. Outside or above a sheath.

Su'ra (su'rah). L. for *Calf of the leg.*

Su'ral. Pertaining to the calf of the leg.

Suralimenta'tion. Over-feeding; gavage.

Surd'itas, Sur'dity. Deafness.

Surdomute (sur-do-mût'). 1. A deaf-mute. 2. Both deaf and dumb.

Sur'geon (sur'je-on). A practitioner of surgery.

Sur'gery (sur'jer-e). That branch of medicine which treats disease by manual and operative procedures. **Antiseptic s., Aseptic s.,** surgery according to antiseptic or aseptic methods. **Major s.,** surgery concerned with the more important and dangerous operations. **Minor s.**, surgery concerned with less important operations, as bandaging, application of splints, dressings, etc. **Operative s.**, surgery dealing with operations. **Orthopedic s.**, surgery dealing with the correction of deformities. **Plastic s.**, the repair of defects by transfer of tissue. **Railway s.**, surgery dealing with railway injuries. **Veterinary s.**, the surgery of domestic animals.

Sur'gical (sur'jik-al). Of, or pertaining to, surgery. **S. fever**, fever that follows an operation or injury. **S. kidney**, kidney affected with nephritis as a result of a surgical operation. **S. neck**, part of shaft of humerus below the tuberosities.

Sur'ra. Disease of domestic animals in India, due to schizomycetes in blood.

Sur'rogate. A substitute or succedaneum.

Sursumduc'tion. Ability to elevate, or the act of elevating, the axis of either eye independently.

Susotox'in. Poisonous ptomain or toxin from hog-cholera cultures.

Suspen'ded animation. A temporary cessation of the vital functions.

Suspen'sion. Treatment of spinal disorders by suspending the patient by the chin and shoulders.

Suspen'sory. Serving to hold up a part. **S. bandage**, bandage or sling for supporting the testes.

Sustentac'ular. Supporting; sustaining.

Sustentac'ulum ta'li. A process of the calcaneum which supports the astragalus.

Susur'rus. L. for *Murmur*.

Sutu'ra. L. for *Suture*. **S. denta'ta**, interlocking of bones by saw-like processes. **S. harmo'nia**, simple apposition of bones. **S. limbo'sa**, an interlocking by bevelled surfaces. **S. no'tha**, an apparent, but not true, suture of bones. **S. serra'ta.** See *S. dentata*. **S. squamo'sa**, the overlapping of edges of bones.

Su'tural. Of, or pertaining to, a suture.

Sutura'tion. Process or act of suturing.

Su'ture. 1. A surgical stitch or seam. 2. Line of junction of adjacent cranial or facial bones. **Basilar s.** separates in part the occipital and sphenoid bones. **Buried s.**, a stitch concealed by the skin. **Catgut-s.**, one in which catgut is employed. **Cobblers' s.**, one in which two threads are employed. **Continuous s.**, a suture in which the stitches are made with one unbroken thread. **Coronal s.**, union of frontal and parietal bones transversely across vertex of skull. **Czerny s., Czerny-Lembert s.** See *Czerny s.*, etc. **Dry s.**, suturation of lips of wound through adhesive plaster. **Ethmofrontal s.**, union between frontal and ethmoid bones. **Ethmolacrimal s.**, between ethmoid and lacrimal bones. **Ethmosphenoid s.**, between ethmoid and sphenoid bones. **False s.**, bony suture without interlocking of the bones. **Frontal s.** in early infancy separates the two frontal bones. **Frontomalar s.**, union between frontal and malar bones. **Frontonasal s.**, between the superior maxillary and frontal bones. **Frontosphenoid s.**, union between alæ of sphenoid and frontal bone. **Frontotemporal s.**, between frontal and temporal bones. **Hare-lip s.**, a twisted suture for hare-lip. **Intermaxillary s.**, between superior maxillary bones. **Internasal s.**, between nasal bones. **Interparietal s., Jugal s., Longitudinal s.**, the sagittal s. **Interrupted s.**, series of stitches each separately tied. **Jobert's s.**, a suture for transverse intestinal wounds. **Lambdoid s.**, between the upper borders of occipital and parietal bones. **Lembert's s.**, a peculiar suture for intestinal wounds. **Mattress s.**, continuous suture applied back and forth through the wound. **Maxillo-lacrimal s.**, between upper maxilla and lacrimal bone. **Metopic s.**, the frontal s. **Nasomaxillary s.**, union between nasal and maxillary bones. **Occipital s.** Same as *Lambdoid s.* **Palatine s.**, between palate bones. **Parietomastoid s.**, between mastoid and parietal bones. **Petro-occipital s.**, between petrous and occipital bones. **Petrosphenoid s.**, between petrous bone and great wing of sphenoid. **Pin-s.**, the hare-lip suture. **Quilled s.**, double thread suture tied over quills. **Relaxation-s.**, a secondary line of stitches to relieve tension on wound-suture. **Sabatier's s.**, insertion of a piece of oiled cardboard into the intestines for the approximation of intestinal wounds. **Sagittal s.**, between upper borders of parietal bones. **Shotted s.**, both ends of the stitch pass through a shot. **Sphenomalar s.**, between malar bone and great wing of sphenoid. **Sphenoparietal s.**, between great wing of sphenoid and parietal bone. **Sphenotemporal s.**, union between temporal and sphenoid bones. **Squamoparietal s.**, **Squamosal s.**, between parietal bone and squamosa. **Squamo-sphenoid s.**, between great wing of sphenoid and squamous portion of temporal bone. **Subcutaneous s.**, a form of continuous buried s. **Tension s.** See *Relaxation s.* **Tongue-and-groove s.**, a peculiar suture for plastic operations.

Suzanne's gland (su-zanz'). A mucous gland of the mouth beneath the alveolingual groove.

Swab. 1. A device for moistening the lips of a helpless patient. 2. A wire with a tuft of sterilized cotton at the end used in collecting material for bacteriologic study.

Swal'low's nest. Same as *Nidus hirundinis.*

Sweat. Perspiration; liquid excreted by the sudoriparous glands.

Sweat'ing fever, S. sickness. Same as *Anglicus sudor.*

Swine-erysipelas. A contagious disease of young hogs, with fever and formation of red blotches on neck and belly. **S.-plague**, epidemic, infectious disease of swine, affecting the respiratory and alimentary tracts.

Syceph'alus (sis-ef'al-us). Same as *Syncephalus.*

Syco'ma. A wart; a condyloma.

Syco'siform (si-ko'sif-orm). Like or resembling sycosis.

Syco'sis (si-ko'sis). Pustular inflammation of hair-follicles, especially of the beard. **S. parasita'ria.** Same as *Tinea sycosis.*

Syd'enham's chorea. Ordinary and uncomplicated chorea. **S.'s laudanum.** wine of opium.

Syllab'ic blindness. An inability to form syllables. **S. utterance.** Same as *Scanning speech.*

Syl'vian aqueduct. See *Aqueduct of Sylvius.* **S. artery**, middle cerebral artery in the Sylvian fissure. **S. fissure**, the large fissure which separates the anterior and middle lobes of the cerebrum. **S. line.** line on exterior of cranium defining the direction of the Sylvian fissure.

Sym'bion. An organism which lives in a state of symbiosis.

Symbio'sis (sim-bi-o'sis). The necessary association of two diverse organisms, neither of which is parasitic.

Symbleph'aron (sim-blef'ar-on). Adhesion of the lids to the eyeball.

Sym'elus (sim'el-us). Same as *Symmelus.*

Syme's amputation. Disarticulation of the foot with removal of both malleoli.

Sym'melus. Monster fetus with legs fused.

Symmet'ric gangrene. Gangrene of fingers, toes, ears, etc., due to a nervous disorder with vascular disturbance.

Sympathconeuri'tis. Inflammation of the sympathetic nerve.

Sympathet'ic. 1. Pertaining to, or caused by, sympathy. 2.

Same as *Sympathetic system.* **S. nerve, S. system,** a system of ganglia, nerves, and plexuses going to the muscular apparatus of blood-vessels and viscera. **S. ophthalmia,** inflammation of one eye following or due to inflammation of the other.

Sympatheticoparalyt'ic. Caused by paralysis of the sympathetic nervous system.

Sympatheticoton'ic. Caused by tonic contraction of arteries due to overaction of the sympathetic.

Sym'phorol (sim'for-ol). Caffein-sulphonic acid: a diuretic. Its salts are also diuretic.

Symphys'eal (sim-fiz'e-al). Of, or pertaining to, a symphysis.

Symphyseot'omy, Symphysiot'omy. Division of the symphysis pubis in order to facilitate delivery.

Symphys'ion (sim-fiz'e-on). The middle point of the outer border of the alveolar process of the lower jaw.

Sym'physis (sim'fis-is). Line of junction and fusion of bones originally distinct. **S. pu'bis,** the junction of the pubic bones.

Sympo'dia. Condition in which the lower extremities are fused together.

Symp'tom (simp'tom). Any evidence of disease or of a patient's state. **S.-complex, S.-grouping.** Same as *Complex of symptoms.* **Constitutional s., General s.,** a symptom produced by the effect of the disease on the whole body. **Local s.,** a symptom caused by localization of the disease in some special part. **Objective s.,** a symptom observed by the physician. **Subjective s.,** a symptom observed by the patient only.

Symptomat'ic. Pertaining to, or of the nature of, a symptom.

Symptomatol'ogy. Branch of medicine which treats of symptoms; systematic discussion of symptoms.

Sym'pus (sim'pus). Monster fetus with feet and legs fused.

Synadel'phus (sin-ad-el'fus). Monster fetus with one body and eight limbs.

Synæsthe'sia (sin-es-the'ze-ah). See *Synesthesia.*

Synal'gia (sin-al'je-ah). Pain experienced in one place, but caused by lesion or stimulation in another.

Synal'gic (sin-al'jik). Characterized by synalgia.

Synanastomo'sis. The anastomosis of several vessels.

Synanthe'ma (sin-an-the'mah). A local or grouped eruption.

Synap'tase (sin-ap'tās). Same as *Emulsin.*

Synarthro'dia. A joint in which adjacent surfaces are connected by an intervening tissue.

Synarthro'dial. Pertaining to synarthrosis.

Synarthro'sis. An immovable joint; joint with no intervening tissue between the bones.

Syneeph'alus. Twin fetus with fused heads.

Synchei'lia. Congenital adhesion of the lips.

Synchondro'sis. Union of bones by intervening fibrous or elastic cartilage.

Synchondrot'omy. Same as *Symphyseotomy.*

Syn'chronism (sin'kro-nizm). Occurrence at the same time.

Syn'chronous (sin'kron-us). Occurring at the same time.

Syn'chysis (sin'kis-is). Derangement or confusion. **S. scintil'lans,** abnormally soft state of the vitreous, with presence of floating particles of cholesterin.

Syn'ciput (sin'sip-ut). See *Sinciput.*

Syn'clitism. Position of fetal head when the planes are parallel with those of the pelvis.

Syn'clonus (sin'klo-nus). Muscular tremor or successive clonic contraction of various muscles together.

Syn'copal. Pertaining to, or characterized by, syncope.

Syn'cope (sin'ko-pe). A swoon; fainting, or a faint. **Local s.,** local asphyxia. See *Asphyxia.*

Syncytio'ma malig'num. A tumor formed at the placental site during pregnancy.

Syncyt'ium (sin-sit'e-um). 1. A large cell with many nuclei. 2. The outermost fetal layer of the placenta, composed of epithelial cells.

Syndac'tylism (sin-dak'til-ism). Union of the toes or fingers.

Syndac'tylus. Monster fetus with toes or fingers blended.

Syndec'tomy (sin-dek'to-me). Same as *Peritomy.*

Syndel'phus (sin-del'fus). Same as *Synadelphus.*

Syndesmi'tis. Inflammation of a ligament or of the conjunctiva.

Syndesmog'raphy. Description of the ligaments.

Syndesmol'ogy. Scientific study of the ligaments.

Syndesmo'ma. A tumor of connective tissue.

Syndesmo'sis. The union of bones by ligaments or by a membrane.

Syndesmot'omy. Dissection or cutting of ligaments.

Syn'drome. Same as *Complex of symptoms.* **S. of Weber,** paralysis of the limbs and hypoglossal nerve on one side and of the oculomotor nerves on the other.

Syndrom'ic. Occurring as a syndrome.

Syne'chia (sin-e'ke-ah). Adhesion, as of the iris to the cornea or lens.

Synechot'omy (sin-ek-ot'om-e). Surgical division of a synechia.

Synecten'terotome. A form of enterotome.

Syner'gic (sin-er'jik). Acting together or in harmony.

Syn'ergist (sin'er-jist). A muscle or agent which acts with another.

Synergy (sin'er-je). Correlated action or co-operation.

Synesthe'sia (sin-es-the'ze-ah). Sensation experienced in one place, but caused by stimulation in another.

Syngen'esis. Theory which holds that each germ contains in itself the germs of every generation that may be derived from it.

Syngig'noeism (sin-jig'no-sizm). Hypnotism or hypnotic suggestion.

Synize'sis (sin-iz-e'sis). Contraction of the pupil of the eye.

Synkine'sis (sin-kin-e'sis). Associated reflex movement.

Synneuro'sis (sin-u-ro'sis). See *Syndesmosis.*

Syn'ocha, Syn'ochus. Old names for a continued fever.

Syn'onym (sin'o-nim). A word which has the same meaning as another word.

Synophthal'mus. Monster fetus with one orbit; a cyclops.

Syn'orchism. Union or blending of the testes.

Synosteol'ogy. The study of joints and articulations.

Synosteot'omy. Dissection of the joints.

Synosto'sis. The union of bones by means of osseous matter.

Syn'otus. Monster fetus with fused ears.

Synovec'tomy. Excision of a synovial membrane.

Syno'via (sin-o've-ah). The viscid fluid of joint-cavities.

Syno'vial. Of, or pertaining to, or secreting, synovia. **S. membrane,** lining membrane of joints, bursæ, and tendon-sheaths.

Syno'vin (sin-o'vin). Mucin found in synovia.

Synovip'arous. Producing synovia.

Synovi'tis. Inflammation of synovial membrane.

Synther'mal (sin-ther'mal). Of the same temperature.

Syn'thesis. The building up of a chemical compound by the union of its elements.

Synthet'ic (sin-thet'ik). Pertaining to, or of the nature of, synthesis.

Syn'tonin. A proteid formed by the action of acids on myosin.

Syntrop'ic (sin-trop'ik). Turned in the same direction.

Synulot'ic. An agent favoring cicatrization.

Syphilelco'sis. Syphilitic ulceration.

Syphilel'cus. A syphilitic ulcer.
Syph'ilide (sif'il-id). Any skin-affection of syphilitic origin.
Syphili'num. A homeopathic preparation of syphilis-poison.
Syphilion'thus. A copper-colored scaly syphilide.
Syphilipho'bia. Same as *Syphilophobia*.
Syph'ilis (sif'il-is). A contagious venereal disease leading to many structural and cutaneous lesions. It has three stages, *primary*, *secondary*, and *tertiary*. **Congenital s., Hereditary s.,** syphilis existing at birth, either hereditary or due to infection from the mother. **S. innocen'tium, S. inson'tium,** syphilis not acquired by coitus.
Syphilit'ic. Affected with, caused by, or pertaining to syphilis.
Syphiliza'tion. Inoculation with syphilis; attempted immunization against syphilis.
Syph'ilized (sif'il-izd). Affected with syphilis.
Syphilocerebro'sis. Any syphilitic disease of the brain.
Syph'iloderm. A syphilitic skin-disease.
Syphilogen'esis, Syphilog'eny. The development of syphilis.
Syphilog'rapher. A writer about syphilis.
Syphilog'raphy. A treatise on, or the bibliography of, syphilis.
Syph'iloid (sif'il-oid). 1. Resembling syphilis. 2. A disease like syphilis.
Syphilol'ogist. An expert in regard to syphilis.
Syphilol'ogy (sif-il-ol'o-je). Sum of knowledge regarding syphilis.
Syphilo'ma (sif-il-o'mah). A tumor of syphilitic origin.
Syphiloma'nia. See *Syphilophobia*.
Syphilopho'bia. Morbid fear of syphilis, or unwarranted belief on the part of a patient that he is suffering from syphilis.
Syphilopho'bic. Affected with syphilophobia.
Syphilon'thus. Same as *Syphilionthus*.
Syphitox'in (sif-it-ok'sin). An antisyphilitic serum.
Syr'iac ulcer. Diphtheria; also oriental sore.
Syrigmopho'nia. A high, whistling sound of the voice.
Syr'inge (sir'rinj). Instrument for injecting fluids.
Syringi'tis. Inflammation of the Eustachian tube.
Syrin'gocele, Syringocœ'le. The central canal of the myelon.
Syringocystadeno'ma. Adenoma of sweat-glands.
Syringomye'lia. Existence of abnormal cavities filled with liquid in spinal cord: sometimes a form of true leprosy.
Syringomyeli'tis. Inflammation of spinal cord with formation of cavities.
Syringomy'elocele. Spina bifida in which the cavity of the protruding part is connected with the central canal of the spinal cord.
Syringomy'elus. Dilatation of central canal of spinal cord, the gray matter being converted into connective tissue.
Syrin'gotome. A knife for cutting a fistula.
Syringot'omy (sir-ing-got'o-me). The cutting of a fistula.
Syrs'ki's organ (sērs'kēz). The male organ of the eel.
Syr'up (sēr'up). A solution of sugar in water, often medicated.
Syssarco'sis. The joining of bones by means of muscles.
Ysso'mus. Twin monster with two heads and bodies united.
Systal'tic. Alternately contracting and dilating.
Sys'tem. 1. The bodily organism. 2. A set or series of parts or organs which unite in a common function. **S.-disease, S.-lesion,** a lesion or disease of the cord affecting those tissues which have a common function. **Muscular s.,** all the muscles of the body considered together. **Pedal s.,** one of the systems of ganglia and fibers of the brain.
Systemat'ic. Pertaining to, or according to, a system.

Systen'ic. Pertaining to the whole organism or to any particular system. **S. circulation,** the general circulation as distinguished from the pulmonary circulation.

Sys'temoid. Resembling a system: said of tumors made up of several tissues.

Sys'tole (sis'to-le). The period of the heart's contraction; also the contraction itself.

Systol'ic (sis-tol'ik). Pertaining to the systole.

Systolom'eter. Instrument for measuring quality of heart-sounds.

Systrem'ma. Cramp in the muscles of a leg.

Syzig'ium Jambola'num (siz-ij'e-um). Jambol, a tree of the East Indies: the seeds are used in diabetes.

Syz'ygy (siz'ij-e). Conjunction and fusion of organs without loss of identity.

T.

T. Abbreviation for *Temperature* and *Tension*.

T-bandage. Bandage like the letter T, single or double. **T-fiber.** a fiber given off at right angles from the axis-cylinder process of a unipolar ganglion-cell.

Tabaco'sis (tab-ak-o'sis). Poisoning by tobacco, chiefly by inhaling tobacco-dust.

Tab'acum (tab'ak-um). L. for *Tobacco*.

Taban'idæ (ta-ban'id-e). Horse-flies.

Tabatière anatomique (tah-bah-te-ār an-at-o-mēk'). Hollow in back of hand at base of thumb.

Tabefac'tion. A wasting of the body.

Tabel'la. A medicated tablet or troche.

Ta'bes (ta'bēz). Any wasting disorder, especially locomotor ataxia. **T. dorsa'lis,** locomotor ataxia. **Hereditary t.,** Friedreich's ataxia. **T. mesenter'ica, T. mesara'ica,** tuberculosis of mesenteric glands in children. **Spasmodic t.,** lateral sclerosis of myelon.

Tabet'ic. Affected with, or pertaining to, tabes. **T. foot,** distortion of the foot in locomotor ataxia.

Tabet'iform. Resembling tabes.

Tab'id (tab'id). Same as *Tabetic*.

Tabifica'tion. Wasting of the body.

Ta'ble (ta'bl). A flat bony plate or lamina.

Tab'let. A medicated troche or disk.

Tab'loid. A form of medicated tablet.

Tab'ule. A medicinal tablet.

Tac [Fr.]. A contagious fever that ravaged Paris in 1411. It was severe, but never fatal.

Tac'amahac. A resin from species of *Calophyllum*, *Fragara*, and *Populus*.

Tache blanche (tahsh blahsh). White spot on liver in infectious disease. **T. bleuatre,** bluish spot on skin in typhoid fever. **T. cérébrale.** Same as *Meningitic streak*. **T. motrice,** motor nerve-ending in which the nerve-fibril passes to a muscle-cell, ending in a slight enlargement.

Tachycar'dia. Excessive rapidity of heart's action. **Essential t.** is paroxysmal and is a neurosis of cardiac nerves.

Tachycar'diac. Pertaining to, or affected with, tachycardia.

Tachypne'a (tak-ip-ne'ah). Very rapid respiration.

Tac'tile, Tac'tual. Pertaining to the touch. **T. corpuscles,** oval or rounded bodies connected with nerve-fibers in the papillæ of the corium. **T. irritability,** negative chemotaxis. See *Chemotaxis*. **T. sense,** sense of touch.

Tactom'eter. Instrument for measuring tactile sensibility.

Tac'tual (tak'tu-al). See *Tactile.*

Tac'tus erudi'tis. Delicacy of touch acquired by practice.

Tæ'nia (te'ne-ah). 1. A flat band or tape. 2. A tapeworm. **T. Demerarien'sis,** a tapeworm of South America, rarely found in man. **T. echinococ'cus,** a tapeworm from the intestines of dogs whose cyst-worms occur in man. **T. for'nicis,** one of the upper peduncles of the pineal gland. **T. hippocam'pi.** Same as *Corpus fimbriatum.* **T. Madagascarien'sis,** a tapeworm of Madagascar. **T. mediocanella'ta, T. sagina'ta,** the beef-tapeworm. **T. semicircula'ris,** a band on wall of third ventricle between the corpus striatum and thalamus. **T. so'lium,** the common species of tapeworm. **T. tu'bæ,** a thickening sometimes observed in the upper border of the perisalpinx. **T. viola'cea,** bluish stripe on the floor of the fourth ventricle.

Tæ'niacide (te'ne-as-Id). See *Teniacide.*

Tæ'niafuge (te'ne-af-ūj). See *Teniafuge.*

Tage'tes. A genus of plants (marigold) with properties of calendula.

Tagliaco'tian operation (tah-lyah-ko'she-an). Same as *Rhinoplasty.*

Tag'ma. Ultimate molecular mass of protoplasm.

Tail-fold. A fold in the early embryo ensheathing the hind-gut. **T.-gut,** prolongation of the archenteron into the tail of the early embryo.

Tail'ors' spasm. Spasm of arm, hand, and fingers in tailors.

Tait's law. In every case of abdominal or of pelvic disease in which life is threatened or health destroyed, and which is due to malignant disease, exploratory laparotomy should be made. **T.'s operation.** See *Salpingo-oöphorectomy.*

Tak'a-diastase (tak'kah). A proprietary ferment from action of Japanese rice-fungus: digestant, etc. **T.-koji,** a diastatic fungus used in the preparation of taka-diastase: it is developed by the culture of taka-moashi. **T.-moashi,** a Japanese rice-fungus, *Eurotium oryzæ,* used in the preparation of diastase as a digestant.

Talal'gia (tal-al'je-ah). Pain in the heel.

Tal'bot's law (tawl'buts). When complete fusion occurs, and the sensation is uniform, the intensity is the same as would occur were the same amount of light spread uniformly over the disk.

Talc, Tal'cum. A soft greasy powder of magnesium silicate.

Tal'ipes (tal'ip-ēz). L. for *Club-foot.* **T. calca'neus,** that in which the patient walks on the heel. **T. ca'vus,** exaggeration of the plantar arch of the foot. **T. equi'nus,** that in which the patient walks on his toes. **T. perca'vus,** extreme plantar curvature. **T. pla'nus,** flat-foot or splay-foot. **T. val'gus,** talipes in which the patient walks on the inner border of the foot. **T. va'rus,** that in which the patient walks on the outer border of the foot.

Talipom'anus (tal-ip-om'an-us). Same as *Club-hand.*

Talocalca'nean. Pertaining to the astragalus and calcaneum.

Talocru'ral. Pertaining to the astragalus and the leg-bones.

Ta'lus. 1. The astragalus. 2. The ankle.

Ta'mar indien (tah-mar' an-de-ahn'). A proprietary laxative confection.

Tam'arind. Tree of tropical countries, *Tamarindus indica,* and its cooling laxative fruit.

Tam'bour. A drum-shaped appliance used in transmitting movements in a recording instrument.

Tam'pon. A plug made of cotton, sponge, or oakum, variously used in surgery.

Tamponade (tam-pon-ād'). Surgical use of the tampon.

Tanace'tum. See *Tansy*.

Tan'ghin (tahn'geen). Exceedingly poisonous seed of *Cerbera Tanghin*, a tree of Madagascar.

Tan'nagen. See *Tannigen*.

Tan'nal. Aluminum tannate: good in throat- and nose-diseases.

Tannal'bin. A proprietary combination of tannin with albumin.

Tan'nate. Any salt of tannic acid.

Tan'nic acid, Tan'nin. Astringent acid, $C_{14}H_{10}O_9$, from tan-bark and many plants: there are several varieties.

Tan'nigen. Diacetyl-tannin, $C_{14}H_8(CH_3CO)_2O_9$; a tasteless astringent powder.

Tan'noform. A preparation of gallotannic acid and formaldehyd, $C_{29}H_{20}O_{18}$: used for bed-sores.

Tannopu'milin. A proprietary preparation containing oil of *Pinus pumilio* and digallic acid: used in skin-diseases.

Tannopumil'lo. A compound of digallic acid with the terpene of *Pinus pumilio:* used in skin-diseases.

Tan'nosal. The tannic-acid extract of creasote: used in tuberculosis.

Tan'sy (tan'ze). The herb *Tanacetum vulgare:* its oil is emmenagogue, anthelmintic, and poisonous.

Tap. To puncture; to empty by paracentesis.

Tape'tum. A band of fibers passing from the callosum to the temporal lobe. **T. lu'cidum,** the iridescent epithelium of the chorioid of cats, etc.

Tape'worm. A parasitic intestinal cestode worm. **Armed t., Pork t.,** *Tænia solium:* the commonest species. **Beef-t., unarmed t.,** *Tænia saginata:* its cysticercus is found in beef. **Broad-t., Fish-t.,** *Bothriocephalus latus:* its larvæ are found in fish. **Dog t., Hydatid t.,** *Tænia echinococcus:* the above are not infrequent parasites in the human subject: several other species occur for the most part locally. See *Tænia*.

Taphepho'bia. Insane fear of being buried alive.

Tapinocephal'ic. Characterized by tapinocephaly.

Tapinoceph'aly. Condition of having a flattened or depressed skull.

Tapio'ca. Starch from the root of *Jatropha manihot:* used as a food.

Tapotement (tah-pōt-maw'). A tapping manipulation in massage.

Tap'ping (tap'ing). See *Paracentesis*.

Tar. A viscid substance obtained mainly by roasting the wood of various species of pine; another kind is obtained from bituminous coal.

Tar'antism. A variety of dancing mania.

Tarax'acin. Bitter principle from taraxacum.

Tarax'acum. A genus of plants with tonic roots; dandelion.

Tardieu's spots (tar-de-uz'). Spots of ecchymosis under the pleura following death by suffocation.

Taren'tula. The poisonous spider *Lycosa tarentula;* also its homeopathic preparations.

Tarnier's sign (tar-ne-āz'). Obliteration of angle between upper and lower uterine segments of pregnant uterus: a sign of abortion.

Tar'sal. Of, or pertaining to, the tarsus. **T. arches,** arches of the palpebral arteries above and below the t. cartilages. **T. canal,** a canal for vessels and nerves beneath the head of the abductor hallucis. **T. cartilages, T. plates,** thin cartilages of the eyelids. **T. cyst, T. tumor.** Same as *Chalazion*.

Tarsal'gia (tar-sal'je-ah). Pain in a tarsus.

Tarsa'lia. The tarsal bones.

Tarsec'tomy. Excision of a tarsus or of a part of it.

Tarsi'tis (tar-si'tis). Inflammation of a tarsus.

Tarsomala'cia. Softening of the tarsal cartilage.
Tarsometatar'sal. Pertaining to the tarsus and metatarsus.
Tarsophy'ma (tar-so-fi'mah). Any tarsal tumor.
Tar'soplasty. Plastic surgery of eyelid or tarsus.
Tarsor'rhaphy (tar-sor'af-e). Same as *Blepharorrhaphy.*
Tarsot'omy (tar-sot'om-e). The operation of incising or removing the tarsus.
Tar'sus. 1. The instep with its seven bones. 2. The firm framework of plates which give shape to the eyelid.
Tar'tar. 1. The sediment of wine-casks: crude potassium bitartrate. 2. Incrustation formed on neglected teeth. **T. emetic,** tartrate of antimony and potassium. See *Cream of tartar.*
Tartar'ic acid. Acid, $C_4H_6O_6$, from lees of wine, forming tartrates.
Tartariza'tion. The treatment of syphilis by inoculation with tartarized antimony.
Tar'tarized. Charged with tartaric acid.
Tartarlith'in. A salt of lithium: used as a uric-acid solvent in rheumatism and gout.
Tar'trate (tar'trāt). Any salt of tartaric acid.
Tash'kend ulcer. Sartian disease or oriental boil.
Taste-buds, T.-bulbs. Certain end-organs in the tongue. **T.-cells,** gustatory cells within the taste-bulbs.
Tattoo'ing. The permanent coloring of the skin or of the cornea, chiefly to cover leukomatous spots.
Tau'rin. A crystalline principle, $C_2H_7SNO_3$, from bile.
Taurochol'ic acid. One of the acids of the bile, $C_{26}A_{45}NSO_7$.
Tautom'erism. Metamerism in which two formulæ are possible, but only one stable substance is obtainable.
Tax'in. Alkaloid from yew: used in epilepsy.
Tax'is. Manual replacement of displaced parts. **Bipolar t.,** treatment of retroverted uterus by upward pressure through rectum, the cervix being pulled down in vagina.
Taxon'omy (tak-son'o-me). Principles of classification.
Te. Symbol of *Tellurium.*
Tea (te). Leaves of *Thea chinensis:* conservant, stimulant, and exhilarant. **T.-mixture.** See *Species.* **Team'ster's t.,** the plant *Ephedra antisyphilitica,* and its decoction: antisyphilitic.
Tea'berry. See *Gaultheria.*
Teale's amputation. Amputation with short and long rectangular flaps.
Tears (tērz). The watery secretion of the lacrimal glands.
Tease (tēz). To pull apart for microscopic examination.
Teat (tēt). The pap or nipple of the mammary gland.
Technique (tek-nēk'). The method of procedure and details of any mechanical process or surgical operation.
Tectoceph'alous (tek-to-sef'al-us). See *Scaphocephalous.*
Tecto'rial. Of the nature of a roof or covering.
Tecto'rium. The membrane of Corti.
Teel oil. The oil of sesame seed.
Teeth. The organs of mastication.
Teeth'ing. Cutting of the teeth; dentition.
Teg'men. A covering or shelter. **T. mastoi'deum,** bony cover of the mastoid cells. **T. tym'pani,** bony layer between the tympanum and the cranial cavity.
Tegmen'tal. Of, or pertaining to, the tegmentum. **T. nucleus.** Same as *Red nucleus.* **T. radiation,** fibers diverging from posterior part of internal capsule to the cortex.
Tegmen'tum. Posterior portion of crus cerebri and pons.
Teg'ument (teg'u-ment). The integument or skin.
Tegumen'tal, Tegumen'tary. Pertaining to the tegument.
Teich'mann's crystals. Crystals of hemin.

Teichop'sia (ti-kop'se-ah). A luminous appearance before the eyes, with a zig-zag, wall-like outline.

Teinodyn'ia (ti-no-din'e-ah). Pain in the tendons.

Te'la (te'lah). A web-like tissue. **T. choroi'dea.** Same as *Velum interpositum.*

Telangiecta'sia, Telangiec'tasis. Dilation of capillaries and minute arteries.

Telangio'sis. Any disease of the capillaries.

Teleg'ony. The reproduction in the offspring of one sire of characteristics of a previous sire by whom the mother has produced offspring.

Teleg'raphers' cramp. Painful spasm of the hand and fingers in telegraphers.

Teleneu'ron (tel-e-nu'ron). A nerve-termination.

Telep'athist. A professed mind-reader.

Telep'athy (te-lep'ath-e). The alleged transfer of thought.

Tellu'ric acid. The dibasic acid, H_2TeO_4, forming tellurates.

Tel'lurism. Disease-producing influence of the soil.

Tellu'rium. An element, by some considered metallic: its symbol is Te, and it is used homeopathically.

Teloden'dron (tel-o-den'dron). Terminal arborescence; a form of nerve-ending occurring in the ciliary body.

Telolec'ithal (te-lo-les'ith-al). Having a yolk concentrated at one of the poles.

Telolem'ma. The covering of a motorial end-plate.

Tem'perament. Peculiar physical character and mental cast of an individual.

Tem'perature. Degree of sensible heat or cold. **Absolute t.** is reckoned from the absolute zero of 273° C. **Normal t.,** that of the human body in health, 98.8° F. **T.-sense,** the faculty which appreciates differences in temperature; eryesthesia and thermesthesia.

Tem'ple. Lateral region of the head above the zygoma.

Tem'poral. Pertaining to a temple. **T. bone,** bone at either side and base of skull containing the hearing apparatus. **T. crest,** ridge on the frontal bone which attaches the temporalis muscle. **T. muscle.** See *Muscles, Table of.*

Tempora'lis muscle. See *Muscles, Table of.*

Temporofa'cial nerve. See *Nerves, Table of.*

Temporomax'illary. Situated between the temporal and the lower maxillary bones.

Temporo-occip'ital. Pertaining to the temporal and occipital bones.

Temporosphe'noid. Pertaining to the temporal and sphenoid bones.

Tem'ulence (tem'u-lens). Drunkenness.

Tena'cious (te-na'shus). Adhesive; tough.

Tenac'ulum. A hook-like instrument for seizing and holding parts.

Te'nax. An oakum specially prepared for surgical uses.

Ten'derness. Cutaneous sensitiveness to pain.

Tendini'tis (ten-din-i'tis). Same as *Tenonitis.*

Tendinosu'ture. The suturing of a tendon.

Ten'dinous (ten'din-us). Pertaining to, or made up of, tendons. **T. spot,** a white thickening of a serous membrane due to a deposit of fibrin.

Ten'do (ten'do). L. for *Tendon.* **T. Achil'lis,** the tendon of the soleus and gastrocnemius muscles at the back of the heel.

Ten'don. The fibrous cord by which a muscle is attached. **T.-cells,** peculiar cells occurring in white fibrous tissue. **T.-reflex,** contraction of a muscle caused by percussion of the tendon. **T.-spindle,** an elliptic or fusiform nerve-ending in a tendon.

Ten'doplasty. Plastic surgery of a tendon.
Tendosynovi'tis. Inflammation of a tendon and its sheath.
Tendovag'inal. Of, or pertaining to, a tendon and its sheath.
Tendovagini'tis. Inflammation of a tendon and its sheath.
Tenes'mus. Ineffectual and painful straining at stool or in urinating.
Te'nia (te'ne-ah). See *Tænia.*
Te'niacide. A medicine that destroys tapeworms.
Te'niafuge. A medicine for expelling tapeworms.
Ten'nis-elbow. Lameness of the elbow due to a strain incurred in playing lawn tennis.
Ten'nysin. An alkaloid or leukomain from brain-substance.
Tenodyn'ia. Pain in a tendon.
Tenoni'tis. Inflammation of Tenon's capsule or of a tendon.
Ten'on's capsule. The capsular non-bony socket of the eye. **T.'s space,** a lymph-space between the sclera and Tenon's capsule.
Tenonta'gra. A gouty affection of the tendons.
Tenonti'tis. Inflammation of a tendon.
Tenontog'raphy. The written description of tendons.
Tenontol'ogy. Sum of what is known regarding the tendons.
Ten'ophyte (ten'o-fīt). An osseous growth in a tendon.
Ten'oplasty (ten'op-las-te). Plastic surgery or repair of tendons.
Tenor'rhaphy. The suturation of a cut tendon.
Tenosto'sis. Conversion of a tendon into bone.
Tenosu'ture. The suturing of a cut tendon.
Tenosynovi'tis. The inflammation of a tendon and its sheath.
Ten'otome (ten'ot-ōm). A knife for performing tenotomy.
Tenot'omist. An expert in tenotomy.
Tenot'omy (ten-ot'om-e). The operation of cutting a tendon.
Ten'sion (ten'shun). The condition of being stretched or tense. **T. of gas,** tendency of a gas to expand. **Intra-ocular t.,** pressure of ocular contents on sclera. **T.-suture,** a stitch inserted to reduce the tension on the lips of a wound.
Ten'sor (ten'sor). See *Muscles, Table of.*
Tent. Conical and expansible plug for dilating an orifice. **Laminaria t.,** made of sea-tangle. **Sponge t.,** made of compressed sponge. **Tupelo t.,** made of wood of tupelo.
Tenth nerve. See *Pneumogastric,* in *Nerves, Table of.*
Tenti'go. Morbid or insane lasciviousness.
Tento'rium. A sheet or process of the dura which roofs in the cerebellum.
Tephromyeli'tis. Inflammation of the gray substance of the spinal cord.
Tephro'sis (tef-ro'sis). Incineration or cremation.
Tepida'rium (tep-id-a're-um). A warm bath.
Ter'as (ter'as), pl. *ter'ata.* L. for a *Monster.*
Terat'ic (ter-at'ik). Monstrous; having the characters of a monster.
Ter'atism. 1. Monstrosity. 2. A fetal monster.
Teratogen'esis. The development of monstrosities.
Terato'geny. The development of fetal monsters.
Ter'atoid (ter'at-oid). Like a monster. **T. tumor,** a teratoma.
Teratol'ogy. The science of monstrosities.
Terato'ma. A tumor containing fetal remains.
Teratopho'bia. Morbid dread of monsters; a morbid expectation of giving birth to a teratism.
Terato'sis (ter-at-o'sis). The condition of a monster.
Terchlo'rid. Compound of three atoms of chlorin with one of another element.
Te're (te're). L. for *Rub.*

29

Ter'ebene. A hydrocarbon, $C_{10}H_{16}$, from turpentine oil: antiseptic.
Ter'ebinth. 1. The tree which affords Chian turpentine. 2. Turpentine.
Terebin'thina. See *Turpentine.*
Terebin'thinate. Resembling or containing turpentine.
Terebin'thinize. To charge with turpentine oil or its vapor.
Ter'ebrant pain, Ter'ebrating pain. A boring or piercing pain.
Terebra'tion. The process of boring.
Te'res ma'jor, T. mi'nor. See *Muscles, Table of.*
Ter in die. L. for *Three times a day.*
Term. 1. A limit or boundary. 2. A definite period.
Ter'ma. The lamina terminalis of the cerebrum.
Ter'minal. Forming, or pertaining to, an end.
Ter'nary. Made up of three elements or radicals.
Terox'id (ter-ok'sid). Same as *Trioxid.*
Ter'pene. Any hydrocarbon of the formula, $C_{10}H_{16}$.
Ter'pin hydrate. A crystalline remedy useful in hay-fever.
Ter'ra. L. for *Earth.* **T. al'ba,** white clay; absorbent. **T. Japon'ica,** pale catechu or gambir.
Ter'rol. A proprietary hydrocarbon used like cod-liver oil.
Ter'tian (ter'shan). Recurring every second (third) day. **T. parasite,** a form of malarial hematozoon.
Ter'tiary (ter'she-a-re). Third in order. **T. current,** electric current induced by an induced or secondary current. **T. degeneration,** degeneration of a nerve from long disuse. **T. syphilis,** syphilis in its third stage.
Tertip'ara. A woman who has borne three children.
Tess'ellated. Checkered: marked by little squares. **T. epithelium.** Same as *Pavement epithelium.*
Test. 1. An examination or trial. 2. A chemical reaction or reagent. **T.-card,** a device used in testing for color-blindness or other eye-defect. **T.-meal,** one given for diagnostic purposes in stomach-disease. **T.-paper,** litmus-paper, or other similarly stained paper. **T.-solution,** any standard solution used in testing. **T.-tube,** tube of thin glass closed at one end: used in chemical tests. **T.-types,** letters of various sizes and shapes used in testing visual power.
Tes'ta. Shell; oyster-shell. **T. o'vi,** egg-shell.
Tes'tes (tes'tēz), pl. of *testis.* The testicles.
Testibra'chium. Superior peduncle of cerebellum.
Tes'ticle. One of the two glands which produce semen.
Tes'ticond. Having undescended testicles.
Testic'ular. Pertaining to a testicle. **T. sensation,** the peculiar variety of pain caused by striking the testis. **T. therapy,** therapeutic use of juice or extract prepared from the animal testis.
Testic'ulin. A preparation of the testicle of animals: sometimes administered as a medicine.
Tes'tidin. An alcoholic extract of the testes of cattle.
Tes'tin. A proprietary preparation of the testes of cattle.
Tes'tis. 1. A testicle. 2. Either posterior tubercle of the corpus quadrigeminum.
Testi'tis (tes-ti'tis). Same as *Orchitis.*
Tetan'ic. Pertaining to, or of the nature of, tetanus.
Tetan'iform. Like or resembling tetanus.
Tetanil'la. Same as *Tetany.*
Tet'anin. A poisonous ptomain, $C_{14}H_{20}N_2O_4$, from cultures of tetanus bacillus.
Tetaniza'tion. The induction of tetanic symptoms or conditions.
Tet'anize. To induce tetanoid movements in the organism or in a muscle.

Tet'anoid. Like tetanus; tetaniform. **T. fever.** Same as *Cerebrospinal meningitis.* **T. paraplegia.** See *Spastic paraplegia.*

Tetanomo'tor. Device for the mechanical production of tetanic motor-spasm.

Tetanotox'in. A poisonous ptomain, $C_5H_{11}N$, from cultures of the bacillus of tetanus.

Tet'anus. 1. An acute disease in which there is a state of persistent tonic spasm of voluntary muscle. 2. Continuous tonic spasm of a muscle; steady contraction of a muscle without distinct twitching. **Idiopathic t.,** that which does not follow a lesion. **T. neonato'rum** usually is due to infection of the infant at the umbilicus. **Puerperal t.** occurs in childbed. **Traumatic t.** follows wound-poisoning.

Tet'any. A disease characterized by painful tonic and symmetric spasm of the muscles of the extremities.

Tet'mil. Ten millimeters as a unit of measurement.

Tetrabra'chius. A monster fetus having four arms.

Tetrachei'rus. A monster fetus having four hands.

Tetra'cid. Capable of replacing four atoms of hydrogen in an acid; or having four atoms of hydrogen replaceable by acid radicals.

Tet'rad. 1. An element with a valence or combining power of four. 2. A group of four similar bodies.

Tetrago'num lumba'le. A quadrangle bounded by four lumbar muscles.

Tetrama'zia. Condition of having four mammary glands.

Tetramethylenediam'in. Same as *Putrescin.*

Tetranop'sia. Obliteration of one-fourth of the field of vision.

Tet'rapus (tet'rap-us). Monster fetus having four feet.

Tetras'celus. Monster fetus having four legs.

Tetras'ter. A figure in karyokinesis produced by quadruple division of the nucleus.

Tetrasto'ma. Genus of trematodes found in urine.

Tetratom'ic. 1. Consisting of four atoms. 2. Having four replaceable hydrogen atoms.

Tetrav'alent (te-trav'al-ent). Having a valence of four.

Tet'ronal. A hypnotic material resembling sulphonal.

Tetrox'id. A compound of an element with four oxygen atoms.

Tet'ter. Popular name for various skin-diseases.

Tex'as fever. An infectious cattle-disease due to insect-poisoning.

Text-blindness. Same as *Word-blindness.*

Text'ural. Pertaining to the texture or constitution of tissues.

Thalamenceph'alon. The interbrain; one of the embryonic structures produced from the posterior part of the anterior cerebral vesicle.

Thalam'ic. Pertaining to the thalamus. **T. epilepsy,** sensory epilepsy ascribed to disease of the thalamus.

Thal'amocele, Thal'amocœle (thal'am-o-sēl). The third ventricle.

Thalamocor'tical. Joining the optic thalamus and the cerebral cortex.

Thalamolentic'ular. Between the optic thalamus and the lenticular nucleus.

Thal'amus. A mass of gray matter at the base of the brain projecting into and bounding the third ventricle: it is called also the *Optic thalamus.*

Thalassopho'bia. Morbid dread or fear of the sea.

Thalassother'apy. Treatment of disease by sea-bathing, sea-voyages, or sea-air.

Thal'lin. An antiseptic and antipyretic substance from coal-tar.

Thalliniza'tion. Treatment by frequent doses of thallin.

Thal'lium (thal'le-um). A rare metal; symbol Tl, atomic weight, 203.7: its sulphate is medicinal.
Thanatognomon'ic. Indicating the approach of death.
Than'atoid. Like or resembling death.
Thanatoma'nia. Suicidal mania.
Thanatom'eter. A thermometer used to prove the occurrence of death.
Thanatopho'bia (than-at-o-fo'be-ah). Unfounded apprehension of imminent death.
The'a (the'ah). See *Tea*.
The'aism. Excess in tea-drinking and its consequences.
Theba'in. A poisonous and anodyne alkaloid, $C_{19}H_{21}NO_3$, from opium.
The'baism. Opium-poisoning.
Thebe'sius's foramina. Venous passages opening into the right auricle of the heart. **T.'s veins,** minute cardiac veins.
The'ca. A case or sheath. **T. vertebra'lis,** the membranes or meninges of the spinal cord.
The'cal. Of, or pertaining to, a sheath. **T. abscess,** an abscess of the theca of a tendon.
Theci'tis. Inflammation of the theca of a tendon.
The'in. The alkaloid of tea, $C_8H_{10}N_4O_2$, isomeric with caffein.
The'ism. Tea-drinking in excess and its ill consequences.
Thelal'gia (the-lal'je-ah). Pain in the nipples.
Theli'tis. Inflammation of a nipple.
The'lium (the'le-um). A papilla.
Thel'yblast (thel'e-blast). The feminonucleus.
The'nad. Toward the thenar eminence or toward the palm.
The'nal. Pertaining to the palm.
The'nar (the'nar). The palm of the hand. **T. eminence,** mound on the palm at the root of the thumb. **T. muscles,** flexor and abductor muscles of thumb.
Theobro'ma caca'o. Tropical plant that affords chocolate.
Theobro'min. An alkaloid from *Theobroma*, $C_7H_8N_4O_2$. **T. salicylate,** a serviceable diuretic, more stable and useful than diuretin. **T. sodiosalicylate.** Same as *Diuretin*.
The'oform (the'o-form). An iodoform substitute.
Theoma'nia (the-o-ma'ne-ah). Religious insanity.
Theophyl'lin. Alkaloid from tea, $C_7H_8N_4O_2$, isomeric with theobromin.
Therapeu'tic, Therapeu'tical. Pertaining to therapeutics.
Therapeu'tics. Scientific account of the treatment of disease.
Therapeu'tist. A person expert in therapeutics.
Ther'apol (ther'ap-ol). A proprietary ozonized oil.
Ther'apy (ther'ap-e). The treatment of disease; therapeutics. **Nuclein-t.,** treatment of disease by nucleins from blood-serum and from various glands. **Serum-t.** See *Serotherapy*.
Theri'aca. An antidote; also, a cure for snake-bite.
Therm. Amount of heat needed to raise one gram of water through one degree centigrade.
Ther'mal (ther'mal). Pertaining to heat.
Thermalge'sia. Condition in which the application of heat produces pain.
Thermanesthe'sia. Lack of ability to recognize sensations of heat.
Thermesthe'sia. Ability to recognize heat or cold.
Thermesthesiom'eter. Instrument for measuring sensibility to heat.
Ther'mic. Of, or pertaining to, heat. **T. fever,** sunstroke or insolation.
Ther'min. Tetrahydronaphthylamin, $C_{10}H_{11}NH_2$, a mydriatic.
Thermo-anesthe'sia. Inability to detect heat-variations.

Thermocauterec'tomy. Same as *Igniextirpation.*

Thermocau'tery. Cauterization by a heated wire or point.

Thermochem'istry. Science of the chemical relations of heat.

Ther'modin. A crystalline analgesic and antipyretic.

Thermo-electric'ity. Electricity generated by heat.

Thermogen'esis. The production of heat in organisms.

Thermogenet'ic, Thermogen'ic. Generating animal heat.

Ther'mograph. An instrument for the registration of heat-variations.

Thermohyperalge'sia. Extreme thermalgesia.

Thermohyperesthe'sia. Abnormal sensitiveness to heat.

Thermo-inhib'itory. Retarding the generation of bodily heat.

Thermol'ysis. 1. Dissociation by means of heat. 2. Dissipation of bodily heat by radiation, etc.

Thermom'eter. An instrument for ascertaining temperatures. [See *Table of the Equivalents*, p. 454.] **Air-t.**, one whose expansible material is air. **Alcohol t.**, one whose tube contains alcohol. **Celsius's t.**, the centigrade t. **Centigrade t.**, one with 100° between the melting-point of ice and the boiling-point of water. **Clinical t.**, one for use at the bedside. **Differential t.**, one for measuring very small variations of temperature. **Fahrenheit t.**, one which registers 180° in place of the 100° of the centigrade. **Fever t.**, ordinary clinical t. **Maximum t.** registers the maximum heat to which it has been exposed. **Mercurial t.** has mercury for its expansible column. **Metallic t.** has some metal other than mercury. **Minimum t.** registers the lowest temperature to which it is exposed. **Réaumur's t.** has 80° in place of the 100° of the centigrade scale. **Self-registering t.** records variations of temperature. **Surface t.**, clinical t. for taking temperature of the surface of the body.

Thermom'etry. Ascertainment of temperature by means of the thermometer.

Thermoneuro'sis. Pyrexia of vasomotor origin.

Thermophil'ic. Not able to grow without a high degree of heat.

Ther'mopile. A thermo-electric battery used in measuring small amounts of radiant heat.

Thermople'gia. Heatstroke or sunstroke.

Thermopolypne'a. Quickened breathing due to great heat.

Ther'mostat. A device for regulating the temperature.

Thermosystal'tic. Contracting under the stimulus of heat.

Thermotac'tic, Thermotax'ic. Regulating or controlling the bodily temperature.

Thermotax'is. 1. Normal adjustment of bodily temperature. 2. The attraction of micro-organisms to a warm body.

Thermotherapeu'tics. Same as *Thermotherapy.*

Thermother'apy. Therapeutic use of heat.

The'sis. An essay prepared by a candidate for a degree.

Thiersch's method. A method of skin-grafting.

Thigh (thi'). The portion of leg above knee. **T-bone.** Same as *Femur*. **T.-friction**, a form of masturbation by rubbing the genitals between the thighs.

Thil'anin. A compound of lanolin and sulphur.

Thio-al'cohol. Same as *Mercaptan.*

Thi'oform. Basic bismuth dithiosalicylate: an antiseptic.

Thiogen'ic (thi-o-jen'ik). Able to convert sulphuretted hydrogen into higher sulphur-compounds.

Thi'ol. A substance prepared from coal-tar oil and sulphur: used in skin-diseases.

Thiolin'ic acid. A substance derived from linseed oil and sulphur: used in skin-diseases.

Thi'onin hydrochlorate. Lanthic violet, a purple dye.

TABLE OF EQUIVALENTS OF CENTIGRADE AND FAHRENHEIT THERMOMETRIC SCALES.

Cent.	Fahr.	Cent.	Fahr.	Cent.	Fahr.
°	°	°	°	°	°
-40	-40.0	9	48.2	57	134.6
-39	-38.2	10	50.0	58	136.4
-38	-36.4	11	51.8	59	138.2
-37	-34.6	12	53.6	60	140.0
-36	-32.8	13	55.4	61	141.8
-35	-31.0	14	57.2	62	143.6
-34	-29.2	15	59.0	63	145.4
-33	-27.4	16	60.8	64	147.2
-32	-25.6	17	62.6	65	149.0
-31	-23.8	18	64.4	66	150.8
-30	-22.0	19	66.2	67	152.6
-29	-20.2	20	68.0	68	154.4
-28	-18.4	21	69.8	69	156.2
-27	-16.6	22	71.6	70	158.0
-26	-14.8	23	73.4	71	159.8
-25	-13.0	24	75.2	72	161.6
-24	-11.2	25	77.0	73	163.4
-23	-9.4	26	78.8	74	165.2
-22	-7.6	27	80.6	75	167.0
-21	-5.8	28	82.4	76	168.8
-20	-4.0	29	84.2	77	170.6
-19	-2.2	30	86.0	78	172.4
-18	-0.4	31	87.8	79	174.2
-17	+1.4	32	89.6	80	176.0
-16	3.2	33	91.4	81	177.8
-15	5.0	34	93.2	82	179.6
-14	6.8	35	95.0	83	181.4
-13	8.6	36	96.8	84	183.2
-12	10.4	37	98.6	85	185.0
-11	12.2	38	100.4	86	186.8
-10	14.0	39	102.2	87	188.6
-9	15.8	40	104.0	88	190.4
-8	17.6	41	105.8	89	192.2
-7	19.4	42	107.6	90	194.0
-6	21.2	43	109.4	91	195.8
-5	23.0	44	111.2	92	197.6
-4	24.8	45	113.0	93	199.4
-3	26.6	46	114.8	94	201.2
-2	28.4	47	116.6	95	203.0
-1	30.2	48	118.4	96	204.8
0	32.0	49	120.2	97	206.6
+1	33.8	50	122.0	98	208.4
2	35.6	51	123.8	99	210.2
3	37.4	52	125.6	100	212.0
4	39.2	53	127.4	101	213.8
5	41.0	54	129.2	102	215.6
6	42.8	55	131.0	103	217.4
7	44.6	56	132.8	104	219.2
8	46.4				

Thionu'ric acid. A compound derivable from uric acid.

Thi'ophene. A liquid, C_4H_4S, from benzene: its compounds have a limited therapeutic use.

Thioresor'cin. Phenylbisulphydrate, $C_6H_4(SH_2)_2$: used like iodoform.

Thiosa'pol. A soap in which sulphur forms an important ingredient.

Thiosinnam'in. A substance, $C_4H_8N_2S$, from oil of mustard and ammonia.

Thiou'rea. Urea with its oxygen replaced by sulphur, $CS(NH_2)_2$; sulfocarbamide.

Third pair. See *Motor oculi*, in *Nerves, Table of.* **T. ventricle,** space between the thalami representing the cavity of the fore-brain.

Thirst. Desire for drink, especially for water.

Thi'ry's fistula. An artificial opening into the intestines for the purpose of staining intestinal juice.

Thi'uret. Crystalline powder, $C_8H_7N_3S_2$: its salts are antiseptic.

Thlipsenceph'alus. Fetal monster with a defective skull.

Tho'ko. A skin-disease endemic in Fiji.

Thoma-Zeiss. An instrument for counting the red and white corpuscles of the blood.

Thom'sen's disease. See *Myotonia congenita.*

Thomso'nianism. An empiric system recognizing only vegetable medicines.

Thoracente'sis. Surgical puncture or tapping of the chest-wall.

Thorac'ic. Of, or pertaining to, the chest. **T. cage,** the musculature of the chest. **T. duct,** principal duct for the lymph and chyle. **T. girdle,** the girdle formed by the scapulæ and clavicles. **T. limbs,** upper limbs; arms and hands.

Thoracocente'sis (tho-rak-o-sen-te'sis). Same as *Thoracentesis.*

Thoracocyllo'sis (tho-rak-o-sil-o'sis). Deformity of the thorax.

Thoracodid'ymus. Double monster united at the thorax.

Thoracodyn'ia (tho-rak-o-din'e-ah). Pain in the thorax.

Thoracogastros'chisis. Fissure of the abdomen and thorax.

Thoracom'eter (tho-rak-om'et-er). Same as *Stethometer.*

Thoracomyodyn'ia. Pain in the muscles of the chest.

Thoracop'agus. Same as *Thoracodidymus.*

Thorac'oplasty. Plastic surgery of the thorax.

Thoracos'chisis. Fissure of chest-wall.

Tho'racoscope (tho'rak-o-skōp). A stethoscope.

Thoracos'copy. Diagnostic examination of the chest.

Thoracosteno'sis. Abnormal contraction of the thorax; wasp-waist.

Thoracot'omy. Surgical incision of the chest.

Thoradel'phus. Twin fetus joined above the navel.

Tho'rax. The chest; part of body between neck and abdomen.

Tho'rium. A rare gray metal.

Thorn-apple. A plant. See *Stramonium.*

Thorn'waldt's disease. Purulent inflammation of Luschka's tonsil.

Thor'oughwart. See *Eupatorium perfoliatum.*

Thread-worm. Same as *Oxyuris.*

Three-day fever. See *Dengue.*

Threpsol'ogy (threp-sol'o-je). Scientific view of nutrition.

Thresh'old. That degree of stimulus that just produces a sensation. **Auditory t.,** the minimum audible or slightest perceptible sound. **T. of visual sensation,** the minimum visible or slightest possible vision of any object.

Thrida'cium. Same as *Lactucarium.*

Thrill. Tremor perceived in auscultation or palpation.

Throat. 1. Pharynx. 2. Fauces. 3. Anterior part of neck.

Throb. A pulsating movement or sensation.
Throe (thro). A severe pain.
Throm'bin. Same as *Fibrinogen.*
Thrombo-arteri'tis. Thrombosis conjoined with arteritis.
Thrombocys'tis. The sac which sometimes forms around a clot or thrombus.
Throm'boid. Like or resembling a thrombus.
Thrombolymphangi'tis. Inflammation of a lymph-vessel due to a thrombus.
Thrombophlebi'tis. Thrombosis conjoined with phlebitis. **T. purulen'ta,** purulent softening of a venous plug with infiltration of the vessel-wall.
Throm'bosed. Affected with thrombosis.
Thrombo'sin. A substance derived from the splitting up of fibrinogen under the influence of the nucleoproteids of broken-down leukocytes.
Thrombo'sis. The formation of a thrombus.
Thrombot'ic. Pertaining to, or affected with, thrombosis.
Throm'bus. A plug in a vessel found at the point of its formation. **Ball-t.,** a rounded antemortem clot in the heart. **Milk-t.,** mammary tumor due to an accumulation of curdled milk.
Through-illumina'tion. See *Transillumination.*
Thrush. Disease of infants with aphthous spots in the mouth.
Thryp'sis. A comminuted fracture.
Thu'ja occidenta'lis. The arbor vitæ or white cedar with medicinal oil and leaves.
Thu'lium. A rare metallic element.
Thumb. The radial or first digit or dactyl of the hand.
Thus. Olibanum or frankincense.
Thylaci'tis. Inflammation of the oil-glands of the skin.
Thymace'tin. A thymol derivative, $C_{14}H_{20}NO_2$: antineuralgic.
Thyme. The plant *Thymus vulgaris:* aromatic and antiseptic.
Thymeleo'sis. Ulceration of the thymus gland.
Thy'mic. Pertaining to the thymus. **T. acid.** Same as *Thymol.* **T. asthma.** Same as *Laryngismus stridulus.*
Thym'ion (thim'e-on). A small cutaneous wart.
Thymi'tis. Inflammation of the thymus gland.
Thy'mol. A stearopten, $C_{10}H_{14}O$, from the oils of thyme and horsemint; it is antiseptic.
Thymop'athy. Any disease of the thymus gland.
Thy'mus. Two-lobed closed gland in the neck of children.
Thy'raden. Thyreoid extract, used therapeutically.
Thyreo-antitox'in. A thyreoid preparation, theoretically $C_6H_{11}N_3O_5$, said to have all the curative properties of the thyreoid extract.
Thyreo-aryte'noid. Pertaining to the thyreoid and arytenoid cartilages. See also *Muscles, Table of.*
Thy'reocele (thi're-o-sēl). Same as *Goiter.*
Thyreo-epiglot'tic. Pertaining to thyreoid and epiglottis.
Thyreo-epiglottid'eus. See *Muscles, Table of.*
Thyreoglan'din. A preparation of thyreoid gland, said to be extremely effective.
Thyreoglos'sal duct. A channel in the fetus between the thyreoid gland and tongue.
Thyreohy'al. A fetal bone which becomes one of the major cornua of the hyoid.
Thyreohy'oid. Pertaining to the thyreoid cartilage and the hyoid bone. **T. muscle.** See *Muscles, Table of.*
Thyreoid, T. body, T. gland. A large ductless gland in front of the trachea. **T. cachexia.** See *Exophthalmic goiter.* **T. cartilage,** the shield-shaped cartilage of the larynx. **T. der'-moid,** a congenital sacrococcygeal tumor probably a relic of the

post-anal gut. **T. extract,** a preparation of sheep's thyreoid, used therapeutically. **T. treatment,** the therapeutic use of thyreoid extract.

Thyreoidec'tomy. Surgical removal of the thyreoid.

Thyreoi'din. 1. A proprietary extract of the thyreoid gland of an animal. 2. An alleged essential secretion of the thyreoid.

Thy'reoidism. 1. Poisoning, or injury, from using thyreoid extract. 2. The ill-effect of removal of the thyreoid.

Thyreoidi'tis. Inflammation of the thyreoid gland.

Thyreoidiza'tion. Treatment by the thyreoid extract.

Thyreoidot'omy. Surgical incision of the thyreoid gland.

Thyreoi'odin. Same as *Iodothyrin.*

Thyreon'cus (thi-re-ong'kus). See *Thyreocele.*

Thyreopri'val. Due to suspension of the function or to the removal of the thyreoid gland.

Thyreopro'teid. 1. A proteid derived from the thyreoid gland: used therapeutically. 2. The substance whose excess is supposed to cause myxedema.

Thyreopro'tein. A protein from the thyreoid gland.

Thyreot'omy. Surgical division of a thyreoid cartilage.

Thyro-. For words beginning thus, see those beginning *Thyreo-.*

Thy'roid (thi'roid). See *Thyreoid.*

Tib'ia. The larger and inner bone of the leg below the knee.

Tib'ial (tib'e-al). Of, or pertaining to, the tibia.

Tibia'lis (tib-e-a'lis). See *Muscles, Table of.*

Tibiofem'oral. Pertaining to the tibia and femur.

Tibiofib'ular. Pertaining to the tibia and fibula.

Tibiotar'sal. Pertaining to the tibia and tarsus.

Tic. A twitching, as of the face. **Convulsive t.,** spasm of the facial muscles. **T. douloureux** (doo-loo-ro'), a spasmodic facial neuralgia.

Tick'ling. Light stimulation of a sensitive surface and its reflex effect, such as involuntary laughter, etc.

T. i. d. Abbreviation for L. *ter in die*, three times a day.

Ti'dal-air. See under *Air.* **T.-wave,** sphygmographic wave next after the percussion-wave.

Tig'lium. See *Croton oil.*

Tigre'tier. A dancing mania endemic in Tigre, Abyssinia.

Til'mus. The pulling out of the hair.

Tim'bre. Musical quality of a tone or sound.

Tin. A white metal, some of whose salts are reagents, others stains; symbol Sn.

Tinctu'ra. L. for *Tincture.*

Tinc'ture. A medicinal solution, usually less strong than a fluid extract. **Ammoniated t.,** a t. made with ammoniated alcohol. **Ethereal t.,** a t. made with ether.

Tin'ea. Ringworm, or other similar microphytic skin-disease. **T. amianta'cea.** See *Seborrhagia.* **T. decal'vans.** See *Alopecia areata.* **T. furfura'cea,** a dry scaly seborrhea. **T. imbrica'ta,** an aggravated form of *T. tricophytina.* **T. syco'sis,** sycosis or barber's itch. **T. tar'si,** ulcerous blepharitis. **T. ton'surans,** ringworm of the scalp. **T. tricophyti'na,** ringworm, a contagious disease of the skin. **T. versic'olor,** a contagious skin-disease caused by *Microsporon furfur.*

Tin'gible (tinj'ib-l). Stainable.

Tinni'tus au'rium. A ringing in the ears. **Telephone t.,** tinnitus due to use of the telephone.

Tipu'lidæ (tip-u'lid-e). Gnats; insects provided with a stinging and sucking apparatus.

Tire (tīr). Exhaustion due to over-exercise.

Tirefond (tĕr-faw'). Instrument like a corkscrew for raising depressed portions of bone.

Tisane (te-zahn'). Same as *Ptisan*.

Tis'ic. Same as *Phthisic*.

Tis'sue (tis'u). An aggregation of fibers and cells composing a structural element. **Adenoid t.,** connective t. with meshes which lodge lymphoid cells. **Adipose t.,** connective t. made of fat-cells in meshwork of areolar tissue. **Areolar t.,** connective t. made up largely of interlacing fibers. **Bony t.** Same as *Bone*. **Cancellous t.,** the spongy tissue of bone. **Cartilaginous t.** Same as *Cartilage*. **Connective t.,** general name for stromatous or non-parenchymatous tissues. **Elastic t.,** connective t. made up of yellow elastic fibers. **Embryonal t.,** connective tissue in its primitive state. **Endothelial t.,** peculiar connective t. which lines serous and lymphoid spaces. **Epithelial t.,** a general name for tissues not derived from the mesoblast. **Erectile t.,** spongy t. that becomes expanded and hard when filled with blood. **Fibrous t.,** the common connective tissue of the body, composed of yellow or white parallel fibers. **Gelatinous t.,** mucous tissue. **Glandular t.,** a specialized form of epithelial t. **Granulation t.,** new tissue formed in the process of granulation and ultimately forming the cicatrix. **Interstitial t.,** the connective tissue between the cellular elements of a structure. **Intertubular t.,** dense tissue of dentin in which dentinal tubes are embedded. **Lymphoid t.** Same as *Adenoid t.* **Mucous t.,** a tissue which represents the embryonic connective tissue. **Muscular t.** See *Muscle*. **Nervous t.** See *Nerve*. **Osseous t.** See *Bone*. **Retiform t.,** adenoid tissue.

Tita'nium. A metallic element: symbol Ti.

Titilla'tion. The act or sensation of tickling.

Titra'tion. Volumetric analysis by means of solutions of standard strength.

Tituba'tion. A stumbling or staggering gait.

Tl. Symbol of *thallium*.

Tn. Symbol of *normal intra-ocular tension*.

Toad'head. A form of nearly aborted head in certain so-called acephalous fetuses.

Tobac'co. The prepared leaves of *Nicotianum taba'cum*: antispasmodic and heart-depressant. **T.-heart,** cardiac disturbance from excessive use of tobacco.

Tobac'coism. Ill-health due to excessive use of tobacco.

Tocodynamom'eter. Instrument for measuring expulsive force of uterine contractions in childbirth.

Tocog'ony (to-kog'o-ne). Parental generation.

Tocol'ogy. Science of reproduction and art of obstetrics.

Tocom'eter (to-kom'et-er). Same as *Tocodynamometer*.

To'cus. Parturition; childbirth.

Toe. A digit or dactyl of the foot. **T.-clonus,** flexion of the great toe in response to the sudden passive extension of its first phalanx. **T.-reflex.** See under *Reflex*.

Toi'let. The cleansing and dressing of an operation wound.

To'kelau ringworm. See *Tinea imbricata*.

Toko-. For words beginning thus, see those beginning *Toco-*.

Tol'erance. Ability to endure the continued use of a drug.

To'lu (to'loo). See under *Balsam*.

Tol'uene (tol-u-ēn). The hydrocarbon C_7H_8; methyl-benzene.

Tolu'ric acid. A crystalline acid sometimes discoverable in urine after the administration of toluic acid.

Tolypy'rin. An antipyretic principle, $C_{12}H_{14}N_2O$; methyl-antipyrin. **T. salicylate.** See *Tolysal*.

Toly'sal. Tolypirin salicylate: useful in rheumatism.

Tomen'tum cer'ebri. Network of minute blood-vessels of the pia and cortex cerebri.

Tomes's fibers (tōmz'ez). Branched processes of odontoblasts which fill the dentinal tubules.

Tomoma'nia. 1. A craze for performing needless surgical operations. 2. Hysteric desire to be operated upon surgically.

Tomoto'cia. Cesarean section.

Tone. Normal degree of vigor and tension. **T.-deafness.** Same as *Amusia, sensory.*

Ton'ga. A mixture of medicinal barks from Fiji: used in neuralgia.

Ton'galine. A proprietary anodyne medicine.

Tongue (tung). A movable muscular organ on the floor of the mouth. **Black t.,** glossophytia; condition in which dorsum of tongue has a dark coat. **T.-depressor,** spatula for pushing down the tongue. **Fern-leaf-pattern t.,** a t. with central furrow and lateral branches. **Filmy t.,** one with symmetric whitish patches. **Furred t.,** coated t. with furred papillæ, giving the mucous membrane the appearance of whitish fur. **Geographic t.** has denuded patches surrounded by thickened epithelium. **Hairy t.,** tongue whose papillæ have a hair-like appearance. **Parrot t.,** dry horny t. of low fevers, which cannot be protruded. **Strawberry t.,** tongue with enlarged red fungiform papillæ. **T.-tie,** congenital shortness of frenum, interfering with its mobility. **Wooden t.,** one affected with actinomycosis.

Ton'ic. 1. Producing and restoring normal tone. 2. Characterized by continuous tension. 3. An agent which tends to restore normal tone. **Cardiac t.,** one which strengthens the heart's action. **General t.,** one which braces up the whole system. **Hematic t.,** one that improves the blood. **Intestinal t.** gives tone to intestinal tract. **Nervine t.** improves the tone of nervous system. **T. spasm.** See under *Spasm.* **Stomachic t.** aids stomachic functions. **Vascular t.,** one which improves the tone of blood-vessels.

Tonic'ity (to-nis'it-e). Normal condition of tone or tension.

Tonk'a bean. The seed of *Dipteryx odorata:* it affords coumarin.

Ton'ograph. A recording tonometer.

Tonom'eter. An instrument to measure tension.

Ton'ophant. An instrument for rendering acoustic vibrations visible.

Ton'oplast (ton'o-plast). A small intracellular body.

Ton'oscope (ton'o-skōp). A device for examining the head or brain by means of sound.

Ton'quinol. White crystalline substance, $C_{11}H_{13}N_3O_6$, used as a substitute for musk.

Ton'sil. 1. A small almond-shaped mass between the pillars of the fauces on either side. 2. A lobe on either side of lower surface of the cerebellum. **Lingual t.,** lymphadenoid mass at base of tongue. **Luschka's t, Pharyngeal t.** See *Luschka's tonsil.* **Third t.,** Luschka's tonsil.

Ton'sillar. Of, or pertaining to, a tonsil.

Tonsilli'tis. Inflammation of a tonsil. **Follicular t.** especially affects the follicles. **Herpetic t.,** a local manifestation of herpes on the tonsil. **Mycotic t.,** a form due to fungi. **Pustular t.** is characterized by formation of pustules. **Suppurative t.** Same as *Quinsy.*

Tonsil'lolith. A concretion or calculus in a tonsil.

Tonsil'lotome. An instrument for cutting off a tonsil.

Tonsillot'omy. Surgical removal of a tonsil.

To'nus (to'nus). Tone or tonicity.

Toot'-poison. A poison from *Conaria sarmentosa* of New Zealand.

Tooth. One of a set of small bone-like structures of the jaws for masti-

eating food. **Deciduous t., Milk-t., Temporary t.,** a tooth of the first dentition. **Permanent t.,** a tooth of the second dentition. See *Bicuspid, Canine, Eye, Hutchinson, Incisor, Molar, Stomach,* and *Wisdom t.* **T.-rash.** See *Strophulus.*

Tooth-ache. Pain in a tooth; odontalgia.

Topesthe'sia. Determination of locality by touch.

Topha'ceous (to-fa'se-us). Of a gritty or sandy nature.

To'phus (to'fus). 1. Same as *Chalk-stone.* 2. Tartar or salivary calculus. **T. syphilit'icus,** a syphilitic node.

Top'ical. Pertaining to a particular spot; local.

Topoal'gia (to-po-al'je-ah). Fixed or localized pain.

Topograph'ic. Describing special regions.

Topog'raphy (to-pog'raf-e). A special description of a part or region.

Toponeuro'sis. Neurosis of a limited region.

Topopho'bia. Morbid dread of particular spots.

Tor'cular Heroph'ili. A depression in the occipital bone at the confluence of a number of venous sinuses.

Tor'men, pl. *tor'mina.* A severe griping or colicky pain.

Tormen'til. The plant *Potentilla tormentilla:* an astringent.

Torn'waldt's disease. See *Thornwaldt's disease.*

Tor'pent. An agent which modifies irritative motions.

Tor'pid (tor'pid). Not acting with vigor.

Torpid'ity. Sluggishness; inactivity; slowness.

Tor'por ret'inæ. Slackened or dulled response of retina to the stimulus of light.

Torrefac'tion (tor-e-fak'shun). The act of roasting or parching.

Tor'refy. To parch, roast, or dry by aid of heat.

Tor'sion. Act of twisting; state of being twisted.

Torsoclu'sion. Acupressure combined with torsion of the bleeding vessel.

Torticol'lis. Wry-neck; a contracted state of cervical muscles, with torsion of the neck. **Fixed t.,** unnatural position of head due to actual and persistent organic muscular shortening. **Rheumatic t.** is due to rheumatism. **Spasmodic t.** is due to spasm of certain neck-muscles.

Tor'ula. Genus of micro-organisms including the yeast-plant.

To'tal aphasia. See under *Aphasia.*

Touch (tutsh). 1. The sense by which contact gives evidence as to their qualities; tactile sense. 2. Palpation with the finger.

Tour de maître (toor deh mâtr). A method of passing a catheter or sound.

Tourette's disease (too-rets'). Convulsive tic, with coprolalia, echolalia, and loss of co-ordination of movements.

Tour'niquet (toor'ne-ket). Instrument for the compression of blood-vessels. Tourniquets are of various kinds, named from the inventors, as *Dupuytren's, Esmarch's, Skey's,* or *Signorini's.* **Field-t.,** padded strap to be buckled on so as to compress the artery. **Horseshoe-t.,** one shaped like a horseshoe, to press at two points. **Provisional t.,** one loosely applied, to be tightened when occasion may require.

Tow. The coarser parts or fibers of flax.

Towelette. A small towel for surgeon's or obstetrician's use.

Tow'elling. Friction with a towel.

Toxalbu'min. Any poisonous albumin, whether of bacterial or other origin.

Toxal'bumose (tok-sal'bu-mōs). A poisonous albumose.

Toxane'mia. Anemia due to a poison.

Toxe'mia. Blood-poisoning; poisoning by toxins produced in the body-cells or by the influence of micro-organisms.

Toxen'zyme (tok-sen'zim). Any poisonous enzyme.

Tox'ic, Tox'ical. Of, pertaining to, or due to, poisoning.

Tox'icant. 1. Poisonous. 2. A poison.
Toxic'ity (tok-sis'it-e). The quality of being poisonous.
Toxicoden'drol. A poisonous, non-volatile oil found in *Rhus toxicodendron.*
Toxicoden'dron (tok-sik-o-den'dron). See under *Rhus.*
Toxicoder'ma. Any skin-disease due to a poison.
Toxicogen'ic (tok-sik-o-jen'ik). Giving origin to poisons.
Toxicohe'mia (tok-sik-o-he'me-ah). Same as *Toxemia.*
Tox'icoid (tok'sik-oid). Resembling a poison.
Toxicol'ogy. The science or study of poisons.
Toxicoma'nia. 1. Intense desire for poisons or intoxicants. 2. Same as *Toxiphobia.*
Toxicomu'cin. A poisonous substance derived from the tubercle-bacillus.
Toxicopath'ic (tok-sik-o-path'ik). Pertaining to toxicopathy.
Toxicop'athy (tok-sik-op'ath-e). Any disease induced by a poison.
Toxicophid'ia (tok-sik-o-fid'e-ah). Venomous serpents collectively.
Toxicopho'bia. Morbid dread of poisons.
Toxicophylax'in. Any phylaxin which destroys the poisons produced by micro-organisms.
Toxico'sis. A diseased condition due to poisoning.
Toxidermi'tis. Any skin-disease due to skin-poisoning.
Toxif'erous (toks-if'er-us). Conveying or producing a poison.
Tox'in. Any poisonous albumin or base of bacterial origin.
Toxine'mia. Blood-intoxication.
Toxinfec'tion (tok-sin-fek'shun). Infection of system by toxins or other poisonous agents.
Toxin'icide (tok-sin'is-id). Agent destructive to toxins.
Toxipho'bia. Insane or morbid fear of being poisoned.
Toxomu'cin (tok-so-mu'sin). See *Toxicomucin.*
Toxopep'tone (tok-so-pep'tōn). A poisonous peptone.
Toxophylax'in (tok-so-fi-lak'sin). See *Toxicophylaxin.*
Toxoso'zin. Any sozin which destroys the poisons produced by micro-organisms.
Tra'bal. Pertaining to the trabs cerebri.
Trabec'ula. A septum which extends from an envelop into the enclosed substance.
Trabs cer'ebri. Same as *Callosum.*
Tra'chea (tra'ke-ah). The tube descending from the larynx to the bronchi; windpipe.
Tra'cheal. Of, or pertaining to, the trachea. **T. tugging,** pulling sensation of the trachea due to aneurysm of arch of the aorta.
Trachea'lis. System of transverse muscle-fibers in the trachea.
Trachei'tis. Inflammation of the trachea.
Trachelag'ra (tra-kel-ag'rah). Gout in the neck.
Trachelectom'opexy. Fixation and excision of the neck of the uterus.
Trachelemato'ma. A hematoma seated on the sternomastoid muscle.
Trachelis'mus. Spasm of the neck-muscles.
Tracheli'tis (tra-kel-i'tis). Same as *Cervicitis.*
Trachelobregmat'ic diameter. One from the center of the bregma to the anterior point of the foramen magnum.
Trachelol'ogy. The study of the neck and its diseases and injuries.
Trachelomas'toid. See *Muscles, Table of.*
Trach'elopexy (trak'el-o-pek-se). Fixation of the neck of the uterus to some other part.
Trach'eloplasty. Plastic surgery of the uterine neck.
Trachelor'rhaphy. Suturation of a lacerated cervix uteri.

Trachelot'omy. The operation of cutting the neck of the uterus.

Tracheo-a'ërocele. Tracheal hernia containing air.

Tra'cheocele (tra'ke-o-sēl). 1. Hernial protrusion of tracheal mucous membrane. 2. Goiter.

Tracheo-esopha'geal (tra-ke-o-e-so-fa'je-al). Pertaining to the trachea and esophagus.

Tracheolaryngot'omy. Incision of the larynx and trachea.

Tracheos'copy (tra-ke-os'ko-pe). Inspection of interior of trachea.

Tracheosteno'sis (tra-ke-o-ste-no'sis). Contraction or narrowing of the trachea.

Tra'cheotome (tra'ke-o-tōm). Instrument for incising the trachea.

Tracheot'omy (tra-ke-ot'om-e). The formation of an artificial opening into the trachea. **Inferior t.** is performed below, and **Superior t.** above, the isthmus of the thyroid. **T.-tube,** tube to be inserted into the opening made in tracheotomy.

Trachi'tis (tra-ki'tis). Inflammation of the trachea.

Tracho'ma (tra-ko'mah). Contagious granular conjunctivitis. **T. defor'mans,** vulvitis with cicatricial deformity.

Trachypho'nia. Roughness of the voice.

Tract (trakt). A region, especially one of some length, principally in the nervous system. **Alimentary t., Digestive t.,** the alimentary canal, or passage from the mouth to the anus. **Direct cerebellar t.,** an ascending tract of fibers at the periphery of the posterior portion of the lateral column of the cord. **Genito-urinary t.,** the genito-urinary organs in continuity. **Habenular t.,** tract of fibers passing from the habenula to the mesial side of the red nucleus. **Intermediolateral t.,** tract of nerve-fibers in lateral column of spinal cord, midway between anterior and posterior gray horns. **Motor t.,** the path of a motor impulse from the brain to a muscle. **Olfactory t.,** the narrow portion of the olfactory lobe of the brain. **Ophthalmic t., Optic t.,** fibers between the visual centers and the optic chiasm. **Pyramidal t.,** the continuation in the spinal cord of the ventral pyramids of the oblongata. **Respiratory t.,** the respiratory organs in continuity. **Sensory t.,** tract of fibers conducting sensation to the brain.

Tractel'lum. An anterior locomotive flagellum.

Trac'tion (trak'shun). The act of drawing or pulling. **Aneurysm-t.,** aneurysm of aorta due to imperfect atrophy of ductus Botalli. **Axis-t.,** traction along an axis, as of the pelvis in obstetrics. **T.-diverticulum,** a sacculation of esophagus due to traction of adhesions. **Elastic t.,** traction by an elastic force, or by means of an elastic appliance.

Trac'tus (trak'tus). *L.* for *Tract.* **T. spira'lis foraminulen'tus,** the maculosa cribrosa quarta.

Trag'acanth (trag'ak-anth). A gum from species of *Astragalus*: much used in pharmacy.

Tra'gal (tra'gal). Pertaining to the tragus.

Trag'icus (traj'ik-us). See *Muscles, Table of.*

Tra'gus (tra'gus). Cartilaginous projection before the external meatus of the ear.

Trance. A profound or abnormal sleep. **T.-coma,** hypnotic lethargy.

Transec'tion. A section made across a bony axis.

Trans'fer, Trans'ference. The passage of a symptom or affection from one part to another; a kind of metastasis.

Transfix'. To pierce through or impale.

Transfix'ion. A cutting through, as in amputation.

Transfora'tion. The perforation or piercing of the fetal skull.

Trans'forator. Instrument for making a transforation.

Transforma'tion. Change of form or structure; degeneration.

Transfu'sion. Transfer of blood from one person to another: the introduction of blood or other fluid into the circulation. **Arterial t.,** transfer of blood into an artery. **Direct t., Immediate t.,** transfer of blood from one person to another without exposure to the air. **Indirect t., Mediate t.,** the transfer of blood from a cup to a blood-vessel. **Venous t.,** transfer of blood to a vein.

Tran'sic. Pertaining to a state of trance.

Transil'iac. Across or between the two ilia.

Transillumina'tion. The inspection of the interior of a cavity by means of a strong light made to pass through its walls: the inside of bodily cavities may also be made visible by means of the Röntgen rays.

Transit'ional zone. The posterior part of the lens-sac during the stage of growth.

Transla'tion. A removal, or change of place.

Translu'cent. Somewhat transparent; diaphanous.

Transmigra'tion. 1. Diapedesis. 2. Change of place from one side of the body to the other. **External t.,** passage of an ovum from one ovary to the other tube without going through its adjacent oviduct. **Internal t.,** the passage of an ovum from one ovary to the uterus through its own oviduct.

Transmis'sion (trans-mish'un). The transfer, as of a disease.

Trans'pirable. Permitting the passage of perspiration.

Transpira'tion. Discharge of air, vapor, or sweat through the skin.

Transplanta'tion. The grafting of tissues taken from the same body or from another.

Transposi'tion. Displacement of viscera to the opposite side.

Tran'sudate. A substance which has passed through a membrane.

Transuda'tion. Passage of serum or other fluid through a membrane.

Transversa'lis (trans-ver-sa'lis). See *Muscles, Table of.*

Transverse (trans-vers'). Extending from side to side, or crosswise.

Transversec'tomy. Excision of a vertebral transverse process.

Transversospina'lis. Series of muscles forming deeper layer of extensor dorsi communis muscle.

Transver'sus. See *Muscles, Table of.*

Trape'zium. 1. The first carpal bone in the distal row. 2. A transverse band of fibers in lower part of the pons.

Trape'zius (tra-pe'ze-us). See *Muscles, Table of.*

Trap'ezoid. The second carpal bone in the distal row.

Trapp's formula. To find the number of grains of solids in 1000 c.c. of urine, multiply the last two figures of the specific gravity by two (Trapp's co-efficient), or by 2.33, according to others.

Trau'be's curves. Long curves in a sphygmogram, made by holding the breath.

Trau'ma (traw'mah). A wound or injury.

Traumat'ic (traw-mat'ik). Of, pertaining to, or caused by, an injury.

Traumat'icin. Gutta-percha dissolved in chloroform (10 per cent.), and used like collodion.

Trau'matism. Condition of system resulting from an injury or wound.

Trau'matol (traw'mat-ol). Same as *Iodocresol.*

Traumatol'ogy (traw-mat-ol'o-je). The science of wounds.

Traumatopne'a, Traumatopnœ'a. Condition in which air passes in and out of a wound in the chest-wall.

Treat'ment. The management and care of a patient or the combatting of his disorder. **Active t.**, treatment directed immediately to a disease. **Expectant t.** See *Expectant.*

Trefu'sia. Red powder prepared from defibrinated blood, and used in chlorosis.

Tre'halose. A sugar, $C_{12}H_{22}O_{11}$, from manna or ergot.

Trem'atode. Any parasitic worm of the class trematoda; a fluke.

Trem'bles. Milk-sickness in cattle.

Tre'mor. An involuntary trembling or quivering. **Arsenical t.**, tremor resulting from arsenical poisoning. **Continuous t.**, a tremor resembling that of paralysis agitans. **Fibrillary t.** See *Fibrillation.* **Forced t.**, movements persisting after voluntary motion, due to intermittent irritation of the nerve-centers. **Intention-t.**, tremor on attempting voluntary motion. **Volitional t.**, trembling of entire body during voluntary effort: seen in multiple sclerosis.

Trem'ulous (trem'u-lus). Trembling or quivering.

Tren'delenburg's position. The patient on the back, body and thighs elevated to about 45 degrees, the legs hanging over the edge of a table.

Trepan'. An obsolete form of the trephine.

Trepana'tion, Trephina'tion. The use of the trephine.

Trephine (tre-fin'). 1. A crown-saw for removing a circular disk or button of bone, chiefly from the skull. 2. To operate on with the trephine.

Trepida'tion. 1. A trembling or oscillatory movement. 2. Nervous anxiety and fear.

Triac'etin (tri-as'et-in). An oily liquid, $C_3H_5(C_2H_3O_2)_3$, from cod-liver oil, fats, etc.

Tri'acid. Having three atoms of hydrogen replaceable by a base.

Tri'ad. 1. Any trivalent element. 2. Trivalent.

Triakaidekapho'bia (tri-ak-i-dek-af-o'be-ah). Morbid fear of the number thirteen.

Tri'al-case. A box or frame with duly arranged trial-lenses. **T.-frame**, a device used in testing for color-blindness. **T.-lenses**, sets of lenses used in testing vision.

Triallylam'in. An oily volatile base, $(C_3H_5)_3N$.

Tri'angle. A three-cornered area or figure. **Bryant's t.**, the iliofemoral t. **Carotid t., inferior, T. of necessity**, between median line of neck in front, the sternomastoid, and anterior belly of omohyoid. **Carotid t., superior, T. of election**, has anterior belly of omohyoid in front, posterior belly of digastric above, and sternomastoid behind. **Cephalic t.**, on anteroposterior plane of skull, between lines from occiput to forehead and to chin, and from chin to forehead. **Digastric t.**, the submaxillary t. **T. of elbow**, in front, the supinator longus on the outside and pronator teres inside, the base toward humerus. **Facial t.**, its angles—basion, and alveolar and nasal points. **Frontal t.**, bounded by maximum frontal diameter and lines to glabella. **Hesselbach's t.**, deep epigastric artery below Poupart's ligament on outside, and margin of rectus muscle on inside. **Iliofemoral t.**, formed by Nélaton's line, another line through superior iliac spine, and a third from this to great trochanter. **Infraclavicular t.** has the clavicle above, upper border of pectoralis major on inside, anterior border of deltoid on outside. **Inguinal t., Scarpa's t.**, has the sartorius outside, adductor longus within, and Poupart's ligament above. **Lesser's t.** has the hypoglossal nerve above, and the two bellies of digastricus on the two sides. **Lumbocosto-abdominal t.** lies between the obliquus externus, the serratus posticus inferior, the erector spinæ, and the obliquus internus. **Macewen's t., Suprameatal t.,** is between lower posterior edge of root of zygoma and superior posterior edge of external auditory canal. **T. of neck, anterior,** the two carotid and the submaxillary t's, together. **T. of neck, posterior,** the occipital and subclavian t's. together. **Occipital t.** has the sternomastoid in front, the trapezius behind, and omohyoid below. **Occipital t., inferior,** the bimastoid line is its base and inion its apex. **Petit's t.,** crest of ilium below and obliquus externus and latissimus dorsi on either side. **Scarpa's t.** Same as *Inguinal t.* **Subclavian t.,** posterior belly of omohyoid above, clavicle below, and sternomastoid at the base. **Submaxillary t.,** lower jaw-bone above, posterior belly of digastric and the stylohyoid below, and median line of neck in front. **Suboccipital t.** lies between the rectus capitis posticus major and superior and inferior oblique muscles.

Triangula'ris (tri-ang-u-la'ris). See *Muscles, Table of.*

Trian'gular ligament. A slip running up from Poupart's ligament behind inner pillar of the external abdominal ring. **T. nucleus.** Same as *Cuneate nucleus.*

Triatom'ic. Containing three atoms, or three replaceable hydrogen atoms.

Trib'adism (trib'ad-ism). Same as *Sapphism.*

Tribromhy'drin. A yellowish antiseptic and sedative liquid, $C_3H_5Br_3$.

Tribro'mid of gold. $AuBr_3$; used in various antiluetic preparations.

Tribrom'methane. Same as *Bromoform.*

Tribromphe'nol (tri-brōm-fe'nol). Same as *Bromol.*

Triceph'alus. A monster fetus with three heads.

Tri'ceps. See *Muscles, Table of.* **T. reflex,** tapping the elbow-tendon produces extension of the forearm.

Trichangiec'tasis. Dilatation of the capillaries.

Trichau'xe. Hypertrichosis; excessive hairiness.

Trichi'asis. 1. Condition of ingrowing hairs about an orifice, or of ingrowing eyelashes. 2. Appearance of hair-like filaments in the urine.

Trichi'na spira'lis. A nematode parasite which sometimes infests the muscles.

Trichini'asis, Trichino'sis. Disease caused by the presence of trichina.

Trichiniza'tion. Infection with trichinæ.

Trichinopho'bia. Morbid dread of trichiniasis.

Trichin'oscope. Apparatus for determining the presence of trichinæ in muscles or in food.

Trich'inous. Containing, or affected with, trichinæ.

Trichi'tis. Inflammation of the hair-bulbs.

Trichloracet'ic acid. A crystalline acid, $C2H_2Cl_3(OH)$: caustic.

Trichlorhy'drin. An anesthetic and hypnotic compound, $C_3H_5Cl_3$.

Trichlo'rid. Combination of three atoms of chlorin with one of another element.

Trichlorphe'nol. A disinfectant and external antiseptic.

Trichocar'dia (tri-ko-kar'de-ah). Same as *Hairy heart.*

Trichocephali'asis. State of being infested with trichocephalus dispar.

Trichoceph'alus (tri-ko-sef'al-us). A genus of intestinal worms, the thread-worms or whip-worms. **T. dis'par** is a harmless parasite of the cecum and neighboring sections of the intestine.

Trichocla'sia (tri-ko-kla'se-ah). Brittleness of the hair.

Tricho-epithelio'ma. A skin-tumor whose cell-growth starts in the follicles of the hairs of the lanugo.

30

Trichoglos'sia (tri-ko-glos'e-ah). Same as *Hairy tongue.*
Tri'choid (tri'koid). Like, or resembling, hair.
Trichol'ogy. Sum of knowledge regarding the hair.
Tricho'ma (tri-ko'mah). See *Entropion.*
Trichomato'sis. Same as *Plica polonica.*
Tricho'matous. Affected with trichoma, or with plica polonica.
Trichom'onas vagina'lis. A protozoön from leukorrheal discharges.
Trichomyco'sis. Any disease of the hair caused by fungi.
Trichon'osus, Trichop'athy. Any disease of the hair.
Tricophha'gia. The insane habit of eating hair.
Trichophyt'ic (tri-ko-fit'ik). Pertaining to trichophyton.
Trichoph'yton. Genus of fungi. **T. ton'surans,** the fungus causing ringworm.
Trichophyto'sis. State of being infested with trichophyton fungi.
Trichoptilo'sis. The splitting of hairs at the end.
Trichorrhex'is nodo'sa. State in which the hair becomes nodose and breaks off.
Tricho'sis. Any disease of the hair; trichiasis.
Trichothe'cium ro'seum. A variety of mould-fungus found in the human ear.
Trichotilloma'nia. The morbid habit of pulling out the hair, accompanied by excessive itching.
Trichro'ic. Exhibiting three different colors in three different aspects.
Tri'chroism. Condition or quality of being trichroic.
Tricip'ital. 1. Three-headed. 2. Relating to the triceps.
Tricor'nic, Tricor'nute. Having three horns, cornua, or processes.
Tricre'sol. A combination of the three cresols: antiseptic.
Tricresolam'in. A disinfectant and antiseptic preparation.
Tricrot'ic. Having three sphygmographic waves or elevations to one beat of the pulse.
Tri'crotism (tri'krot-izm). Quality of being tricrotic.
Tricus'pid (tri-kus'pid). Having three points or cusps. **T. disease,** disease of the tricuspid valve. **T. valve,** the valve which closes the passage between the right cardiac auricle and the right ventricle.
Tricl'con. Instrument for extracting foreign bodies from wounds.
Triencph'alus (tri-en-sef'al-us). See *Triocephalus.*
Triethylam'in. A ptomain, $C_6H_{15}N$, from putrefying fish.
Trifa'cial nerve (tri-fa'shal). See *Nerves, Table of.*
Trifor'mal. Paraformaldehyd, an antiseptic compound.
Trigem'inal (tri-jem'in-al). Pertaining to the trigeminus.
Trigem'inus (tri-jem'in-us). See *Nerves, Table of.*
Trig'ger-finger. Condition in which a finger snaps into place in flexion or extension.
Trigoceph'alus. A monster with fore part of the head triangular.
Tri'gone, Trigo'num. A triangle; especially the smooth surface on the inside of the base of the bladder. **Olfactory t.,** triangular area of gray matter between the roots of the olfactory tract.
Trigonocephal'ic. Having a triangle-shaped head.
Tri'labe (tri'lāb). A three-pronged lithotrite.
Trill. A tremulous utterance.
Triman'ual. Accomplished by the use of three hands.
Trimethylam'in. A ptomain, C_3H_9N, from vegetable and animal tissues.
Trimethylendiam'in. A deadly ptomain, $C_3H_{10}N_2$, from cultures of the cholera-spirillum.

Trimor'phous. Crystallizing in three different forms.
Trineu'ric (tri-nu'rik). Having three neurons.
Trini'trin (tri-ni'trin). Nitroglycerin.
Trinitrophe'nol (tri-ni-tro-fe'nol). Same as *Picric acid.*
Triocepli'alus. Monster fetus with no organs of sight, hearing, or smell.
Tri'onal. A crystalline hypnotic, $C_8H_{18}S_2O_4$: used like sulphonal.
Tri'onym. A name consisting of three parts.
Trior'chid (tri-or'kid). A person having three testicles.
Triox'id. A combination of three oxygen atoms with one of another element.
Trip'ara (trip'ar-ah). Same as *Tertipara.*
Tripha'sic. Triply varied, or triply phasic: used in the record of experiments regarding the electromotive actions of muscle.
Triphe'nin. An antipyretic and analgesic, $C_{11}H_{15}O_2N$: used like phenacetin.
Tripier's amputation (trip-e-āz'). Amputation of a foot through the calcaneum.
Triple phosphate. Ammonium and magnesium phosphate.
Trip'let. 1. Any one of three infants born at one birth. 2. A combination of three lenses.
Tri'plex (tri'pleks). Triple or threefold. **T. pills,** pills of three active ingredients.
Triplo'pia. State in which an object is seen as threefold.
Trique'trous bone, Os trique'trum. 1. Any Wormian bone. 2. The cuneiform bone of the carpus.
Trira'diate lines. The stars of the embryonic lens. **T. sulcus,** the orbital fissure.
Tris'moid (triz'moid). Variety of trismus nascentium: said to be due to pressure on occipital bone during delivery.
Tris'mus. Tetanic spasm of the jaw-muscles.
Trisplanch'nic. Pertaining to the three great visceral cavities. **T. nervous system,** the sympathetic nervous system.
Tristima'nia. Melancholia.
Trisul'phate. A sulphate with three sulphuric-acid radicals.
Tritic'eous nodule, Tritic'eum (trit-ish'e-us, trit-is'e-um). A nodule in the thyrohyoid ligament.
Trit'icin (trit'is-in). A proprietary food preparation.
Trit'icum. A genus of grasses including wheat. **T. re'pens,** couch-grass; diuretic.
Trit'urable. Susceptible of being triturated.
Trit'urate. 1. To reduce to powder by rubbing. 2. A substance powdered fine by rubbing.
Tritura'tion. 1. Reduction to powder by friction or grinding. 2. A triturated substance.
Triv'alent. Uniting with, or replacing, three hydrogen atoms.
Tro'car. Sharp-pointed instrument used with a cannula for tapping.
Trochan'ter. Either one of the two processes below the neck of the femur.
Trochanter'ic, Trochante'rian. Pertaining to a trochanter.
Trochan'tin. The lesser trochanter.
Tro'che, Trochis'cus. A medicated tablet or disk.
Tro'chin. The lesser tuberosity of the humerus.
Troch'lea. A pulley-shaped part or structure.
Troch'lear. Pertaining to a trochlea. **T. nerve,** the fourth cranial.
Trochlea'ris. See *Muscles, Table of.*
Trochocepha'lia, Trochoceph'aly. Abnormal or premature union of frontal and parietal bones.
Tro'choid (tro'koid). Pivot-like or pulley-shaped.
Trochoi'des. A pivot-joint or pulley-joint.

Trol'ley sickness. Peculiar illness said to be caused by riding in electric cars.

Trom'mer's test. Test for sugar, made with a copper-solution.

Tropacoca'in. Alkaloid from a Javanese coca: anesthetic and non-mydriatic.

Troph'esy. Derangement of nutrition from failure of motor-nerve influence.

Troph'ic. Of, or pertaining to, nutrition. **T. center,** a nerve-center which regulates nutrition.

Troph'oblast. The epiblastic layers lining the chorionic villi in the fetal placenta.

Trophoneuro'sis. 1. Any functional nervous disease due to a trophic disorder. 2. Same as *Trophesy.*

Trophoneurot'ic. Pertaining to a trophoneurosis.

Troph'onine. Proprietary food from beef, eggs, and gluten.

Trophop'athy. Any derangement of the nutrition.

Troph'oplast (trof'o-plast). A granular protoplasmic body.

Trophot'ropism. A kind of chemotaxis for the nutritive matter of cells.

Tro'pic acid. An acid, $C_9H_{10}O_3$, derived from atropin.

Trop'ical chlorosis. Anchylostomiasis.

Tro'pin. A crystalline base, $C_8H_{15}NO$, derived from atropin.

Tropom'eter. Instrument for measuring the twist or torsion of a long bone; also, instrument for measuring the movements of the eye.

Trousseau's spots (tru-sōz'). Same as *Meningitic streak.* **T.'s symptom,** muscular spasm in tetany upon pressing the nerves or arteries of the parts affected.

Troy weight. See *Weight.*

Trun'cal (trung'kal). Pertaining to the trunk.

Trun'cate (trung'kāt). To amputate; to deprive of limbs.

Trunk. The body considered apart from the head and limbs.

Truss. Device for retaining a reduced hernia in its place.

Tryp'sase. Trypsin considered as an enzyme, or non-organized ferment.

Trypse'sis (trip-se'sis). Trephination.

Tryp'sin. The main protolytic ferment of the pancreatic secretion.

Trypsin'ogen. The zymogen from which trypsin is formed.

Tryp'tone. Any peptone produced by digestive action of trypsin.

Tryptone'mia. Presence of tryptones in the blood.

Tub. To use the cold bath in fever.

Tu'bal. Pertaining to a tube or oviduct. **T. nephritis,** inflammation of the kidney-tubes. **T. pregnancy,** pregnancy occurring in an oviduct.

Tube. A hollow cylindric organ or instrument. **Air-t.,** any tubular passage of respiratory apparatus. **Auscultatory t.,** instrument used in testing the sense of hearing. **T.-cast,** cast of renal tubule. **Crooke's t.,** exhausted vacuum-tube used in obtaining Röntgen rays. **Drainage-t.,** tube used in surgery to facilitate escape of fluids. **Eustachian t.,** canal from naso-pharynx to tympanum. **Fallopian t.** See *Oviduct.* **Feeding-t.,** a tube for introducing food into the stomach. **Geissler's t.,** a tube containing a highly rarefied gas. **Intubation-t., Tracheotomy-t.,** breathing-tube used after laryngotomy or tracheotomy. **Stomach-t.,** a tube for feeding or washing stomach.

Tu'ber. An enlargement, knob, or swelling. **T. cinere'um,** an eminence of gray substance on floor of third ventricle.

Tu'bercle. 1. Any mass of small rounded nodules produced by the bacillus of tuberculosis. 2. A nodule or small eminence. **Adductor t.,** eminence on femur which attaches tendon of adductor magnus. **Amygdaloid t.,** nodule on roof of descending cornu of lateral ventricle. **Anatomic t.,** warty growth on dissector's hand. **Carotid t., Chassaignac's t.,** nodule on transverse process of sixth cervical vertebra. **Conoid t.,** on clavicle for attachment of conoid ligament. **Darwinian t.** See *Darwinian.* **Deltoid t.** on clavicle attaches part of deltoid muscle. **Fibrous t.,** tubercle of bacillary origin which contains connective-tissue elements. **Genial t.,** tubercle on either side of middle line on inner surface of lower jaw-bone. **Genital t.,** eminence of fetal life in front of cloaca: it becomes the penis or clitoris. **Lacrimal t.,** on upper jaw-bone where lacrimal groove reaches the orbital surface. **Laminated t.,** nodule of cerebellum. **Lower's t.,** within right auricle, between orifices of venæ cavæ. **Miliary t.,** the typical form of bacillary, or true disease-tubercle; especially a form of minute tubercle formed in great numbers and sometimes found in various parts and organs. **Pterygoid t.,** on inner surface of inferior maxilla: attaches internal and pterygoid muscles. **T. of Rolando,** rounded gray mass under the surface of lateral column of the oblongata. **Scalene t.,** on first rib, for attaching anterior scalene muscle. **Zygomatic t.,** on the zygoma, at the junction of its anterior root.

Tuber'cular. Of, or pertaining to, tubercle.

Tuber'culin. A therapeutic and diagnostic preparation from cultures of the bacillus of tuberculosis. **T. R.,** tuberculin prepared by pounding in a mortar dried cultures of tubercle-bacilli and adding distilled water. It is then centrifugalized. It is preserved in 20 per cent. of glycerin. It is said to induce no reaction.

Tuber'culinose. A modified form of tuberculin.

Tuberculi'tis. Inflammation of, or near, a tubercle.

Tuber'culocele. Tuberculous disease of the testicle.

Tuberculoci'din. An albumose used like tuberculin.

Tuberculofi'broid. Characterized by tubercle that has undergone a fibroid degeneration.

Tuberculo'ma (tu-ber-ku-lo'mah). A tuberculous mass.

Tuberculo'sis. An infectious disease caused by *Bacillus tuberculosis*, and characterized by formation of tubercle in the tissues. **Cestodic t.,** a disease simulating tuberculosis, but due to excessive infestation with cestode parasites.

Tuber'culous. Pertaining to, or affected with, tubercles or tuberculosis.

Tuber'culum (tu-ber'ku-lum). A tubercle. **T. acus'ticum,** collection of nerve-cells behind the accessory auditory nucleus.

Tuberos'ity. A broad eminence situated on a bone.

Tubo-abdom'inal pregnancy. Pregnancy in fimbriated end of Fallopian tube, so that the fetus is partly in the tube and partly in the abdomen.

Tuboligamen'tous. Pertaining to the oviduct and broad ligament.

Tubo-ova'rian. Of, or pertaining to, an oviduct and ovary.

Tuboperitone'al. Pertaining to the oviduct and peritoneum.

Tubotym'panal canal. A tube of the embryonic hypoblast whence the tympanum and Eustachian tube are formed.

Tu'bular. Of, or pertaining to, a tubule. **T. breathing,** bronchial respiration. **T. gestation.** See *Tubal pregnancy.* **T. membrane.** Same as *Perineurium.*

Tu'bule (tu'būl). Any small tube. **Dentinal t's.,** the tubular structures of the teeth. **Segmental t's.,** the tubules of the Wolffian body. **Seminiferous t's.,** the tubules of the testicle. **Uriniferous t's.,** the minute winding canals making up the substance of the kidney.

Tubuloder'moid. A dermoid tumor due to the persistence of a fetal tube.

Tufnell's method. The treatment of aneurysm by light feeding and rest.

Tuft, Malpighian. A Malpighian body.

Tumefa'cient. Producing, or tending to produce, tumefaction.

Tumefac'tion. A swelling; puffiness.

Tu'menol. A substance from petroleum; used like ichthyol.

Tu'mor. A swelling, especially one due to morbid growth of a tissue not normal to the part. **T. al'bus,** white swelling; tuberculosis of a bone or joint. **Benign t.,** one not likely to recur after removal. **Cystic t.,** one not solid. **False t.,** one due to extravasation, exudation, echinococcus, or retained sebaceous matter. **Fibroid t.,** a fibroma. **Gubler's t.,** on back of wrist, when extensors of hand are paralyzed. **Gummy t.** See *Gumma.* **Heterologous t.** is made up of tissue which differs from that in which it grows. **Histioid t.** is formed of a single tissue. **Homologous t.,** one whose substance resembles that on which it grows. **Malignant t.,** one which is likely to recur and eventually to destroy life. **Mixed t.,** one which combines characters of two or more classes. **Mucous t.,** a myxoma. **Muscular t.,** a myoma. **Organoid t.,** from complex tissues, and resembling an organ. **Phantom t.,** abdominal or other swelling not due to structural change, but usually to a neurosis. **Sebaceous t.,** tumor of a sebaceous gland; atheroma. **Splenic t.,** enlarged spleen. **Teratoid t.,** formed by combination of various organs. **True t.,** any tumor produced by proliferation.

Tumul'tus. Excessive organic action.

Tung'sten. A heavy brittle metal: calcium tungstate is used in skiagraphy.

Tu'nic. A lining membrane or coat.

Tu'nica. Same as *Tunic.* **T. adna'ta,** the portion of conjunctiva that comes in contact with the eyeball. **T. adventi'tia,** outer coat of an artery. **T. albugin'ea,** the sclera; also, the fibrous coat of the testis or ovary. **T. ex'tima, in'tima, me'dia,** the outer, inner, and middle coats of an artery. **T. Ruyschia'na.** Same as *Entochoroidea.* **T. vagina'lis,** the serous covering of the testis. **T. vasculo'sa.** 1. Same as *Mesochoroidea.* 2. The vascular coat of the testis.

Tu'nicin (tu'nis-in). Substance resembling cellulose, from the tissues of certain low forms of animal life.

Tun'nel-anemia. Same as *Actinomycosis.* **T.-disease.** Same as *Caisson-disease.*

Tu'pelo. The tree *Nyssa grandidentata:* its root is used in making surgeons' tents.

Tur'binal. 1. Turbinated. 2. A turbinated bone.

Tur'binated bodies. Masses formed by the turbinated bones with their covers of vascular tissue. **T. bones,** the three bones situated on the outside of the nasal fossæ.

Turbinec'tomy. Surgical removal of a turbinated bone.

Turbin'otome. A cutting-instrument for surgical removal of a turbinated bone.

Turbinot'omy. Surgical cutting of a turbinated bone.

Türck's column. Anterior or direct pyramidal tract of spinal cord.

Turges'cence. Distention or swelling of a part.

Turges'cent (ter-jes'ent). Swelling or beginning to swell.

Tur'gid (ter'jid). Congested and swollen.

Tur'gor (ter'gor). Condition of being turgid; normal, or other fulness.

Tur'meric (ter'mer-ik). Rhizome of *Curcuma longa.*

Tur'merol. An oily alcohol from turmeric.

Turn'ing. Version in obstetric practice.

Turn of life. Same as *Menopause.*

Tur'pentine. An oleoresin, chiefly from coniferous trees. **Canada t.** See *Balsam, Canada.* **Chian t.,** oleoresin from *Pistacia terebinthus.* **Common t.,** from *Pinus sylvestris*, etc. **T., oil of,** volatile oil of common turpentine; diuretic, stimulant, and rubefacient. **Venice t.,** from *Larix Europæa.* **White t.,** from *Pinus palustris*, etc.

Tur'peth. The plant *Ipomœa turpethum* of India: purgative. **T. mineral,** yellow subsulphate of mercury, $H_2SO_4.2HgO$.

Turun'da. A surgeon's tent.

Tus'sal. Pertaining to a cough.

Tussila'go. Leaves of *T. farfara*, coltsfoot: tonic, demulcent, and antibechic.

Tus'sis. L. for *Cough.* **T. convulsi'va,** whooping-cough or pertussis.

Tus'sive. Of, or pertaining to, a cough.

Tus'sol. Antipyrin mandilate, a proprietary whooping-cough remedy.

Tutam'ina oc'uli. The protecting appendages of the eye, as lids, lashes, etc.

Twelfth nerve. See *Hypoglossal*, in *Nerves, Table of.*

Twin. One of two individuals born at one birth.

Twinge. A keen, darting pain.

Twisted suture. The ordinary hare-lip suture.

Twitch. A simple unit of muscular effort.

Tyl'ion. Point on anterior edge of optic groove in median line.

Tylo'ma (ti-lo'ma). A callus or callosity.

Tylo'sis. Formation of callosities, or a condition marked by the occurrence of callosities.

Tym'panal. Pertaining to the tympanum.

Tympanec'tomy. Excision of the membrana tympani.

Tympan'ic. Of, or pertaining to, the tympanum. **T. bone, T. plate, T. ring,** body-wall which surrounds the tympanum and external canal. **T. membrane.** Same as *Membrana tympani.* **T. nerve.** See *Nerves, Table of.*

Tympani'tes. Distention of the abdomen with gas or air.

Tympanit'ic. 1. Characterized by tympanites. 2. Bell-like or tympanic. **T. resonance,** resonance produced by percussion over a cavity containing air or gas.

Tympani'tis (tim-pan-i'tis). Same as *Otitis media.*

Tympanohy'al. Part of the embryonic hyoid arch becoming fused with the styloid process.

Tympanot'omy. Surgical puncture of the membrana tympani.

Tym'panum. The middle ear, or ear-drum.

Tym'pany. 1. Tympanites. 2. A tympanic or bell-like percussion-note.

Typh-fever. Typhus and typhoid fever viewed together.

Typhin'ia (tif-in'e-ah). Relapsing fever.

Typhlenteri'tis. Appendicitis.

Typhli'tis. Inflammation of the cecum.

Typhlo-empye'ma. An abdominal abscess accompanying appendicitis.

Typhlol'ogy. A treatise on blindness.

Typhlo'sis (tif-lo'sis). Blindness.

Typhlot'omy. The operation of cutting into the cecum.

Typhobacillo'sis. The symptoms due to poisoning by the toxins of the *Bacillus typhosus.*

Ty'phoid (ti'foid). 1. Pertaining to, or resembling, typhus. 2. Typhoid fever. **T. condition, T. state,** a condition of weakness, feeble pulse, and low delirium. **T. fever.** See under *Fever.* **T. spine,** a painful state of the vertebral region after typhoid fever.

Typhoid'al. Resembling typhoid.

Typhoidette (ti-foi-det'). A mild form of typhoid fever.

Typhomala'rial fever. Malarial fever with typhoidal symptoms.

Typhoma'nia (ti-fo-ma'ne-ah), **Typho'nia.** The delirium accompanying typhus or typhoid fever.

Typhopneumo'nia. Pneumonia with typhoid fever or pneumonia with typhoid state.

Typhosep'sis. The septic poisoning which occurs in typhus.

Typhotox'in. A deadly ptomain, $C_7H_{17}NO_2$, from cultures of typhoid bacillus.

Ty'phous (ti'fus). Pertaining to, or like, typhus.

Ty'phus. A contagious fever characterized by petechial eruption, high temperature, and great prostration. **Petechial t.,** true typhus. **T. recur'rens.** Same as *Relapsing fever.* **T. sid'erans,** a malignant and quickly fatal form.

Typ'ical. Presenting the distinctive features of any type.

Tyran'nism. Insane or morbid cruelty; also, cruelty with sexual perversion.

Ty'rein. Coagulated casein of milk.

Tyrem'esis. Infantile vomiting of curd.

Tyri'asis (tir-i'as-is). A variety of true leprosy.

Ty'roid. Of cheesy consistence; caseous.

Tyroleu'cin. Substance, $C_{14}H_{22}N_2O_4$, from decomposition of albumin.

Tyro'ma (ti-ro'mah). A caseous mass.

Tyromato'sis (ti-ro-mat-o'sis). Caseous degeneration.

Tyro'sin. A crystalline amido-acid, $C_9H_{11}NO_3$, a product of the decomposition of proteids.

Tyro'sis. Cheesy degeneration or caseation.

Ty'rothrix. A genus of bacteria resembling *Bacillus.*

Tyrotox'icon. A poisonous ptomain sometimes occurring in milk, cheese, and ice-cream.

Tyr'rel's fascia. Fascia between the bladder and rectum. **T.'s hook,** blunt hook for drawing the iris through a hole in the cornea.

Ty'son's glands. Sebaceous glands about the foreskin and vulva.

U.

U. Symbol of *Uranium.*

Uf'felman's test (oof'el-mahnz). Test for hydrochloric acid or lactic acid in the stomach.

Ukam'bin. An African arrow-poison somewhat resembling digitalis.

Ulatro'phia (oo-lat-ro'fe-ah). Shrinkage of the gums.

Ul'cer (ul'ser). An open sore other than a wound. **Amputating u.,** ulceration encircling a part and destroying the tissue to the bone. **Atheromatous u.,** loss of substance in the wall of an artery or the endocardium from breaking down of an atheromatous patch. **Chancroidal u.** See *Chancroid.* **Curling's u.,** an ulcer of the duodenum seen after severe burns of the body. **Follicular u.,** small ulcer on mucous membrane, having origin in a lymph-follicle. **Fungous u.,** one covered by fungous granulations. **Indolent u.,** one with an indurated, elevated edge and a non-granulating base, usually occurring on the leg. **Inflamed u.,** one surrounded by marked inflammation. **Jacob's u.** See *Rodent u.* **Marjolin's u.,** an ulcer having for its seat an old cicatrix. **Peptic u.,** ulcer of mucous membrane of stomach or duodenum. **Perforating u.,** an ulcer that perforates the tissues of a part, especially the foot or the stomach. **Phagedenic u.,** one which rapidly eats away the tissues. **Phlegmonous u.** Synonym of *Inflamed u.* **Rodent u.,** ulcer which gradually involves and eats away soft tissues and bones.

Round u., the peptic ulcer of the stomach. **Serpiginous u.**, one healing in one place and spreading in another. **Tuberculous u.**, one due to the tubercle-bacillus. **Varicose u.**, an ulcer due to varicose veins.

Ul'cerate (ul'ser-āt). To produce a sore or to become affected with an ulcer.

Ulcera'tion (ul-ser-a'shun). Formation of an ulcer.

Ul'cerative (ul'ser-a-tiv). Characterized by ulceration.

Ulceromem'branous tonsillitis. That which is characterized by herpetic vesicles which ulcerate and become covered with a membranous film.

Ul'cerous (ul'ser-us). Of the nature of an ulcer.

Ul'cus. L. for *Ulcer.* **U. ventric'uli**, ulceration of the stomach.

Ulemorrha'gia. Bleeding from the gums.

Ulerytli'ema. An erythematous disease with formation of cicatrices.

Ulet'ic (u-let'ik). Pertaining to the gums.

Ulex'in. Diuretic and tonic alkaloid, $C_{11}H_{14}NO_2$, from seeds of European furze.

Uli'tis. Inflammation of the gums.

Ul'mus. The inner bark of *Ulmus fulva;* slippery elm.

Ul'na. The inner and larger bone of forearm.

Ul'nad (ul'nad). Toward the ulna.

Ul'nar. Pertaining to the ulna.

Ulna'ris (ul-na'ris). See *Muscles, Table of.*

Ulnocar'pal. Of, or pertaining to, the carpus and ulna.

Ulnora'dial. Pertaining to the ulna and radius.

Ulocarcino'ma. Carcinoma of the gums.

U'loid. Resembling a scar, but not due to any lesion of the skin.

Ulon'cus. Swelling of the gums.

Ulorrha'gia (u-lo-ra'je-ah). Free hemorrhage from the gums.

Ulorrhe'a (u-lo-re'ah). Bleeding from the gums.

Ulot'richous (u-lot'rik-us). Having woolly hair.

Ul'timate (ul'tim-āt). Final or most remote. **U. analysis**, resolution of a substance into its component elements.

Ul'timum mo'riens. 1. Last part of the body to die; the right auricle. 2. Upper portion of the trapezius muscle.

Ultrabrachycephal'ic. Having a cephalic index of more than 90.

Ultz'mann's test (oolts'mahnz). A test for bile-pigments in the urine.

Umbil'ical. Of, or pertaining to, the umbilicus. **U. arteries**, the arteries which accompany the umbilicus. **U. cord**, the cord which connects the placenta with the navel of the fetus *in utero.* **U. duct.** Same as *Omphalomesenteric duct.* **U. fissure**, the part of longitudinal fissure of liver which lodges the umbilical vein. **U. hernia.** See *Hernia.* **U. souffle**, hissing sound supposed to arise from the umbilical cord. **U. vesicle**, portion of yolk-sac of embryo bending from the umbilicus.

Umbil'icated. Marked by the presence of depressed or navel-like spots.

Umbilica'tion. A navel-like depression or pit.

Umbili'cus. The navel; cicatrix which marks the site of entry of the umbilical cord.

Um'bo. The apex of the membrana tympani.

Umbras'copy (um-bras'ko-pe). Same as *Skiascopy.*

Unavoid'able hemorrhage. Hemorrhage due to detached placenta prævia.

Un'cia (un'se-ah). L. for *Ounce.*

Un'ciform. Hooked or shaped like a hook. **U. bone**, bone at the ulnar edge of carpus and in the distal row. **U. fasciculus**, the fasciculus which connects the temporosphenoid and frontal lobes of the cerebrum. **U. process,** a process of the ethmoid bone.

Un'cinate (un'sin-āt). Shaped like a hook; hooked. **U. convolution, U. gyrus,** a convolution of the occipital lobe of the cerebrum near temporal lobe.

Uncina'tum (un-sin-a'tum). The unciform bone.

Un'cipressure. Pressure with a hook to stay hemorrhage.

Uncon'scious. Insensible.

Unc'tion. An ointment; the application of an ointment.

Unc'tuous (unk'chu-us). Greasy or oily.

Un'cus. A hook or hook-shaped structure. **U. gy'ri fornica'-ti.** See *Uncinate convolution.*

Un'dulant fever. Mediterranean fever. See *Fever.*

Undula'tion. A wave-like motion in any medium.

Un'dulatory theory. Doctrine that light, electricity, and heat are propagated by undulations in an ether which pervades all space.

Un'finished cough. A peculiar cough, commonly due to, and pathognomonic of, aneurysm of the arch of aorta.

Un'gual. Of, or pertaining to, the nails. **U. bone.** Same as *Lacrimal bone.*

Un'guent (un'gwent). An ointment, salve, or cerate.

Unguen'tum (ung-gwen'tum). L. for *Ointment.*

Unguic'ulate. Having claws or resembling a claw.

Un'guinal (ung'gwin-al). Pertaining to an unguis.

Un'guis. 1. A nail. 2. An onyx of the cornea.

Un'gula. An instrument for extracting a dead fetus.

Uniax'ial (u-ne-ak'se-al). Having but one axis.

Unicel'lular (u-nis-el'u-lar). Made up of a single cell.

U'nicism. The obsolete doctrine that there is but one venereal virus.

U'nicorn-root. See *Aletris.* **U.-uterus,** a uterus with but one horn or oviducal process.

Unicor'nous. Having but one cornu.

Unilat'eral (u-nil-at'er-al). Affecting but one side.

Uniloc'ular. Having but one loculus or compartment.

Uninu'cleated (u-nin-u'kle-a-ted). Having a single nucleus.

Unioc'ular. Of, or pertaining to, only one eye.

U'nion. See *Healing.*

Unio'val. Arising from one ovum: used of certain twin pregnancies.

Unip'ara. A woman who has borne but one child.

Unip'arous. Having given birth to but one child.

Unipo'lar (u-nip-o'lar). Having but a single pole.

U'nitary. Composed of, or pertaining to, a single individual.

Univ'alent. Having a valence of one; replacing one hydrogen atom.

Univer'sal joint. A ball-and-socket joint.

Unof. Abbreviation for *Unofficial.*

Unoffi'cial. Not authorized by the established dispensatories and formularies.

Unor'ganized. Not organized. **U. ferment,** a chemical ferment. See *Ferment.*

Unsex'. To spay or deprive of the ovaries.

Un'striated muscle. Muscle without transverse striations; involuntary muscle.

Un'well. 1. Sick, or not well. 2. Menstruating.

Up'siloid (up'sil-oid). V-shaped.

U'rachal. Of, or pertaining to, the urachus.

U'rachus (u'rak-us). Cord which connects the bladder to the navel.

Uræ'mia, Ure'mia. Accumulation of urinary matters in the blood.

U'ral, Ura'lium (u'ral, u-ra'le-um). Crystalline compound of chloral and urethane with hypnotic properties.

U'ramil (u'ram-il). A compound from uric acid.

U'ramin. Guanidin; a poisonous base derivable from guanin.

Uranal'ysis (u-ran-al'is-is). The analysis of urine.

Uranisconi'tis. Inflammation of the palate.

Uranis'coplasty. Plastic operation for cleft palate.

Uraniscor'rhaphy. Same as *Staphylorrhaphy.*

Uranis'cus. The palate; the roof of the mouth.

Ura'nium. A hard metal; symbol U; sparingly used in medicine.

Uran'oplasty (u-ran'o-plas-te). Same as *Uraniscoplasty.*

Uranos'chisis. Cleft palate; congenital fissure of the palate.

Ura're. 1. See *Curare.* 2. A South American arrow-poison like curare, but distinct from it.

Ura'rize. To put under the influence of urare.

U'rate. Any salt of uric acid.

Urat'ic. Pertaining to the urates, or to gout.

Urato'ma. A concretion made up of urates; tophus.

Urato'sis. The deposit of urates in the tissues.

Uratu'ria (u-rat-u're-ah). Same as *Lithuria.*

U'rea (u're-ah). A white crystalline substance, CON_2H_4, from urine, etc.

U'real. Pertaining to urea.

Uream'eter. Apparatus for measuring the urea present in urine.

Uream'etry (u-re-am'et-re). Measurement of the urea present in urine.

Urech'ysis. An effusion of urine into areolar tissue.

Urede'ma, Urœde'ma. Swelling from extravasated urine.

Ure'do (u-re'do). Same as *Urticaria.*

U'reid (u're-id). Any compound urea; urea with its hydrogen variously replaced.

Urelco'sis. 1. Ulceration in the urinary tract. 2. Ulceration due to disease of the urinary apparatus.

Ure'mic (u-re'mik). Caused by, or pertaining to, uremia.

Ureom'eter (u-re-om'et-er). Same as *Ureameter.*

Ureom'etry (u-re-om'et-re). Same as *Ureametry.*

Urer'ythrin (u-rer'ith-rin). Same as *Uroerythrin.*

Ure'sis (u-re'sis). The act of passing urine.

Ure'ter. One of the tubes through which the urine goes from the kidney to the bladder.

Ureteral'gia (u-re-ter-al'je-ah). Pain in the ureter.

Ureterec'tomy (u-re-ter-ek'to-me). Excision of a ureter.

Ureteri'tis. Inflammation of a ureter.

Ureterocystoneos'tomy. Same as *Ureteroneocystostomy.*

Ureterocystos'tomy. Formation of a communication between a ureter and kidney to the bladder.

Uretero-enteros'tomy. Formation of a communication between the ureter and the bowel.

Ure'terolith. A calculus in the ureter.

Ureterolithot'omy. Excision of a calculus from ureter.

Ureteroneocystos'tomy. Formation of a communication between the ureter and a new portion of the bladder.

Ureteropyeli'tis. Inflammation of a ureter and the pelvis of the kidney.

Ureteropyeloneos'tomy. Formation of artificial passage from pelvis of kidney to ureter.

Ureterot'omy. Operation of cutting into a ureter; uretero-ureterostomy.

Uretero-ureteros'tomy. Formation of a passage from one ureter to the other.

Ureterovag'inal. Of, or pertaining to, a ureter and the vagina.

U'rethane. 1. A substance antipyretic and hypnotic, $C_3H_7NO_2$. 2. Any ester of carbamic acid.

Ure'thra. The passage through which urine is discharged from the bladder. It consists of a *prostatic portion*, one and one-half inches long; a *membranous portion*, one-half to four-fifths of an inch long; and a *spongy* or *penile portion*, enclosed in the corpus spongiosum.

Ure'thral. Of, or pertaining to, the urethra.

Urethral'gia (u-re-thral'je-ah). Pain in the urethra.

Urethrec'tomy. Surgical resection of the urethra.

Ure'thrism, Urethris'mus. Chronic spasm of the urethra.

Urethri'tis (u-re-thri'tis). Inflammation of the urethra.

Ure'throcele. Prolapse of the female urethra through the meatus urinarius.

Urethrom'eter. Apparatus for measuring the urethra.

Urethrope'nile. Pertaining to the urethra and penis.

Urethroperine'al. Pertaining to the urethra and perineum.

Urethroperineoscro'tal. Pertaining to the urethra, perineum, and scrotum.

Ure'throplasty. Plastic surgery of the urethra.

Urethrorec'tal. Pertaining to the urethra and rectum.

Urethrorrha'gia. Flow of blood from the urethra.

Urethror'rhaphy. Suturation of a urethral fistula.

Urethrorrhe'a (u-reth-ro-re'ah). A flow from the urethra.

Ure'throscope. Instrument for viewing interior of urethra.

Urethroscop'ic. Pertaining to the urethroscope.

Urethros'copy. Visual inspection of the urethra.

Ure'throspasm. Spasm of the urethral muscular tissue.

Urethrosteno'sis. Stricture or stenosis of the urethra.

Urethros'tomy. Formation of an opening into the urethra in cases of incurable stricture.

Ure'throtome. Instrument for cutting a urethral stricture.

Urethrot'omy. Cutting operation for curing a urethral stricture.

Urethrovag'inal. Of, or pertaining to, the urethra and vagina.

Uret'ic. Promoting the secretion of urine.

U'ric acid. See *Acid*.

Uricacide'mia. Accumulation of uric acid in the blood.

Urice'din. A proprietary gout medicine. A mixture of sodium sulphate, chlorid, and citrate with lithium citrate.

Urice'mia (u-ris-e'me-ah). Same as *Uricacidemia*.

Uridro'sis. Escape of urinous matter in the sweat.

Uriesthe'sis. Normal impulse to pass the urine.

Uri'na (u-ri'nah). L. for *Urine*.

U'rinal (u'rin-al). A receptacle for urine.

Urinal'ysis (u-rin-al'is-is). Analysis of the urine.

U'rinary. Of, or pertaining to, the urine.

U'rinate (u'rin-āt). To void the urine.

Urina'tion. The discharge or passage of urine.

U'rine. The fluid secreted by the kidneys, stored in the bladder, and discharged by the urethra.

Urine'mia (u-rin-e'me-ah). Same as *Uremia*.

Urinif'erous. Transporting or conveying urine. **U. tubules,** minute passages in substance of the kidney.

Urinip'arous (u-rin-ip'ar-us). Secreting urine.

Urinogen'ital (u-rin-o-jen'it-al). Same as *Urogenital*.

Urinol'ogy (u-rin-ol'o-je). Same as *Urology*.

Urinom'eter. Instrument for finding the specific gravity of the urine.

Urinom'etry. Ascertainment of the specific gravity of the urine.

Urinos'copy (u-rin-os'ko-pe). Same as *Uroscopy*.

U'rinose, U'rinous. Containing, or of the nature of, urine.

Urisol'vin. A proprietary uric-acid solvent.
Urn'ing (oor'ning) [Ger.]. A sexual pervert.
Urobacil'lus. Any microbe from decomposing urine.
Urobi'lin. A pigment found in urine. **U. jaundice,** jaundice probably due to urobilin in the blood.
Urobilin'ogen. A chromogen which decomposes into blood.
Urobilinu'ria. An excess of urobilin in the urine.
Uroca'nin. A base, $C_{11}H_{10}N_4O$, derivable from urocaninic acid.
Urocanin'ic acid. A crystalline acid, $C_{12}H_{12}N_4O_4$, from dog's urine.
U'rocele (u'ro-sēl). Distention of scrotum with extravasated urine.
Uroche'sia (u-ro-ke'ze-ah). Discharge of urine through the rectum.
Urochloral'ic acid. An acid found in the urine after the exhibition of chloral.
Urochlor'ic acid. A substance sometimes found in urine after the exhibition of chloral.
U'rochrome (u'ro-krōm). A yellow pigment or coloring-matter of urine.
Urocri'sis. A crisis marked by copious discharge of urine.
Urocris'on. Diagnosis by observing the urine.
Urocrite'rion. A symptom observed in the inspection of urine.
Urocyan'ogen. A blue pigment of urine, especially of cholera patients.
Urocyano'sis. Blue urine; indicanuria.
U'rocyst, Urocys'tis. The urinary bladder.
Urocysti'tis. Inflammation of the urinary bladder.
Urodial'ysis. Partial suppression of the urine.
Uroer'ythrin. A reddish coloring-matter of urine in rheumatism.
Urofuscohem'atin. A red-brown color from urine in certain diseases.
Urogas'ter. The urinary intestine; a part of the allantoic cavity of the embryo.
Urogen'ital. Pertaining to urinary apparatus and to the genitalia. **U. ducts,** the Wolffian duct and duct of Müller. **U. sinus,** the anterior portion of the fetal cloaca which receives the urogenital sinus.
Urog'enous (u-roj'en-us). Producing urine.
Uroglau'cin. Indigo-blue occurring in the urine.
Urogravim'eter. Same as *Urinometer*.
Urohem'atin. The pigmentary substance of the urine.
Urohematopor'phyrin. Hematoporphyrin in the urine.
U'rolith. A calculus or gravel in the urine.
Urolithi'asis. Formation of urinary calculi.
Urolithol'ogy. Sum of knowledge regarding urinary calculi.
Urol'ogy. Sum of knowledge regarding the urine.
Urolu'tein. A yellow pigment of the urine.
U'romancy (u'ro-man-se). Same as *Uroscopy*.
Uromel'anin. A black pigment, $C_{18}H_{43}N_7O_{10}$, from urine.
Urom'elus. A monster fetus with fused limbs.
Urom'eter (u-rom'et-er). Same as *Urinometer*.
Uron'cus (u-rong'kus). A urinary swelling.
Uronol'ogy. A treatise on the urine.
Uropha'ein. An odoriferous pigment in the urine.
Urophan'ic (u-ro-fan'ik). Appearing in the urine.
Uroph'erin (u-rof'er-in). Lithium diuretin, a proprietary diuretic mixture.
Uropit'tin. A resinous substance, $C_9H_{10}N_2O_3$, from urochrome.
Uropla'nia. The secretion of urine from abnormal parts.
Uropoie'sis (u-ro-poi-e'sis). The secretion or formation of urine.
Uropoiet'ic (u-ro-poi-et'ik). Pertaining to the formation of urine.
Uropsam'mus. Urinary gravel.
Urorrha'gia. An excessive secretion of urine.

Urorrhe'a. An involuntary flow of urine; enuresis.
Uror'rhodin. A rosy pigment from urine.
Uroru'bin. A red pigment derivable from urine.
Urorubrohem'atin. A red pigment rarely found in the urine.
Urosa'cin (u-ro-sa'sin). Same as *Urorrhodin.*
Uros'cheocele (u-ros'ke-o-sēl). See *Urocele.*
Uros'copy. Examination or inspection of the urine.
Urosep'sin. A septic poison from urine in the tissues.
Urosep'sis. Septic poisoning from retained and absorbed urinary substances.
Uro'sis. Any disease of the urinary organs.
Urospec'trin. A pigment of normal urine.
Uroste'alith. A fatty material from urinary calculi.
Urotox'ic (u-ro-tok'sik). Same as *Toxemic.*
Urot'ropin (u-rot'ro-pin). A proprietary solvent, $(CH_2)_6N_4$, for uric-acid concretion.
U'rous. Having the nature of urine.
Uroxan'ic acid. A principle derivable from uric acid.
Uroxan'thin. A yellow coloring-matter of the urine.
Urox'in (u-rok'sin). See *Alloxantin.*
Urti'ca. Genus of plants; the true nettles.
Urtica'ria. Nettle-rash or hives; a skin-disease marked by transient eruption of wheals.
Urtica'rial, Urtica'rious. Pertaining to, or of the nature of, urticaria.
Urtica'tion. 1. Flogging of a part with nettles. 2. Burning sensation, as of the sting of nettles.
Ustila'go ma'ydis. Corn-smut; a fungus with the action of ergot.
Ustula'tion. The drying of a substance by heat.
Us'tus (us'tus). L. for *Burnt.*
U'terine (u'te-rin). Of, or pertaining to, the uterus. **U. extract,** an animal extract sometimes prescribed therapeutically. **U. milk,** the white milky substance between the villi of the placenta of the gravid uterus.
Uteri'tis. Inflammation of the uterus.
Uterocer'vical. Pertaining to the ureter and the cervix uteri, as *ureterocervical* fistula.
Uterogesta'tion. Uterine gestation.
Uteroma'nia (u-ter-o-ma'ne-ah). See *Nymphomania.*
Utero-ova'rian. Pertaining to the uterus and the ovary.
Uteropex'ia, U'teropexy. Same as *Hysteropexia.*
Uteroplacen'tal. Pertaining to the placenta and uterus.
Uterosa'cral. Pertaining to the uterus and sacrum.
U'terotome. Same as *Hysterotome.*
Uterot'omy (u-ter-ot'o-me). Same as *Hysterotomy.*
Uteroton'ic (u-ter-o-ton'ik). Giving muscular tone to the uterus.
Uterovag'inal. Pertaining to the uterus and vagina.
Uterove'sical. Pertaining to the uterus and the bladder.
U'terus. The womb; a hollow organ, the abode and place of nourishment of the embryo and fetus. **U. bicor'nis,** one with two horns. **U. cordifor'mis,** a heart-shaped uterus. **U. du'plex,** a double uterus. **Gravid u.,** the uterus in pregnancy. **Irritable u.,** one affected with neuralgia. **U. masculi'nus,** sinus pocularis of prostate. **Unicorn u.,** one with a single cornu.
U'tricle (u'trik-l). 1. The expanded part of the membranous labyrinth of the ear. 2. The uterus masculinus.
Utric'ular. 1. Bladder-like. 2. Pertaining to the utricle.
Utriculi'tis. Inflammation of the sinus pocularis.
Utric'ulus. Same as *Utricle.* **U. hom'inis.** Same as *Sinus pocularis.*
Uvæfor'mis (u-ve-for'mis). The middle coat of the chorioid.

U'va ur'si. The leaves of *Arctostaphylos uva ursi*, or **bearberry**: tonic, astringent, and anthelmintic.
U'vea. The iris, ciliary body, and chorioid together.
U'veal. Pertaining to the uvea. **U. tract.** See *Uvea*.
Uveit'ic (u-ve-it'ik). Of the nature of uveitis.
Uvei'tis (u-ve-i'tis). Inflammation of the uvea; iritis.
U'viform (u' vif-orm). Shaped like a grape.
U'vula. A small fleshy body hanging from the soft palate above root of the tongue. **U. cerebel'li**, lobule, the posterior limit of fourth ventricle. **U. ves'icæ**, a small eminence at the base of the bladder projecting into the urethra.
Uvulapto'sis. See *Uvuloptosis*.
U'vular (u' vu-lar). Pertaining to the uvula.
Uvula'ris. The azygos uvulæ muscle.
U'vulatome (u'vu-lat-ōm). Instrument for cutting the uvula.
Uvulat'omy. Excision of a part of the uvula.
Uvuli'tis. Inflammation of the uvula.
Uvulopto'sis. A relaxed, pendulous state of the uvula.
U'vulotome. See *Uvulatome*.
Uvulot'omy. See *Uvulatomy*.

V.

V. Abbreviation for *Vision*; symbol of *Vanadium*.
Vaccig'enous (vak-sij'en-us). Producing vaccine-virus.
Vac'cin (vak'sin). Any material for preventive inoculation.
Vac'cina. Same as *Vaccinia*.
Vac'cinal. Pertaining to vaccinia, or to vaccination. **V. fever**, the fever that sometimes follows vaccination.
Vac'cinate. To inoculate, especially with vaccine-virus.
Vaccina'tion. Act or process of vaccinating; protective inoculation against small-pox.
Vaccina'tionist. One who defends the practice of vaccination.
Vaccina'tor. 1. One who vaccinates. 2. Instrument for vaccinating.
Vac'cine. 1. Vaccinal. 2. Pertaining to the cow. 3. The virus of cow-pox. **V.-farm**, establishment for the production of vaccine-virus from the heifer. **V.-point**, bit of quill or bone charged with vaccine-virus. **V.-rash**, erythema following vaccination. **V.-virus**, virus of cow-pox used in vaccination.
Vaccinel'la. A spurious and ineffective form of vaccinia.
Vaccin'ia (vak-sin'e-ah). Cow-pox; a disease of man and animals, regarded as a modified small-pox.
Vaccin'iform. Resembling vaccinia, or cow-pox.
Vac'cinin (vak'sin-in). The inoculable principle by which cow-pox is communicated.
Vaccinl'ola. Secondary eruption of vesicles after vaccination.
Vaccinliza'tion. Vaccination persistently repeated until the virus has no appreciable effect.
Vaccinosyph'ilis. Syphilis following inoculation with impure vaccine.
Vacuola'tion. The process of forming vacuoles.
Vac'uole (vak'u-ōl). A space or cavity formed in the protoplasm of a cell.
Vac'uum. A space devoid of air or other gas. **V.-treatment**, enclosure of a limb in a partial vacuum. **V.-tube**, a tube of glass nearly devoid of any gaseous contents.
Vag'abonds' disease. Pigmentation of skin due to lice.
Va'gal (va'gal). Pertaining to the vagus nerve.
Vagi'na (va-ji'nah). Canal from slit of vulva to cervix uteri.

Vag'inal (vaj'in-al). Of, or pertaining to, the vagina or to any sheath.

Vaginali'tis. Inflammation of the tunica vaginalis testis.

Vag'inate (vaj'in-āt). Sheathed.

Vaginis'mus (vaj-in-iz'mus). Painful spasm of the vagina due to local hyperesthesia.

Vagini'tis (vaj-in-i'tis). Inflammation of the vagina.

Vaginodyn'ia (vaj-in-o-din'e-ah). Pain in the vagina.

Vaginofixa'tion. Suturing of the fundus of the uterus to the vaginal peritoneum in cases of retroflexion.

Vaginoperitone'al. Pertaining to the vagina and to the peritoneum.

Vaginot'omy (vaj-in-ot'o-me). Incision into the vagina.

Vaginoves'ical (vaj-in-o-ves'ik-al). Pertaining to the vagina and bladder.

Vagi'tus (va-ji'tus). The cry of an infant. **V. uteri'nus,** a cry at or just before birth.

Vagot'omy (va-got'om-e). The operation of cutting the vagus.

Va'gus. See *Pneumogastric nerve,* in *Nerves, Table of.* **V.-pneumonia,** pneumonia due to injury of the pneumogastric nerve.

Va'lence, Va'lency. Same as *Quantivalence.*

Val'erene. Same as *Amylene.*

Vale'rian. The root of *Valeriana officinalis,* an antispasmodic and nerve-stimulant plant.

Vale'rianate. Any salt of valerianic acid.

Valerian'ic acid, Vale'ric acid. See *Acid.*

Valetudina'rian. An invalid; a feeble person.

Val'gus (val'gus). 1. Same as *Talipes valgus.* 2. A bow-legged person.

Vallec'ula. A depression. **V. cerebel'li,** a longitudinal fissure of the cerebellum. **V. Syl'vii,** a depression made by the fissure of Sylvius at base of brain. **V. un'guis,** the socket for the root of a nail.

Valleix's points (val-lāz'). Tender spots (puncta dolorosa) in neuralgia.

Vallet's mass (val-lāz'). Mass of iron carbonate or ferrous carbonate.

Val'ley of the cerebellum. Longitudinal cerebellar fissure.

Valsal'va's experiment. Auto-inflation of the tympanic cavity. **V.'s sinuses,** pouches in aorta and pulmonary artery behind each semilunar valve.

Valve. A fold in a canal or passage which prevents reflux of its contents. **Aortic v.,** semilunar valve at aortic entrance. **Bauhin's v.,** fold at junction of ileum and cecum. **Bicuspid v.** See *Mitral v.* **Coronary v.,** a valve at entrance of coronary sinus into right auricle. **Hasner's v.,** kind of valve at lower meatus of nose. **Heister's v.,** fold inside of neck of gall-bladder. **Ileocecal v.** See *Bauhin's v.* **Ileocolic v.,** fold between ileum and colon. **Kerkring's v's.,** the valvulæ conniventes. **Mitral v.,** valve between left auricle and left ventricle. **Pulmonary v.,** valve at junction of pulmonary artery and right ventricle. **Pyloric v.,** mucous fold at the pylorus. **Semilunar v's.,** valves which guard entrances to aorta and pulmonary artery. **Thebesius's v.** See *Coronary v.* **Tricuspid v.** controls opening from right auricle to right ventricle. **V. of Varolius,** the ileocecal valve. **V. of Vieussens,** white layer that connects superior peduncles of cerebellum and roofs the fourth ventricle.

Val'vula (val'vu-lah). A small valve.

Val'vulæ conniven'tes. Transverse mucous folds in small intestine.

Val'vular. Of, or pertaining to, a valve.

Val'zin (val'zin). Same as *Dulcin*.

Vana'dium. A white and rare metal: symbol V.

Van Bu'ren's disease. Chronic inflammation of the corpora cavernosa.

Van Hook's operation. Uretero-ureterostomy.

Vanil'la. A genus of climbing orchids. Fruit of *V. planifolia* is a stimulant and flavoring agent.

Vanil'lin. Aromatic principle, $C_8H_8O_3$, from vanilla.

Vanil'lism. Dermatitis and pruritus from handling vanilla.

Van Swie'ten's solution. Solution of one part of mercury perchlorid in 900 parts of water and 100 parts of alcohol.

Va'por. A gas which at ordinary temperatures is a liquid or solid. **V.-bath,** immersion in a vapor, usually hot. **V.-douche,** treatment by a jet of hot vapor.

Vapo'rium. A device for treating disease by the local application of heat or cold.

Vaporiza'tion. Conversion into vapor; treatment by a vapor.

Vap'orole. A glass capsule containing a single dose of a volatile drug.

Varicel'la. Chicken-pox; an infectious eruptive disease of childhood.

Var'iciform. Having the form of a varix.

Varicobleph'aron (var-ik-o-blef'ar-on). A varicose tumor of the eyelid.

Var'icocele (var'ik-o-sēl). Enlargement of the scrotal and spermatic veins.

Varicocelec'tomy. Removal of a part of scrotum for varicocele.

Varicom'phalos (var-ik-om'fal-os). A varicose tumor of the umbilicus.

Var'icose aneurysm. See *Aneurysm*. **V. vein,** a greatly enlarged and contorted vein.

Varicos'ity. 1. A varix. 2. Quality of being varicose.

Varicot'omy. Excision of a varix or varicose vein.

Varic'ula. A varix of the conjunctiva.

Vari'ola. Small-pox; an acute infectious fever characterized by a general eruption and followed by pitting. **Black v.** See *Hemorrhagic v.* **Coherent v.,** the pustules coalesce at edges, but do not become confluent. **Confluent v.,** severe form with pustules becoming more or less confluent. **Discrete v.,** the pustules remain distinct. **Hemorrhagic v.,** hemorrhage occurs into the vesicles, or from mucous surfaces. **Malignant v.,** severe and fatal form of hemorrhagic v. **Modified v.** See *Varioloid*. **V. ve'ra,** simple and unmodified small-pox.

Vari'olate. Of the nature of variola.

Variola'tion, Varioliza'tion. Inoculation with unmodified small-pox.

Varioloid'. A modified and mild form of small-pox.

Vari'olous. Of, or pertaining to, small-pox.

Variolovac'cine. Virus obtained by inoculating a heifer with small-pox.

Variolovaccin'ia. Cow-pox in the heifer caused by inoculation with small-pox.

Va'rix. An enlarged and tortuous vein. **V. lymphat'icus,** an enlarged and tortuous lymphatic vessel.

Var'nish. A resinous solution in oil or alcohol: it is of limited use in surgery.

Varo'lian. Pertaining to the pons Varolii. **V. bend,** the third fetal cerebral flexure.

Va'rus. 1. Having the legs bowed in; in-kneed. 2. See *Talipes varus*.

Vas, pl. *va'sa*. A vessel. **V. aber'rans.** 1. A blind tube sometimes connected with the epididymis or vas deferens. 2. Any anomalous or unusual vessel. **V. def'erens,** excretory duct of the testicle passing from the testis to the ejaculatory duct.

Va'sa, pl. of *vas.* **V. afferen'tia,** the lymphatic vessels which enter a gland. **V. bre'via,** the small branches of the splenic artery going to the stomach. **V. efferen'tia,** lymphatics which leave a gland. **V. rec'ta,** straight tubes formed by the seminiferous tubules. **V. vaso'rum,** the arteries and veins in the walls of the larger blood-vessels. **V. vortico'sa,** the stellate veins of the choroid.

Va'sal. Pertaining to a vas, or vessel.

Vasa'lium. True vascular tissue.

Vas'cular. Pertaining to, or full of, vessels.

Vascular'ity (vas-ku-lar'it-e). Condition of being vascular.

Vasculariza'tion. The process of becoming vascular; a furnishing with new vessels.

Vas'cularize. To supply with vessels; to render vascular.

Vas'culum aber'rans. The *Vas aberrans.*

Vasec'tomy. Surgical removal of the vas deferens.

Vas'elin (vas'el-in). A variety of petrolatum.

Vas'icin (vas'is-in). An alkaloid from *Adhatoda vasica.*

Vasifac'tive. Producing new vessels.

Vas'iform. Resembling a vas, or vessel.

Vasoconstric'tive. Contracting the blood-vessels.

Vasoconstric'tor. 1. Causing constriction of blood-vessels. 2. A vasoconstrictive nerve.

Vasocoro'na. The assemblage of arteries which pass radially into the spinal cord from its periphery.

Vasoden'tin. Dentin provided with blood-vessels.

Vasodila'tor. 1. Causing dilatation of blood-vessels. 2. A nerve thus acting.

Vasofac'tive, Vasofor'mative. Same as *Vasifactive.*

Vasogan'glion. Any vascular ganglion or rete.

Vas'ogene. A proprietary petrolatum preparation.

Vasohyperton'ic (va-zo-hi-per-ton'ik). Same as *Vasoconstrictor.*

Vasohypoton'ic (va-zo-hi-po-ton'ik). Same as *Vasodilator.*

Vaso-inhib'itor. A vasodilator nerve.

Vaso-inhib'itory. Same as *Vasodilator.*

Va'sol. A proprietary form of atomizer.

Vasomo'tion. The contraction or dilatation of a vessel.

Vasomo'tor. 1. Either vasoconstrictor or vasodilator. 2. Any agent that effects vasomotion.

Vasomo'tory. Effecting vasomotion.

Vasosen'sory. Supplying sensory filaments to the vessels.

Vasoton'ic. Regulating the tone of a vessel.

Vasotroph'ic. Affecting nutrition through alteration of the caliber of the blood-vessels.

Vas'tus (vas'tus). See *Muscles, Table of.*

Va'ter's ampullæ (vah'ters). Dilatation at junction of common bile-duct and pancreatic duct. **V.'s corpuscles,** tactile subcutaneous end-organs.

Vec'tis. A curved lever for making traction on the fetal head in labor.

Veg'etal (vej'et-al). Common to plants and animals alike.

Vegeta'rian. One whose food is exclusively of vegetable origin.

Vegeta'rianism. The opinion and practice which restricts man's food to substances of vegetable origin.

Vegeta'tion. A plant-like neoplasm.

Veg'etative. Concerned with growth and nutrition. **V. pole,** that pole of an ovum which contains food-matter.

Vegeto-an'imal. Common to plants and animals.

Ve'hicle (ve'hik-l). An excipient.

Veil (vāl). 1. A caul or piece of amniotic sac occasionally covering the face of a new-born child. 2. Slight huskiness of the voice.

Vein (vān). A vessel which conveys blood to or toward the heart. **Angular v.**, downward extension of frontal going to facial v. **Auditory v's.** accompany the ear arteries. **Axillary v.**, large v. which receives the brachial v's. **Azygos v's.**, three veins which connect the precava and postcava. **Basilar v.**, large v. which goes to Galen's v. **Basilic v.**, on palmar side of forearm. **Brachial v's.** accompany brachial artery. **Brachiocephalic v.**, the innominate v. **Breschet's v's.**, v's. of the diploë. **Cephalic v.**, a great v. of the arm. **Coronary v.** goes to coronary sinus of the heart. **Emissary v's.**, veins connecting cerebral sinuses with external veins of head. **Facial v.**, extension of angular v. to internal jugular. **Femoral v., common**, accompanies femoral artery and becomes the external iliac. **Femoral v., deep**, accompanies femoral artery and goes to superficial femoral. **Femoral v., superficial**, joins with deep femoral to form common femoral v. **Galen's v's.**, two v's. of brain going to the straight sinus. **Gastric v.** accompanies gastric artery. **Hemiazygos v's.**, veins accessory to azygos v's. **Hemorrhoidal v's.**, plexus around the rectum. **Iliac v., common**, vein formed by confluence of external and internal iliac v's. **Iliac v., external**, upward extension of common femoral. **Iliac v., internal**, joins the external to form common iliac. **Innominate v.**, great v., formed by internal jugular and subclavian, going to the precava. **Jugular v., anterior**, a branch of external jugular. **Jugular v., external**, a branch of the subclavian. **Jugular v., internal**, goes from lateral sinus to the innominate v. **Marshall's v.** See *Oblique v.* **Median basilic v.** joins superficial ulnar and forms basilic. **Median cephalic v.** joins superficial radial to form cephalic. **Median v's., deep** and **superficial**, veins of the forearm. **Oblique v.**, on dorsal aspect of left auricle. **Ophthalmic v.** goes from eye to cavernous sinus. **Popliteal v.** of leg and thigh becomes the femoral v. **Portal v.** takes blood of superior mesenteric and portal v's. to liver. **Pulmonary v's.**, four v's., two from either lung to left auricle. **Radial v.**, from dorsum of wrist to cephalic vein. **Renal v.** accompanies renal artery. **Salvatella v.**, vein from little finger. **Saphenous v., external**, or **short**, of foot, leg, and calf to popliteal. **Saphenous v., internal**, or **long**, long v. on inner aspect of thigh to femoral v. **Spermatic v.** returns the blood of the testis on the right to postcava, on the left to left renal. **Splenic v.** goes from spleen to portal v. **Subclavian v.**, from axillary v. to innominate v. **Temporomaxillary v.**, from temporal and internal maxillary v's. to external jugular. **Trolard's v.** runs along posterior branch of fissure of Sylvius to superior petrosal sinus. **Ulnar v.**, principal v. of anterior and ulnar aspect of forearm. **Umbilical v.** conveys blood from placenta to fetus. **V. of Vesalius**, vein going from the pterygoid plexus to the cavernous sinus. **Vitelline v's.**, fetal veins from yolk-sac to sinus venosus.

Vela'men. Any membrane, meninx, or tegument. **V. vul'væ**, the Hottentot apron.

Ve'lar. Pertaining to a velum.

Vellica'tion. A twitching of the muscle.

Velpeau's bandage. A bandage for fracture of the clavicle.

Ve'lum. Any veil or veil-like organ. **Anterior** or **superior v.** See *Valve of Vieussens.* **Inferior** or **posterior v.**, **V. of Tari'nus**, the commissure of the flocculi of the cerebellar hemisphere. **V. interpo'situm**, membranous roof of the third ventricle. **V. pal'ati**, the soft palate.

Ve'na, pl. *ve'næ*. L. for *Vein*.

Ve'næ ca'væ. The precava (vena cava descendens) and postcava (vena cava ascendens). **V. com'ites**, veins which accompany an artery. **V. Gale'ni**, two veins of the cerebrum which discharge themselves into the straight sinus. **V. stella'tæ.** See *Stars of Verheyen*. **V. Thebe'sii.** See *Thebesius's foramina*. **V. vortico'sæ**, the venous network of the choroid.

Venena'tion. Poisoning; a poisoned condition.

Veneno'sa. Venomous snakes collectively.

Ven'enous (ven'en-us). Poisonous or toxic.

Vene'real. Due to, or propagated by, sexual intercourse.

Ven'ery (ven'er-e). Sexual commerce; coitus.

Venesec'tion. The opening of a vein for the letting of blood.

Ven'iplex (ven'ip-lex). A venous plexus.

Ven'om. A poison, especially one normally produced by an animal. **V.-globulin**, a globulin from snake-poison. **V.-peptone**, a peptone from snake-poison.

Venos'ity. Excess of venous blood in a part.

Ve'nous (ve'nus). Of, or pertaining to, the veins. **V. blood**, the blood which is contained in the veins. **V. hum**, the murmur which is heard over the larger veins in anemia.

Vensto'ria. A proprietary food preparation.

Vent. 1. An outlet, as for pus. 2. The anus. 3. Free discharge.

Ven'ter. The belly; any belly-like part.

Ventila'tion. The process of supplying with fresh air.

Ven'tose (ven'tōs). A cupping-glass.

Ven'trad. Toward a belly, venter, or ventral aspect.

Ven'tral. Pertaining to the abdomen. **V. zone of His**, the ventral thickening of the embryonic dorsal spinal cord projecting into the central canal.

Ven'tricle. Any cavity; either one of the two lower and larger cavities (right and left ventricles) of the heart, or of the various cavities of the brain. **V. of Arantius**, lower end of fourth ventricle. **Callosal v.**, space between either labium cerebri and the callosum. **Fifth v.**, narrow space between layers of septum lucidum. **Fourth v.** represents primitive cavity of the hindbrain. **V. of the larynx**, space between the true and false vocal cords. **Lateral v.**, space in each cerebral hemisphere representing the cavity of original cerebral vesicle. **V. of the myelon**, the central canal of spinal cord. **Pineal v.**, the cavity beneath or within the pineal body. **Third v.**, space which represents the cavity of embryonic forebrain. **Verga's v.**, occasional space between the callosum and fornix.

Ventricor'nu. The ventral horn of gray matter in the spinal cord.

Ventricor'nual. Pertaining to the ventricornu.

Ventric'ular. Of, or pertaining to, a ventricle. **V. aqueduct.** See *Aqueductus Sylvii*. **V. ligament**, a false vocal cord. **V. muscle**, the thyreo-epiglottideus.

Ventric'ulus. L. for *Ventricle*.

Ventricum'bent. Prone; lying on the belly.

Ven'triduct. To bring or carry ventrad.

Ventrifixa'tion. Same as *Ventrofixation*.

Ventrifixu'ra u'teri. Fixation of uterus to the wall of the abdomen.

Ventrimeson. The median line on the ventral surface.

Ventripyr'amid. The ventral pyramid of the oblongata.

Ventrocystor'rhaphy. The stitching of a cyst to the abdominal wall.

Ventrofixa'tion. The stitching of a viscus to the abdominal wall.

Ven'trose (ven'trōs). Having a belly.

Ventrosuspen'sion. The cure of uterine retroposition by fixing the uterus to the abdominal wall.

Ventrot'omy. Same as *Celiotomy* or *Laparotomy.*

Ventrovesicofixa'tion. The fixation of the uterus and bladder to the abdominal wall.

Ven'ule. A venous radicle or little vein.

Vera'trin. Poisonous alkaloidal mixture from sabadilla: irritant, stimulant, and heart-depressant.

Vera'trinize, Ver'atrize. To bring under the influence of veratrin.

Vera'trol. A medicine, $C_8H_{10}O_2$, which when used externally lowers the temperature, and is safer than guaiacol.

Vera'trum. A genus of plants: *V. viride* is a vasomotor depressant, and is used in sthenic inflammations.

Ver'bal agraphia. See *Agraphia.*

Verbas'cum thap'sus. Mullein, a plant whose leaves and flowers are demulcent and stimulant.

Ver'dea. A variety of Italian wine.

Ver'digris. A mixture of basic copper acetates: used for ringworm, etc.

Ver'ga's ventricle. See *Ventricle.*

Verhey'en's stars. See *Stars of Verheyen.*

Ver'juice. A preparation of the juice of unripe grapes.

Ver'micide. A remedy that destroys intestinal worms.

Vermic'ular. Worm-like. **V. movements,** peristaltic movements.

Vermicula'tion. Peristaltic motion; peristalsis.

Ver'miform. Worm-shaped. **V. appendix.** See under *Appendix.* **V. process,** either surface (superior or inferior) of the median lobe of the cerebellum, or the lobe itself.

Vermif'ugal (ver-mif'u-gal). Expelling intestinal worms.

Ver'mifuge (ver'mif-ūj). An anthelmintic medicine.

Vermina'tion. Infestation with worms or with other vermin.

Ver'minous. Pertaining, or due, to worms.

Ver'mis. 1. L. for *Worm.* 2. Median lobe of the cerebellum.

Ver'muth. A liqueur prepared with wine and aromatic herbs.

Ver'nal catarrh, V. conjunctivitis. Conjunctivitis recurring with the spring.

Ver'nin. Alkaloid or base, $C_{16}H_{20}N_8O_8$, from clover, vetches, and ergot.

Ver'nix caseo'sa. Unctuous substance which covers the skin of the fetus.

Verno'nin. A cardiant principle, $C_{10}H_{24}O_7$, from *Vernonia nigritiana,* an African plant.

Verru'ca. A wart. **V. acumina'ta,** pointed condyloma of the genitals or anus. **V. men'strua,** homeopathic preparation of the menses of a woman with warts. **V. necrogen'ica,** node of the skin due to dissection-poisoning; dissection-tubercle. **V. Perua'na,** Peruvian wart; an endemic disease of Peru.

Verru'ciform (ver-u'sif-orm). Shaped like a wart.

Verru'cose, Verru'cous. Warty; like a wart.

Verru'gas. Same as *Verruca Peruana.*

Ver'sion. The act of turning; especially the manual turning of the fetus in delivery. **Bipolar v.** is effected by acting upon both poles of fetus. **Cephalic v.,** turning of fetus so that the head presents. **Combined v.,** external and internal versions together. **External v.** is effected by outside manipulation. **Internal v.** is done by the hand within uterus. **Pelvic v.,** version by manipulation of the breech. **Podalic v.,** that which brings down one or both feet. **Spontaneous v.,** one which is effected without aid from without.

Ver'tebra. Any one of the thirty-three bones of the spinal column; also, any one of the segments of which the cranium and facial bones are made up.

Ver'tebral. Of, or pertaining to, a vertebra, or the vertebræ. **V. arch,** the neural arch. **V. canal,** the tube which encloses the spinal cord. **V. column,** the backbone. **V. foramen.** 1. The hollow space enclosed by a vertebral arch. 2. A vertebrarterial foramen. **V. groove,** the groove lying outside of the laminæ of the vertebræ. **V. ribs,** the last two, or floating ribs.

Vertebra'rium. The spinal column.

Vertebrarte'rial foramen. A foramen in the transverse processes of the cervical vertebræ for the vertebral artery.

Ver'tebrate, Ver'tebrated. Having a vertebral column or resembling one.

Vertebrochon'dral. Connected with a vertebra and a costal cartilage.

Vertebrocos'tal. Pertaining to a vertebra and a rib.

Vertebromam'mary diameter. The anteroposterior diameter of the chest.

Vertebroster'nal. Connected with a vertebra and the sternum.

Ver'tex. The summit or top; crown of the head. **V.-presentation.** See under *Presentation.*

Vertig'inous. Affected with, or pertaining to, vertigo.

Verti'go (ver-ti'go, but usually called ver'tig-o). Giddiness or dizziness. **Auditory v., Aural v.,** is due to ear-disease. **Cerebral v.** is due to some brain-disease. **Epileptic v.** attends or follows an epileptic attack. **Essential v.** is without discoverable cause. **Gastric v.** is associated with disease of stomach. **Hysterical v.,** form associated with hysteria. **Labyrinthine v.** See *Menière's disease.* **Lithemic v.** is associated with gout and lithemia. **Objective v.,** objects seem to patient to be moving around him. **Ocular v.** is caused by eye-disease. **Organic v.,** caused by lesion of brain or cord. **Paralyzing v.** See *Gerlier's disease.* **Peripheral v.** is due to non-central irritation. **Special-sense v.,** aural or ocular v. **Subjective v.,** that in which the patient seems to himself to be turning round and round. **Toxemic v.** is due to some poison in the blood.

Verumonta'num. A rounded projection on the floor of the prostatic portion of the urethra.

Vesa'lius, foramen of. See *Foramen.* **V., vein of.** See *Vein.*

Vesa'nia. Strict insanity with neither coma nor pyrexia.

Vesan'ic. Pertaining to strict or pure insanity.

Vesi'ca (ves-i'kah). L. for *Bladder.*

Ves'ical. Of, or pertaining to, the bladder. **V. crises,** paroxysms of pain in the bladder in locomotor ataxia.

Ves'icant, Ves'icatory. 1. A blistering drug or agent. 2. Blistering.

Vesica'tion. Act of blistering; a blister.

Ves'icle. A small blister or bladder. **Allantoic v.,** internal hollow portion of allantois. **Auditory v.,** a part of cerebral v. whence percipient parts of ear are formed. **Blastodermic v.,** sac formed by blastoderm. **Cerebral v.,** embryonic expansion of neural canal whence the brain is formed. **Compound v.,** one which has more than one chamber. **Germinal v.,** nucleus of an ovum. **Graafian v.,** structure which holds the ovum while still within the ovary. **Olfactory v.,** vesicle in the embryo developing into olfactory bulb and tract. **Optic v.,** process of cerebral vesicle whence percipient parts of eye are formed. **Otic v.** See *Auditory v.* **Seminal v.,** either one of two réservoirs for semen. **Umbilical v.** See *Yolk-sac.*

Ves'icocele. Hernia of bladder.

Vesicocer'vical. Pertaining to the bladder and cervix uteri.

Vesicofixa'tion. The stitching of the uterus to the bladder.
Vesicoprostat'ic. Of, or pertaining to, the bladder and prostate.
Vesicopu'bic. Pertaining to the bladder and pubes.
Vesicospi'nal. Pertaining to the bladder and spine.
Vesicot'omy. Incision of the bladder.
Vesico-u'terine. Of, or pertaining to, the bladder and uterus.
Vesicovag'inal. Of, or pertaining to, the bladder and vagina.
Vesic'ula. L. for *Vesicle.* **V. germinati'va.** See *Germinal vesicle.* **V. semina'les.** See *Seminal vesicles.*
Vesic'ular. Of, pertaining to, or of the nature of, a vesicle. **V. breathing, V. respiration,** breathing characterized by soft low murmur of normal respiration. **V. column, V. cylinder,** a column of nerve-cells in the dorsal gray horn of the spinal cord. **V. eczema,** vesicular eruption of the scalp. **V. murmur.** Same as *V. breathing.* **V. râle.** Same as *Crepitant râle.*
Vesicula'tion. Presence or formation of vesical râle.
Vesic'uliform. Shaped like a vesicle.
Vesiculi'tis. Inflammation of a vesicle.
Vesiculocav'ernous. Both vesicular and cavernous.
Vesiculotympan'ic. Both vesicular and tympanic.
Vespa'jus. Suppurative inflammation of the hairy part of the scalp.
Ves'sel. Any canal for carrying a fluid, as blood or lymph. **Absorbent v's.,** the lymphatics and lacteals. **Hemorrhoidal v's.,** varicose veins of the rectum. **Nutrient v's.,** vessels supplying the interior of bones.
Vestib'ular. Of, or pertaining to, the vestibule.
Ves'tibule. The oval cavity of the internal ear forming the approach to the cochlea. **V. of aorta,** small space at root of aorta. **V. of ear,** cavity at entrance to cochlea in the internal ear. **V. of nose,** anterior part of the nostrils. **V. of pharynx,** the fauces. **V. of vagina,** space below clitoris and between nymphæ.
Vestibulo-ure'thral. Pertaining to the vestibule of the vulva and to the urethra.
Vestib'ulum. L. for *Vestibule.*
Ves'tige. A rudimentary or degenerate part which, either in the embryo or in some other species or organism, is well developed.
Vestig'ial. Of the nature of a vestige or trace. **V. fold,** a fibrous band of the pericardium representing the obliterated left innominate vein.
Vesu'vin. Bismarck brown: used as a microscopic stain.
Vet. Popular name for a veterinary surgeon.
Ve'ta. A form of mountain-sickness in the Andes.
Veterina'rian. A veterinary surgeon.
Vet'erinary. Pertaining to domestic animals.
Viabil'ity. Ability to live after birth.
Vi'able (vi'ab-l). Able to live or likely to live.
Vi'al (vi'al). A small bottle.
Vi'bex. A linear ecchymosis or streak of effused blood.
Vi'bratile (vi'brat-il). Swaying or moving to and fro.
Vibra'tion. The act of swaying or undulating.
Vi'brator. An apparatus used in vibratory treatment.
Vi'bratory. Having a vibrating or to-and-fro movement.
Vib'rio. A genus of microbes. **V. of Metschnikoff,** a species which causes a fatal form of septicemia.
Vibris'sæ. The hairs within the nostrils; also, the whiskers of a cat.
Vibrom'eter, Vi'brophone. Devices used in the treatment of deafness due to deposits of plastic material or inspissated mucus: they act by producing vibrations which tend to break up adhesions.

Vibrotherapeu'tics. The therapeutic use of vibrating appliances.

Vibur'num. Genus of shrubs. **V. op'ulus** and **V. prunifo'lium** are medicinal species.

Vica'rious. Taking the place of something else. **V. menstruation,** habitual monthly discharge from an abnormal situation.

Vichy water (ve-she'). A mineral water from Vichy, in France: diuretic.

Vic'ious cicatrix. A cicatrix which causes a deformity.

Vi-co'coa. A preparation of malt, hops, kola, and cocoa.

Vicq-d'Azyr's bundle. Band of nerve-fibers going from the thalamus to the corpus albicans.

Vid'ian artery. Branch of internal maxillary running along the Vidian nerve. **V. canal,** foramen in sphenoid bone for Vidian nerve and artery. **V. nerve.** See *Nerves, Table of.*

Vien'na caustic, V. paste. Paste of quicklime and caustic potash.

Vie'rin. A substance from a tropical American tree, not unlike quinin.

Vieussens, valve of (ve-uh-sounz'). See *Valve.*

Vigfutinor'mal. Having one-twentieth of what is normal.

Vi'go plaster (ve'go). Plaster of turpentine, wax, lead-plaster, mercury, etc.

Vig'oral. A proprietary beef food preparation.

Villa'ti's solution (vil-lah'tēs). Solution of 6 parts each of zinc sulphate and copper sulphate, 12 of solution of lead subacetate, and 70 of vinegar.

Vil'li (vil'i). The plural of *villus.*

Villi'tis. Inflammation of the villous tissue of the coronet and of the plantar substance of the horse's foot.

Vil'lose, Vil'lous. Shaggy with soft hairs.

Villos'ity. 1. Condition of being covered with villi. 2. A villus.

Vil'lus, pl. *vil'li.* 1. A vascular chorionic tuft. 2. A minute club-shaped projection from the mucous membrane of the intestine.

Vin'cula ten'dinum. Filaments which connect the phalanges with the flexor tendons.

Vin'culum (ving'ku-lum), pl. *vincula.* A band or frenum.

Vin'egar. 1. A weak and impure dilution of acetic acid. 2. A medicinal preparation of dilute acetic acid. **Aromatic v.,** a refreshing restorative preparation of alcohol with various aromatic oils.

Vino'lia. A proprietary toilet and healing preparation.

Vi'nous. Pertaining to, or of the nature of, wine.

Vi'num (vi'num). L. for *Wine.*

Vi'olet-blindness. Inability to distinguish violet tints.

Vir'gin. A woman or girl who has had no sexual intercourse.

Virgin'ity. Maidenhood; condition of being a virgin.

Vir'idin. An alkaloid of *Veratrum viride.*

Vir'ile. Peculiar to man, or the male sex; procreative. **V. reflex,** retraction of the accelerator urinæ muscle on tapping the penis.

Viriles'cence. Manifestation of male qualities in women of advanced age.

Viril'ia (vir-il'e-ah). Male generative organs.

Viril'ity. Normal reproductive power in the male sex.

Virip'otent (vir-ip'o-tent). Marriageable; nubile.

Vir'ol. A preparation of malt and marrow.

Vi'rose, Vi'rous. Having poisonous qualities.

Vir'tual cautery. See *Cautery, Potential.*

Vir'ulence. Extreme poisonousness or acrimony.

Vir'ulent. Exceedingly noxious or deleterious.

Viruliferous. Conveying a virus or infectious germ.

Vi'rus. An animal poison, especially one produced by, and capable of transmitting, a disease. **V. anima'tum,** a living bacterial poison.

Vis, pl. *vi'res.* L. for *Force* or *Energy.* **V. a fron'te,** a force that draws or attracts. **V. a ter'go,** force that pushes. **V. formati'va,** energy which manifests itself in the formation of new tissue. **V. medica'trix natu'ræ,** the healing power of unaided nature.

Vis'cera (vis'ser-ah), pl. of *viscus.*

Vis'cerad (vis'ser-ad). Toward the viscera.

Vis'ceral (vis'ser-al). Of, or pertaining to, viscera. **V. arches,** the postoral or pharyngeal arches; a series of four lateral folds of the anterior walls of the embryo in the neck-region. **V. clefts,** fissures between the visceral arches.

Visceral'gia. Pain in the viscera.

Vis'ceralism. The opinion that the viscera are the main seats of disease.

Viscerimo'tor. Conveying motor stimulus to a viscus.

Visceropto'sis. Prolapse or downward displacement of a viscus.

Vis'cid, Vis'cous. Glutinous; adhesive; sticky.

Viscid'ity, Viscos'ity. The property of being adhesive.

Vis'cus, pl. *vis'cera.* Any large interior organ in any of the four great bodily cavities, especially those in the abdomen.

Vis'ion (vizh'un). The faculty or act of seeing; sight. **Binocular v.,** use of both eyes together without diplopia. **Central v., Direct v.,** that performed by macula lutea. **Chromatic v.** See *Chromatopsia.* **Double v.,** diplopia. **Half-v.,** hemianopia. **Indirect v., Peripheral v.,** that performed by parts of retina outside the macula lutea. **Multiple v.,** polyopia. **Solid v., Stereoscopic v.,** is that which gives perception of relief, or of depth of objects.

Vis'ual (viz'u-al). Pertaining to vision or sight. **V. angle,** angle made at the eye by lines joining the extremities of objects and the nodal point. **V. axis,** line through nodal point and center of cornea to object of vision. **V. field,** space containing all objects visible while the eye is in a fixed position. **V. purple,** purple pigment in the retinal rods, bleached by action of light; rhodopsin.

Visuo-au'ditory. Pertaining to both sight and hearing.

Vi'tal (vi'tal). Of, or pertaining to, life. **V. capacity,** the quantity of air a person can breathe out after a full inspiration. **V. signs,** temperature, pulse, and respiration.

Vi'talism. The opinion that bodily functions are produced by a distinct principle called vital force.

Vi'talist (vi'tal-ist). A believer in vitalism.

Vi'tals. The parts and organs necessary to life.

Vi'tamalt. A proprietary malt-extract.

Vi'tapath. A vitapathic practitioner.

Vi'tapathic. Pertaining to vitapathy.

Vitap'athy. A so-called school of quack medicine.

Vit'ellary (vit'el-a-re). Same as *Vitelline.*

Vitel'lin. A globulin from the yolk of egg.

Vit'elline. Resembling, or pertaining to, the vitellus or yolk. **V. artery,** a fetal artery from the primitive aorta to the yolk-sac. **V. duct,** the omphalomesenteric duct. **V. membrane,** the outer membrane lining the ovum. **V. veins,** fetal veins from the yolk-sac to the sinus venosus.

Vitelloin'tein. Yellow pigment obtainable from lutein.

Vitelloru'bin. A reddish pigment obtainable from lutein.

Vitili'go. A skin-disease with formation of smooth patches Same as *Xanthoma* and *Leukoderma.*

Vitiligoid'ea. See *Leukoderma.*

Vitodynam'ic. Pertaining to vital force.

Vitreocapsuli'tis. Inflammation of membrane which enfolds the vitreous body.

Vitreoden'tin. A dense and glass-like form of dentin.

Vit'reous. 1. Glassy or hyaline. 2. Same as *V. body*. **V. body, V. humor,** transparent semifluid mass between the lens and the retina. **V. chamber,** the largest and most posterior of the chambers of the eye. **V. degeneration,** hyaline degeneration. **V. electricity,** positive static electricity. **V. membrane.** 1. The inner membrane of the choroid. 2. A membrane of hair-follicles separating outer root-sheath from internal layer. **V. table,** the inner table of a cranial bone.

Vit'riol. Any crystalline sulphate. **Blue v.,** copper-sulphate. **Green v.,** iron-sulphate; copperas. **Oil of v.,** sulphuric acid. **White v.,** zinc-sulphate.

Vi'trum. L. for *Glass*.

Vit'ular. Pertaining to a calf.

Vit'ulary fever. A puerperal brain-affection of cows.

Vivifica'tion. The conversion of lifeless into living proteid matter in the process of assimilation.

Viviperception. The study of the vital processes of a living organism.

Viv'isect. To dissect while yet alive.

Vivisec'tion. Dissection or cutting operation upon a living animal.

Vivisec'tionist. One who practises or defends vivisection.

Vivisec'tor. One who vivisects or practises vivisection.

Vivisecto'rium. A place for the performance of vivisections.

Vlem'inckx's solution (flem'ingz). Solution of lime and sulphur in water or in petroleum.

Vo'cal. Of, or pertaining to, the voice. **V. area,** that part of the glottis which lies between the vocal cords. **V. cords,** the thyreo-arytenoid ligaments of the larynx: the inferior are called *true*, and the superior *false*, vocal cords. **V. fremitus,** a vibration or thrill of the chest-wall in speaking. **V. ligaments,** the true vocal cords, or thyreo-arytenoid ligaments. **V. muscle.** See *Thyreo-arytenoideus*, in *Muscles, Table of*. **V. process,** a process of the arytenoid cartilage to which the vocal cords are attached. **V. signs,** indications of disease shown by changes of voice, as in fremitus or resonance.

Vod'ka. A variety of whiskey made in Russia.

Voice. A sound uttered by the mouth.

Void. To cast out as waste matter.

Vo'la (vo'lah). The sole or palm.

Vo'lar. Pertaining to a palm or sole.

Vol'atile (vol'at-il). Tending to evaporate rapidly.

Volatiliza'tion. Conversion or change into a vapor.

Voli'tion. The act or power of willing.

Volk'mann's canals (fōlk'mahnz). Passages in the subperiosteal layer of bones communicating with the Haversian canals.

Vol'ley. A rhythmic succession of muscle-twitches artificially induced.

Volsel'la. Forceps with double-toothed blades.

Volt. The unit of electromotive force; one ampere of current against one ohm of resistance.

Vol'tage. Electromotive force measured in volts.

Volta'ic. Pertaining to Volta, an electrician. **V. electricity,** electricity developed through chemical action. **V. irritability,** responsiveness of muscle to galvanic stimulus.

Vol'taism (vōl'ta-izm). Same as *Galvanism*.

Voltam'eter. Apparatus for measuring strength of a galvanic current.

Volt'meter. Instrument for measuring electromotive force in volts.

Voltoli'ni's disease. Purulent labyrinthic otitis.

Volumet'ric analysis. See *Analysis.*

Vol'untary. Accomplished in accordance with the will.

Voluntomo'tory. Subject to voluntary motor influence.

Vo'lupty. Sensual pleasure.

Vol'vulus. Intestinal obstruction due to a knotting and twisting of the bowel.

Vo'mer. Bone which forms the lower and posterior portion of the septum of the nose.

Vo'merine. Of, or pertaining to, the vomer.

Vomerobas'ilar canals. Canal formed at junction of the sphenoid bone and vomer.

Vom'ica. 1. Abnormal cavity in an organ, especially in the lung. 2. Profuse and sudden expectoration of pus or putrescent matter.

Vom'it. 1. Matter expelled from the stomach by the mouth. 2. An emetic. **Bilious v.,** vomit stained with bile. **Black v.,** darkened blood cast up from the stomach in yellow fever. **Coffee-ground v.,** bloody vomit of malignant stomach-disease.

Vom'iting. Forcible ejection of contents of stomach through the mouth. **Dry v.,** nausea with attempts at vomiting, but with the ejection of nothing but gas. **Incoercible v.,** vomiting that cannot be controlled. **Pernicious v.,** vomiting in pregnancy so severe as to threaten patient's life. **Stercoraceous v.,** vomiting of fecal matter.

Vom'ito ni'gro. Black vomit; also, yellow fever.

Vom'itory (vom'it-o-re). An emetic.

Vomituri'tion. Repeated ineffectual attempt to vomit; retching.

Vom'itus. Vomiting; also, matter vomited. **V. matuti'nus,** the morning vomiting of chronic gastric catarrh.

Von Grae'fe's sign (fŏn gra'fez). Failure of lid to move downward with eyeball in exophthalmic goiter.

Vor'tex. Whorled arrangement of muscle-fibers in the heart.

Vox. L. for *Voice.* **V. choler'ica,** the peculiar suppressed voice of true cholera.

Vul'canite. Vulcanized caoutchouc, or India rubber.

Vul'nerary. An agent which promotes the healing of wounds.

Vul'nerating (vul'ner-a-ting). Inflicting wounds.

Vul'nus (vul'nus), pl. *vul'nera.* L. for *Wounds.*

Vulsel'la, Vulsel'lum. Same as *Volsella.*

Vul'va. The external female genitalia or pudenda.

Vul'var (vul'var). Of, or pertaining to, the vulva.

Vulvis'mus (vul-viz'mus). Same as *Vaginismus.*

Vulvi'tis. Inflammation of the vulva.

Vulvo-u'terine. Pertaining to the vulva and uterus.

Vulvovag'inal. Pertaining to the vulva and the vagina. **V. anus.** See *Anus.* **V. glands.** See *Glands of Bartholini.*

Vulvovagini'tis. Inflammation of the vulva and the vagina.

W.

W. The chemical symbol of *Tungsten.*

Wach'endorf's membrane. 1. The pupillary membrane. 2. The membrane which invests a cell.

Wachs'muth's mixture. Anesthetic mixture of 1 part of oil of turpentine with 5 parts of chloroform.

Wade's balsam. Compound tincture of benzoin.

Wa'fer. A thin layer or paste used to enclose a dose of medicine; also, a flat vaginal suppository.

Wag'ner's corpuscles. The oval-shaped bodies at the termination of certain nerve-fibers; tactile corpuscle.

Wahoo'. See *Euonymus.*

Wal'cheren fever (wol'ker-en). A severe form of remittent fever.

Wal'cher's position. A position in labor in which the woman is in the dorsal posture, with hips at edge of table and lower extremities hanging.

Wal'king typhoid. Typhoid fever in which the patient refuses to go to bed.

Walle'rian degeneration. See under *Degeneration.*

Wall-eye. Leukoma of the cornea; also, divergent strabismus.

Wal'nut. See *Juglans.*

Walpur'gis oil. A petroleum from Eichstädt, Germany: a popular polychrest remedy.

Wan'dering. Moving about; abnormally movable. **W. abscess,** one which burrows and points at a place distant from its original seat. **W. cell,** a leukocyte. **W. kidney, W. spleen.** Same as *Floating kidney* or *spleen.*

Wank'lynize. To treat with Wanklyn's test, as in testing bread for alum.

War'burg's tincture. A powerfully antiperiodic and sudorific mixture.

Ward. A large room in a hospital.

War'drop's operation. Distal ligation of an artery for aneurysm.

Ware'housemen's itch. Palmar eczema among workmen in warehouses.

War'ming plaster. Plaster of pitch with cantharides.

Wart. An elevation of the skin, and sometimes of the mucous membrane, formed by hypertrophy of the papillæ. **Anatomic w.,** warty growth on hands of dissectors.

Wash (wash). A lotion.

Wash'erwomen's itch. Eczema on the hands of laundresses.

Wash'ing soda. Sodium carbonate.

Wash-leath'er-skin. Condition in which silver makes a black mark on the skin.

Wasp. Any stinging hymenopterous insect of the family of which the genus *Vespa* is a type. Wasp-venom has a limited use in homeopathic practice. **W.-waist,** a deformity of the waist due to certain myopathies.

Was'ter (wās'ter). An ox or a cow affected with tuberculosis.

Was'ting palsy. Progressive muscular atrophy.

Watch'makers' cramp. Spasm of the finger-muscles in watchmakers.

Wat'er. A tasteless, inodorous liquid, H_2O. **W.-bag,** a bag for holding hot or cold water for therapeutic application. **W.-bed,** a rubber mattress containing water. **W. on the brain.** See *Hydrocephalus.* **W.-brash.** See *Pyrosis.* **W. on the chest,** hydrothorax. **W.-cure,** hydrotherapy. **W.-dressing,** treatment of wounds by water. **W.-glass,** aqueous solution of sodium silicate: used in surgery, etc. **W.-gruel,** thin porridge containing no milk. **W.-hammer pulse.** See under *Pulse.* **W.-jug, W.-pox,** varicella, or chicken-pox. **W.-rigor,** the state of rigor in a muscle induced by the action of water: a term used in electromotor experiments.

Wat'ers. Same as *Liquor amnii.*

Watt. Amount of pressure developed by one volt of potential with one ampere of current.

Wave-theory. The undulatory theory.

Wa'vy respiration. See *Interrupted respiration.*

Wax. One of a series of plastic substances deposited by insects or obtained from plants. **Shoemakers' w.**, a compound used by cobblers: a popular remedy for cuts and punctures.

Wax'ing kernels. Enlarged lymph-glands on the neck or in the groin of a child.

Wax'y. Resembling or pertaining to wax. **W. degeneration.** See *Degeneration.*

Wean. To cause an infant to cease to take food by sucking.

Wean'ing-brash. Diarrhea occurring as a result of weaning.

Wea'zand. The trachea, or windpipe.

Webbed. Having a membrane which connects with adjacent organs. **W. fingers, W. toes**, the union of toes or fingers by a thin band of tissue.

We'ber. Same as *Coulomb.*

Web'er's law. See *Law.* **W.'s paradox**, a muscle so over-stretched that it cannot contract may become still longer. **W.'s syndrome.** See *Syndrome.*

Weep'ing-eczema. See under *Eczema.* **W.-sinew**, cystoma on a tendon or aponeurosis.

Wei'del's reaction. The murexid-test.

Wei'gert's method. Use of hematoxin for staining nerve-fiber.

Weight. Downward pressure due to gravity. [See *Table of Weights and Measures*, pp. 494–498.] **Atomic w.**, weight of an atom of an element as compared with the weight of an atom of hydrogen. **Molecular w.**, the weight of a molecule of a substance as compared with the weight of an atom of hydrogen.

Weil's disease (wilz). Acute infectious jaundice.

Weir-Mitchell's treatment. Treatment of neurasthenia by liberal feeding, massage, and rest.

Weit'brecht's retinacula (vit'brektz). Ligaments on the neck of the great trochanter.

Wen. A sebaceous cyst; also, a goiter.

Werl'hoff's disease. See *Purpura hemorrhagica.*

Wer'nicke's reaction. A peculiar reaction of the pupil in hemianopia when exposed to light.

West'phal's nucleus. A group of nerve-cells posterior to the proper nucleus of the trochlear nerve. **W.'s symptom**, absence of knee-jerk in locomotor ataxia.

Wet'cup. A cupping-glass to be used after scarification.

Wet-nurse. A nurse who gives suck to her charge.

Wet-pack. The wrapping of a patient in wet sheets.

Whar'ton's canal. W.'s duct. The duct of the submaxillary gland. **W.'s jelly**, the jelly-like tissue of the umbilical cord.

Wheal. A white or pinkish ridge on the skin, as in urticaria or after the stroke of a whip.

Wheel'house's operation. A variety of external urethrotomy.

Wheeze. A sound made by suddenly forcing the breath through the glottis.

Wheez'ing. Difficult breathing attended with a whistling sound.

Whelk. A wheal, or protuberance, on the face.

Whey. The thin serum of milk after the curd and cream are separated.

Whif'fing murmurs. Certain systolic murmurs characteristic of some cases of chlorosis.

Whip-snap action. Sudden spasm of the cremaster, which may bruise and wound the testicle.

Whip-worm. See *Trichocephalus.*

Whirl-bone. 1. The patella, or knee-cap. 2. The head of the femur.

Whish'ing sound. The placental souffle.

Whis'key. Whis'ky. A distilled alcoholic liquor from barley, corn, and potatoes. **W.-nose**, acne rosacea.

TABLE OF WEIGHTS AND MEASURES.

APOTHECARIES' WEIGHT.

Grains.		Scruples.		Drams.		Troy ounces.		Pound.
gr. 20	=	℈ 1						
60	=	3	=	ʒ 1				
480	=	24	=	8	=	℥ 1		
5760	=	288	=	96	=	12	=	℔ 1

AVOIRDUPOIS WEIGHT.

Grains.		Drams.		Ounces.		Pound.
gr. 27.34375	=	dr. 1				
437.5	=	16	=	oz. 1		
7000	=	256	=	16	=	℔ 1

SOLID MEASURE.

Cubic inches.		Cubic feet.		Cubic yard.
1728	=	1		
46656	=	27	=	1

DRY MEASURE.

Pints.		Quarts.		Gallons.		Pecks.		Bushels.		Quarter.
2	=	1								
8	=	4	=	1						
16	=	8	=	2	=	1				
64	=	32	=	8	=	4	=	1		
512	=	256	=	64	=	32	=	8	=	1

APOTHECARIES' (WINE) MEASURE.

Minims.		Fluidrams.		Fluidounces.		Pints.		Gallon.
♏ 60	=	fʒ 1						
480	=	8	=	f℥ 1				
7680	=	128	=	16	=	O 1		
61440	=	1024	=	128	=	8	=	G. 1

IMPERIAL MEASURE.

Minims.		Fluidrams.		Fluidounces.		Pints.		Gallon.
60	=	1						
480	=	8	=	1				
9600	=	160	=	20	=	1		
76800	=	1280	=	160	=	8	=	1

Table for Converting Apothecaries' into Imperial Measure.

APOTHECARIES' MEASURE.		IMPERIAL MEASURE.			
		Pints.	Fluidounces.	Fluidrams.	Minims.
1 minim	=				1.04
1 fluidram	=			1	2.5
1 fluidounce	=		1	0	20
1 pint	=		16	5	18
1 gallon	=	6	13	2	23

Table for Converting Imperial into Apothecaries' Measure.

IMPERIAL MEASURE.		APOTHECARIES' MEASURE.				
		Gallon.	Pints.	Fluidounces.	Fluidrams.	Minims.
1 minim	=					0.96
1 fluidram	=					58
1 fluidounce	=				7	41
1 pint	=		1	3	1	38
1 gallon	=	1	1	9	5	8

METRIC WEIGHTS AND MEASURES.

The *meter*, or unit of length, at 32° F., = 39.370432 inches.
The *liter*, or unit of capacity, = 33.816 fluidounces.
The *gram*, or unit of weight, = 15.43234874 troy grains.

Comparative Values of Apothecaries' and Metric Fluid Measures.

Minims.		Cubic Centimeters.	Minims.		Cubic Centimeters.	Fluid-ounces.		Cubic Centimeters.	Fluid-ounces.		Cubic Centimeters.
1	=	0.06	25	=	1.54	1	=	30.00	21	=	621.00
2	=	0.12	30	=	1.90	2	=	59.20	22	=	650.00
3	=	0.18	35	=	2.16	3	=	89.00	23	=	680.00
4	=	0.24	40	=	2.50	4	=	118.40	24	=	710.00
5	=	0.30	45	=	2.80	5	=	148.00	25	=	740.00
6	=	0.36	50	=	3.08	6	=	178.00	26	=	769.00
7	=	0.42	55	=	3.40	7	=	207.00	27	=	798.50
8	=	0.50				8	=	236.00	28	=	828.00
9	=	0.55				9	=	266.00	29	=	858.00
10	=	0.60	Fluidrams.			10	=	295.70	30	=	887.25
11	=	0.68	1	=	3.75	11	=	325.25	31	=	917.00
12	=	0.74	1¼	=	4.65	12	=	355.00	32	=	946.00
13	=	0.80	1½	=	5.60	13	=	385.00	48	=	1419.00
14	=	0.85	1¾	=	6.51	14	=	414.00	56	=	1655.00
15	=	0.92	2	=	7.50	15	=	444.00	64	=	1892.00
16	=	1.00	3	=	11.25	16	=	473.11	72	=	2128.00
17	=	1.05	4	=	15.00	17	=	503.00	80	=	2365.00
18	=	1.12	5	=	18.50	18	=	532.00	96	=	2839.00
19	=	1.17	6	=	22.50	19	=	562.00	112	=	3312.00
20	=	1.25	7	=	26.00	20	=	591.50	128	=	3785.00

Comparative Values of Apothecaries' and Metric Weights.

Grains.		Grams.	Grains.		Grams.	Grains.		Grams.	Drams.		Grams.
$\frac{1}{100}$	=	0.00065	1	=	0.065	24	=	1.55	1	=	3.90
$\frac{1}{64}$	=	0.00101	2	=	0.130	25	=	1.62	2	=	7.80
$\frac{1}{60}$	=	0.00108	3	=	0.195	26	=	1.70	3	=	11.65
$\frac{1}{50}$	=	0.00130	4	=	0.260	27	=	1.75	4	=	15.50
$\frac{1}{48}$	=	0.00135	5	=	0.324	28	=	1.82	5	=	19.40
$\frac{1}{40}$	=	0.00162	6	=	0.400	29	=	1.87	6	=	23.30
$\frac{1}{36}$	=	0.00180	7	=	0.460	30	=	1.95	7	=	27.20
$\frac{1}{32}$	=	0.00202	8	=	0.520	31	=	2.00	Ounces.		
$\frac{1}{30}$	=	0.00216	9	=	0.600	32	=	2.10	1	=	31.10
$\frac{1}{25}$	=	0.00259	10	=	0.650	33	=	2.16	2	=	62.20
$\frac{1}{24}$	=	0.00270	11	=	0.715	34	=	2.20	3	=	93.30
$\frac{1}{20}$	=	0.00324	12	=	0.780	35	=	2.25	4	=	124.40
$\frac{1}{18}$	=	0.00360	13	=	0.845	36	=	2.30	5	=	155.50
$\frac{1}{16}$	=	0.00405	14	=	0.907	37	=	2.40	6	=	186.60
$\frac{1}{15}$	=	0.00432	15	=	0.972	38	=	2.47	7	=	217.70
$\frac{1}{12}$	=	0.00540	15.5	=	1.000	39	=	2.55	8	=	248.80
$\frac{1}{10}$	=	0.00648	16	=	1.040	40	=	2.60	9	=	280.00
$\frac{1}{8}$	=	0.00810	17	=	1.102	42	=	2.73	10	=	311.00
$\frac{1}{6}$	=	0.01080	18	=	1.160	44	=	2.86	11	=	342.14
$\frac{1}{5}$	=	0.01296	19	=	1.240	48	=	3.00	12	=	373.23
$\frac{1}{4}$	=	0.01620	20	=	1.300	50	=	3.25	14	=	435.50
$\frac{1}{3}$	=	0.02160	21	=	1.360	52	=	3.40	16	=	497.60
$\frac{1}{2}$	=	0.03240	22	=	1.425	56	=	3.65	24	=	746.40
$\frac{3}{4}$	=	0.04860	23	=	1.460	58	=	3.75	48	=	1492.80
									100	=	3110.40

Comparative Values of Metric and Apothecaries' Weights.

Grams.		Grains.	Grams.		Grains.	Grams.		Grains.	Grams.		Grains.
0.0010	=	1/64	0.065	=	1.003	1	=	15.43	100	=	1543.23
0.0020	=	1/32	0.100	=	1.543	2	=	30.86	125	=	1929.04
0.0040	=	1/16	0.130	=	2.006	3	=	46.30	150	=	2314.85
0.0065	=	1/10	0.150	=	2.315	4	=	61.73	175	=	2700.65
0.0081	=	1/8	0.180	=	2.778	5	=	77.16	450	=	6944.55
0.0108	=	1/6	0.200	=	3.086	6	=	92.60	550	=	8487.78
0.0162	=	1/4	0.300	=	4.630	7	=	98.02	650	=	10031.01
0.0324	=	1/2	0.500	=	7.716	8	=	123.46	750	=	11574.26
0.0486	=	3/4	0.700	=	10.803	9	=	138.90	850	=	13117.49
0.0567	=	7/8	0.900	=	13.890	10	=	154.32	1000	=	15432.35

Comparative Values of Avoirdupois and Metric Weights.

Avoir. Ounces.		Grams.	Avoir. Ounces.		Grams.	Avoir. Ounces.		Grams.	Avoir. Pounds.		Grams.
1/16	=	1.772	5	=	141.75	13	=	368.54	3	=	1360.78
1/8	=	3.544	6	=	170.10	14	=	396.90	4	=	1814.37
1/4	=	7.088	7	=	198.45	15	=	425.25	5	=	2267.96
1/2	=	14.175	8	=	226.80	Avoir. Pounds.			6	=	2727.55
1	=	28.350	9	=	255.15	1	=	453.60	7	=	3175.14
2	=	56.700	10	=	283.50	2	=	907.18	8	=	3628.74
3	=	85.050	11	=	311.84	2.2	=	1000.00	9	=	4082.33
4	=	113.400	12	=	340.20				10	=	4535.92

Comparative Values of Metric Fluid and Apothecaries' Measures.

Cubic Centimeters.		Fluid-ounces.	Cubic Centimeters.		Fluid-ounces.	Cubic Centimeters.		Fluidrams.	Cubic Centimeters.		Minims.
1000	=	33.81	400	=	13.53	25	=	6.76	4	=	64.8
900	=	30.43	300	=	10.14	10	=	2.71	3	=	48.6
800	=	27.05	200	=	6.76	9	=	2.43	2	=	32.4
700	=	23.67	100	=	3.38	8	=	2.16	1	=	16.00
600	=	20.29	75	=	2.53	7	=	1.89	0.09	=	1.46
500	=	16.90	50	=	1.69	6	=	1.62	0.07	=	1.14
473	=	16.00	30	=	1.00	5	=	1.35	0.05	=	0.81

Comparative Values of Standard and Metric Measures of Length.

Inches.		Centimeters.	Inches.		Centimeters.	Inches.		Millimeters.	Inches.		Millimeters.
12	=	30.48	6	=	15.24	1/25	=	1.00	5/8	=	15.85
11	=	27.94	5	=	12.70	1/12	=	2.11	2/3	=	16.92
10	=	25.40	4	=	10.16	1/8	=	3.17	3/4	=	19.05
9	=	22.86	3	=	7.62	1/4	=	6.35	5/6	=	21.15
8	=	20.32	2	=	5.08	1/3	=	8.46	7/8	=	22.19
7	=	17.78	1	=	2.54	1/2	=	12.70	11/12	=	23.28

White arsenic. Same as *Arsenic trioxid.* **W. atrophy.** See *Atrophy.* **W. cell, W. corpuscle.** See *Blood-corpuscle.* **W. commissure,** anterior commissure of spinal cord. **W. gangrene.** See under *Gangrene.* **W. lead,** basic lead carbonate. **W. line,** linea alba. **W. matter, W. substance,** that part of brain, spinal cord, and other nervous structures which is composed of white medullated nerve-fibers. **W. precipitate.** See *Precipitate.* **W. softening,** fatty degeneration of brain-substance in which the affected area has become white and anemic. **W. substance of Schwann.** See *Myelia.* **W. swelling,** tuberculous arthritis. **W. vitriol,** zinc sulphate.

Whites (hwits). Same as *Leukorrhea.*

White's operation. Castration for cure of enlarged prostate.

Whit'low. A felon; panaris, or paronychia.

Whoop (hoop). The sonorous and convulsive inspiration of pertussis.

Whoop'ing-cough. Pertussis; an infectious disease characterized by coryza, bronchitis, and violent spasmodic cough.

Wick'ersheimer's fluid. An arsenical fluid for preserving anatomic preparations.

Wi'dal's serum-test (ve'dahls). A test for typhoid fever made by adding one part of blood-serum from a suspected case to ten parts of a bouillon-culture of typhoid bacilli. If the person has typhoid a reaction occurs, consisting of gradual loss of motility in the bacilli after their coagulation into groups.

Wilde's cords (wildz). Bands which cross the callosum transversely. **W.'s incision** or **operation,** incision of skin, subcutaneous tissue, and periosteum covering the mastoid process for relief of mastoid-disease.

Wil'lis, circle of. See *Circle.* **W.'s cords,** bands which cross the superior longitudinal sinus transversely. **W.'s nerve.** See *Spinal accessory,* in *Nerves, Table of.*

Wil'low. A tree of the genus *Salix:* the barks of many species are tonic and antiperiodic.

Wil'son's disease. Acute exfoliative dermatitis.

Winck'el's disease. Epidemic hemoglobinuria of young infants.

Wind'age. Supposed lesion caused by missiles which do not really strike.

Wind'pipe. The trachea.

Wine. Fermented grape-juice; an alcoholic stimulant. **W.-glass,** a measure nearly equal to two fluidounces. **Red w.,** wine of a dark color, like Bordeaux, claret, and especially port. **White w.,** wine of a light color, like Madeira, and especially sherry.

Wing. See *Ala.*

Wins'low, foramen of. See *Foramen.* **W.'s ligament.** See *Ligament.*

Win'tergreen. See *Gaultheria.*

Win'ter-itch. Same as *Pruritus hiemalis.*

Win'trich's sign. See *Sign.*

Wir'sung's canal, W.'s duct. The pancreatic excretory duct.

Wis'dom-tooth. The last molar tooth on either side of each jaw.

Witch-hazel. See *Hamamelis.*

Wolf'fian body. Same as *Mesonephros.* **W. duct,** a canal, the main element of the mesonephros. **W. tubules,** a set of small tubes joining the Wolffian duct at right angles.

Wolfs'bane. Same as *Aconite.*

Womb. See *Uterus.*

Wood-alcohol. Same as *Methyl-alcohol.* **W.-flour,** very fine saw-dust: used in surgical dressings. **W.-naphtha,** hydrocarbon mixture distilled from wood. **W.-oil.** Same as *Gurjun-balsam.*

W.-tar. See *Tar.* **W.-wool,** a proprietary wood-fiber fabric for surgeons' and obstetricians' wadding, sheets, napkins, etc.

Wool. The hair of sheep and lambs: lambs' wool is used in surgery. **W.-fat,** lanolin or agnin; prepared suint of sheeps' wool. **W.-sor'ters' disease.** True anthrax.

Woora'li, Woora're. See *Curare* and *Urari.*

Word-blindness. See *Blindness.* **W.-center,** the center which controls the recognition of the meaning of words. **W.-deafness.** See *Deafness.*

Working distance. The distance of the objective of a microscope from the object.

Worm. See *Helminth.* **W.-abscess,** abscess due to the presence of worms. **Bladder-w.,** tænia echinococcus. **W.-fever,** fever in children due to worms in the intestine. **Guinea-w.** See *Filaria.* **Pin-w.** See *Oxyuris.* **Round-w.** See *Ascaris.* **Tapew.** See *Tapeworm.* **Whip-w.** See *Trichocephalus.*

Wor'mian bones. Supernumerary bones in the sutures of the skull.

Worm-seed. See *Chenopodium* and *Santonica.*

Worm'wood. See *Absinthium.*

Wors'ted-test. See *Holmgren's test.*

Wort-gel'atin. A bacterial culture-medium prepared from beer-wort and gelatin.

Woul'fe's bottle (vool'fiz). A three-necked bottle used in saturating liquids with gases, or in washing gases.

Wound. Any solution of the continuity of an external or internal surface caused by violence; a traumatism. **Contused w.,** one made by a blunt object. **Incised w.,** one caused by a cutting instrument. **Lacerated w.,** one in which the tissues are torn. **Open w.,** one having a free outward opening. **Penetrating w.** lays open an important cavity of the body. **Poisoned w.,** one into which septic matter has been introduced. **Punctured w.,** one made by a pointed instrument. **Subcutaneous w.,** one with a very small external opening in the skin.

Wris'berg's ansa. The nerve connecting the great splanchnic and right pneumogastric. **W.'s cartilage.** See *Cartilage.* **W.'s ganglion.** See *Ganglion.* **W.'s nerve.** 1. Small nervous cord accompanying facial and auditory nerves within internal auditory canal. 2. The lesser internal cutaneous nerve supplying the skin of the arm.

Wrist (rist). The carpus; the part which connects the forearm and hand. **W.-clonus.** See under *Clonus.* **W.-drop,** a paralysis of the extensor muscles of the hand and fingers, mainly due to metallic poisoning.

Wri'ters' cramp. Pain and spasm of the arm, hand, and fingers, due to writing.

Wri'ting hand. A condition in paralysis agitans in which the hand assumes that position in which the pen is commonly held.

Wry-neck. See *Torticollis.*

Wura'ri. Same as *Curare.*

Wur'ras. An anthelmintic drug from Africa, resembling kamala.

Wy'man's strap. An arrangement of straps for restraining violent insane patients.

X.

Xanthæm'atin. See *Xanthematin.*

Xan'thalin. An alkaloid, $C_{37}H_{36}N_2O_9$, of opium.

Xan'thein (zan'the-in). The soluble part of the yellow coloring-matter of flowers.

Xanthelas'ma (zan-thel-az'mah). See *Xanthoma.*

Xanthem'atin. A yellow substance derivable from hematin.

Xan'thic (zan'thik). 1. Yellow. 2. Pertaining to xanthin. **X. calculus.** See *Calculus.* **X. oxid.** See *Xanthin.*

Xan'thin (zan'thin). A leukomain, $C_5H_4N_4O_2$, from most of the bodily tissues.

Xanthinu'ria. Excess of xanthin in the urine.

Xanthochro'mia. Any yellowish discoloration.

Xanthocreat'inin. A poisonous yellow leukomain, $C_5H_{10}N_4O$, from muscle.

Xanthoc'rous. Having a yellowish complexion.

Xanthocyano'pia. Inability to perceive red and green tints.

Xanthocys'tin (zan-tho-sis'tin). Substance found in tubercles of a corpse.

Xanthoder'ma, Xanthoder'mia. A yellowish discoloration of the skin.

Xanthodon'tous (zan-tho-don'tus). Having yellowish teeth.

Xanthokyan'opy (zan-tho-ki-an'o-pe). Same as *Xanthocyanopia.*

Xantho'ma (zan-tho'mah). A disease with formation of yellow neoplastic growths on the skin, in form of either smooth plates (*X. pla'num*) or nodules (*X. tubero'sum*). **X. diabetico'rum,** skin-disease associated with diabetes mellitus. **X. mul'tiplex,** xanthoma distributed over the whole body. **X. palpebra'rum,** xanthoma affecting the eyelids. **X. tubercula'tum,** or **X. tubero'sum,** rare disease, with formation of tubercular lesions on the soles, palms, and extensor surfaces of the extremities.

Xanthomel'anous. Having black hair and a yellowish skin.

Xanthop'athy (zan-thop'ath-e). Same as *Xanthoderma.*

Xan'thophane. A yellow pigment from the retinal cones.

Xanthoplas'ty (zan-tho-plas'te). Same as *Xanthoderma.*

Xanthoprote'ic reaction. Orange color produced by heating proteids with nitric acid.

Xanthopro'tein. An orange pigment produced by heating proteids with nitric acid.

Xanthop'sia. Condition in which objects appear yellow.

Xanthop'sin. Visual purple partially discolored.

Xanthop'sis. Yellow pigment, or pigmentation, in cancers.

Xanthopuc'cin. An alkaloid from *Hydrastis canadensis.*

Xantho'sis. A yellowish discoloration.

Xan'thous. Belonging to, and of, the yellow races of mankind.

Xanthox'ylum. Prickly-ash; a genus of rutaceous trees: the bark is medicinal.

Xanthu'ria. Excess of xanthin in the urine.

Xenogen'esis. Alternation of generation, or heterogenesis.

Xenog'enous. Caused by a foreign body, or origination outside the organism.

Xenophthal'mia. Traumatic conjunctivitis.

Xerocollyr'ium. A dry collyrium; eye-salve.

Xeroder'ma. Disease marked by roughness and dryness of the skin. **X. of Kaposi,** diffuse idiopathic atrophy of the skin. **X. pigmento'sum,** a fatal disease, marked by brown spots and ulcers of the skin, with muscular atrophy.

Xe'roform. Compound of tribromphenol and bismuth; used in cholera.

Xero'ma (ze-ro'mah). Abnormally dry condition of the conjunctiva.

Xeromeni'a. Vicarious menstruation.

Xeropha'gia (ze-ro-fa'je-ah). The eating of dry food.

Xerophthal'mia. Conjunctivitis with atrophy and no liquid discharge.

Xero'sis. Abnormal dryness, as of the eye or skin.

Xerosto'mia. Dryness of the mouth from lack of the normal secretion.

Xerot'ic (ze-rot'ik). Characterized by dryness.

Xerotrip'sis. Treatment by friction; dry rubbing.

Xiphister'num. Same as *Xiphoid cartilage.*

Xiphocos'tal. Pertaining to the xiphoid cartilage and the ribs.

Xiphod'ymus (zi-fod'im-us). Same as *Xiphopagus.*

Xiphodyn'ia (zi-fo-din'e-ah). Pain in the xiphoid appendix.

Xi'phoid (zi'foid). Sword-shaped; ensiform. **X. appendix, X. cartilage.** Same as *Ensiform cartilage.* **X. ligament,** ligament which connects the x. appendix with the seventh rib.

Xipoph'agus (zi-pof'ag-us). A double monster joined at the thorax and pelvis.

X-ray dermatitis. Inflammation of skin caused by exposure to X-rays.

X-rays. Same as *Röntgen rays.*

Xy'lene (zi'lēn). Same as *Xylol.*

Xyloi'din. An explosive prepared from starch by action of nitric acid.

Xy'lol. Dimethyl-benzene, C_8H_{10}: used in medicine, and as a solvent in microscopy.

Xy'lose (zi'lōs). A sugar, $C_5H_{10}O_5$, from leek-wood and jute.

Xys'ma (zis'mah). Bits of membrane in stools of diarrhea.

Xys'ter (zis'ter). A surgeon's raspatory, or file.

Xys'tus (zis'tus). Scraped lint.

Y.

Y. Symbol of *Yttriane.* **Y-angle,** the angle between the radius fixus and line joining lambda and inion. **Y-cartilage,** Y-shaped cartilage in the acetabulum at the place of union of the ischium, ilium, and os pubis. **Y-ligament.** 1. Part of the capsular ligament of the hip-joint. 2. A ligament of the ankle connecting the scaphoid, cuboid, and calcaneal bones.

Yab'in. An alkaloid from the bark of *Andira excelsa.*

Yam, wild. See *Dioscorea.*

Yard. 1. A measure of three feet. See *Weights and Measures, Table of.* 2. The penis.

Yar'row (yar'o). See *Achillea.*

Ya'va-skin. A kind of elephantiasis caused by the habitual use of kava.

Yaw'ey. Affected with yaws.

Yawn'ing. A deep involuntary inspiration with open mouth.

Yaws (yawz). See *Framboesia.*

Yeast. A ferment consisting of various species of *Saccharomyces:* antiseptic, and useful in poultices.

Yelk. See *Yolk.*

Yellow fever. A dangerous bacterial infective fever, chiefly of tropical America, characterized by jaundice, hemorrhage, and bloody vomiting. **Y. precipitate,** yellow mercuric oxid, HgO. **Y. softening,** a true softening of the brain, of a yellow tint. **Y. spot.** See *Macula lutea.* **Y. wash,** a lotion of 18 grains of mercuric chlorid in 10 fluidounces of lime-water; also, a wash of yellow mercuric oxid.

Yen'omal. A proprietary remedy: said to be a coal-tar derivative.

Yer'ba san'ta. Same as *Eriodictyon.*

Yer'bin. Alkaloid from *Ilex paraguayensis,* resembling caffein.

Yolk. 1. The nutritive part of the ovum. 2. The yellow portion of a bird's egg. 3. Crude wool-fat, or suint. **Y.-cavity,** an open space within the yolk. **Y.-cells, Y.-granules,** granular elements composing the yolk. **Y.-sac.** See *Umbilical vesicle.* **Y.-stalk,** the umbilical duct.

Young-Helmholtz theory. Doctrine that color-vision depends on three sets of retinal fibers, corresponding to the colors red, green, and violet.

Young's rule. For the dosage of children, divide the age by the age plus twelve, which will give the proper fraction of the adult dose. See *Table of Doses*, p. 506.

Ytter'bium (it-ter'be-um). A very rare metal: symbol Yb.

Yt'trium (it're-um). A rare metal allied to cerium; symbol Y.

Yuc'ca. Genus of plants: the wood of some species is used for surgeons' splints.

Z.

Zacatil'la (zah-kah-tēl'yah). The choicest quality of cochineal.

Zanal'oin. The aloin of Zanzibar aloes.

Zaran'than. Hardening of the breast.

Ze'a mays. Maize, or Indian corn: the styles and stigmas are diuretic.

Zed'oary. The rhizome of *Curcuma zedoaria:* much like ginger.

Zeis'mus (ze-is'mus). Skin-disease, said to be due to excessive diet of maize.

Zeis'sian glands (zis'e-an). Sebaceous glands with ducts on edge of eyelid. **Z. stye.** See under *Stye.*

Zelotyp'ia. Morbid or insane zeal; insane jealousy.

Zen'ker's degeneration, Zenk'erism. A glassy degeneration and abnormal brittleness of a muscle.

Ze'oscope (ze'o-skōp). Apparatus for determining the alcoholic strength of a liquid by means of its boiling-point.

Ze'ro. The point on a thermometer-scale at which the graduation begins. The zero of the Centigrade and Reaumur thermometer is the melting-point of ice. That of the Fahrenheit is 32° below the melting-point of ice.

Ziehl-Neelson stain. The staining of microscopic specimens in the carbol-magenta solution, followed by treatment in dilute sulphuric acid, and by a further staining with methyl-blue: used for tubercle-bacilli.

Zinc. A blue-white metal, many of whose salts are medicinal and poisonous; symbol Zn.

Zin'giber (zin'jib-er). L. for *Ginger.*

Zinn's ligament. The annular ligament whence arise the recti muscles of the eye. **Zonule of Z.,** the suspensory ligament of the eye-lens.

Zitt'mann's decoction. Compound decoction of sarsaparilla.

Zn. Symbol of *Zinc.*

Znak. A badge worn in Russia by members of the medical profession.

Zoan'thropy. Maniacal belief of a patient that he has become a beast.

Zo'etrope. Apparatus which affords pictures of objects apparently moving as in life.

Zo'midin (zo'mid-in). A constituent of meat-extract.

Zo'na (zo'nah). 1. A girdle or belt. 2. Herpes zoster. **Z. arcua'ta,** the tunnel formed by the combined arches of Corti. **Z. cartilagin'ea,** limbus of spiral lamina. **Z. cilia'ris,** ciliary processes taken together. **Z. denticula'ta,** inner zone of basilar membrane with z. cartilaginea. **Z. facia'lis,** herpes zoster of face. **Z. fascicula'ta,** the central part of the cortex of a suprarenal capsule. **Z. glomerulo'sa,** the outermost layer of the cortex of a suprarenal capsule. **Z. incer'ta,** anterior portion of a network beneath the thalamus. **Z. ophthal'mica**, herpes of ophthalmic nerve. **Z. orbicula'ris**, thick ring of capsular ligament around the acetabulum. **Z. pectina'ta**, the outer part of the basilar membrane of the cochlea. **Z. pellu'-cida, Z. radia'ta**, the more inward of the two lining membranes of the ovum. **Z. perfora'ta**, outer section of the basilar membrane of the cochlea. **Z. reticula'ris**, the inner layer of the cortex of a suprarenal capsule. **Z. tec'ta**, part of the basilar membrane which lodges the organ of Corti.

Zo'nal stratum. A layer of white fibers on the surface of the thalamus.

Zone. A girdle or belt. **Cornuradicular z.**, outer part of Burdach's column. **Hysterogenous z.**, region of body whereon pressure may elicit a hysteric attack.

Zonesthe'sia. A sensation as of constriction, as by a girdle.

Zo'nular cataract. See *Cataract.*

Zo'nule of Zinn. See *Zinn's zonule.*

Zonuli'tis. Inflammation of Zinn's zonule.

Zoobiol'ogy. The biology of animals.

Zoochem'istry (zo-o-kem'is-tre). Chemistry of the animal tissues.

Zoog'enous (zo-oj'en-us). Acquired from animals.

Zoo'geny, Zoo'gony. The production or generation of animals.

Zooglœ'a. A colony of certain microbes embedded in a jelly-like matrix.

Zo'ograft (zo'o-graft). A graft of tissue from an animal.

Zoograft'ing. Grafting of animal tissue onto the human body.

Zo'oid (zo'oid). A form which resembles an animal.

Zool'ogy (zo-ol'o-je). A science of the form, nature, and classification of animals.

Zoon'omy (zo-on'o-me). Same as *Zoobiology.*

Zoopar'asite (zo-o-par'as-It). Any animal parasite.

Zoopathol'ogy. Veterinary medicine, or the science of the diseases of the lower animals.

Zooph'agous (zo-of'ag-us). Subsisting upon animal food.

Zoopho'bia (zo-o-fo'be-ah). Insane dread of animals.

Zo'ophyte (zo'of-It). Any plant-like animal.

Zo'osperm (zo'o-sperm). Same as *Spermatozoön.*

Zo'ospore (zo'o-spōr). Any spore moving by means of cilia.

Zoot'omy (zo-ot'o-me). The dissection or anatomy of animals.

Zos'ter (zos'ter). Shingles, or herpes zoster. **Z. auricula'ris**, herpes zoster of the ear. **Z. brachia'lis**, herpes zoster of the arm and forearm. **Z. ophthal'micus**, herpes along the course of the ophthalmic nerve.

Zos'teriform. Resembling zoster.

Zumo-ana'na. A digestant, tonic, and stimulant prepared from pine-apple juice.

Zwets'chen-wasser. A liqueur prepared in Germany from prunes.

Zy'gal fissure. Any cerebral fissure consisting of two branches connected by a stem or zygon.

Zygapoph'ysis. The articular process of a vertebra.

Zyg'ion (zij'e-on). Craniometric point at either end of bizygomatic diameter.

Zygo'ma. An arch formed by the zygomatic process of the temporal bone and by the malar bone.

Zygoma'tic arch. Same as *Zygoma.* **Z. process**, projection at base of the squamous portion of the temporal bone.

Zygomatico-auricula'ris. The attrahens aurem muscle.

Zygomat'icus. See *Muscles, Table of.*

Zygomaxilla're (zi-go-mak-sil-a're). A craniometrical point at the lower end of the zygomatic suture.

Zy'gon (zi'gon). The bar or stem connecting the two branches of a zygal fissure.

Zy'goneure (zi'go-nūr). A nerve-cell containing other nerve-cells.

Zy'lonite (zi'lo-nīt). A form of celluloid used in dentistry and surgery.

Zy'mase (zī'mās). See *Enzyme*.

Zyme (zīm). Any ferment that may be pathogenic.

Zy'mic (zi'mik). Pertaining to organized ferments.

Zy'min (zī'min). Same as *Zyme*.

Zy'mogen (zī'mo-jen). Any substance which may give rise to a ferment.

Zy'mogene. A microbe which causes a fermentation.

Zymogen'ic (zi-mo-jen'ik). Causing a fermentation.

Zy'moid (zī'moid). Any poison from decaying tissue.

Zymol'ogy (zi-mol'o-je). The science of, or sum of, knowledge regarding fermentation.

Zymol'ysis. Digestion by means of an enzyme.

Zymolyt'ic. Pertaining to, or caused by, zymolysis.

Zymom'eter (zi-mom'et-er). Same as *Zymosimeter*.

Zy'mophyte (zī'mo-fīt). A bacterium causing fermentation.

Zymosim'eter, Zymosiom'eter. Instrument for measuring the degree of fermentation.

Zymo'sis. 1. Fermentation. 2. The development of any zymotic disease. 3. Any infectious or contagious disease.

Zymot'ic (zi-mot'ik). Caused by, or pertaining to, zymosis. **Z. disease,** any disease due to a ferment; an infectious disease.

Zy'motoid. A proprietary preparation for affections of the skin and mucous membranes.

Zy'murgy (zi'mer-je). The art of brewing, distilling, and wine-making.

A TABLE OF DOSES

IN BOTH APOTHECARIES' AND METRIC SYSTEMS.

The following doses are intended for adults. The dose for a child may be obtained approximately by Young's rule: Divide the age by the age plus 12, which will give the fraction of the adult dose to be used for the child. Thus, for a child of four years, $\frac{4}{4+12} = \frac{1}{4}$, and the dose is $\frac{1}{4}$ that for an adult.

Narcotics should be given in only one-half this proportion, while cathartics may be employed in two or three times this proportion.

For *hypodermic* use the dose should be one-half of that by the mouth; by the *rectum*, five-fourths of the same.

In the following table gr. = grains, dr. = drams, m. = minims, oz. = ounces. The doses in the metric system are either grams or cubic centimeters.

Medicine.	Apoth. Dose.	Metric Dose.	Medicine.	Apoth. Dose.	Metric Dose.	Medicine.	Apoth. Dose.	Metric Dose.
Absinthin . .	15–30 gr.	1.000–2.000	Acid, sulphuric			Ammonia, spir-		
Acaroid resin . .	6–12 gr.	0.400–0.800	arom. . . .	5–15 m.	0.333–1.000	itus fœtid. .	$\frac{1}{2}$– 1 dr.	2.000–4.000
Acetal	1 dr.	4.000	dil.	5–15 m.	0.333–1.000	Ammoniac . . .	2–10 gr.	0.133–0.666
Acetanilid. See			sulphurous . .	5–30 m.	0.333–2.000	Ammonium ace-		
Antifebrin.			tannic	1–10 gr.	0.066–0.666	tat., liquor .	1– 8 dr.	4.000–32.00
Acetone	15–20 m.	1.000–1.23	tartaric	10–20 gr.	0.666–1.333	benzoate . . .	5–15 gr.	0.333–1.000
Acetophenone .	3–10 m.	0.200–0.666	trichloracetic .	2– 4 gr.	0.133–0.266	bromid	5–20 gr.	0.333–1.333
Acetphenetidin.			Aconite, abst. . .	$\frac{1}{4}$– $\frac{1}{2}$ gr.	0.016–0.033	carbonate . . .	3–10 gr.	0.200–0.666
See *Phenace-*			ext.	$\frac{1}{6}$– $\frac{1}{3}$ gr.	0.011–0.022	chlorid	1–20 gr.	0.066–1.333
tin.			fl.	$\frac{1}{2}$– 2 m.	0.033–0.133	iodid	2–10 gr.	0.133–0.666
Acetyltannin.			tinct.	1– 5 m.	0.066–0.333	phosphate . . .	5–20 gr.	0.333–1.333
See *Tannigen.*			Fleming's . .	$\frac{2}{3}$– 2 m.	0.044–0.133	picrate	$\frac{1}{8}$– $\frac{1}{2}$ gr.	0.008–0.033
Achillea, extrac-			Aconitin	$\frac{1}{200}$–$\frac{1}{50}$ gr.	0.000335–0.0013	valerianate . .	1– 5 gr.	0.066–0.333
tive	1– 3 dr.	4.000–12.000	Adonidin	$\frac{1}{4}$– $\frac{1}{3}$ gr.	0.016–0.022	Amygdala amar.,		
oil	5–15 m.	0.333–1.000	Agaricin	$\frac{1}{24}$– $\frac{1}{6}$ gr.	0.0027–0.011	aqua . . .	2– 4 dr.	8.000–16.000

Acid, acetic dil. .	60–90 m.	4.000–6.000
agaric	1/10– 3/4 gr.	0.004–0.049
anticyclic . . .	1/100 gr.	0.00066
arsenous . . .	1/64–1/12 gr.	0.00101–0.0054
benzoic	5–15 gr.	0.333–1.000
boric	5–15 gr.	0.333–1.000
camphoric . .	10–30 gr.	0.666–2.000
carbolic	1/4– 1 gr.	0.016–0.066
cathartinic . .	4– 6 gr.	0.260–0.400
chrysophanic .	1/8–10 gr.	0.008–0.666
cinnamic . . .	1–10 m.	0.066–0.666
citric	10–30 gr.	0.666–2.000
di-iodosalicylic	5–10 gr.	0.333–0.666
fluoric dil. . .	15–20 m.	1.000–1.333
gallic	3–15 gr.	0.200–1.000
gynocardic . .	1/2– 3 gr.	0.032–0.194
hydriodic, syr.	1/2– 3 dr.	2.000–12.00
hydrobrom. dil.	20 m.–2 dr.	1.333–8.000
hydrochlor. dil.	3–10 m.	0.200–0.666
hydrocyan. dil.	1– 5 m.	0.066–0.333
iodosalicylic .	5–10 gr.	0.324–0.666
lactic	15–30 gr.	1.000–2.000
nitric dil. . . .	3–15 m.	0.200–1.000
nitrohydrochloric	1–10 m.	0.066–0.666
dil.	5–20 m.	0.333–1.333
osmic	1/60 gr.	0.00108
oxalic	1/4– 1 gr.	0.016–0.066
paracresotic . .	2 gr.–2 dr.	0.133–8.000
phenylaceric .	1– 3 gr.	0.066–0.200
phosphoric dil.	5–30 m.	0.333–2.000
picric	1– 5 gr.	0.066–0.333
salicylic	5–20 gr.	0.333–1.333
sclerotic . . .	1/2–1 1/2 gr.	0.033–0.100

Agathin	8–10 gr.	0.520–0.666
Agave Americana, ext. fl. . .	2 oz.	64.000
Agrimony . . .	1 dr.	4.000
Ailanthus, ext. fl.	10–60 m.	0.666–4.000
tinct.	10 m.–2 dr.	0.666–8.000
Aletrin	1/4– 2 gr.	0.016–0.133
Allium, syrup. .	1– 4 dr.	4.000–16.00
Alnuin	2–10 gr.	0.133–0.666
Aloe, ext. aq. . .	1/2– 3 gr.	0.033–0.200
pilulæ	1– 3	
et asaf. . . .	2– 5	
et ferri. . . .	1– 3	
et mast. . . .	1– 2	
et myrrh. . .	2– 5	
pulvis, et canellæ	5–20 gr.	0.333–1.133
purif.	1– 5 gr.	0.066–0.333
tinct.	1/2– 2 dr.	2.000–8.000
et myrrh. . .	1/2– 2 dr.	2.000–8.000
vinum	1– 2 dr.	4.000–8.000
Aloin	1– 3 gr.	0.066–0.200
Alphol	8–15 gr.	0.520–1.000
Alum	10–15 gr.	0.666–1.000
Aluminum hydrate	3–15 gr.	0.200–1.000
Alveloz succus .	15–30 gr.	1.000–2.000
Amber, oil of . .	5–10 gr.	0.324–0.666
Ambergris . . .	5 gr.–1 dr.	0.324–4.000
Ammonia, aqua.	5–30 m.	0.333–2.000
mist.	4– 8 dr.	16.000–32.00
spiritus	5–30 m.	0.333–2.000
arom.	15–60 m.	1.000–4.000

mist.	2– 4 dr.	8.000–16.000
oleum . . .	1/4– 1 m.	0.0165–0.066
Amylene hydrat.	1–1 1/2 dr.	4.000–6.000
Amyl nitrite . .	1/4– 1 m.	0.0165–0.066
Amylum iodatum	3–30 gr.	0.200–2.000
Analgene	7–15 gr.	0.460–1.000
Analgesin. See *Antipyrin.*		
Anemonin . . .	1/50–1/10 gr.	0.0013–0.0065
Angelica, root or seeds	30 gr.-1 dr.	2.000–4.000
Anhalonium Lewini, ext. fl.	1– 3 m.	0.066–0.200
Anilin	1– 3 gr.	0.066–0.200
camphorate . .	8–12 gr.	0.520–0.800
sulphate . . .	3– 5 gr.	0.200–0.333
Anisum, oleum .	1– 5 m.	0.066–0.333
spiritus	1– 2 dr.	4.000–8.000
Anthemis, infus. or ext. fl. . .	15–60 gr.	1.000–4.000
Antifebrin . . .	2–10 gr.	0.133–0.666
Antihydropin .	10–15 gr.	0.648–0.97
Antikamnia . .	4–10 gr.	0.266–0.666
Antimonium oxid	1– 2 gr.	0.066–0.133
pil. comp. . . .	1– 3	
et potas. tart.; diaph. .	1/20– 1/8 gr.	0.003–0.008
emet. . . .	1– 2 gr.	0.066–0.133
pulv.	1– 5 gr.	0.066–0.333
sulphid pur. .	1/4– 1 gr.	0.016–0.066
sulphuret . . .	1/2– 3 gr.	0.033–0.200
wine	1– 5 m.	0.066–0.333

A TABLE OF DOSES (*continued*).

Medicine.	Apoth. Dose.	Metric Dose.	Medicine.	Apoth. Dose.	Metric Dose.	Medicine.	Apoth. Dose.	Metric Dose.
Antinervin	10–15 gr.	0.648–0.97	Belladon., abst.	1/10–1 gr.	0.006–0.066	Calomel. See *Hy-*		
Antipyrin	5–10 gr.	0.333–0.666	ext. alc.	1/10–½ gr.	0.006–0.033	*drarg. chlor.*		
amygdalate	¾–6 gr.	0.049–0.400	fol., ext. fl.	3–6 m.	0.200–0.400	*mit.*		
Antirheumatin	1–1½ gr.	0.066–0.100	rad., ext.	⅛–¼ gr.	0.008–0.016	Calumba, ext.	3–10 gr.	0.200–0.666
Antisepsin	6–7 gr.	0.400–0.466	fl.	1–3 m.	0.066–0.200	fl.	5–30 m.	0.333–2.000
Antiseptol	1–3 gr.	0.066–0.200	tinct.	1–20 m.	0.066–1.333	tinct.	½–2 dr.	2.000–8.000
Antispasmin	½–1 gr.	0.033–0.066	Benzanalgin	7½–45 gr.	0.492–2.926	Calx chlorata	3–6 gr.	0.200–0.400
Antithermin	3–8 gr.	0.200–0.520	Benzanilid	1–15 gr.	0.066–0.970	sulphurata	1/10–½ gr.	0.006–0.033
Apiol	3–5 m.	2.000–0.333	Benzoin, tinct.	½–1 dr.	2.000–4.000	Calx, liq.	½–2 oz.	16.000–64.00
Apiolin	3 m.	0.200	comp.	½–2 dr.	2.000–8.000	syr.	½–2 dr.	2.000–8.000
Apocodein hy-			Benzonaphtol	4–8 gr.	0.260–0.520	lac. phos.	1–2 dr.	4.000–8.000
drat.	3–4 gr.	0.194–0.260	Benzoyl-guaiacol.	3–12 gr.	0.194–0.780	Camphora	1–20 gr.	0.066–1.333
Apocynin	¼–½ gr.	0.016–0.033	Berberin	1–10 gr.	0.066–0.666	aqua	1–4 dr.	4.000–16.00
Apomorphin hy-			Berberis, ext. fl.	5–30 m.	0.333–2.000	monob.	1–5 gr.	0.066–0.333
drochl.	1/30–1/10 gr.	0.002–0.006	tinct	10–60 m.	0.666–4.000	Rubini tinct.	2–5 m.	0.133–0.333
Apone	5–10 m.	0.333–0.666	Betin	2–4 gr.	0.133–0.260	spirit	5–20 m.	0.333–1.333
Arbutin	⅙–¼ gr.	0.011–0.016	Betol	15–40 gr.	0.970–2.600	Cannabinone	¾–1¼ gr.	0.050–0.082
Arecalin	1/20–1/10 gr.	0.0032–0.0066	Bismuth et am-			Cannabin tan.	5–10 gr.	0.333–0.666
Argentum, iodid.	¼–1 gr.	0.016–0.066	mon. cit.	1–5 gr.	0.066–0.333	Cannabis ind.,		
nitrate	⅙–¼ gr.	0.011–0.016	naphtolate	15–30 gr.	0.970–2.000	ext.	⅙–½ gr.	0.011–0.033
oxid	½–2 gr.	0.033–0.133	subcarb.	10–30 gr.	0.666–2.000	fl.	1–5 m.	0.066–0.333
phosphate	⅓–½ gr.	0.022–0.033	nit.	10–60 gr.	0.666–4.000	tinct.	15–30 m.	1.000–2.000
Arnica flo., tinct.	5–30 m.	0.333–2.000	Blatta orientalis	2–8 gr.	0.133–0.520	Cantharides,		
rad., ext.	1–3 gr.	0.066–0.200	Boldin	2–4 gr.	0.133–0.266	tinct.	1–20 m.	0.066–1.333
fl.	5–20 m.	0.333–1.333	Boldo, tinct.	5–8 m.	0.133–0.260	Capsicum	2–5 gr.	0.133–0.333
tinct.	5–30 m.	0.333–2.000	Boldoglucin	20–60 gr.	1.333–4.000	ext. fl.	5–30 m.	0.333–2.000
Arsenic et hy-			Brayera	2–8 dr.	8.000–32.00	oleores	1–5 m.	0.066–0.333
drar. iod., liq.	2–10 m.	0.133–0.666	ext. fl.	2–8 dr.	8.000–32.00	tinct.	10–30 m.	0.666–2.000

iodid.	1/20–1/10 gr.	0.003–0.006	infus.	2– 8 oz.	64.000–256.00	Carbo animal.		
Arsenit., liquor			Bromal hydrate	2– 5 gr.	0.133–0.333	purif.	10–60 gr.	0.666–4.000
brom.	1– 4 m.	0.066–0.266	Bromamid	10–15 gr.	0.666–0.970	Carbon bisulph.	1/2– 1 m.	0.033–0.066
Asafœtida	5–20 gr.	0.333–1.333	Bromoform	3–15 gr.	0.194–0.970	Cardam., tinct.	1– 2 dr.	4.000–8.000
mist.	4– 8 dr.	16.000–32.00	Bromol	2– 4 gr.	0.133–0.266	comp.	1– 2 dr.	4.000–8.000
pilulæ	1– 4		Brousnika	2– 4 dr.	8.000–16.000	Cari, oleum	1– 5 m.	0.066–0.333
tinct.	30–60 m.	2.000–4.000	Brucin	1/64–1/16 gr.	0.001–0.004	Carpain (hypoderm.)	1/10–1/6 gr.	0.006–0.011
Asaprol	5–10 gr.	0.333–0.666	Bryonia, tinct.	5–30 m.	0.333–2.000	Caryophyl., ol.	1– 5 m.	0.066–0.333
Asclepiadin	1– 5 gr.	0.066–0.333	Bryonin	2 gr.	0.133	Cascara sagrada,		
Asclepidin	1– 5 gr.	0.066–0.333	Buchu, ext. fl.	10–60 m.	0.666–4.000	ext. fl.	10–20 m.	0.666–1.333
Asepsin. See *Antisepsin.*			infus.	1/2– 2 oz.	16.000–64.00	Cascarin	1 1/2– 3 gr.	0.099–0.198
Asparagin	1– 2 gr.	0.066–0.133	Butyl-chloral-hydrate	2–15 gr.	0.133–0.970	Castanea, ext. fl.	1/2– 2 dr.	2.000–8.000
Aspidium, ext. fl.	1– 2 dr.	4.000–8.000	Buxin. Same as *Bebeerin.*			Castoreum	6–15 gr.	0.400–0.970
oleores	15–60 gr.	1.000–4.000	Cact. grandiflor.,			Catechu	1–30 gr.	0.066–2.000
Aspidospermin	1/2– 3 gr.	0.033–0.200	ext. fl.	15–20 m.	1.000–1.333	tinct. comp.	10–60 m.	0.666–4.000
Atropin	1/100–1/40 gr.	0.00066–0.0016	tinct.	5–10 m.	0.333–0.666	Caulophyllin	1– 4 gr.	0.066–0.266
sulphate	1/100–1/40 gr.	0.00066–0.0016	Caffein	1– 5 gr.	0.066–0.333	Cerium oxal.	1– 5 gr.	0.066–0.333
Aurantium amar.			citrat.	2–10 gr.	0.133–0.666	Cetrarin	1 1/2– 3 gr.	0.099–0.200
ext. fl.	1 1/2– 2 dr.	6.000–8.000	sodiosalicylate.	1– 4 gr.	0.066–0.260	Chaulmoogra oil	2–10 m.	0.133–0.666
tinct.	1– 2 dr.	4.000–8.000	tri-iodid	2– 4 gr.	0.333–0.533	Chenopod., ol.	5–10 m.	0.333–0.666
dulcis, tinct.	1– 2 dr.	4.000–8.000	Cajuput, oleum	1– 5 m.	0.066–0.333	Chian turpentine	7–20 gr.	0.460–1.333
Auri chlorid.	1/50–1/30 gr.	0.0013–0.002	Calam., ext. fl.	15–60 m.	1.000–4.000	Chimaphila, ext. fl.	1/2– 2 dr.	2.000–8.000
et sod. chlorid.	1/30–1/10 gr.	0.002–0.006	Calc. bromid.	5–30 gr.	0.333–2.000	Chinoidin	1–30 gr.	0.066–2.000
Auri monocyani.	1/10– 1/4 gr.	0.006–0.016	carb. precip.	5–20 gr.	0.333–1.333	Chinolin tartrate	5–20 gr.	0.333–1.333
tricyani.	1/10– 1/4 gr.	0.006–0.016	chlorid.	10–20 gr.	0.666–1.333	Chiretta, ext. fl.	15–30 m.	1.000–2.000
Azederach, decoc.	1/2– 1 oz.	16.000–32.000	hippurate	5–10 gr.	0.333–0.666	tinct.	15–60 m.	1.000–4.000
Bals. tolutan., syr.	1– 2 dr.	4.000–8.000	hypophosph.	10–20 gr.	0.666–1.333	Chloral	1–15 gr.	0.066–1.000
tinct.	10–30 m.	0.666–2.000	iodid	1– 3 gr.	0.066–0.200	ammonium	15–30 gr.	1.000–2.000
Baptisia, ext.	1–10 gr.	0.066–0.666	phos. precip.	2–10 gr.	0.133–0.666	butyl-	5–40 gr.	0.333–2.660
fl.	2–20 m.	0.133–1.333	salicylate	8–24 gr.	0.520–1.550	-caffein (hypoderm.)	3–4 1/2 gr.	0.194–0.293
tinct.	5–30 m.	0.333–2.000	santoninate	1/4– 3/4 gr.	0.016–0.050	croton-	10–25 gr.	0.666–1.620
Barm	2– 8 dr.	8.000–32.00	Calendula, tinct.	15–30 m.	1.000–2.000			
Bebeerin	2– 5 gr.	0.133–0.333						

A TABLE OF DOSES (*continued*).

Medicine.	Apoth. Dose.	Metric Dose.
Chloral hydrate.	10–30 gr.	0.666–2.000
Chloralamid . .	10–30 gr.	0.666–2.000
Chloralose . . .	3–14 gr.	0.194–0.907
Chlori, aqua . .	10–20 m.	0.666–1.333
Chlorodyne . . .	10–30 m.	0.666–2.000
Chloroform . . .	2–20 m.	0.133–1.333
mist.	1– 2 dr.	4.000–8.000
spirit	10–60 m.	0.666–4.000
tinct. comp. . .	20–60 m.	1.333–4.000
et morph. . .	5–10 m.	0.333–0.666
Chrysarobin . .	2–20 gr.	0.133–1.333
Cimicifuga, ext. fl.	5–30 m.	0.333–2.000
tinct.	5–30 m.	0.333–2.000
Cinchona	10–60 gr.	0.666–4.000
ext.	1– 5 gr.	0.066–0.333
fl.	10–60 m.	0.666–4.000
tinct.	1/2– 2 dr.	2.000–8.000
comp.	1/2– 2 dr.	2.000–8.000
Huxham's .	1/2– 2 dr.	2.000–8.000
Cinchonidin sulph.	1–30 gr.	0.066–2.000
Cinchonin . . .	1–30 gr.	0.066–2.000
sulph.	1–30 gr.	0.066–2.000
Cinnamomum .	5–20 gr.	0.333–1.333
ext. arom. fl. .	1–30 m.	0.066–2.000
oleum.	1– 5 gtt.	0.066–0.333
pulv. arom. . .	10–30 gr.	0.666–2.000

Medicine.	Apoth. Dose.	Metric Dose.
Copaiba, oleum .	10–15 m.	0.666–1.000
resin	1– 5 gr.	0.066–0.333
Coriandri, ol. . .	2– 5 m.	0.133–0.333
Cornus, ext. fl. .	10–60 m.	0.666–4.000
Cornutin	1/6– 1/4 gr. (daily).	0.011–0.016
Coronilla, powder	15–30 gr. (daily).	1.000–2.000
tinct.	1/2– 1 dr. (daily).	2.000–4.000
Coto, tinct. . . .	1–15 m.	0.066–1.000
Cotoin	1– 4 gr.	0.066–0.266
Creolin	1/2– 1 gr.	0.033–0.066
Creosotum . . .	1– 3 m.	0.066–0.200
aqua	1– 4 dr.	4.000–16.00
Creta præparat. .	5–20 gr.	0.333–1.333
mist.	2– 4 dr.	8.000–16.00
pulv. comp. . .	5–60 gr.	0.333–4.000
Crocus, tinct. . .	1– 2 dr.	4.000–8.000
Croton chloral .	5–10 gr.	0.333–0.666
Cubeba	10–60 gr.	0.666–4.000
ext. fl.	5–30 m.	0.333–2.000
oleores	5–20 m.	0.333–1.333
oleum	5–20 m.	0.333–1.333
tinct.	1– 2 dr.	4.000–8.000
trochisci . . .	1– 3	
Cupri acetas . .	1/10– 1/4 gr.	0.006–0.016
ammon. . . .	1/6– 1 gr.	0.011–0.066

Medicine.	Apoth. Dose.	Metric Dose.
Elaterin, trit. . .	1/8– 1/2 gr.	0.008–0.033
Elenin, ext. . . .	1/8 gr.	0.008
tinct.	5 m.	0.333
Emetin (emetic)	1/10– 1/2 gr.	0.0066–0.033
(expectorant).	1/100– 1/40 gr.	0.00066–0.0015
Ergot	10–60 gr.	0.666–4.000
ext.	1 1/2– 8 gr.	0.099–0.533
fl.	15–60 m.	1.000–4.000
vin.	1– 4 dr.	4.000–16.00
Ergotin	2– 8 gr.	0.133–0.533
Erigeron, oil . .	5–15 m.	0.333–1.000
Eriodictyon, ext.	2– 5 gr.	0.133–0.333
fl.	15–60 m.	1.000–4.000
Erythrox., ext. fl.	1/2– 2 dr.	2.000–8.000
Eserin	1/64– 1/20 gr.	0.001–0.003
Ether fortior. . .	10–60 m.	0.666–4.000
spirit.	10–60 m.	0.666–4.000
comp.	5–60 m.	0.333–4.000
nit.	1/2– 2 dr.	2.000–8.000
Ethoxycaffein .	1– 3 gr.	0.066–0.200
Ethyl bromid . .	10–60 m.	0.666–4.000
Ethylene bromid	6–12 m.	0.399–0.798
Eucalyptol . . .	5–15 m.	0.333–1.000
Eucalyptus, ext. fl.	10–60 m.	0.666–4.000
oleum	5–10 m.	0.333–0.666
tinct.	1/2– 2 dr.	2.000–8.000
Eugenol	10–15 m.	0.666–1.000

spirit	5–30 m.	0.333–2.000	arsenit.	1/100 gr.	0.00066	Euonymin . . .	1/2– 3 gr.	0.033–0.200
tinct.	1/2– 2 dr.	2.000–8.000	sulphas.	1/4– 1/2 gr.	0.016–0.033	Euonymus, ext.	1– 5 gr.	0.066–0.333
Cocain	1/8– 2 gr.	0.008–0.133	Curare	1/32– 1/6 gr.	0.002–0.011	Eupatorium, ext.		
hydrochlorate .	1/6– 1 gr.	0.011–0.066	Curarin	1/100–1/40 gr.	0.00066–0.0015	fl.	10–60 m.	0.666–4.000
phenate	1/12– 1/6 gr.	0.0054–0.011	Cypripedium, ext.			Euphorin	7–15 gr.	0.454–1.000
Cocculus, ext. fl.	1– 3 m.	0.066–0.200	fl.	10–30 m.	0.666–2.000	Europhen . . .	1/4–1 1/2 gr.	0.016–0.099
tinct.	2–15 m.	0.133–1.000	Cytisin nitrat.			Exalgin	3– 6 gr.	0.200–0.400
Codein	1/2– 1 gr.	0.033–0.066	(hypoderm.) .	1/20–1/12 gr.	0.003–0.0054	Fel bovis inspis.	5–15 gr.	0.333–1.000
Colchicein (hypo-			Damiana, ext. .	2–10 gr.	0.133–0.666	purif.	5–10 gr.	0.333–0.666
derm.) . . .	1/60–1/30 gr.	0.0011–0.0022	fl.	10–60 m.	0.666–4.000	Ferri, albuminas.	10–20 gr.	0.666–1.333
Colchicin	1/100–1/20 gr.	0.00066–0.0032	Daturin	1/120–1/20 gr.	0.0005–0.003	amar., vin. . .	1– 4 dr.	4.000–16.00
Colchicum rad.,			Dendakin . . .	1–10 gr.	0.066–0.666	et ammon. acet.	2– 3 oz.	64.000–96.000
ext. . . .	1/2–1 1/2 gr.	0.033–0.100	Dermatol	5–10 gr.	0.333–0.666	cit.	2– 5 gr.	0.133–0.333
fl.	2– 5 m.	0.133–0.333	Diastase	5–15 gr.	0.333–1.000	mist. . . .	2– 3 oz.	64.000–96.00
vin.	5–15 m.	0.333–1.000	Digitalin	1/64–1/32 gr.	0.001–0.002	sulph. . . .	5–10 gr.	0.333–0.666
sem., ext. fl. . .	1– 5 m.	0.066–0.333	Digitalis	1/2– 2 gr.	0.033–0.133	tart.	5–15 gr.	0.333–1.000
vin.	5–30 m.	0.333–2.000	abstr.	1/4– 2 gr.	0.016–0.133	arom., mist. . .	1/2– 1 oz.	16.000–32.00
tinct.	10–30 m.	0.666–2.000	ext.	1/6– 1/2 gr.	0.011–0.033	arsen.	1/10–1/6 gr.	0.006–0.011
Colocynth, ext. .	1/2– 2 gr.	0.033–0.133	fl.	1– 3 m.	0.066–0.200	benzoas	1– 5 gr.	0.066–0.333
comp.	5–10 gr.	0.333–0.666	infus.	1– 4 dr.	4.000–16.00	bromid	1– 5 gr.	0.066–0.333
Condurango . .	20–30 m.	1.333–2.000	tinct.	5–30 m.	0.333–2.000	syr.	5–30 m.	0.333–2.000
Coniin	1/64–1/32 gr.	0.001–0.002	Digitoxin	1/200–1/100 gr.	0. 00033–0.00066	carb., massa. . .	3– 5 gr.	0.200–0.333
Conium, abst. . .	1/2– 2 gr.	0.033–0.133	Dioscorea, ext. fl.	15–30 m.	1.000–2.000	sacch.	2–10 gr.	0.133–0.666
ext. alc.	1– 5 gr.	0.066–0.333	Diuretin	10–15 gr.	0.666–1.000	chlorid., liq. . .	2–10 m.	0.133–0.666
fl.	2– 5 m.	0.133–0.333	Dover's powder .	5–15 gr.	0.333–1.000	tinct.	5–20 m.	0.333–1.333
tinct.	5–30 m.	0.333–2.000	Dracontium, ext.			citrat.	2– 5 gr.	0.133–0.333
Convallamarin .	1/2– 2 gr.	0.033–0.133	fl.	30–60 m.	2.000–4.000	liq.	5–10 m.	0.333–0.666
Convallaria, ext.	2–10 gr.	0.133–0.666	Duboisia, ext. . .	1/6– 1/4 gr.	0.011–0.016	vin.	1– 2 dr.	4.000–8.000
fl.	2–10 m.	0.133–0.666	tinct.	5–20 m.	0.333–1.333	comp., mist. . .	1/2– 1 oz.	16.000–32.00
infus.	1/2– 2 oz.	16.000–64.00	Duboisin, sulph.	1/100–1/60 gr.	0.00066–0.001	pil.	2– 5	
Convallarin . .	2– 4 gr.	0.133–0.266	Dulcamara, ext.			hypophos. . . .	5–10 gr.	0.333–0.666
Copaiba	10–60 m.	0.666–4.000	fl.	1– 2 dr.	4.000–8.000	syr.	1– 2 dr.	4.000–8.000
massa	5–30 gr.	0.333–2.000	Dulcin	2/5 gr.	0.0259	iodid.	1– 5 gr.	0.066–0.333
mist. comp. . .	1– 4 dr.	4.000–16.00	Elaterin	1/60–1/12 gr.	0.001–0.0054	pil.	1– 2	

A TABLE OF DOSES (*continued*).

Medicine.	Apoth. Dose.	Metric Dose.	Medicine.	Apoth. Dose.	Metric Dose.	Medicine.	Apoth. Dose.	Metric Dose.
Ferri iodid. sac.	5–10 gr.	0.333–0.666	Helenin	1/6– 1/3 gr.	0.011–0.022	Iodopyrin	1–15 gr.	0.066–1.000
syr.	5–30 m.	0.333–2.000	Helleborein	1/10– 1/4 gr.	0.0066–0.016	Iodotannin, syr.	1– 4 m.	0.066–0.260
lactas	1– 3 gr.	0.066–0.200	Helleborus			Iodothein	2–15 gr.	0.133–1.000
et mang. carb.			niger, ext.	½– 5 gr.	0.033–0.333	Ipecac (emetic)	15–30 gr.	1.000–2.000
sac.	5–20 gr.	0.333–1.333	fl.	5–15 m.	0.333–1.000	(expectorant)	1/6– 1 gr.	0.011–0.066
iod., syr.	10–30 m.	0.666–2.000	Hemalbumin	15 gr.	1.000	ext. fl.	1– 5 m.	0.066–0.333
phos., syr.	1 dr.	4.000	Hematox., ext.	5–20 gr.	0.333–1.333	pulv., et opii	2–15 gr.	0.133–1.000
oxalas	1– 2 gr.	0.066–0.133	Hemogallol	1½–7½ gr.	0.099–0.493	syr.	½– 2 dr.	2.000–8.000
oxid. hydrat.	½– 1 oz.	16.000–32.00	Hemoglobin	½– 2 gr.	0.033–0.133	tinct., et opii	5–15 m.	0.333–1.000
phosphas	5–10 gr.	0.333–0.666	Hemol	1½–7½ gr.	0.099–0.493	vin.	1–60 m.	0.066–4.000
et pot. tartar.	5–10 gr.	0.333–0.666	Hoang-Nan	3– 5 gr.	0.200–0.333	Iridin	2– 4 gr.	0.133–0.266
pyrophosphas	1– 5 gr.	0.066–0.333	tinct.	1– 5 m.	0.066–0.333	Iris, ext.	1– 5 gr.	0.066–0.333
et quin. cit.	3– 5 gr.	0.200–0.333	Homatropin	1/3 gr.	0.022	fl.	5–30 m.	0.333–2.000
sol.	5–15 m.	0.333–1.000	Humulus,			Jalapa	10–20 gr.	0.666–1.333
quin. et strych.			ext. fl.	5–15 m.	0.333–1.000	abstr.	1– 5 gr.	0.066–0.333
phos. syr.	1– 2 dr.	4.000–8.000	oleores	2– 5 gr.	0.133–0.333	ext. fl.	15–30 m.	1.000–2.000
et strych. cit.	1– 3 gr.	0.066–0.200	tinct.	½– 2 dr.	2.000–8.000	pulv. comp.	10–60 gr.	0.666–4.000
subcarbonas	5–30 gr.	0.333–2.000	Hydracetin	¼– 3 gr.	0.016–0.200	res.	2– 5 gr.	0.133–0.333
sulph. exsic.	½– 2 gr.	0.033–0.133	Hydrang., ext. fl.	30–60 m.	2.000–4.000	tinct.	½– 2 dr.	2.000–8.000
gran.	1– 5 gr.	0.066–0.333	Hydrarg. chlor.			Jambul	5–10 gr.	0.333–0.666
valerianas	1– 3 gr.	0.066–0.200	cor.	1/80–1/10 gr.	0.00075–0.006	Juglans, ext.	5–20 gr.	0.333–1.333
Ferrum dialys.	5–15 m.	0.333–1.000	mit.	1/6– 8 gr.	0.011–0.533	Junip., ext. fl.	30–60 m.	2.000–4.000
reductum	1– 5 gr.	0.066–0.333	cum creta	½–10 gr.	0.033–0.666	oleum	5–20 m.	0.333–1.333
Fœniculum, ol.	2– 5 m.	0.133–0.333	cyan.	1/100–1/10 gr.	0.00066–0.006	spirit.	1– 3 dr.	4.000–12.00
Frangula, ext. fl.	½–2½ dr.	2.000–10.000	iodid. flav.	1/6– 1 gr.	0.011–0.066	comp.	4– 8 dr.	16.000–32.00
Fuchsin	½– 4 gr.	0.033–0.266	rub.	1/50–1/10 gr.	0.0013–0.006	Kairin	3–30 gr.	0.200–2.000
Galbanum, pil.			vir.	1/10– 1/3 gr.	0.006–0.022	Kamala	1– 2 dr.	4.000–8.000
comp.	1–3		massa.	1–10 gr.	0.066–0.666	ext. fl.	30–60 m.	2.000–4.000

Galega, aq. ext. . .	7½–15 gr.	0.492–1.000	oxid. rub. . . .	1/50–1/10 gr.	0.0013–0.006	Kava-kava . . .	15–60 m.	1.000–4.000
Galla, tinct. . . .	½– 2 gr.	2.000–8.000	subsulph. flav. .	¼– ½ gr.	0.016–0.033	Keroform . . .	1– 5 gr.	0.066–0.333
Gallobromol . .	7½ gr.-2 dr.	0.492–8.000	Hydrastin . . .	5–10 gr.	0.333–0.666	Kino	5–30 gr.	0.333–2.000
Gambogia . . .	1– 4 gr.	0.066–0.266	Hydrastinin . . .	1/12– 1/6 gr.	0.0054–0.011	pulv. comp. . .	5–15 gr.	0.333–1.000
Gaultheria, ol. .	3–10 m.	0.200–0.666	Hydrastis canadensis . . .	20 m.	1.333	tinct.	½– 2 dr.	2.000–8.000
Gelsemin	1/60–1/20 gr.	0.001–0.003	ext. fl.	8–30 m.	0.533–2.000	Koussin	30–60 gr.	2.000–4.000
Gelsemium, ext. fl.	5–20 m.	0.333–1.333	tinct.	30–90 m.	2.000–6.000	Krameria, ext. .	5–10 gr.	0.333–0.666
tinct.	8–15 m.	0.533–1.000	Hydrochinone .	5–30 gr.	0.333–2.000	fl.	5–30 m.	0.333–2.000
Gentiana, ext. .	1– 5 gr.	0.066–0.333	Hydrocotyle . .	8–15 gr.	0.533–1.000	syr.	½– 4 dr.	2.000–16.00
fl.	5–60 m.	0.333–4.000	Hydronaphtol .	30–60 m.	2.000–4.000	tinct.	5–60 m.	0.333–4.000
infus. comp. . .	1– 4 dr.	4.000–16.000	Hyoscin, hydrobr. . .	1/100–1/60 gr.	0.00066–0.001	Lactopeptin . .	5–15 gr.	0.333–1.000
tinct.	½– 1 dr.	2.000–4.000				Lactophenin . .	10–15 gr.	0.666–1.000
Geranium, ext. fl.	15–30 m.	1.000–2.000	Hyoscyamin, sulph.	1/128–1/32 gr.	0.0005–0.002	Lactucarium . .	5–15 gr.	0.333–1.000
Glonoin	1/120–1/60 gr.	0.00054–0.001				ext. fl.	8–30 m.	0.533–2.000
Glycyrrhiza, mist. comp. .	1– 4 dr.	4.000–16.000	Hyoscyamus, abs.	2– 5 gr.	0.133–0.333	syr.	1– 3 dr.	4.000–12.00
pulv. comp. . .	30–60 gr.	2.000–4.000	ext. alc.	1– 2 gr.	0.066–0.133	Lactucin	1– 5 gr.	0.066–0.333
Gossypium, ext. fl	15–45 m.	1.000–3.000	fl.	5–15 m.	0.333–1.000	Lantanin	15–30 gr.	1.000–2.000
			tinct.	15–30 m.	1.000–2.000	Laurocerasus, aq.	5–30 m.	0.333–2.000
			Hypnal	½– 1 gr.	0.033–0.066	Lavandulæ, ol. .	1– 5 m	0.066–0.333
Granatum, ext. fl.	½– 2 dr.	2.000–8.000	Hypnone	5–10 m.	0.333–0.666	spirit.	½– 1 dr.	2.000–4.000
Grindel., ext. fl.	10–60 m.	0.666–4.000	Ichthyol	3– 4 gr.	0.200–0.266	comp.	30–60 m.	2.000–4.000
Guaiacol	½– 2 m.	0.033–0.133	Ignatia, abstr. .	½– 1 gr.	0.033–0.066	tinct., comp. . .	½– 2 dr.	2.000–8.000
bi-iodid	5–10 gr.	0.333–0.666	ext.	¼– ½ gr.	0.016–0.033	Leptandra, ext. .	1– 3 gr.	0.066–0.200
carbonate . . .	6– 8 gr.	0.400–0.520	fl.	1– 6 m.	0.066–0.400	fl.	20–60 m.	1.333–4.000
salicylate . . .	5–15 gr.	0.333–1.000	tinct.	2–10 m.	0.133–0.666	Leptandrin . . .	1– 3 gr.	0.066–0.200
Guaiacum, tinct.	5–60 m.	0.333–4.000	Indigo	20–60 gr.	1.333–4.000	Limonis, oleum .	1– 5 m.	0.066–0.333
am.	5–30 m.	0.333–2.000	Ingluvin	10–20 gr.	0.666–1.333	Lipanin	1– 4 dr.	4.000–16.00
Guarana, ext. fl. .	10–30 m.	0.666–2.000	Inulin	1– 3 gr.	0.066–0.200	Lithii benzoas .	5–15 gr.	0.333–1.000
Gulandra	2– 3 gr.	0.133–0.200	Iodin, liq. com.	1–10 m.	0.066–0.666	bromidum . .	5–20 gr.	0.333–1.333
Gurjun, bals. . .	1– 2 dr.	4.000–8.000	tinct.	1– 5 m.	0.066–0.333	carbonas . . .	2–10 gr.	0.133–0.666
Hamamel., ext. fl.	1–60 m.	0.066–4.000	Iodocaffein . . .	2–15 gr.	0.133–1.000	citras	2– 5 gr.	0.133–0.333
Hazelin	1– 5 gr.	0.066–0.333	Iodoform	1– 3 gr.	0.066–0.200	salicylas . . .	5–30 gr.	0.333–2.000
Hedeoma, ol. . .	2– 5 m.	0.133–0.333	Iodol	½– 2 gr.	0.033–0.133	Lobelia, acet. . .	5–30 m.	0.333–2.000
						ext. fl.	1– 5 m.	0.066–0.333

A TABLE OF DOSES (*continued*).

MEDICINE.	APOTH. DOSE.	METRIC DOSE.
Lobelia, infus.	1– 4 dr.	4.000–16.00
tinct.	5–30 m.	0.333–2.000
Lobelin	½– 1 gr.	0.033–0.066
Lugol's sol.	1–10 m.	0.066–0.666
Lupulin	5–10 gr.	0.333–0.666
Lycetol	15 gr.	1.000
Lysidin	15–60 gr.	1.000–4.000
Magnesia	15–60 gr.	1.000–4.000
Magnesii, boro-citras	2– 4 dr.	8.000–16.00
carb.	10–60 gr.	0.666–4.000
citras, gran.	2– 8 dr.	8.000–32.00
mist. et asaf.	½– 4 dr.	2.000–16.00
silic. hydrat.	1– 2 dr.	4.000–8.000
sulphas	1– 8 dr.	4.000–32.00
sulphis	5–30 gr.	0.333–2.000
Malakin	15 gr.	1.000
Maltum, ext.	1–2½ dr.	4.000–10.00
Mangan. binox.	2– 5 gr.	0.133–0.333
iodid. syr.	10–30 m.	0.666–2.000
sulph.	2– 5 gr.	0.133–0.333
Manna	1– 2 oz.	32.000–64.00
Marrub., ext. fl.	1– 2 dr.	4.000–8.000
Matico, ext. fl.	30–60 m.	2.000–4.000
tinct.	½– 2 dr.	2.000–8.000
Matricar., ext. fl.	8–30 m.	0.533–2.000
Meconarcein	1/6– ½ gr.	0.011–0.033
Menthæ pip., ol.	1– 5 m.	0.066–0.333

MEDICINE.	APOTH. DOSE.	METRIC DOSE.
Nitroglycerin	1/200–1/50 m.	0.000335–0.0013
tinct.	½–10 m.	0.033–0.666
Nuclein	30–45 gr.	2.000–3.000
Nux vom.	1– 5 gr.	0.066–0.333
abstr.	¼– ½ gr.	0.016–0.033
ext.	⅛– ½ gr.	0.008–0.033
fl.	1– 5 m.	0.066–0.333
tinct.	5–20 m.	0.333–1.333
Opium	1/6– 1 gr.	0.011–0.066
acet.	5–15 m.	0.333–1.000
ext.	¼– 1 gr.	0.016–0.066
liq. comp.	5–15 m.	0.333–1.000
pil.	1– 2	
pulv.	½– 3 gr.	0.033–0.200
tinct.	5–20 m.	0.333–1.333
camph.	5–75 m.	0.333–5.000
comp.	1–60 m.	0.066–4.000
deod.	5–20 m.	0.333–1.333
vin.	5–20 m.	0.333–1.333
Orexin	3– 9 gr.	0.200–0.600
Orthin	5– 8 gr.	0.333–0.520
Ouabain	1/1000 gr.	0.000066
Oxyspartein	½– 1 gr.	0.033–0.066
Pambotano	18 dr.	70.000
Pancreatic liq.	1– 4 dr.	4.000–16.00
Pancreatin	10–20 gr.	0.666–1.333
Papayotin	1– 5 gr.	0.066–0.333
Paracotoin	1½– 3 gr.	0.099–0.200

MEDICINE.	APOTH. DOSE.	METRIC DOSE.
Phytolac., ext. fl.	5–30 m.	0.333-2.000
tinct.	8–60 m.	0.533–4.000
Pichi, ext.	5–10 gr.	0.333–0.666
Picis liq., syr.	2– 4 dr.	8.000–16.00
Picrin	¼– ½ gr.	0.016–0.033
Picrotoxin	1/120–1/60 gr.	0.0005–0.0011
Piliganin hydrochl.	1/6– ⅓ gr.	0.011–0.022
Pilocarpin hydrochlor.	1/64– ½ gr.	0.001–0.033
Pilocarpus, ext. fl.	5–60 m.	0.333–4.000
Piper, ext. fl.	15–45 m.	1.000–3.000
oleores	¼– 1 gr.	0.016–0.066
Piperazin	15 gr.	1.000
Piperin	1– 8 gr.	0.066–0.533
Piperonal	15 gr.	1.000
Piscidia, ext. fl.	15–60 m.	1.000–4.000
Plumbi acetas	½– 3 gr.	0.033–0.200
iodid	¼– ½ gr.	0.016–0.033
Podophyll. abs.	¼– 1 gr.	0.016–0.066
ext.	½–1½ gr.	0.033–0.100
fl.	5–30 m.	0.333–2.000
res.	⅛– ½ gr.	0.008–0.033
Podophyllotoxin.	1/60–1/10 gr.	0.0011–0.006
Polygonum, ext.	1– 5 gr.	0.066–0.333
fl.	10–60 m.	0.666–4.000
Potassii acetas	5–60 gr.	0.333–4.000

spirit.	1–30 m.	0.066–2.000	Paracresalol . .	3–30 gr.	0.200–2.000	arsen., liq. . . .	2–10 m.	0.133–0.666
Menthol	½– 2 gr.	0.033–0.133	Paraform	7½–15 gr.	0.493–1.000	bicarb.	5–30 gr.	0.333–2.000
Menyanthes . .	20–30 gr.	1.333–2.000	Paraldehyd . . .	30–60 m.	2.000–4.000	bitart.	1– 2 dr.	4.000–8.000
Mercury. See			Pareira, ext. fl. .	30–60 m.	2.000–4.000	brom.	5–60 gr.	0.333–4.000
Hydrargyrum.			Parthenin . . .	10–30 gr.	0.666–2.000	carb.	2–20 gr.	0.133–1.333
Metaldehyd . . .	2– 8 gr.	0.133–0.533	Pelletierin . . .	10–20 gr.	0.666–1.333	chloras.	2–20 gr.	0.133–1.333
Methacetin . . .	2– 5 gr.	0.133–0.333	sulphate . . .	3– 6 gr.	0.200–0.400	citras	15–60 gr.	1.000–4.000
Methoxycaffein .	4 gr.	0.260	tannate	12–24 gr.	0.780–1.560	liq.	2– 4 dr.	8.000–16.00
Methylacetanilid	2– 5 gr.	0.133–0.333	Pental (inhala-			mist.	½– 1 oz.	16.000–32.00
Methylal	2– 5 m.	0.133–0.333	tion)	1½–2½ dr.	5.000–10.000	cyanid	1/16– 1/8 gr.	0.004–0.008
Methylene blue .	1½– 4 gr.	0.099–0.260	Pepo, res.	10–15 gr.	0.666–1.000	ferrocyanid . .	5–10 gr.	0.333–0.666
Migrainin . . .	15 gr.	1.000	Pepsin, liq. . . .	2– 4 dr.	8.000–16.00	hypophosph. .	5–10 gr.	0.333–0.666
Monesin	½ gr.	0.033	pur.	15–30 gr.	1.000–2.000	iodid	2–15 gr.	0.133–1.000
Monobromacet-			sacch.	5–60 gr.	0.333–4.000	liquor	5–30 m.	0.333–2.000
anilid	3–15 gr.	0.200–1.000	Pereirin	10–30 gr.	0.666–2.000	nitras	5–15 gr.	0.333–1.000
Morphin and			Petrolatum . . .	1– 2 dr.	4.000–8.000	permang. . . .	½– 2 gr.	0.033–0.133
salts	1/20– ½ gr.	0.003–0.033	Pheduretin . . .	5–15 gr.	0.333–1.000	et sod. tartras .	½– 1 oz.	16.000–32.00
Morrhuol	4–12 gr.	0.260–0.780	Phenacetin . . .	5–15 gr.	0.333–1.000	sulphas	1– 4 dr.	4.000–16.00
Moschus	2–10 gr.	0.133–0.666	Phenidin	15 gr.	1.000	sulphid	1–10 gr.	0.066–0.666
tinct.	15–60 m.	1.000–4.000	Phenocoll . . .	15 gr.	1.000	sulphis	3–10 gr.	0.200–0.666
Mudar	2– 5 gr.	0.133–0.333	Phenylurethane	7½ gr.	0.554	tartraboras . .	5–15 gr.	0.333–1.000
Muscarin	1/30– 1 gr.	0.002–0.066	Phloridzin . . .	15–30 gr.	1.000–2.000	tartras	1– 4 dr.	4.000–16.00
Mussaenin, pulv. .	1– 2 oz.	32.000–64.00	Phosphorus . .	1/128–1/50 gr.	0.0005–0.0013	tellurate . . .	½– ¾ gr.	0.033–0.049
Myrrh, tinct. . .	10–30 m.	0.666–2.000	oleum	1– 3 m.	0.066–2.000	Propylamin . .	1– 5 m.	0.066–0.333
Myrtol.	2– 4 m.	0.133–0.260	pil.	1– 4		Prun. virg., ext.		
Napellin	½– ¾ gr.	0.033–0.048	syr. comp. . .	1– 2 dr.	4.000–8.000	fl.	30–60 m.	2.000–4.000
Naphtalene . . .	2–10 gr.	0.133–0.666	tinct. (Thomp-			syr.	1– 4 dr.	4.000–16.00
Naphtol	5–15 gr.	0.333–1.000	son's)	1 dr.	4.000	Pseudohyoscya-		
Narcein.	1/6– ½ gr.	0.011–0.033	Physostig., ext. .	1/16– 1/6 gr.	0.004–0.011	min (hypo.) .	1/200–1/10 gr.	0.0005–0.006
Naregam., tinct.	15–30 m.	1.000–2.000	fl.	1– 3 m.	0.066–0.200	Pulsatil., ext. fl.	2– 5 m.	0.133–0.333
Nasrol	1 dr.	4.000	tinct.	5–15 m.	0.333–1.000	Pyoktanin . . .	7½–15 gr.	0.493–1.000
Neurodin	15–30 gr.	1.000–2.000	Physostigmin,			Pyrazol	15–30 gr.	1.000–2.000
Niaouli oil . . .	4 m.	0.260	salicyl. . . .	1/128–1/64 gr.	0.0005–0.001	Pyrethrum . . .	20–60 gr.	1.333–4.000
Nicotin	1/20–1/10 m.	0.003–0.006	sulph.	1/128–1/64 gr.	0.0005–0.001	Pyridin	2–10 m.	0.133–0.666

A TABLE OF DOSES (*continued*).

Medicine.	Apoth. Dose.	Metric Dose.	Medicine.	Apoth. Dose.	Metric Dose.	Medicine.	Apoth. Dose.	Metric Dose.
Quassia, ext. . .	1– 5 gr.	0.066–0.333	Santoninoxim .	¾–2¼ gr.	0.049–0.149	Solanin	1/6– 1 gr.	0.011–0.066
fl.	30–60 m.	2.000–4.000	Sapo	5–30 gr.	0.333–2.000	Somnal	30 m. 2 dr.	2.000–8.000
tinct.	5–60 m.	0.333–4.000	Sarsap., ext. fl. .	½– 1 dr.	2.000–4.000	Sozoiodol	1– 3 gr.	0.066–0.200
Quassiin	1/30– 1/3 gr.	0.0022–0.022	comp.	½– 1 dr.	2.000–4.000	Spartein	½– 2 gr.	0.033–0.133
Quebrachin . . .	1– 2 gr.	0.066–0.133	Sassafras, ext. fl.	½– 2 dr.	2.000–8.000	sulphate . . .	1/10–1½ gr.	0.006–0.099
Quebracho, ext. .	2– 8 gr.	0.133–0.533	oleum	1– 5 m.	0.066–0.333	Spasmotin . . .	⅔–10 gr.	0.0432–0.666
fl.	5–60 m.	0.333–4.000	Scammonium . .	3–10 gr.	0.200–0.666	Spigelia, ext. fl. .	15–60 m.	1.000–4.000
tinct.	1– 4 dr.	4.000–16.00	res.	2–10 gr.	0.133–0.666	infus. comp. . .	1– 3 oz.	32.000–96.00
vin.	1– 4 dr.	4.000–16.00	Scilla	1– 3 gr.	0.066–0.200	et sen., ext. fl. .	½– 2 dr.	2.000–8.000
Quinidin and			acet.	10–30 m.	0.666–2.000	Stillingia, ext. fl.	10–60 m.	0.666–4.000
salts	1–30 gr.	0.066–2.000	ext. fl.	1– 5 m.	0.066–0.333	tinct.	½– 1 dr.	2.000–4.000
Quinin and salts	1–30 gr.	0.066–2.000	comp.	5–30 m.	0.333–2.000	Stramon., ext. .	1/6– ½ gr.	0.011–0.033
Randia, tinct. .	15–60 m.	1.000–4.000	syr.	½– 1 dr.	2.000–4.000	fl.	1– 5 m.	0.066–0.333
Resorcin	2–10 gr.	0.133–0.666	comp.	10–30 m.	0.666–2.000	tinct.	5–20 m.	0.333–1.333
Retinol	1 gr.	0.066	tinct.	5–30 m.	0.333–2.000	Strontium, bro-		
Rheum	2–30 gr.	0.133–2.000	Scillain	1/60 gr.	0.0011	mid	10–60 gr.	0.666–4.000
ext.	5–15 gr.	0.333–1.000	Scillopicrin . . .	1/60 gr.	0.0011	iodid	5–60 gr.	0.333–4.000
fl.	15–45 m.	1.000–3.000	Scoparin	½– 1 gr.	0.033–0.066	lactate	2–2½ dr.	8.000–10.000
mist., et sod. .	2 dr.–1 oz.	8.000–32.00	Scoparius, ext. fl.	½– 1 dr.	2.000–4.000	Stroph., tinct. .	5–10 m.	0.333–0.666
pil.	1– 3		Scopolamin, hy-			Strophanthin . .	1/120–1/60 gr.	0.0005–0.001
comp.	2– 5		drochlorid . .	1/240–1/60	0.00025–0.0011	Strychnin and		
pulv. comp. . .	30–60 gr.	2.000–4.000	Scutellar., ext. fl.	½– 2 dr.	2.000–8.000	salts	1/64–1/12 gr.	0.001–0.0065
syr.	1– 4 dr.	4.000–16.00	Senega, abstr. . .	5–10 gr.	0.333–0.666	Succin., oleum .	5–10 m.	0.333–0.666
arom.	1– 4 dr.	4.000–16.00	ext. fl.	5–15 m.	0.333–1.000	Sulphaminol . .	4 gr.	0.160
tinct.	1– 8 dr.	4.000–32.00	syr.	1– 2 dr.	4.000–8.000	Sulphonal . . .	5–30 gr.	0.333–2.000
arom.	30–75 m.	2.000–5.000	Senegin	¼– 1 gr.	0.016–0.066	Sulphur	10–60 gr.	0.666–4.000
dulc.	1– 4 dr.	4.000–16.00	Senna	5–60 gr.	0.333–4.000	Sumbul, ext. fl. .	15–60 m.	1.000–4.000
vin.	1– 2 dr.	4.000–8.000	confect.	1– 2 dr.	4.000–8.000	tinct.	5–30 m.	0.333–2.000

Rhus glab., ext.			ext. fl.	1– 4 dr.	4.000–16.00	Svapnia	1/2– 2 gr.	0.033–0.133
fl.	30–60 m.	2.000–4.000	infus. comp.	1– 2 oz.	32.000–64.00	Tanacet., ol.	1– 3 m.	0.066–0.200
tox., ext. fl.	1– 6 m.	0.066–0.400	syr.	1– 2 dr.	4.000–8.000	Tannigen	3–7 1/2 gr.	0.200–0.493
tinct.	1/10– 1 m.	0.006–0.066	Serpent., ext. fl.	10–30 m.	0.666–2.000	Taraxac., ext.	5–15 gr.	0.333–1.000
Ricin., oleum	1– 8 dr.	4.000–32.00	tinct.	1/2– 2 dr.	2.000–8.000	fl.	1/2– 2 dr.	2.000–8.000
Rosa, ext. fl.	1/2– 2 dr.	2.000–8.000	Sinapis, ol. vol.	1/8– 1/4 m.	0.008–0.0165	Terebene	5–20 m.	0.333–1.333
syr.	1– 2 dr.	4.000–8.000	Sodii acetas	15–60 gr.	1.000–4.000	Terebinthinæ, ol.	5–30 m.	0.333–2.000
Rubidium-ammo-			arsenas	1/64–1/16 gr.	0.001–0.006	Terpin hydr.	5–10 gr.	0.333–0.666
nium bromid	20–30 gr.	1.333–2.000	liq.	2–15 m.	0.133–1.000	Terpinol	10–15 m.	0.666–1.000
Rubus, ext. fl.	10–60 m.	0.666–4.000	benzoas	5–15 gr.	0.333–1.000	Tetronal	10–20 gr.	0.666–1.333
Rumex, ext. fl.	15–60 m.	1.000–4.000	bicarb.	5–30 gr.	0.333–2.000	Teucrin (hypo-		
Rusot	20–30 gr.	1.333–2.000	bisulph.	3–10 gr.	0.200–0.666	derm.)	10–45 gr.	0.666–2.916
Ruta, ext. fl.	15–30 m.	1.000–2.000	boras	5–30 gr.	0.333–2.000	Thallin	2–15 gr.	0.133–1.000
oleum	1– 5 m.	0.066–0.333	brom.	5–30 gr.	0.333–2.000	sulphate	4– 8 gr.	0.260–0.518
Sabina, ext. fl.	5–15 m.	0.333–1.000	carb.	5–30 gr.	0.333–2.000	Thein (hypo.)	1/6– 1 gr.	0.011–0.066
oleum	1– 3 m.	0.066–0.200	chloras	5–20 gr.	0.333–1.333	Theobromin.		
Saccharin	1/4– 2 gr.	0.016–0.133	liq.	10–60 m.	0.666–4.000	See *Cocain.*		
Safrol	20–30 m.	1.333–2.000	chlorid	10–60 gr.	0.666–4.000	Thermodin	8–10 gr.	0.518–0.666
Salacetol	30–45 gr.	2.000–3.000	dithiosalicylate	3 gr.	0.200	Thiol	2–10 gr.	0.133–0.666
Salicin	5–30 gr.	0.333–2.000	formate	2/5–1 1/5 gr.	0.026–0.080	Thiosinnamin	4 1/2– 7 gr.	0.243–0.454
Salicylamid	3– 5 gr.	0.200–0.333	hypophosph.	5–10 gr.	0.333–0.666	Thymacetin	3– 5 gr.	0.200–0.333
Salipyrin	15 gr.	1.000	hyposulph.	5–20 gr.	0.333–1.333	Thymol	1/2– 2 gr.	0.033–0.133
Salocoll	15–30 gr.	1.000–2.000	iodid	5–15 gr.	0.333–1.000	Thyroidin	1 1/2–4 1/2 gr.	0.099–0.293
Salol	5–15 gr.	0.333–1.000	liquor	5–30 m.	0.333–2.000	Tiglii, oleum	1/2– 2 m.	0.033–0.133
Salophen	1–1 1/2 dr.	4.000–6.000	nitras	1– 2 oz.	32.000–64.00	Tolypyrin	5–15 gr.	0.333–1.000
Sanguin., acet.	10–30 m.	0.666–2.000	nitris	1/2– 3 gr.	0.033–0.200	Tolysal	15–30 gr.	1.000–2.000
ext. fl.	5–15 m.	0.333–1.000	paracresotate	1–20 gr.	0.066–1.333	Tonga, ext. fl.	1/2 dr.	2.000
tinct.	5–60 m.	0.333–4.000	phosphas	2–15 gr.	0.133–1.000	Tribromphenol	1/2– 4 gr.	0.033–0.260
Sanguinarin	1/12– 1/4 gr.	0.005–0.016	salicylas	5–30 gr.	0.333–2.000	bismuth	7 gr.	0.454
Santal., ext. fl.	1– 2 dr.	4.000–8.000	santoninas	2–10 gr.	0.133–0.666	Tricresol	1 1/2 gr.	0.099
oleum	5–30 m.	0.333–2.000	sulphas	5–20 gr.	0.333–1.333	Trillin	2– 4 gr.	0.133–0.260
Santonica	5–60 gr.	0.333–4.000	sulphis	5–20 gr.	0.333–1.333	Trimethylam.,		
ext. fl.	15–60 m.	1.000–4.000	sulphocarb.	10–30 gr.	0.636–2.000	hydrochl.	1– 3 gr.	0.066–0.200
Santonin	1– 5 gr.	0.066–0.333	telluras	2/7– 4/5 gr.	0.018–0.052	Trional	10–30 gr.	0.666–2.000

A TABLE OF DOSES (*continued*).

Medicine.	Apoth. Dose.	Metric Dose.	Medicine.	Apoth. Dose.	Metric Dose.	Medicine.	Apoth. Dose.	Metric Dose.
Triphenin . . .	10–15 gr.	0.666–1.000	Valerian., ext. .	5–10 gr.	0.333–0.666	Zea, ext. fl.	1– 2 dr.	4.000–8.000
Tritic., ext. fl. . .	1– 4 dr.	4.000–16.00	fl.	10–30 m.	0.666–2.000	infus.	ad lib.	
Trypsin	5–10 gr.	0.333–0.666	oleum	2– 5 m.	0.133–0.333	Zedoary	8–30 gr.	0.518–2.000
Tuberculin . . .	1/200–1/130 gr.	0.0003–0.0005	tinct.	½– 2 dr.	2.000–8.000	Zinc, acetate . .	½– 2 gr.	0.033–0.133
Turpent., Chian	3– 5 gr.	0.200–0.333	amm.	½– 2 dr.	2.000–8.000	bromid	½– 2 gr.	0.033–0.133
Tussol	¾– 5 gr.	0.0486–0.333	Verat. vir., ext. fl.	1– 5 m.	0.066–0.333	cyanid	1/16– ⅛ gr.	0.004–0.008
Uloxin	1/20–1/10 gr.	0.003–0.006	tinct.	3–10 m.	0.200–0.666	iodid	½– 2 gr.	0.033–0.133
Upas tieuté, ext.	¼– ½ gr.	0.016–0.033	Veratrin	1/64–1/10 gr.	0.001–0.006	oxid	1–10 gr.	0.066–0.666
Ural, Uralium .	15–45 gr.	1.000–2.916	Viburn., ext. fl. .	½– 2 dr.	2.000–8.000	phosphid . . .	1/50–1/20 gr.	0.0013–0.003
Uranium, nitrate	⅙– 1 gr.	0.011–0.066	Vieirin	1– 3 gr.	0.066–0.200	subgallate . . .	1– 4 gr.	0.066–0.260
Urea	10 gr.	0.666	Viola, ext. fl. . .	2–10 m.	0.133–0.666	sulphate . . .	10–30 gr.	0.666–2.000
Urethane	10–15 gr.	0.666–1.000	Warburg's tinct.	15–60 m.	1.000–4.000	sulpho-ichthy-		
Uricedin	7–15 gr.	0.454–1.000	Xanthium			olate	½– 1 gr.	0.033–0.066
Uropherin . . .	15 gr.	1.000	specios. . . .	10–20 gr.	0.666–1.333	valerianate . .	½– 3 gr.	0.033–0.200
Urotropin . . .	7–30 gr.	0.454–2.000	Xanthoxy., ex. fl.	15–30 m.	1.000–2.000	Zingib., ext. fl. .	5–30 m.	0.333–2.000
Ustilag., ext. fl. .	15–60 m.	1.000–4.000	Xeroform . . .	5– 8 gr.	0.333–0.518	oleores	½– 1 gr.	0.033–0.066
Uva ursi, ext. fl.	10–60 m.	0.666–4.000	Xylol	1– 2 gr.	0.066–0.133	syr.	½– 2 dr.	2.000–8.000
Valerian., abstr.	5–15 gr.	0.333–1.000	Yerba reuma . .	5–10 gr.	0.333–0.666	tinct.	15–60 m.	1.000–4.000

www.ingramcontent.com/pod-product-compliance
Lightning Source LLC
Chambersburg PA
CBHW020856210326
41598CB00018B/1683

* 9 7 8 3 7 4 2 8 3 1 3 4 7 *